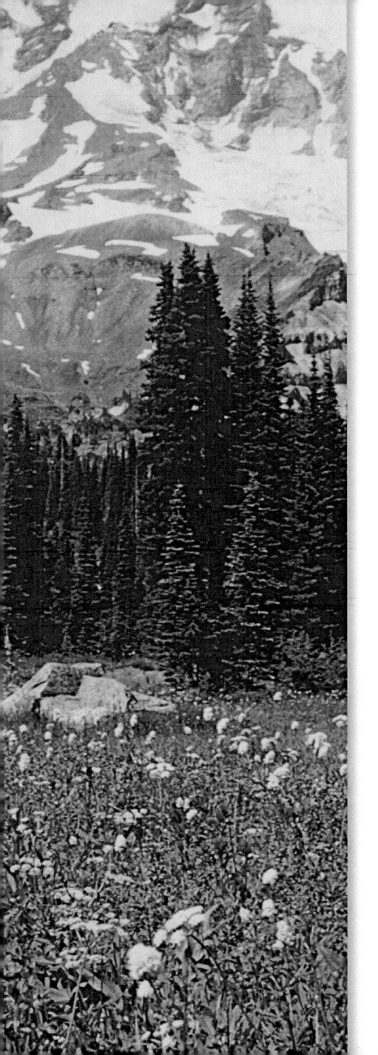

Environmental Health

Ecological Perspectives

Kathryn Hilgenkamp

JONES AND BARTLETT PUBLISHERS

Sudbury, Massachusetts

BOSTON   TORONTO   LONDON   SINGAPORE

World Headquarters

Jones and Bartlett Publishers
40 Tall Pine Drive
Sudbury, MA 01776
978-443-5000
info@jbpub.com
www.jbpub.com

Jones and Bartlett Publishers
Canada
6339 Ormindale Way
Mississauga, ON L5V 1J2
CANADA

Jones and Bartlett Publishers
International
Barb House, Barb Mews
London W6 7PA
UK

Jones and Bartlett's books and products are available through most bookstores and online booksellers. To contact Jones and Bartlett Publishers directly, call 800-832-0034, fax 978-443-8000, or visit our website, www.jbpub.com.

Substantial discounts on bulk quantities of Jones and Bartlett's publications are available to corporations, professional associations, and other qualified organizations. For details and specific discount information, contact the special sales department at Jones and Bartlett via the above contact information or send an email to specialsales@jbpub.com.

ISBN-13: 978-0-7637-2377-4
ISBN-10: 0-7637-2377-0

About the cover image: Zebra mussels washed up on beach, Lake Erie.

Printed on recycled paper.

Production Credits
Acquisitions Editor: Jacqueline Ann Mark-Geraci
Senior Production Editor: Julie Champagne Bolduc
Associate Editor: Nicole L. Quinn
Editorial Assistant: Amy L. Flagg
Associate Marketing Manager: Wendy Thayer
Interactive Technology Manager: Dawn Mahon Priest
Manufacturing Buyer: Therese Connell
Composition: Graphic World
Cover Design: Kristin E. Ohlin
Senior Photo Researcher: Kimberly Potvin
Cover Image: Courtesy Great Lakes Environmental Research Lab, U.S. Environmental Protection Agency
Printing and Binding: Malloy, Inc.
Cover Printing: Malloy, Inc.

Library of Congress Cataloging-in-Publication Data
Hilgenkamp, Kathryn, 1952–
    Environmental health : ecological perspectives / Kathryn Hilgenkamp.
        p. cm.
    Includes bibliographical references and index.
    ISBN 0-7637-2377-0
    1. Environmental health.   2. Human ecology—Health aspects.   3. Ecology.   I. Title.
    RA565.H52 2005
    362.196'98—dc22

6048

Printed in the United States of America   2004022761
15 14 13 12 11   10 9 8 7 6 5 4

Dedication

Dedicated to my dad, LeRoy Thoms (1927–2004), a man who taught me how important each sunrise and sunset is, how to appreciate every breath, every drop of rain, every grain of sand, every speck of dirt, how short life is, and how precious life is.

Contents

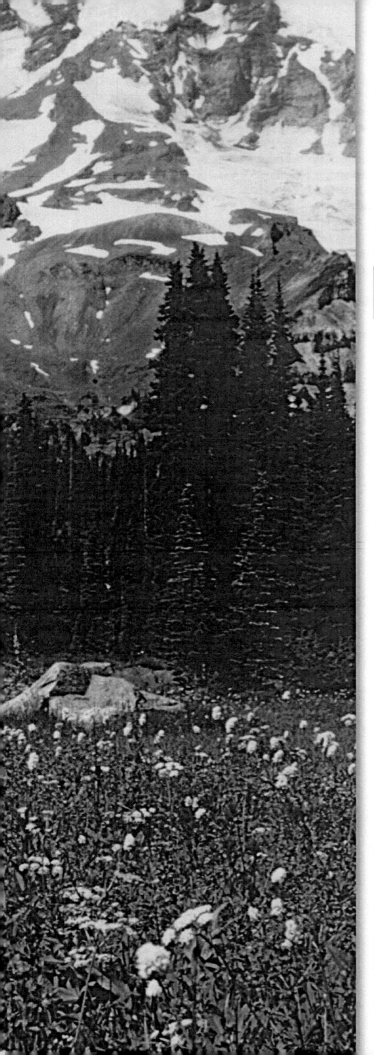

Preface

nvironmental Health takes the reader on a fascinating journey, beginning with curiosity about the environment and ending with a desire to protect it. The text begins with an explanation of the cycles of life and how humans can have a global impact upon nature through seemingly harmless practices. It also explains how human activities increase the presence of harmful pathogens, magnify the effects of chemicals and technological devices, as well as change weather patterns. The mission of this book is to provide an overview of how human habits impact the environment, which, in turn, influence the health of all. Additional information regarding laws designed to suppress harmful activities and prevent environmental problems is provided.

This first edition of *Environmental Health* is a proactive effort to provide historical and background information about the measures that have been implemented to conserve and preserve the environment as a public health effort. *Environmental Health* includes current information regarding issues related to environmental health such as:

- Global efforts to combat global warming

- Public health measures from the Roman Empire to the present

- Emerging and antibiotic-resistant diseases

- Specific information about toxic chemicals

- Risk assessment and public health interventions

- Safety of irradiation and genetically engineered foods

- Land pollution and indoor pollution

- Alternative fuels and alternative fuel vehicles

- The impact of UV and other forms of radiation

- E-waste

- The history of occupational safety

- Emergency preparedness and bioterrorism

The features developed in this text help readers gain the skills to make a difference in this world. Each chapter offers several learning tools that will aid in the understanding and application of key concepts.

Digging Deeper boxes are integrated throughout each chapter. These offer readers more in-depth information related to chapter material such as overpopulation, nutrient recycling, food-borne illnesses, and advances in policy by key scientists and legislators.

Consider the Cost boxes show readers what they as consumers can do to ensure a healthier and safer environment. These feature boxes explore real-life topics such as reducing the possibility of infection, detoxification of one's body, and storing hazardous chemicals in the home. These boxes are based on the idea that once we learn proper methods of preservation, conservation, and prevention, we can take appropriate action.

Healthy People 2010 Objectives are integrated throughout the text. This feature shows the preventive health measures directed toward environmental and public health that are related to the chapter. A listing of all the Healthy People 2010 Objectives that relate to environmental health is also included.

Chapter Assignments give readers the opportunity to analyze their behavior and the toxins affecting our environment.

Summaries provide a focus on the key topics within the chapter.

Chapter glossaries define key terms.

Selected Environmental Laws describe important laws to help readers in their research, writing, and presentations.

A listing of journals is included for further topic exploration.

A text-specific Web site has additional resources for any classroom environment.

Acknowledgments

The writing of a textbook is no small undertaking and requires guidance, encouragement, and scrutiny by several individuals. My gratitude extends to:

Pamela D. Doughty, PhD, CHES, Assistant Professor, Health and Kinesiology Department, Texas A & M at Kingsville, TX

David P. Gilkey, DC, PhD, Assistant Professor, Department of Environmental and Radiological Health Sciences, Colorado State University, Fort Collins, CO

Richard R. Jurin, PhD, Director, Environmental Studies Program, University of Northern Colorado, Greeley, CO

Michael D. Monroe, MPH, CHES, Manager, Air Education and Outreach Section, Bureau of Air Quality, South Carolina Department of Health and Environmental Services, Columbia, SC

Mary H. Ward, PhD, Epidemiologist, Occupational and Environmental Epidemiology Branch, Division of Cancer Epidemiology and Genetics, National Cancer Institute, National Institutes of Health, Bethesda, MD

The editorial staff at Jones and Bartlett Publishers:

Kris Ellis for thinking this was a good idea

Nicole Quinn for providing the framework and suggestions

Jacqueline Mark-Geraci for her enthusiasm and encouragement

Julie Bolduc for her editorial comments

And:

Jason Johnson for rescuing my hard drive when it crashed and smoldered due to a lightning storm

My family for sacrificing family time while the book was being written

The public health officials, government agencies, universities, environmentalists, conservationists, and nature lovers who gave permission to use their photos and illustrations

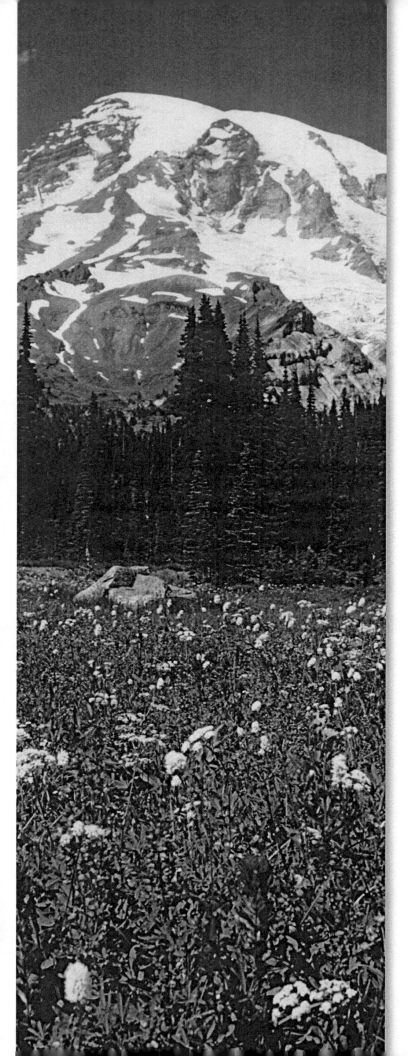

Environmental Principles and Ecology

1

A new type ot thinking is essential if humankind is to survive.

Albert Einstein, 1921 Nobel Prize
in Physics (1879–1955)

OBJECTIVES

1. Define the terms in the glossary at the end of the chapter.

2. Describe the Earth and its layers.

3. Describe the atmospheric layers.

4. Describe the biomes and how they were developed.

5. Describe the term biosystem and the importance of biodiversity.

6. Explain the importance of ecosystems.

7. Describe the impact of humans on ecosystems.

8. Distinguish between extinct, threatened, and endangered species.

9. List and describe the cycles of life known as bio-geochemical cycles.

10. Differentiate preservation from conservation practices.

Introduction

The environment exists from the center of the Earth to the outer reaches of its atmosphere. The world as it is known is made of matter that is created, restored, and changed through natural or unnatural processes (Figure 1-1). It is important to have a basic background in **geology** and earth science to explain dependent and interdependent relationships of all aspects of the **environment** and how the **sustainability** of life is affected. This chapter provides an overview of ecological and environmental principles to help understand how life on the planet is sustained and recycled for future generations to come.

The Earth

The Earth's outer environment consists of several spherical layers above the core and mantle: the lithosphere, the hydrosphere, the **biosphere**, and the atmosphere. The core consists of an inner (solid) and an outer (molten) layer, is about 2,166 miles thick, and composed mostly of iron (Fe) with some nickel (Ni). The outer core is about 1,410 miles thick and about 10% sulphur (S). It is primarily responsible for producing the Earth's magnetic field as it spins around the solid inner core. The inner core, which is under pressure, is solid, about 756 miles thick. The mantle is the largest layer, about 1,800 miles thick, composed mostly of iron (Fe), magnesium (Mg), aluminum (Al), silicon (Si), and oxygen (O) silicate compounds. It is relatively flexible, so it flows instead of fracturing.

LITHOSPHERE

The lithosphere includes the crust and mantle. The crust is the thinnest and coolest layer of the Earth. It is up to 62 miles thick and is thinnest under the oceans (up to 6 miles). It is composed of the least dense calcium (Ca) and sodium (Na) aluminum-silicate minerals. The crust is rocky and brittle because it is relatively cold. This makes it particularly fragile during earthquakes.

Approximately 30% of the Earth's surface is covered by land with seven continental land masses. The highest point on Earth is Mount Everest, located on the border of Tibet and Nepal in the Central Himalayas in Southeast Asia. The lowest point on land is the Dead Sea—1,320 feet below sea level—located on the border between Israel and the West Bank to the west and Jordan to the east. It is so salty that it is unable to support any type of life.

HYDROSPHERE

Without water, the average person would live only a few days (Donatelle, 2001). Bacteria and other organisms also need water to survive and reproduce. Approximately 70% of the Earth's surface is covered by water. Approximately 97% of the hydrosphere is salt water (oceans, estuaries, and seas), while the remaining 3% is found in ice caps, glaciers, freshwater (rivers, streams, lakes, wetlands, groundwater, aquifers), soil moisture, and the atmosphere. Less than 1% of the Earth's water is usable by humans.

BIOSPHERE

Life is possible when there is air, moisture, nutrients, and a temperature conducive to life. Conditions for life extend approximately 5 miles in the atmosphere to 5 miles below the ocean surface. Some life can exist without light, but

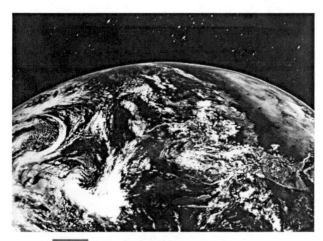

FIGURE 1-1 **Earth** It is a wonder that so much diversity and life can exist on one planet.

> *Geology*
> The study of the physical nature of Earth and its history including the structure and development of the crust, its interior, individual rock types, and fossil formations.
>
> *Environment*
> All conditions, circumstances, and influences surrounding and affecting the development or existence of people or other living things.
>
> *Sustainability*
> The ability to meet the needs of the present without compromising the ability of future generations to meet their own needs; an environmental protection strategy designed to protect Earth's resources.
>
> *Biosphere*
> The part of the Earth's environment in which living organisms are found and interact. The biosphere may also be termed the *ecosphere*.

most forms of life require sunlight and a certain amount of atmospheric pressure to survive. Most life occurs where sunlight is able to penetrate. The biosphere encompasses all life on the planet. The biosphere can be described by describing various biomes, ecosystems, and biosystems.

Biomes

Biomes are specific to certain regions within the biosphere established according to climate. The climate determines the types of vegetation and animals that live there. Biomes may be categorized in various ways (Figure 1-2). Major biomes include:

1. alpine
2. tundra
3. taiga
4. temperate forest
5. deciduous forest
6. grassland
7. deserts
8. tropical biomes

Each biome has a specific soil type, rainfall, growing season, vegetation, and wildlife (Figure 1-3). Biomes also have various forms of **natural resources** (air, water, land, minerals) and life (microorganisms, plants, insects, birds, animals).

> *Biomes*
> Regional ecosystems defined by biogeography and climatic characters.
>
> *Natural resources*
> Natural assets ready for use that can be drawn upon to take care of a need, such as water, wood, coal, and oil.

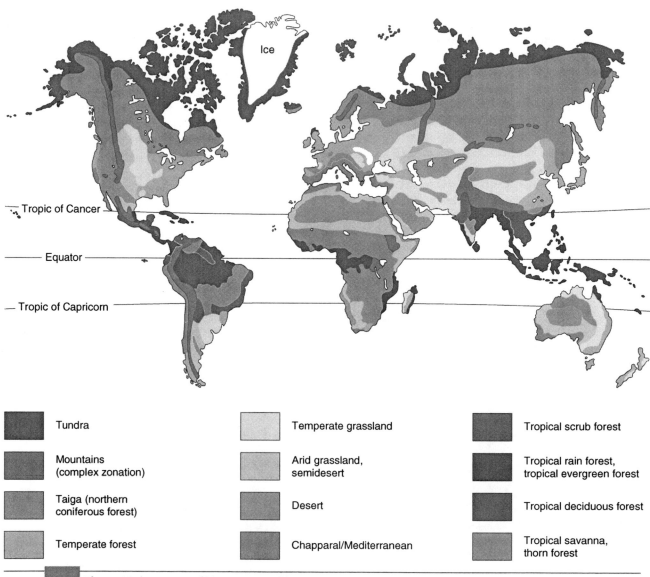

■ Tundra	■ Temperate grassland	■ Tropical scrub forest
■ Mountains (complex zonation)	■ Arid grassland, semidesert	■ Tropical rain forest, tropical evergreen forest
■ Taiga (northern coniferous forest)	■ Desert	■ Tropical deciduous forest
■ Temperate forest	■ Chapparal/Mediterranean	■ Tropical savanna, thorn forest

FIGURE 1-2 Biomes Various types of biosystems and biomes are located all over the Earth.

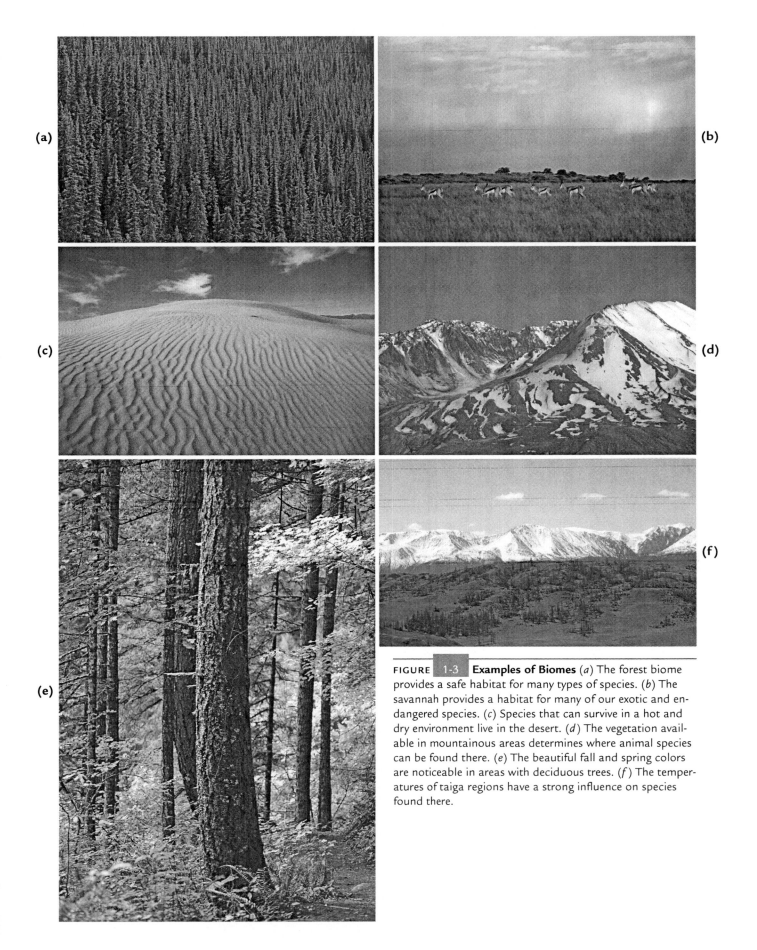

(a)

(b)

(c)

(d)

(e)

(f)

FIGURE 1-3 **Examples of Biomes** (*a*) The forest biome provides a safe habitat for many types of species. (*b*) The savannah provides a habitat for many of our exotic and endangered species. (*c*) Species that can survive in a hot and dry environment live in the desert. (*d*) The vegetation available in mountainous areas determines where animal species can be found there. (*e*) The beautiful fall and spring colors are noticeable in areas with deciduous trees. (*f*) The temperatures of taiga regions have a strong influence on species found there.

ALPINE

This refers to regions just below the snow lines in mountain regions such as the Himalaya Mountains, Andes Mountains, and Rocky Mountains. The altitude is 10,000 feet or more. The average summer temperature is 10 to15°C and the average winter temperature is below freezing. Because of the severe climate and very little carbon dioxide for photosynthesis, there are only 200 known species of plants. Because plants do not decompose quickly, the soil is very poor. There are few animal species because of intense exposure to the sun. Those that remain hibernate.

TUNDRA

Tundras are found in the upper latitudes of the northern hemisphere around the Arctic Ocean. They are somewhat barren and treeless with shrubs and woody bushes. The growing season lasts 6 to 10 weeks and the annual rainfall is less than 10 inches. Winds are dry and strong. Winters are long, dark, and cold, and a permanent layer of ice or frozen soil lies beneath the topsoil, preventing the growth of larger plants and trees. Bogs and marshes are common. Animals include polar bear, arctic hare, arctic fox, caribou, snowy owl, and waterfowl.

TAIGA

Taigra regions consist of a belt of coniferous trees across North America and Eurasia with subpolar temperatures and severe weather. Rainfall averages 15 to 20 inches annually. The area is dry in the winter and humid in the summer. Animals include fur-bearing predators such as large herbivores such as elk and moose, and small herbivores such as beaver and snowshoe hares.

DECIDUOUS FOREST

This area of western and central Europe, eastern Asia, and eastern North American receives 30 to 60 inches per year.

The climate is warm and humid and the winters are often dry. Vegetation includes broadleaf deciduous trees such as oak, maple, beech, hickory, and elm. Herbivores in the area include white-tail deer, gray squirrels, and chipmunks. Omnivores include raccoons, skunks, and black bears. Carnivores include wolves, mountain lions, and bobcats.

GRASSLANDS

The grasslands are found in the central lowlands and high plains of North America, the Ukraine through Russia and Mongolia. The pampas of South America and the Veldt of Africa feature a semiarid, warm to hot summer. Receiving 10 to 20 inches per year, fertile soils bear perennial grasses, sunflowers, woodlands, and legumes. Bison, pronghorn deer, ground squirrels, gophers, coyotes, badgers, and black-footed ferrets reside in the area in North America.

CHAPARRAL

This biome is found on the west coast of the United States, the west coast of South America, the tip of South Africa, the western tip of Australia, and coastal areas of the Mediterranean. A chaparral includes flat plains, rocky hills, and mountain slopes. Plants such as poison oak, yucca, shrubs and cacti have small leaves to hold moisture. The climate is extremely hot and dry, making fires and droughts common. The animals are mainly grassland and desert types and include coyotes, jackrabbits, mule deer, alligator lizards, horned toads, praying mantis, honeybees, and ladybugs.

DESERT AND DESERT SCRUB

Dry lands characteristically have less than 10 inches of precipitation per year, which evaporates rapidly. They are frequently seen in the rain shadow areas of high mountain ranges. Temperatures may rise in the summer but drop to freezing at night. Evergreens

and thorny, spiny, and taprooted plants survive in these dry areas.

TROPICAL RAIN FOREST

With a rainfall averaging 50 to 250 inches a year, trees may become 100 to 120 feet tall with woody vines, air plants, and lush vegetation. Tropical rain forests are seen in Central and South America, Central Africa, and Southeastern Asia. Rainforests are decreasing rapidly, yet more than half of all the world's species are estimated to live there. Species include the African elephant, Bengal tiger, chimpanzee, orangutang, toucan, King cobra, and anaconda, to name a few.

TROPICAL SAVANNAS

These areas in eastern Africa, Venezuela, Columbia, Brazil, and Central America encounter dry seasons with less than 4 inches per month to wet seasons with 30 to 50 inches of rain. Some include dry zones, grassy areas, and wooded areas. Elephants, zebras, antelopes, gazelles, giraffes, lions, leopards, jackals, and hyenas are found in tropical savannas.

AQUATIC BIOMES

There are two types of aquatic biomes: marine and freshwater. The marine or saltwater biome is the largest biotic community covering three fourths of the Earth. The marine biomes are divided between coral reefs, estuaries, and oceans. The ocean biome has the largest and most diverse selection of fish and animals, including sea mammals such as whales, dolphins, sharks, walrus, and seals. There are many species of sea animals, fish, seaweed, coral, plankton, and algae. The ocean biome includes inter-tidal zones, open ocean, and deep sea. The freshwater biomes include species existing in rivers, lakes, and other surface water environments. Animal species include otters, beaver, many types of birds, fish, amphibians, insects, and microorganisms.

Ecosystems

The various types of life forms are defined in terms of **ecosystems.** An *ecosystem* consists of living and nonliving elements in a particular area that are mutually beneficial. Organisms in ecosystems interact with each other and nonliving components to process energy and cycle nutrients. There are five main types or categories of ecosystems comprising most of Earth's surface:

1. agroecosystems
2. coastal ecosystems

TABLE 1-1   Ecosystems

Ecosystems	Resources	Provisions
Agroecosystems	Food, cellulose fiber	Habitat for birds; build organic matter and atmospheric carbon; maintain surface water; production of plants and animals for food
Coastal ecosystems	Fish, seaweed, water, sand, salt	Habitat and biodiversity; waste management; transportation; human habitat; employment; recreation
Forest ecosystems	Timber for fuel and shelter, water for drinking and irrigation, vines, bamboo, leaves, edible plants, game	Removal of air pollutants; oxygen emission; nutrient cycling; watershed (infiltration, purification, flow control, soil stabilization); biodiversity; atmospheric carbon; employment; human and wildlife habitats; recreation
Freshwater systems	Water for drinking and irrigation, fish, hydroelectricity	Water flow buffer; waste distribution; nutrient cycling; biodiversity; aquatic life; transportation; employment; recreation
Grassland ecosystems	Supports domestic livestock, game, fiber, water for drinking and irrigation	Watershed (infiltration, purification, flow control, soil stabilization); nutrient cycling; biodiversity; soil; atmospheric carbon; human and wildlife habitat; recreation

3. forest ecosystems

4. freshwater systems

5. grassland ecosystems

Each of these ecosystems is linked together. Adjacent ecosystems influence each other. See Table 1-1 for additional information on ecosystems.

Some ecosystems are stable and others are dynamic. Stable ecosystems are ones with processes in "dynamic equilibrium" as nutrients revolve within the system (or are recycled) with little overall loss. Minor disruptions occur to most ecosystems, and a true steady state is seldom achieved. Ecosystems change over time. Natural disasters, climate changes, and human activities have changed ecosystems. Succession and retrogression are processes by which ecosystems change.

Ecosystem succession. Succession refers to normal, predictable, and progressive changes in biotic communities leading to the establishment of a climax community. Succession usually begins when a disturbance—such as volcanic eruption, glacier retreat, or meteorite—kills many or all of the life forms within a region. *Primary succession* is the term used when new organisms emerge in a formerly barren area. When all life and topsoil is destroyed, soil must be reestablished with dust, primitive plants, and **organic** material. Spores or seeds from primitive plants such as moss or lichens become anchored in the new soil and discharge minerals. As more organic material is generated by decaying materials, conditions to support insects and invertebrates begin to provide fertile grounds for rooted plants. As plants compete for food, drawing moisture and other nutrients away, smaller plants are succeeded by larger plants. After many years, a greater number of plants emerge and animals that are in search of food move into the area. As a result, a new ecosystem emerges.

Secondary succession describes when dormant species emerge. When soil conditions are disrupted but topsoil and some limited vegetation remain, succession can occur much more quickly. An example of this is the return of an abandoned farm field to a climax forest. Because the fertile soil is already present, seeds and rhizomes present in the soil grow quickly. Plants move in, sprouting from the present seeds or rhizomes or are carried to the site by wind, birds, and grazing animals. These early plants are also known as *native plants* and may include wildflowers, tall grasses, and compact woody bushes. These grasses will eventually crowd out the wildflowers. The native trees may be replaced by new growth trees such as dogwood and sumac. After a time, perhaps a century or two, the climax forest trees will

Ecosystems
Identifiable areas within nature in which the organisms interact within themselves and their environment, exchanging nutrients within the system.

Succession
Predictable changes in biotic communities after an environmental disturbance. Primary succession occurs when new organisms emerge in a barren area. Secondary succession occurs when dormant species emerge.

Organic
Something containing the element carbon, such as plants and animals.

move into a typical temperate forest and include such trees as oak, maple, hickory, and elm, replacing the new-forest trees. Bodies of water can also experience succession when soil erodes into the water and new aquatic organisms emerge.

Ecosystem retrogression. When the climate changes, soils are poisoned or eroded or species are eliminated or introduced, the internal compensating mechanisms of the ecosystem may not be sufficient to return the ecosystem to its previous stable state. **Retrogression** is a negative process that reduces the diversity of an ecosystem placing a number of species at risk. As land is overgrazed or farmed intensively, tropical forests are burned and then farmed, water resources are depleted, or land is mismanaged, these changes in nature destroy species. Even adding new species to an ecosystem can be a threat to environmental stability as complex ecosystems are disturbed. Further, the species remaining may be less desirable from a human point of view. Simple systems in which fewer species exist or diversity reduction takes place are at greater risk of failure. The lack of cross-links in an ecosystem food chain means fewer alternatives for feeding. When a species is reduced in number or dies off, its predators also die off if other alternatives do not exist.

Evolution. Darwin's theory of evolution proposed species survival in terms of survival of the fittest. There is a natural pecking order among species that requires the weak to either become strong or succumb to external forces. Most species need to adapt to stressful and ever-changing environments if they are to survive. An example of how a species can adapt to environmental changes is the emergence of antibiotic resistant strains of bacteria such as tuberculosis. This occurs due to DNA mutations as a result of exposure to outside elements.

Ecosystem dominance. When one species dominates other species and competes more successfully than others for key resources, there is a profound effect on the ecosystem. Overpopulation or the introduction of an invasive species can be destructive. In most cases, the dominant part of an ecosystem is plant life. Plants provide food, shelter, shade, soil preservation, and oxygen for other life; the less plant life, the less animal and human life.

Biosystems. A **biosystem** refers to a collection of living things that depend on one another for existence. The type of biosystem inhabited depends on geographical and weather conditions. Maintenance of the biosystem is important because each living thing directly affects another. An important aspect of biosystems is **biodiversity**. Biodiversity describes the variety of living things in an area or region at a given point in time. It is important that there is a balance between **decomposers**, plant, animal, and human species. Elimination of a plant species may cause birds and animals to migrate to other areas in search of food. Overpopulation of one animal species may destroy vegetation or other animals that help keep the biosystem in a state of balance, particularly the predators. Predatory animals reduce the number of less-aggressive competitors to maintain their population, destroying other important plant and animal life.

 The average surface temperature of the Earth is 61°F. The coldest temperatures are found in Antarctica with an average temperature of −60°F. The hottest temperature on average is in the Sahara Desert with an average temperature of 130°F.

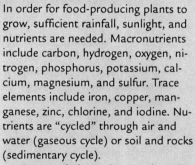 **Digging Deeper** NUTRIENT "RECYCLING"

In order for food-producing plants to grow, sufficient rainfall, sunlight, and nutrients are needed. Macronutrients include carbon, hydrogen, oxygen, nitrogen, phosphorus, potassium, calcium, magnesium, and sulfur. Trace elements include iron, copper, manganese, zinc, chlorine, and iodine. Nutrients are "cycled" through air and water (gaseous cycle) or soil and rocks (sedimentary cycle).

Gases cycled pertain to carbon, hydrogen, oxygen, and nitrogen. Carbon is the most important component of biological systems. It is found in the at-mosphere and dissolved in bodies of water. Carbon is created by plants through photosynthesis and animals receive the carbon they need by eating plants. It is returned back to the environment through respiration and from decay of dead animals or animal waste. The Earth's atmosphere is 78% nitrogen. However, atmospheric nitrogen cannot be absorbed by plants unless it is returned to the soil by lightening or by bacteria that normally lives with leguminous plants (such as soybeans). These methods convert the nitrogen to a form that is accessible to plants. Ani-mal waste is converted to ammonia, which is acted upon by bacteria-producing nitrates that produce free nitrogen back to the atmosphere.

Phosphorus and sulfur are also important to plant and animal life, but the sedimentary process needed to produce it takes a great deal of time—as much as centuries. Phosphorous reservoirs in rocks and soils are washed away when exposed to rainfall. When this rain is absorbed by plants, the energy is transferred to plant-eating animals. Most phosphorus is lost due to erosion.

Atmosphere

The atmosphere is divided into layers: (1) the troposphere; (2) the stratosphere; (3) the mesosphere; (4) thermosphere; and (5) ionosphere (Figure 1-4). The troposphere is where life exists, consisting of oxygen, nitrogen, and other gases. The stratosphere contains ozone (O_3) that absorbs infrared radiation. The mesosphere and thermosphere consists of light nitrogen and oxygen molecules lost to space. The ionosphere (known as Earth's magnetic field) captures protons and electrons emitted by solar storms seen as the *aurora borealis.*

Gravity pulls the atmosphere close to the Earth and gives weight to the atmosphere. *Atmospheric pressure* (the force exerted on objects by the weight of the air) is measured by a barometer. The atmospheric pressure fluctuates according to air density and altitude. At sea level, atmospheric pressure is 14.7 pounds per square inch. The atmospheric pressure decreases above sea level and increases below sea level. Atmospheric pressure and density vary according to thermal radiation and air movement. The energy driving the air movement in the atmosphere is from the sun, which strikes the Earth unevenly. Warmer air is less dense, so it expands and rises. Cooler air is more dense and higher in pressure. Differences in air pressure give rise to wind. The direction of wind is influenced by the rotation of the Earth, friction, and solar warming.

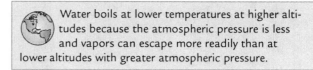

Water boils at lower temperatures at higher altitudes because the atmospheric pressure is less and vapors can escape more readily than at lower altitudes with greater atmospheric pressure.

The Cycles of Life

arious cycles of life on the planet help to regenerate the temperature we need, the air we breathe, the water we drink, the land we use, and the food we eat. It is important to

Retrogression
The reduction of diversity in an ecosystem.

Biosystems
Composites of living organisms living in a particular area governed by climate.

Biodiversity
A variety of living things in a geographical area, region, or particular time dependent on another for existence.

Decomposers
Insects, bacteria, fungi, and protozoan that break down complex organic materials into mineral nutrients to be used by plants.

FIGURE 1-4 **Atmospheric Layers** There are several layers of gases where life can exist. Source: NASA.http://liftoff.msfc.nasa.gov/academy/space/atmosphere.html.

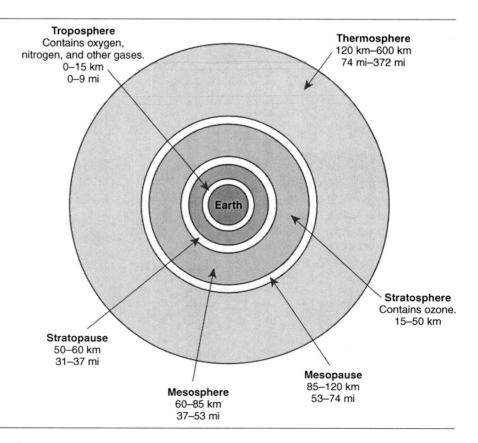

Troposphere
Contains oxygen, nitrogen, and other gases.
0–15 km
0–9 mi

Thermosphere
120 km–600 km
74 mi–372 mi

Earth

Stratosphere
Contains ozone.
15–50 km

Stratopause
50–60 km
31–37 mi

Mesosphere
60–85 km
37–53 mi

Mesopause
85–120 km
53–74 mi

understand how these "cycles of life" work to sustain the planet and influence human health.

THE SOLAR CYCLE

The atmosphere is strongly influenced by the *solar cycle,* which is a term used to describe the cycles of the sun influencing seasons, storms, and activities such as sunspots and flares. Life on Earth requires a continuing source of energy, which is provided by the sun. Solar radiation reaching the Earth's atmosphere is absorbed, scattered, and reflected by clouds and Earth's surface, so about 50% of it reaches the land and ocean.

Clouds are important to the **climate** because they cover a significant part of the Earth, scattering and reflecting solar radiation back into space. When they are present, clouds play an important role in energy transfer, water transfer, and solar heat. Low clouds have a cooling effect because they are thicker and reflect much of the incoming solar radiation out to space. High, thin, cirrus clouds have a warming effect because they only slightly filter the incoming solar radiation while trapping some of Earth's radiation and reflecting back to the surface. Deep convective clouds have neither a warming nor a cooling effect because their reflective and absorptive capabilities neutralize each other.

The balance between incoming solar radiation and outgoing infrared radiation is important to climate. *Climate* is a term used to describe the average weather within a particular area over a long period of time and includes temperature, precipitation, humidity, wind, cloud cover, and solar radiation. Climate is affected most by the position of the Earth with respect to the sun. The intensity or energy from the sun diminishes with the distance from the sun. The seasons are caused by the tilt of the Earth on its axis as it revolves around the sun. The sun impacts the Earth in bands of decreasing energy extending north and south from the equator. Weather changes are influenced by rotation of the Earth. For instance, in North America, winds flow from the west to the east. The amount of solar energy absorbed is important to temperature and moisture distribution. Warmer air can hold moisture; therefore, warmer climates have more rain (such as rainforest areas). Warm dry air absorbs moisture, creating dry land areas (such as desert areas). As a result of stable climate conditions, plants and animals become characteristic of specific areas.

THE ENERGY CYCLE

All energy in the Earth's environment is possible because of the sun (Figure 1-5). Plants absorb radiation from the sun and through a process known as *photosynthesis,* store chemical energy and release energy in the form of carbon dioxide, oxygen, and water. Some of the stored energy is used in respiration, which transfers heat into the environment. The rest of the energy is used for plant growth. Plants are consumed by insects, animals, and humans for energy and nutrients. Energy is transferred through the **food chain** with higher-level organisms feeding on lower-level organisms), and much energy is lost. Organisms eating lower on the food chain, therefore, supply more energy while organisms eating higher on the food chain (consuming more organisms over time) consume energy. *Herbivores* consume only plants. *Omnivores* consume plants and animals. *Carnivores* consume other animals.

> The Gaia hypothesis is the idea, developed by James Lovelock, that Earth's systems behave as a single living entity, striving to maintain health and stability conducive to the existence of life. The term "gaia" means Earth, a live planet with life unique to the atmosphere and conditions of the planet.

Consider the Cost | TRANSFER OF ENERGY AND THE FOOD CHAIN

A way of looking at how much energy is lost when one organism consumes another is to look at energy transfer. All plants and animals contain energy through carbohydrates, proteins, and fats. When an animal eats a plant, less energy is lost than if the animal eats another animal. Consider the following facts:

- It takes 10 pounds of corn to produce 1 pound of beef. When a steer is slaughtered, only 40% of it is eaten.

- It takes 10 pounds of beef to make 1 pound of human weight.

- It takes less grain to produce 1 pound of pork or poultry because it can be produced faster than beef.

- Animals produced for their meat produce faster if they are confined to a place where they cannot move around.

- Compared to beef, pork, or poultry, it takes less energy to produce 1 pound of fish. Fish farms help produce fish quicker for harvest.

Eating lower on the food chain is one way to decrease the demand for meat and lower grocery bills, reduce waste products (manure, urine, and unused body parts) from livestock, reduce noxious odor emissions from slaughterhouse and meat-packing plants, and reduce the incidence of food-borne illnesses due to contaminated meat products. The problem is that no culture has ever willingly given up meat in significant amounts once they have developed a taste for it (Nanavukaren, 1999).

As each type of organism consumes another, it receives nutrients and poisons absorbed by the organism it eats. It is important to know that nutrients absorbed from one organism to another can be recycled.

BIOGEOCHEMICAL CYCLING

The recycling of **inorganic** to organic nutrients is known as **biogeochemical cycling**. Biogeochemical cycling takes place as the atmosphere interacts with life on Earth to transport and transform one type of material to another. Biogeochemical cycling includes hydrological, sedimentary, and gaseous cycles that distribute six elements important to life: hydrogen, carbon, oxygen, nitrogen, phosphorus, and sulfur. These elements, or *macronutrients*, combine in various ways to make up more than 95% of all living things.

THE HYDROLOGIC CYCLE

The **hydrologic cycle** includes evaporation, transpiration, condensation, precipitation, infiltration, and surface and groundwater flow (Figure 1-6). This cycle moves enormous quantities of water around the world. Water first evaporates from surface water, plants, and soil and is transported to the atmosphere as water vapor, liquid water droplets, or ice crystals. When water vapor condenses

as clouds, they reflect harmful solar rays back into the atmosphere, thus cooling temperatures. When atmospheric water vapor condenses due to heat energy, it falls back to the Earth in the form of rain, hail, sleet, or snow. After

Climate
Weather conditions such as temperature, precipitation, and wind typical to an area or region.

Food chain
A succession of organisms in a feeding hierarchy; food energy is transferred from one organism to another as each consumes a lower member and is then preyed upon by a higher member.

Inorganic
Composed of nonanimal or nonvegetable matter, not containing carbon, derived from mineral sources.

Biogeochemical cycling
The natural process of converting inorganic to organic nutrients.

Hydrologic cycle
A series of naturally occurring events in which water is changed from a liquid to a gas, rises into the atmosphere, is condensed, and falls back to Earth; movement of water molecules on a global scale through oceans, atmosphere, surface water, and groundwater.

FIGURE 1-5 **Energy Cycle** How energy is created, used, and recycled is one of the most important facts of life. Source: Rod Nave, Georgia State University. Reprinted with permission.

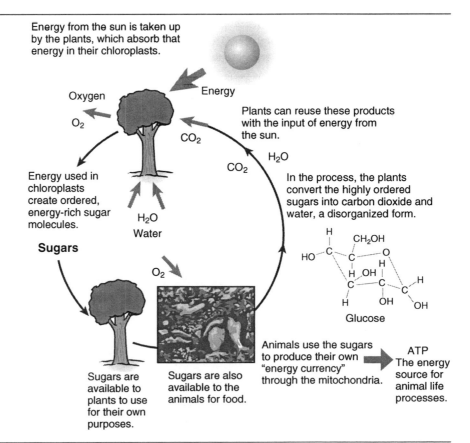

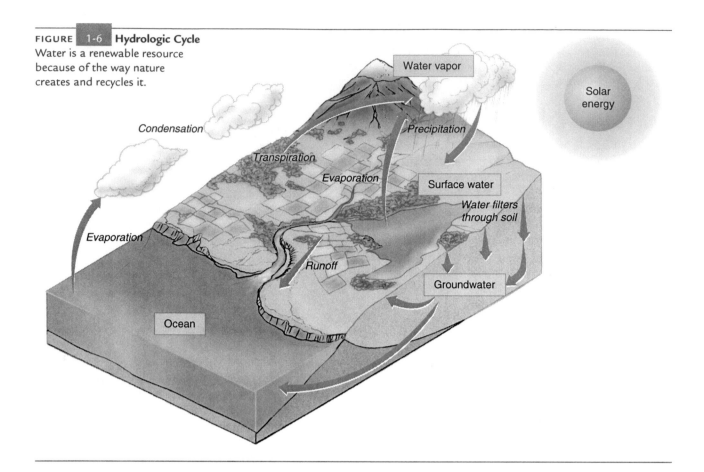

FIGURE 1-6 **Hydrologic Cycle**
Water is a renewable resource
because of the way nature
creates and recycles it.

falling to the Earth, it adds to surface water or filters through the soil to groundwater aquifers. The hydrologic cycle intersects with sedimentary and gaseous cycles.

SEDIMENTARY CYCLE

The **sedimentary cycle** is tied to the hydrological cycle because water carries materials from land to the oceans where nutrients are deposited as sediments. Nutrients such as calcium, iron, and phosphorus are gradually leached from sedimentary rock by rain or erosion. The sedimentary cycle is extremely slow due to the process of weathering.

Phosphorus Cycle

The **phosphorous cycle** consists of the release of phosphorus from sedimentary rock (Figure 1-7). Phosphorous is the main element in compounds such as adenosine triphosphate (ATP), which is important in the transfer of chemical energy in animals. The phosphorous content of soils is important. Most agricultural soils must be enriched by adding phosphate fertilizers. Plants take up released phosphorus in their roots, which are then consumed by animals. Animal wastes and decomposing animal matter release phosphorous back to the soil for reuse by plants. Mining and agriculture can erode soil and carry phosphorous into streams, estuaries, and oceans where it

settles in an insoluble form at the bottom of these waters and becomes a pollutant. Sources of inorganic phosphorous are being depleted rapidly and the Earth faces a future of infertile soils.

Sulfur Cycle

Sulfur plays an important part in the structure and function of proteins. It is also one of the main cycles most disturbed by human activity. The **sulfur cycle** begins with the sulfur dioxide (SO_2) or the particles of sulfate (SO_4) compounds in the atmosphere. Plants take up sulfur and it is returned to land or water after the plants die or are consumed by animals. Bacteria transfer the organic sulfur to hydrogen sulfide gas (H_2S) to re-enter the atmosphere, water, and soil, continuing the cycle. The acid property of sulfur is important to the natural weathering of rocks, acid precipitation, and rates of **denitrification**. When natural sources are combined with man-made sources, smog and acid rain develop and become major pollution problems.

GASEOUS CYCLES

Gaseous cycles represent the flow of energy and nutrients in an ecosystem. They occur when most of the element is found in the form of a gas. Gaseous cycles include the oxygen cycle, carbon cycle, and nitrogen cycle.

FIGURE 1-7 **The Phosphorus Cycle** The phosphorous cycle returns minerals to the soil and is a function of the hydrological cycle. (Source: Marietta College, Department of Biology and Environmental Science. http://www.marietta.edu/~biol/102/ecosystem.html#Energyflowthroughtheecosystem3. Accessed February 18, 2005.)

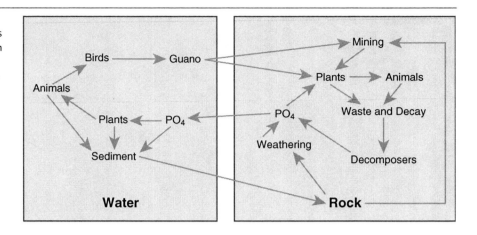

The Oxygen Cycle

Oxygen is present in the atmosphere, in carbohydrates, in water, and in carbon dioxide. Oxygen gas and water are released into the atmosphere by plants through photosynthesis where oxygen is utilized by plants and animals through respiration. The current level of oxygen in the atmosphere today took billions of years to achieve. Without the **oxygen cycle**, higher-level animals and humans would not exist.

Carbon Cycle

Animals and humans depend on carbon for energy. Carbon is available in the environment in gas, liquid, or solid form. The **carbon cycle** is the process in which carbon dioxide is released into the atmosphere, absorbed by water and soil, and then reabsorbed by plants for food. Plants convert inorganic carbon and water to fuel through the process of photosynthesis. When an animal eats the plant, waste is released through respiration and excretion back into the atmosphere. In addition, dead plants and animals decay, releasing carbon back into the soil. Forests act as "carbon sinks" by absorbing and storing carbon dioxide in the atmosphere. Bogs, oceans, and decaying matter below the ground convert decaying materials into **fossil fuels** such as coal, oil, or natural gas. These are recovered and burned to release carbon dioxide back into the atmosphere.

Oceans also operate as carbon sinks because of the capacity to store heat. The top eight feet of ocean water holds as much heat as the Earth's entire atmosphere. Ocean currents transport stored heat and dissolved gases to different parts of the world. As ocean waters circulate, heat is transferred from low altitudes to high altitudes, from north to south, and from the surface to the ocean depths and back. As a result, the ocean is the largest reservoir of carbon, holding 50 times more carbon than the atmosphere and 20 times more than land.

Nitrogen Cycle

The **nitrogen cycle** begins when atmospheric nitrogen becomes fixated in the soil through lightning, bacteria, or rhozobium plant species (Figure 1-8). Usable forms of nitrogen include nitrates (NO_{3-}), nitrites (NO_{2-}), and ammonia (NH_{4+}). Nitrates are produced

Sedimentary cycle
The breakdown of rock and transportation of sediment and nutrients by water through erosion or weathering.

Phosphorus cycle
A sedimentary cycle that releases phosphorus with assistance from the hydrologic cycle.

Sulfur cycle
The release and production of sulfur that involves the production of acid rain.

Denitrification
The process of changing nitrogen from a solid to a gas that is discharged into the atmosphere.

Oxygen cycle
The transformation of oxygen from plants to the atmosphere due to photosynthesis; for respiration of animals.

Carbon cycle
Movement of carbon on a global scale through oceans, atmosphere, and biological organisms.

Fossil fuels
Coal, oil, and natural gas; carbon-based sources of energy derived from the fossilized remains of dead plants and animals; a nonrenewable energy source.

Nitrogen cycle
The continuous, cyclic progression of chemical reactions in which atmospheric nitrogen is compounded, dissolved in rain, deposited in the soil, assimilated and metabolized by bacteria and plants, and returned to the atmosphere following decomposition.

FIGURE   1-8   **Nitrogen Cycle**
Nitrogen is an important soil
nutrient replenished by storms
and decomposition.

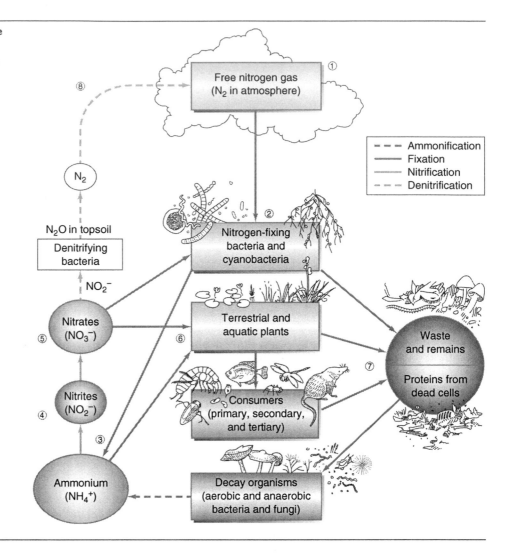

from combustion of fossil fuels and the erosion of nitrate-rich rocks. Nitrates are released into soil and water and absorbed by plants. Nitrogenous ammonium compounds are released from animal wastes and decomposition of dead organisms by microbes in the soil. The ammonia is then converted to nitrites and nitrates by nitrifying bacteria to be absorbed by plants through the soil. Nitrates and ammonia are used to create agricultural fertilizers that increase soil fertility. Organic nitrogen may be recycled back to the atmosphere by denitrifying bacteria living in mud and sediment of lakes, ponds, streams, and estuaries.

Examining biogeochemical cycles provides a way to understand how nutrients get into soils in order to make the soil productive and how water resources are replenished. Biogeochemical cycles also explain depletion of the ozone layer, global climate change, droughts, acid precipitation, and disruption of ecosystems by the use of synthetic chemicals.

Human Interaction Problems with the Environment

The human species dominates most ecosystems on Earth. Its dominance is related to intelligence and population numbers. The domestication of plants and animals, the creation of new habitats, and the ability to alter genetic material are just some of the ways humans have changed nature's course. On the other hand, humans have done more damage to the Earth than any other species. In fact, humans are considered to be the "dirty species" because they pollute their own habitat with dirty technology, pollution, and land degradation, becoming a danger to themselves and others. As human populations increase, ecosystems change, climate changes, and natural resources are used at a rate far greater than they can ever be replaced (Figures 1-9 through 1-15).

When North American muskrats were brought to the Netherlands in 1906, they had no natural enemies that kept the population under control. Millions of muskrats inhabited the canals, weakening the dikes that protected the low country from flooding.

In the Mediterranean, seaweed from the Pacific that was released from aquarium tanks of the Oceanographic Museum in Monaco grew out of control. From the French Riviera to Croa-tia, the seaweed crowded out native plant and animal species.

A species known as Leidy's comb jellyfish was discharged by a ship into the Black Sea in the 1980s and multiplied so rapidly that zooplankton were unavailable as sources of food for many fish species (Bright, 1998).

Other foreign species that have posed problems include red imported fire ant (*Solenopsis invicta*), Africanized honeybee (*Apis mellifera scutellata*), Formosan subterranean termite (*Coptotermes formosanus*), European gypsy moth (*Lymantria dispar*), Asian tiger mosquito (*Aedes albopictus*), water hyacinth (*Eichhornia crassipes*), musk thistle (*Carduus nutans*), Russian olive (*Elaeagnus angustifolia*), zebra mussel (*Dreissena polymorpha*), bullfrog (*Rana catesbeiana*), brown tree snake (*Boiga irregularis*), kudzu (*Pueraria Montana*), and nutria (*Myocastor coypus*). For additional invasive species, see www.invasivespecies.gov.

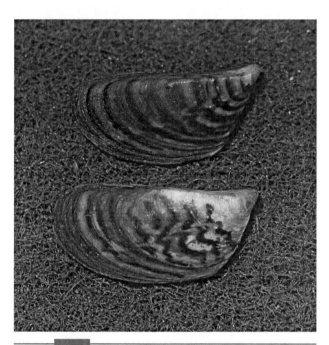

FIGURE 1-9 **Zebra Mussels** Originally from the Balkans and Soviet Union, they are a major problem in the Great Lakes of the U.S.

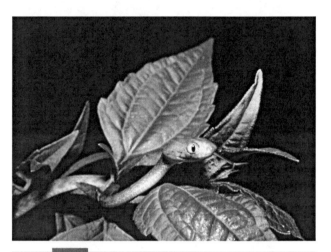

FIGURE 1-10 **Brown Tree Snake** Originally from Australia, the brown tree snake has done considerable ecological damage to Guam.

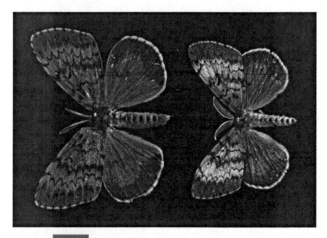

FIGURE 1-11 **Gypsy Moth** Brought from France by a naturalist, they escaped and have plagued Massachusetts since 1869.

OVERPOPULATION

The more people there are, the greater the demand on resources and the more waste. The global human population continues to multiply in logarithmic proportions and to develop energy intensive technologies, resulting in the discharge of dramatic levels of toxic substances into the air, water, and land (see Chapter 2). Before the Industrial Revolution (see Chapter 3 for an historical account), environmental degradation was gradual, occurring over hundreds or thousands of years. Since then, the scale, speed, and long-term threat on

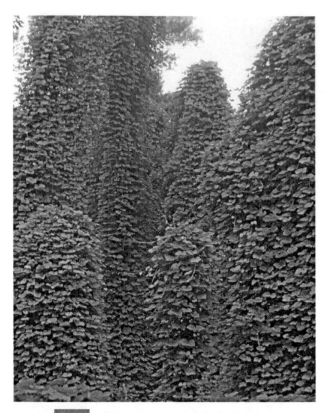

FIGURE 1-12 **Kudzu** Originally from China this plant takes over land and vegetation from the Midwest to the East and Southern states.

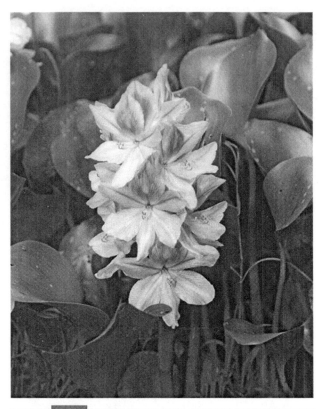

FIGURE 1-13 **Water Hyacinth** A native of South America, it clogs up waterways and canals in Southern and South-western states.

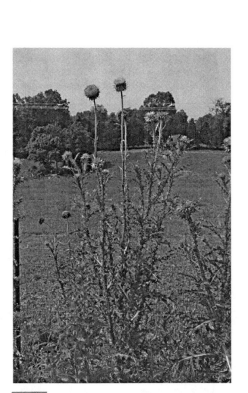

FIGURE 1-14 **Musk Thistle** A native plant of Eurasia, it can be dense enough to crowd out grass in pastures in the U.S. and Canada.

ecosystems is a global priority. Human interactions threaten the climate, sea levels, the atmosphere, water, soil, species, and more.

DEMAND ON NATURAL RESOURCES

The constant population growth and desire for improved living standards has increased the demand for natural resources, land, water, and air. These are **nonrenewable resources**, yet humans are consuming them as if there were an endless supply. Scarce resources have always prompted competitiveness, greed, and a lack of vision for the future. Scientists have been concerned for years that these resources will become depleted. In 1961, scientists assessed human use of the Earth and estimated that 70% of the biospheric capacity had already been used (Kirby, 2002). Some suggested that by the year 1999 humans had already absorbed 120% of the Earth's natural ability to regenerate its ecological capacity.

Nonrenewable resources
Natural resources that are considered finite in amounts; predicted to become scarce due to their rapid depletion.

FIGURE 1-15 **Nutria**
Trapped in South America for their fur coats, they have created problems in Louisiana and other Southern states because they reproduce quickly and destroy wetlands vegetation.

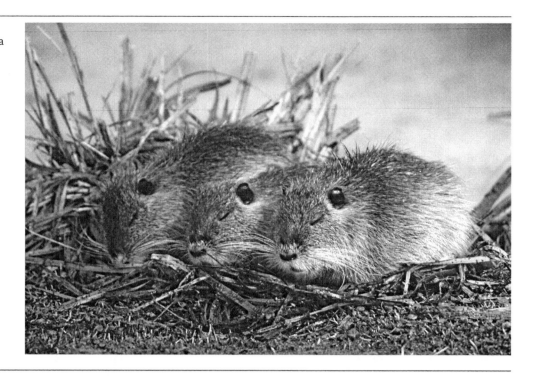

Consider the Cost

PRESERVATION

Destruction, abuse, and misuse of environmental resources required for life is detrimental to the health of the world and its environment. There are many ways that individuals can help preserve, conserve, and maintain the environment. Each member of society needs to develop respectful attitudes, a sense of control over environmental issues, and to modify behaviors that threaten or endanger the environment and human health. This may require forethought, a sense of responsibility, and extra time, but can have major impacts. Community leaders and public health professionals must express a concern for other citizens, practice responsible behaviors, solicit collaborative efforts from others, and generate a sense of community.

Preservation strategies include respect for the air, water, land, and other natural resources. Preservation includes developing an attitude of respect for the environment and all living things in it. Spend more time outdoors; plan family outings in public parks, national forests, and at historical monuments

rather than amusement parks. Develop an historical view for all inhabited areas and nurture an appreciation for that land. Form futuristic behaviors so that others may enjoy what is enjoyed today. Take on a new awareness of plants and animals that share the Earth's environment and a sense of harmony with other living things. Dispose of trash responsibly and encourage laws that ask others to do the same. Visit the natural wonders and be in awe at their greatness. Donate monies to help preserve natural beauty. There are many organizations dedicated to the preservation of national parks, beaches, wildlife, and other environmental concerns. It is always a good idea to belong to groups with similar interests to further a cause about which one feels strongly.

CONSERVATION

Conservation strategies can be directed toward the prudent use of air, water, and land. In order to preserve air quality, plant trees, shrubs, and other vegetation to keep the oxygen in the

environment. Limit outdoor burning and have automobile emissions systems inspected annually. To conserve water, use it prudently indoors and outdoors. Turn down the thermostats in cold weather and turn them up in warm weather to conserve electricity. Require less personal space for living, parking vehicles, and in other ways. Consider the number of pets or children for which one can responsibly care. Purchase fuel-efficient homes, automobiles, and appliances. Purchase less disposable items and generate less trash. Purchase biodegradable soaps and be careful about how waste is disposed in water and on the land. Minimize the use of pesticides, chemical fertilizers, and do not pour harmful chemicals or petroleum products on the ground. Encourage employers to reduce, reuse, recycle, and use recycled products. Ask communities to offer recycling and collections programs. Lobby for returnable deposits on bottles and cans.

Human activities sometimes destroy forests and wetlands, threatening ecosystems. Deforestation, soil erosion, desertification, and loss of biodiversity were problems even in ancient times. Natural disasters, climate changes, and disease further threaten ecosystems, but these changes are usually confined within a specific area. Most biotic communities are proving unable to respond to the unrelenting pressures of disruption, thus causing major species loss, water contamination, climatic changes, and other changes to the global ecosystems. These are not in the best interests for human survival or the quality of life. The entire Earth is affected by **greenhouse gas** emissions, ozone depletion, acid rain, toxic waste, and large-scale industrial accidents.

Plants and animals have become extinct over the centuries that Earth has existed. Some of the extinctions (e.g., dinosaurs) occurred due to mass extinction episodes caused by climate change, extreme geological activity, huge meteors colliding with the Earth, or other natural factors that took thousands of years to occur. It is believed that the natural rate of extinction would be 1 to 10 species lost per year. Since the 1500s when humans and their domestic animals began to colonize various parts of the Earth, as many of 811 species have disappeared. Activities causing the loss of species today include the destruction of habitat, illegal hunting (known as *poaching*), overfishing, and pesticide poisoning. According to the World Resources Institute (2000), 100 species become extinct every day due to tropical deforestation.

Digging Deeper

In the Rocky Mountain region, the gray wolf, kit fox, grizzly bear, black-footed ferret, and wolverine are all considered to be endangered mammals. Endangered birds include the bald eagle, whooping crane, piping plover, lesser prairie chicken, and burrowing owl. The boreal toad, greenback cutthroat trout, pike minnow, humpback chub, and the razorback sucker are also endangered due to the growing numbers of humans inhabiting the area.

During the nineteenth century, the numbers of grizzly bear decreased as ranchers and government trappers increased. The black-footed ferret is considered to be the rarest mammal in North America. It is dependent on the prairie dog for food and when prairie dog populations were controlled by poisoning, the black-footed ferret population also decreased (Gompper and Williams, 1998). The boreal toad numbers have declined dramatically in the last 20 to 25 years due to habitat destruction, a fungus (*Batrachochytrium dendrobatitis*), increasing ultraviolet radiation, the introduction of nonnative species, and contaminants (Blaustein et al., 2003).

Digging Deeper — PARTIAL LIST OF EXTINCT SPECIES OF THE U.S.

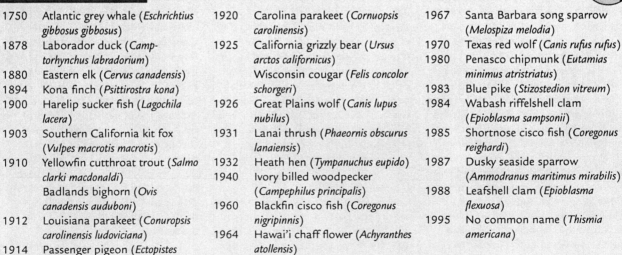

Year	Species	Year	Species	Year	Species
1750	Atlantic grey whale (*Eschrichtius gibbosus gibbosus*)	1920	Carolina parakeet (*Cornuopsis carolinensis*)	1967	Santa Barbara song sparrow (*Melospiza melodia*)
1878	Laborador duck (*Camptorhynchus labradorium*)	1925	California grizzly bear (*Ursus arctos californicus*)	1970	Texas red wolf (*Canis rufus rufus*)
1880	Eastern elk (*Cervus canadensis*)		Wisconsin cougar (*Felis concolor schorgeri*)	1980	Penasco chipmunk (*Eutamias minimus atristriatus*)
1894	Kona finch (*Psittirostra kona*)	1926	Great Plains wolf (*Canis lupus nubilus*)	1983	Blue pike (*Stizostedion vitreum*)
1900	Harelip sucker fish (*Lagochila lacera*)	1931	Lanai thrush (*Phaeornis obscurus lanaiensis*)	1984	Wabash riffelshell clam (*Epioblasma sampsonii*)
1903	Southern California kit fox (*Vulpes macrotis macrotis*)	1932	Heath hen (*Tympanuchus eupido*)	1985	Shortnose cisco fish (*Coregonus reighardi*)
1910	Yellowfin cutthroat trout (*Salmo clarki macdonaldi*)	1940	Ivory billed woodpecker (*Campephilus principalis*)	1987	Dusky seaside sparrow (*Ammodranus maritimus mirabilis*)
	Badlands bighorn (*Ovis canadensis auduboni*)	1960	Blackfin cisco fish (*Coregonus nigripinnis*)	1988	Leafshell clam (*Epioblasma flexuosa*)
1912	Louisiana parakeet (*Conuropsis carolinensis ludoviciana*)	1964	Hawai'i chaff flower (*Achyranthes atollensis*)	1995	No common name (*Thismia americana*)
1914	Passenger pigeon (*Ectopistes migratorius*)				

The current rate of extinction is estimated to be extremely high because many species have never been identified. Over 11,000 species of plants and animals are known to be endangered or threatened. Estimates are that one-third of all U.S. animals (971 species) are at risk of extinction (The Nature Conservancy, 2002).

Human Solutions to Environmental Problems

There is no doubt that where there are environmental concerns, humans are part of the problem. Fortunately, humans can also develop ways of measuring and monitoring demands on the environment. If necessary, laws have been created to stop the abuse and misuse of human rights and privileges (read the Endangered Species Act of 1973) (Figures 1-16, 1-17, and 1-18). Increased knowledge and ability created techniques to produce food using new methods that require less land, create new landscapes, breed new species, and ways to reuse waste materials for the purpose of creating new landscapes and producing energy.

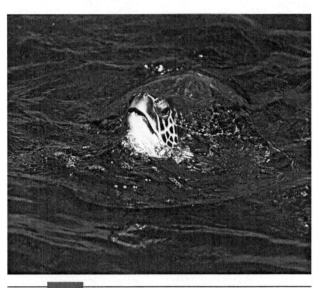

FIGURE 1-16 **Green Sea Turtle** Native to Florida and the Pacific coast of Mexico, they have been listed as endangered/threatened since 1978.

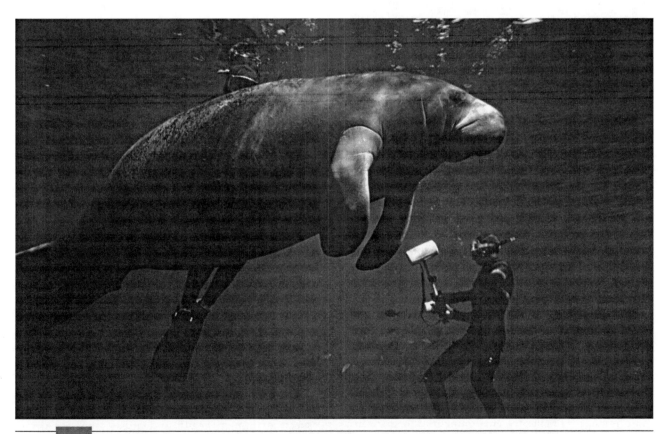

FIGURE 1-17 **West Indian Manatee** After being hunted extensively, there are only about 2,000 manatee on the coast from Florida to Brazil.

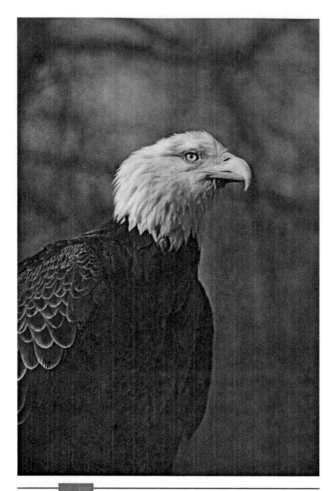

FIGURE 1-18 **Bald Eagle** Once an endangered species because of pesticides and predators, it was moved to the "threatened species" list in 1994.

may have long-term negative consequences to the natural environment. The goal of human ecology is to enable humans to progress and prosper without disrupting the environment in which they live. Growing populations in developing and industrialized countries contribute to events that impoverish and threaten ecosystems. Land development is not controlled, natural resources are depleted, pollution affects food and water supplies, and new diseases and disease patterns emerge. No human, plant, animal, or insect is immune to exposure from toxic substances or the effects of uncontrolled progress and technology.

Public Health and Environmental Health Strategies

ecause humans have a profound impact on the environment and the environment has a strong effect on health and the quality of life, it is important to study ecological balances that sustain environmental quality. It is also important to study factors that adversely impact human health as well as the degree to which human health is affected.

Public health efforts attempt to prevent human illnesses and premature death. As the demand for public health services increases, the need for trained personnel and educational programs becomes increasingly important. Public health strategies are orchestrated by organizations interested in public health at the international, national, state, and local levels. Public health priorities include population control, emissions control, sanitation, waste management, immunizations, and disaster preparation.

The term *environmental health* was defined by the World Health Organization (WHO) in 1989 as "those aspects of human health and disease that are determined by factors in the environment" (Pan American

Ecology is the study of interrelationships of organisms and their environment, while **bioecology** is the science dealing with interrelations of plant and animal communities with their environment. Ecologists monitor ecosystems for the **conservation** and **preservation** of the natural environment so that important resources important to human, animal, and plant existence are not lost. Major concerns among ecologists include global warming, deforestation, **habitat** loss, water **pollution** and available drinking water supplies, air pollution, energy resources, human population growth, species protection and diversity, land use, and food production.

Human ecology is the study of the complex and varied systems of interaction between people and their environment. Anthropologists, biologists, geographers, sociologists, and psychologists have studied the reciprocal effects of humans and the environment for a long time. Humans have the remarkable ability to adapt to their environment in positive ways, however, the tendency for most humans is to alter the environment to their advantage. The concern then becomes that those tendencies

Health Organization, 2004). This definition asserted that environmental factors influenced quality of life, human health, and disease states. By 1993, the WHO expanded the definition to name biological, physical, chemical, social, and psychological environmental factors in an environment, including indoor as well as outdoor factors. The 1989 WHO definition also referred to environmental health as "the theory and practice of assessing, controlling factors in the environment that can potentially affect health." The practice of environmental health includes the assessment, correction, control, and prevention of environmental factors adversely affecting the health of present and future generations. In 1998 the U.S. Department of Health and Human Services Environmental Health Policy Committee considered 28 definitions from state, national, and international agencies for adoption without resolution until 2000 when the U.S. Department of Health and Human Services specifically defined environmental health as

> . . . those aspects of human disease, and injury that are determined or influenced by factors in the environment. This includes the study of both direct pathological effects of various chemical, physical, and biological agents, as well as the effects on health of the broad physical and social environment, which includes housing, urban development, land-use and transportation, industry, and agriculture. (USDHHS, 2000).

At the local level, *environmental health* is a term used to describe services that assess and evaluate potential environmental risks to human populations to prevent disease and exposure to toxic substances. Environmental health is not just a governmental or nonprofit organization responsibility. It requires collaboration and cooperation among businesspeople and private citizens as well. The need for individuals to work together and assist with environmental problems is imperative, particularly in the twenty-first century. Individuals need to collectively practice conservation for the good of all. Ecology and environmental health are everyone's business and essential to the quality and longevity of life.

Summary

Relationships between the environment, population growth, ecology, and conservation are important to quality of life and human health. Natural geological processes and corresponding "cycles of life" are important to replenishing nutrients needed for plant growth, animal species, and human survival.

The evolution and prosperity of the human species has progressed to include concerns about depletion of natural resources, pollution, misuse of land, and endangerment of species.

Many sciences and professions devote substantial time and effort to prevent, control, and regulate human activities so that the environment can be preserved. Environmental health professionals and environmental health services include the study of the effects of various agents on health, assessing risk to human health, and applying ecological principles to minimize or control short-term and long-term effects on humans. Environmental health is a concern and a responsibility for everyone.

REFERENCES

Annan, K. (2002). Beyond the horizon. Special report: How to save the earth. *Time Magazine*, 160, A18–A19.

Aron, J. L., & Patz, J. A. (Eds.). (2001). *Ecosystem change and public health: A global perspective*. Baltimore, MD: The Johns Hopkins University Press.

Ecology
The scientific study of the relations of living things to one another and to their environment.

Bioecology
The science dealing with interrelation of plant and animal communities with their environment.

Conservation
Planned management to prevent the loss, destruction, or waste of natural resources; includes preservation or restoration.

Preservation
To keep what is already present intact as long as possible.

Habitat
A place where a plant or animal normally lives; part of an ecosystem.

Pollution
Harmful substances deposited in the air, water, or on land leading to contamination of the environment.

Human ecology
The study of interactions between people and their environment.

Endangered species
Any species in danger of becoming extinct.

Threatened species
A species that is rare and may incur harm or distress; likely to become an endangered species within the foreseeable future.

Ayyad, M. A. (2003). Case studies in the conservation of biodiversity: Degradation and threats. *Journal of Arid Environments, 54,* 165–183.

Blaustein, A., Romansic, J., Kiesecker, J., & Hatch, A. (2003). Ultraviolet radiation, toxic chemicals and amphibian population declines. *Diversity and Distributions, 9,* 123–141.

Bright, C. (1998). *Life out of bounds: Bioinvasion in a borderless world.* New York: W. W. Norton.

Colborn, T., Dumanowski, D., & Peterson Myers, J. (1996). *Our stolen future: Are we threatening our fertility, intelligence, and survival?* New York: Penguin Books.

Donatelle, R. (2001). Water: A critical nutrient. In A. Author, & B. Author, *Health: The basics* (p. 222). Boston: Allyn & Bacon.

Donatelle, R. J. (2001). *Health: The basics.* (4th ed.). Boston: Allyn & Bacon.

De Groot, N. (2001). Water resources management. In J. Aron & J. Patz *Ecosystem change and public health: A global perspective.* Baltimore: The Johns Hopkins University Press.

Gompper, M., & Williams, E. (1998). Parasite conservation and the black-footed ferret recovery program. *Conservation Biology, 12,* 730–732.

Irvin, J. (1999). How long can a human live without water and food? Ohio State University. Retrieved February 19, 2005 from http://www.madsci.org/posts/archives/sep99/937540022.Gb.r.html.

Kaufman, L., & Mallory, K. (Eds.) (1993). *The last extinction,* (2nd ed.). Cambridge, MA: MIT Press.

Kirby, A. (2002). Human use exhausts the Earth: Humanity's footprint on the planet. *GMT, 22,* 43.

Moore, G. (1999). *Living with the Earth: Concepts in environmental health science.* Boca Raton, FL: Lewis Publishers.

Nadakavukaren, A. (2000). *Our global environment: A health perspective.* Prospect Heights, IL: Waveland Press, Inc.

Ruttenber, A. J., & Ragsdale, H. L. (1995). The ecologic basis of health and disease. In D. Blumenthal & A. J. Ruttenber, *Introduction to Environmental Health* (2nd ed.). (pp. 3–32). New York: Springer Publishing Company.

Shabecoff, P. (2000). *Earth rising: American environmentalism in the 21st century.* Washington, DC: Island Press.

Tokar, B. (1997). *Earth for sale: Reclaiming ecology in the age of corporate greenwash.* Cambridge, MA: South End Press.

U.S. Department of Health and Human Services. (1998). An ensemble of definitions of environmental health, November 20, 1998. Retrieved November 2, 2004, from http://www.health.gv/environment/DefinitionsofEnvHealth/ehdef1.htm.

U.S. Department of Health and Human Services. (2000). Defining environmental health and environmental health indicators. Retrieved November 2, 2004, from http://www.fep.paho.org/english/env/Indicadores/Page 06.asp?Valida=ok.

Wallace, R. (1950). The miracle of the Copper Basin. *The Tennessee Conservationist, 15,* 8–9.

Wilford, J. N. (1991). The gradual greening of Mt. St. Helens. *New York Times,* Oct. 8, B9.

Woodward, S. (1998). Introduction to biomes, *Geography, 235,* June. http://www.runet.edu/~swoodwar/classes/geog235/biomes.

World Resources Institute. (2000). *World resources: 2000–2001: People and ecosystems: The fraying web of life.* Washington, DC: World Resources Institute.

ASSIGNMENTS

1. Determine which biome you live in and provide a list of trees, plants, and animals native to the area and their ability to thrive and survive.

2. Select one of the cycles of life and develop a poster or presentation that explains how that cycle utilizes natural processes to replace life-giving resources.

3. Develop a 5-minute speech explaining why natural forces in the atmosphere and on land cannot support the demands that current human populations impose upon them.

4. Look up information concerning endangered and threatened species in the area in which you live. Find out how they became extinct.

5. Write an essay about the relevance of natural sciences and ecology to human health.

6. Visit three Web sites of agencies involved in the practice of environmental health and write about the mission, function, and activities associated with these agencies or organizations.

7. Use a science or health database on your library home page and search for a full-text article related to an environmental health concern. A partial listing of potential journals follows.

8. Consider the responsibility an individual has in preserving the environment.

9. Read one of the following recommended journals or books and write a two-paragraph review.

10. Use the Internet to locate the U.S. government site for an environmental law (see below).

SELECTED ENVIRONMENTAL LAWS

1973 Endangered Species Act (ESA) (PL 93-205)
Conserve the various species of fish, wildlife, and plants facing extinction.

SELECTED PROFESSIONAL JOURNALS

Basic and Applied Ecology
Climatic Change
Ecosystem Health
Ecosystem

Environmental Health Perspectives
Environmental History
Environmental Science and Technology
Estuaries
Global Change and Human Health
Human Ecology: An Interdisciplinary Journal
Journal of Ecology
Journal of Environmental Quality
Nature
Public Health and the Environment
Science
Scientific American
The New Environmentalist
World Health Report

ADDITIONAL READING

Bush, M. M. (2003). *Ecology of a changing planet* (3rd ed.). Upper Saddle River, NJ: Prentice-Hall.

Durning, A., & Starke, L. (eds.). (1992). *How much is enough? The consumer society and the future of the Earth.* New York: Norton.

Ehrlich, P. R., & Ehrlich, A. H. (1996). *Betrayal of science and reason: How anti-environment rhetoric threatens our future.* Washington, DC: Island Press.

Jeffries, M. (1997). *Biodiversity and conservation.* New York: Routledge.

Lappe, F. (1991). *Diet for a small planet.* New York: Ballantine Books.

McConnell, R. L., & Abel, D. C. (2001). *Environmental issues: Measuring, analyzing, and evaluating.* Upper Saddle River, NJ: Prentice Hall.

Tivy, J., & O'Hare, G. (1982). *Human impact on the ecosystem.* Edinburg, NY: Oliver & Boyd.

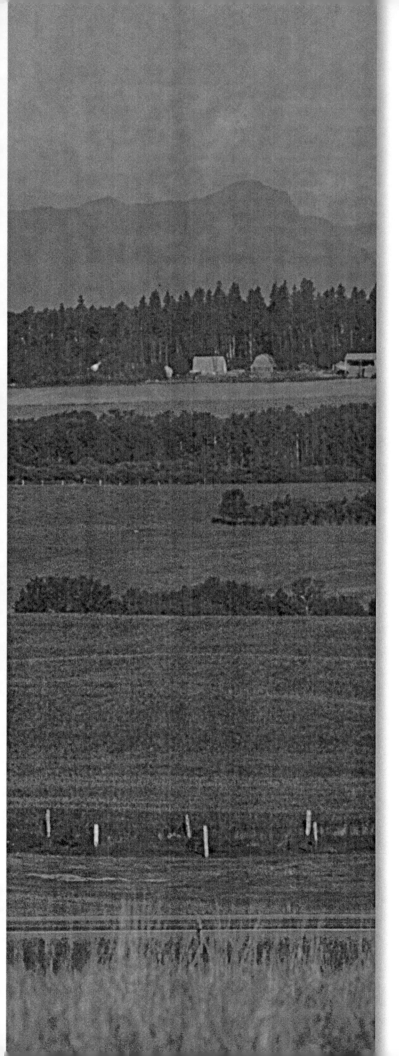

Humans and Global Issues

2

Should the whole frame of Nature round him break,
In ruin and confusion hurled,
He, unconcerned, would hear the mighty crack,
And stand secure amidst a falling world.

Joseph Addison (1672–1719)

OBJECTIVES

1. Contrast environmental concerns between a developing and industrialized country.

2. Explain why population growth is a global concern.

3. Give examples of natural and man-made disasters that occur around the world.

4. Give examples of how air pollution in one country affects another.

5. Explain where acid rain comes from and the damage it does.

6. Describe the phenomenon of global warming and its cause.

7. Explain Darwin's theory of evolution.

8. List several ways in which global environmental concerns have been addressed.

9. Describe an international initiative to reduce threats of global warming and other environmental concerns.

10. Apply the three "Es" to the three "Ps" of global health concerns.

Introduction

Experts from around the world have examined past, continuing, and escalating problems associated with changes in the environment and environmental quality (National Environmental Health Association, 1998). This chapter provides an overview of environmental issues of global concern.

Most of the literature concerning global environmental health issues distinguishes concerns of industrialized nations from that of developing nations (United Nations Development Programme, 2000). Both contribute to global problems. **Industrialized countries**, with an emphasis on affluence and the "good life," have made some important trade-offs in advances in agriculture, industry, and transportation, imposing new environmental health threats on urban and rural populations. **Developing countries** often lack the technology to progress without damage to the environment. Affluent countries sometimes rob poor countries of their **natural resources** and are also known to dump toxic and other waste on their land. All nations then experience devastating effects from new diseases that spread quickly.

There is no doubt that uncontrolled exploitation of the environment leads to immediate and long-term health problems. No one can be shielded from its effects. Some of the environmental changes, such as natural disasters and climate changes, cannot be controlled. Some can be predicted so that one can be prepared and encounter less damage. Other changes, such as uncontrolled population growth, deforestation, misuse of land, air pollution and ozone depletion, and the exportation of toxic waste, can be prevented, but not without substantial effort. Trends in human activities demand attention so that problems of large communities are not worsened. Living conditions; air, water, and food quality; and exposure to toxic substances are rural as well as urban issues. Waste management, pest control, disease control, exposure to toxic substances, energy demand, and safety concerns are just some of the concerns impacted by the environment. This chapter is devoted to the discussion of global environmental health problems and the collaborative efforts to address them.

Global Environmental Concerns

UNCONTROLLED POPULATION GROWTH

From 1950 to 1975, the world's population increased 64%. Today the world is home to 6.2 billion people, growing at a rate of about 80 million people per year (Ashford, 2004) (Figure 2-1). The largest population growth is in

> The Pew Charitable Trust is probably the biggest contributor to environmental causes. This organization has funded the National Environmental Trust, formerly known as the Environmental Information Center, since 1993.

Industrialized countries
Countries based economically on large-scale businesses, dependent upon production or manufacturing.

Developing countries
Growing or expanding economically, socially, and politically from an undeveloped condition.

Natural resources
Products naturally present that are ready for use; sources that can be used to their advantage such as soil, water, wildlife, or minerals; resources found in the natural environment.

FIGURE 2-1 **Annual Increases in World Population** Source: U.S. Census Bureau, International Data Base, April 2005. http://www.census.gov/ipc/www/world.html.

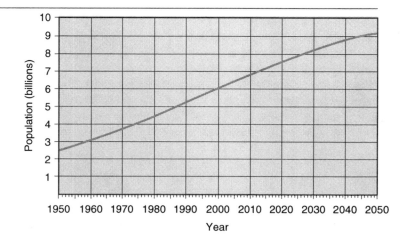

CHAPTER TWO HUMANS AND GLOBAL ISSUES 23

When population grew by 2% for more than 25 years and eventually passed the 800 million mark, finally growing to nearly 1 billion people, Chinese national leaders initiated "Strategic Demographic Initiatives" (SDI) that advocating later marriage, longer intervals between pregnancies, and fewer children per mother. The effect was minimal until economic incentives were provided. By the mid-1980s 16% of Chinese couples had signed the "Only Child Glory Certifi-

cates" that entitled them to preferred housing, education, and employment opportunities.

Despite these strategies, the legal age for marriage was lowered and many women born in the 1960s became of child-bearing age. Population rates continued to rise in rural areas where farming families needed more children to produce additional labor. In 1974, the Chinese government, aided by financial

assistance from the United Nations, began to distribute free contraceptives to married couples. By 1999, 83% of Chinese married couples were practicing contraception, compared to 76% in the United States and 44% in developing nations (Tobias, 1998). Chinese leaders believe that they can create a "sustainable population size" with increased efforts at producing more effective contraceptive alternatives.

countries with large numbers of young people and where large families are the norm, such as India, China, Pakistan, Nigeria, Bangladesh, and Indonesia. These and other less developed countries account for 81% of the world's population and 90% of the world's births per year (Haub, 2002). India and China alone account for one third of births worldwide; if India does not curtail population growth, by 2050 it will surpass China as the world's most populous nation (Kluger & Dorfman, 2002). It is also projected that by the year 2150, Africa will have quadrupled its population.

On the other side of the globe, Latin American populations have also increased substantially. At the end of the twentieth century, there were 500 million people in Latin America (Martin & Midgley, 2003). Today the population has reached nearly one billion. Immigration and migration to coastal and other desirable areas place a strain on resources. Many people from Mexico and Latin America have migrated to the United States in search of work and homes for their families, increasing the need for food, education, jobs, housing, and medical care.

The United States population growth contributes to 3% of world population growth. The population of the United States has also increased due to immigration and declining death rates due to improved sanitation, increased food production, and improved medical care. The highest birth rate in the United States was from 1946 to 1961 (known as the post–World War II "baby boom") (Population Reference Bureau, 2004). Since then, birth rates have declined as women have become more educated, sought careers, and waited longer before getting married. Also, better contraceptives are available to de-

lay having children. Families have become smaller due to the expense of raising larger families. Recently birth rates among Anglo-European Americans declined while birth rates among Hispanic, African American, and Asian Americans increased. By the year 2050, less than half of the children in the United States will be of Anglo-European descent (U.S. Census Bureau, 1999).

Not all countries have experienced population growth. Countries such as Italy, Spain, Portugal, Greece, Slovenia, Sweden, Japan, Poland, and the Ukraine have achieved **zero population growth** (ZPG). Today, the majority of countries have some type of family planning program. Unfortunately, family planning efforts constitute a small part of some national budgets.

Japan and Western Europe have experienced a phenomenon known as **demographic drift**. *Demographic drift* is a stabilization in population that occurs when the economy improves and standards of living rise. Russia has experienced a decline in population due to infant mortality rates, poor health, high fat diets, cigarette smoking, alcoholism, and high levels of stress (National Research Council, 1997). In the past 25 years Europe has experienced population decline (Carnell, 2004). Some believe that global population growth will eventually cease, but by the time population growth in all countries has stabilized, however, the world's population is expected to reach 12 billion or more (Population Reference Bureau, 2002). It is not known if the Earth will have enough resources to support a population of 12 billion

In prehistoric times, the average life span was about 18 years. Before 1900, the average life expectancy in the United States was 47 years. Today, the average life expectancy is 80 years for women and 78 years for men.

Immigration has contributed to population growth in the United States because it has one of the most liberal immigration policies in the world. Immigration adds at least 850,000 to 1.2 million people to the U.S. population each year (Camarata, 2001). The majority of immigrants to the United States for the last 30 years has been from Latin America and Asia.

or more because the 6 billion people currently on the planet have already exceeded the capacity of natural resources in many areas.

Food sources, adequate housing, jobs, and finances are problems in all countries as population growth increases. Access to health services, especially among the poor, children, and in rural areas, has become more important now than ever. Some industrialized countries with dense populations have attempted to slow population growth by providing status and monetary incentives. These efforts appear to be futile.

LAND POLLUTION

Increasing population growth means an increased need for food and waste disposal. Food is consumed faster than it is grown, taking 14.4 months to replenish what is consumed in 12 months (Kluger & Dorfman, 2002). To provide enough food for large numbers of people, additional land must be cleared and water supplies must be used to irrigate crops. As the need for more farm land and housing developments increase, rainforests and wetlands are destroyed in industrialized as well as developing countries. Removing them takes away natural processes for maintaining oxygen and water supplies in the environment. As nutrients in topsoil are depleted by growing crops, chemical replacements are preferred over conser-

Most individuals would attribute declining death rates in the United States to specialized medical training, advancements in pharmaceutical medications, and expensive diagnostic and treatment technologies. The primary factor, however, is improved sanitation and other public health strategies. Pasteurization of milk and chlorinated water supplies has decreased food-borne illnesses. Mechanized agricultural practices and increased use of fertilizers and pesticides have made it possible to produce increased amounts of foods. The discovery and use of antibiotics and vaccines have also contributed significantly to the increased life expectancy.

vation efforts such as crop rotation. Pesticides and herbicides are used abundantly to increase food productivity. More than ever before, the use of hazardous substances has outgrown efforts to control them.

More people also means more human waste and garbage (Figure 2-2). The disposal of human excrement

Zero population growth (ZPG)
When the population growth rate is equal to or less than zero.

Demographic drift
The stabilization of population drift as the economy improves and standard of living increases.

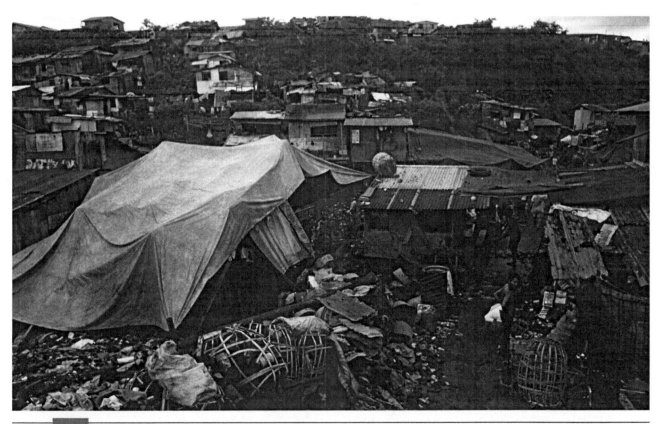

FIGURE 2-2 This photo from Manilla, the Phillippines, illustrates the effect that poverty has on housing, food sanitation, and waste management.

has become a problem in many areas of the country, subjecting residents to foul smells when it is processed for drying. Sewers overflow, particularly during rainstorms, discharging contents into creeks and streams within city limits. Landfills fill quickly as more convenience items are used. Cities such as New York have resorted to hauling garbage away by barge to be dumped in ocean waters. Toxic wastes are shipped to other countries for disposal.

As people move from the inner city to suburban areas, the need for transportation increases as well as the need for more multiple-lane highways. Uncontrolled growth in communities results in **urban sprawl**, destroying important habitats for animals and native vegetation. Litter abounds on roadsides everywhere.

INCREASED ENERGY NEEDS

As populations and technology increases, energy needs and problems due to ravaged land and the discharge of by-products become more prevalent. Energy needs consume natural resources such as coal, oil, and uranium. Fossil fuels are not replaceable—at least not in a lifetime! Coal must be mined and coal mining leaves behind trenches and residues harmful to water supplies. Oil drilling on land and off-shore can produce oil spills, contaminating land and water supplies. Oil slicks on water surfaces kill fish, fowl, and mammals. The threat that oil sources may be depleted creates an urgency to find fuel sources on foreign soils or in formerly inaccessible areas. Because the need for energy is so great, power plants cannot create enough electrical power and the need to generate energy using hydroelectric and nuclear sources has increased. History has dictated that the damming of water sources has proved inefficient and detrimental to local residents and their biosystem. In addition, the more nuclear power plants there are, the greater the likelihood of nuclear accidents such as Chernobyl and Three Mile Island.

AIR POLLUTION

Automobiles and industries use fossil fuels that cannot be burned completely. The process of incomplete combustion leaves by-products such as carbon dioxide, nitrous dioxide, carbon monoxide, and particulate matter. Air pollutants cause rainfall to become acidic, destroying plant life, damaging building materials, and making the soil toxic. More people have allergies, asthma, and other respiratory problems due to air pollution (Figure 2-3). The thinning of the ozone layer due to the use of propellants, refrigerants, and combustible fuels containing chlorofluorocarbons has increased the long-term effects of ultraviolet (UV) radiation from the sun, especially in mountainous regions. Scenic views are obstructed by smog and the effects of thermal inversion. Air pollution from one country travels to another and further into the atmosphere. Canadians estimate that nearly one-third of their **acid rain** deposition is from U.S. emissions. Pollutants are being carried from the United Kingdom to Sweden and Germany. Japan suffers from the effects of industry in China (Figure 2-4).

CLIMATE CHANGES

Air pollution causes increases in atmospheric temperature known as **global warming** (Figure 2-5). Because of this global warming effect, summer and winter temperatures are higher than they were in previous centuries. Polar ice caps are melting and sea levels are rising. Unusual weather patterns and storms created by El Niño threaten coastal populations. There is an increase in droughts and flooding. Droughts mean a significant decrease in crop yields, affecting food supplies for many.

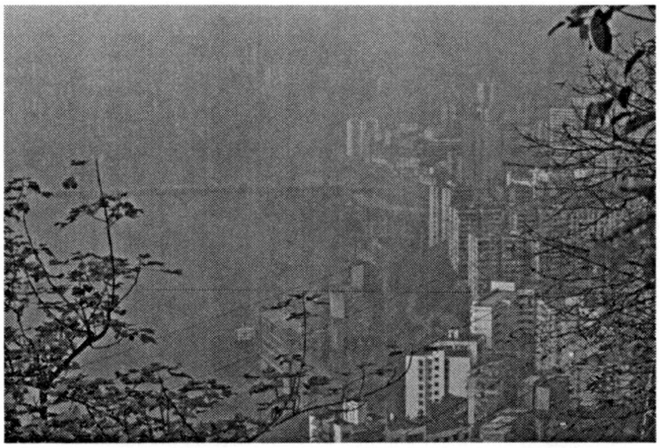

FIGURE 2-3 Smog over Chongqing, China.

Acid rain was first noted in 1872 in England. A product of the industrial revolution, acid rain develops when sulfur dioxide (SO_2) and nitrous oxide (N_2) from the burning of fossil fuel combine and is deposited to the Earth. Acid "rain" falls in the form of rain, snow, or ice and has a pH value of 5.6. Acid rain is found all over the world as emissions are carried by wind and air masses.

In 1984, chemicals were released from an explosion at a Union Carbide pesticide plant in Bhopal, India. Approximately 3,000 people were killed and 200,000 were injured from the methyl isocyanate gas that was discharged.

In addition to climatic changes, the effects of global warming include an increase in human illnesses because of the emergence of new diseases and the reemergence of old ones.

DISEASE PREVENTION AND CONTROL

Throughout the history of humankind, plagues and other communicable diseases have wiped out entire populations. **Pandemics** threaten all nations because global travel makes it easier for diseases to be transmitted from place to place. Many strains of the flu originate in Asia and eventually reach other parts of the world. Diseases such as malaria, dengue fever, HIV/AIDS, and Ebola have become major health concerns around the globe. Diseases such as smallpox, tuberculosis, and cholera, once thought to be eradicated, are now reemerging. The threat of bioterrorism also has prompted national

Urban sprawl
The building of new housing developments and subdivisions, strip malls for retail and commercial areas, and other uses of large tracts of land with large areas between increasing dependence on the automobile.

Acid rain
Rain with an acidic quality (pH of less than 5.6, normal pH is 7.0) due to the accumulation of sulfur dioxide (SO_2) and nitrogen dioxide (NO_2) from incomplete combustion emissions. The rain damages vegetation, kills fish, harms humans, and erodes stone, marble, metal, and paint.

Global warming
An increase in the average temperature of the atmosphere that causes changes in climate.

Pandemic
An epidemic extending beyond the confines of a wide area, typically a continent, such as HIV/AIDS; a widespread problem.

FIGURE 2-4 **Power Plant Emissions** The generation of power creates air pollution problems according to the type of fuel used.

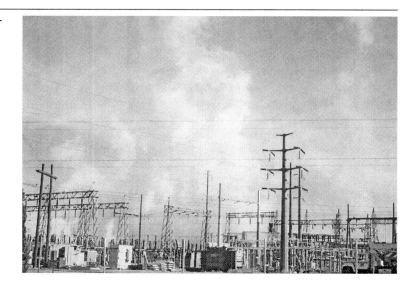

FIGURE 2-5 **Global Temperature Changes** Environmental changes are evidenced by changes in global temperature known as "global warming." Source: United States National Climactic Data Center, 2001.

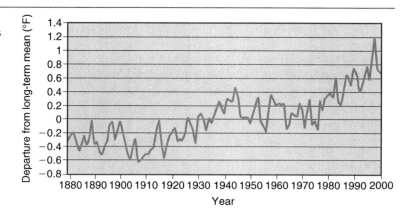

> Crowded living conditions provide a breeding ground for acute infections that often have serious complications. In Bombay, India, the world's third largest city, many citizens lack toilet facilities and are exposed to human waste (Brown et al., 1998). In Rajkot, a city of 600,000, tap water only runs for 20 minutes per day (Bhart, 1994).
>
> From 1992–1997 in New York City, a tuberculosis epidemic with antibiotic-resistant strains generated public health and ethical concerns as noncompliant patients were detained to contain the disease (Coker, 2000).

efforts to be on alert for unusual instances of deadly and dangerous diseases to thwart an **epidemic.**

Living conditions are important to good health. Increased exposure to outdoor environmental contaminants decreases immunity to ward off diseases. Air, land, and water pollution provide opportunities for bacteria and other pathogens to breed. The decrease in atmospheric ozone increases the susceptibility to skin cancer. Chemicals dumped without regulation pose risks of immediate and long-term exposure. Indoor recreational and social events, urban transportation systems, office buildings, and school environments provide ample indoor opportunities to spread contagious diseases. However, public health efforts such as water sanitation and waste management have removed many disease-causing agents and have improved the health of populations in nearly every country. Nothing has done more to increase life expectancy than improved air, water, food, and other environmental interventions. Sustaining optimal environmental conditions is an ongoing struggle.

DISASTERS AND WAR

Natural disasters have always been a global concern. Volcanic eruptions, explosions caused by earthquakes, and forest fires are just some of the events that leave particulate matter and noxious gases in the atmosphere. These residual substances travel many miles and affect many people. Hurricanes, tornados, and other storms create water run-off problems, straining urban sewers, polluting surface water, and eroding farmlands. Homes are flooded and water supplies are contaminated. Molds infiltrate living quarters and disease carriers multiply, requiring emergency efforts to control possible harm to humans and animals. National and international efforts often are needed to aid areas of the country requiring disaster assistance.

In addition to natural disasters, man-made disasters have created many problems. Oil spills from drilling and transporting oil have damaged land, polluted water, destroyed habitats, and killed animals (see Chapter 8). Nuclear accidents such as Chernobyl and others have contaminated environments and injured people. Military training leaves land mines, unusable land, and air pol-

lution behind. Wars have utilized nuclear and chemical weapons that damage land, vegetation, and human health. Many veterans of wars are still suffering the repercussions of exposure to **defoliants**, pesticides, and nerve gases.

TOXIC SUBSTANCES

Industrialization has contributed substantially to the emission of toxic substances in the environment. Modern office equipment, housing materials, and home appliances distribute various types of energy in a way that can be harmful to human health (see Chapter 11). Exposure to harmful chemicals is a major concern, particularly for pregnant women and the young. Toxic substances pose a special environmental hazard because they remain in the environment for an extended period of time and the effects can be cumulative with repeated exposure.

Saving the Planet

Like most primitive animals, humans are resistant to change. When threatened, we usually revert to our instinctual or primitive ways of reacting to danger. Yet we can intuitively agree that if "old" methods do not work, it is time to try another approach. However, unlike other animals, humans have the capability to find new ways of coping with changes. The process, though, might require cooperation, collaboration, and change. Efforts of representatives around the world have addressed global environmental health issues and include family planning, reduction in world hunger, land conservation, energy conservation, and technology.

POPULATION CONTROL

Nearly all countries have encouraged their populations to practice some form of birth control to decrease infant mortality and improve maternal health. Industrialized countries such as China have promoted zero population growth, although the concept of having only one child was not expressly followed by all Chinese citizens according to the Law on Population and Family Planning (2002). Experts agree that the less education a woman has, the more babies she will have. Women who do not have a basic education typically do not know about the use of condoms to prevent sexually transmitted diseases and pregnancy, and have babies earlier than more educated women do (Bertini, 2003). For every four years of education, the number of births drop by one infant per mother. In many countries, economic development and the establishment of a more educated workforce has been encouraged to enable a greater number of people access to educational opportunities, health care, and family planning services.

Digging Deeper   MARGARET SANGER

Margaret Sanger was educated and worked as a maternity nurse on the lower east side of New York. Her mother had 11 children and her health suffered; she died at the age of 49. Margaret was the sixth child. In 1912, Sanger gave up nursing to distribute birth control information in spite of the fact that The Comstock Act of 1873 forbade the distribution of birth control devices and information. In 1913, she was indicted in the United States for mailing obscenities. She fled to Europe and the indictment was withdrawn. In 1914, she founded the National Birth Control League. In 1916, Margaret, her sister

Ethel Byrne, and Fania Mindell, set up the first birth control clinic in the United States in Brooklyn. They were sent to a workhouse for creating a public nuisance. Her many arrests helped change laws giving doctors the right to give birth control advice to patients. During the 1920s, she traveled, lectured, and tried to persuade government leaders to support birth control efforts in Japan, China, India, and the Soviet Union. Sanger helped organize the first World Population Conference in Geneva in 1927. Her efforts eventually merged to form the Planned Parenthood Federation.

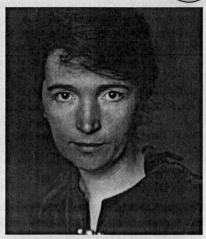

REDUCTION IN WATER DEMANDS

Water management systems in many urban areas are becoming antiquated and must be redeveloped to regulate household consumption. The average person requires 50 quarts of water per day for drinking, bathing, cooking, and other basic needs. In most cases, this consumption of water could be reduced. Urban areas encountering drought seasons have banned using large amounts of water for washing cars, lawn sprinkling, and filling swimming pools on certain days of the week.

The United Nations has long recognized the need for drinkable water. Twenty-eight government and other non-governmental agencies from the United Nations have encouraged an effort known as Water, Sanitation, and Hygiene for All (WASH) to provide water services and hygiene training by the year 2015 to everyone who lacks them (WASH, 2004).

REDUCTION IN WORLD HUNGER

The majority of the world's food supply is provided by grain production. The development of hybrid species, genetically engineered seeds needing less nitrogen from the soil, and pest-resistant plants demonstrates the human's adaptation to environmental concerns.

In some areas, the manner in which foods are distributed to various populations contributes to famine. War and disintegration of social order can lead to uneven food distribution and starvation. Because food is a perishable item, it must be transported before it spoils. Increased transportation, refrigerated units, improved food packaging, and dehydration procedures have increased food availability to millions worldwide. Many organizations (such as the Peace Corps) have been formed to help provide food for hungry nations through financial aid, advisement, in-

 In many cases, the problem of world hunger is not attributed to just overpopulation and poverty. Doubling the current food production capacities will not change conditions of poverty and starvation. In some areas of the globe, lack of good agricultural techniques and nutrient-depleted top soils limits the types of food that can be grown. Lack of water, a harsh climate, and lack of labor force to help with the planting and harvesting of foods are also contributing factors.

struction, and personnel to help nations become self-sufficient in providing food. The solution to world hunger is to break the cycle of stagnant agricultural productivity, poverty, high birth rates, unemployment, and poor health.

LAND PRESERVATION

Deforestation presents economic, environmental, and recreational concerns. Tropical rain forests provide an important habitat for more species than any other biosystem in the world, including plants used for medicinal purposes. Tropical rain forests are cleared by burning off trees and vegetation to increase land for grazing animals to produce meat. As heavy rainfall continues, minerals such as iron and aluminum oxide leach from the soil. In mountainous areas logging operations clear trees and erosions occurs. In some areas mud slides destroy

Epidemic
A marked increase in the incidence of disease within a limited area affecting increasing numbers of people.

Defoliants
A chemical agent used to kill plant growth.

campgrounds and homes. Preservation of forests is especially important to environmental concerns.

In rural and agricultural areas of the United States, efforts to prevent soil erosion such as using terraces and planting grassy waterways have been effective. Rotation of crops such as corn and soybeans replace nitrogen and other nutrients back into the soil for the next crop. Fertilizers and topsoil seep into groundwater and surface water supplies causing disruptions to natural biosystems. While some species of plant and animal life can tolerate variations in temperature, sunlight, and moisture, it is much better to conserve a thriving habitat than to destroy one and attempt to create another through artificial means.

NEW SOURCES OF ENERGY

Not all areas of the globe have access to modern energy sources. Power demands are expected to increase from developing countries by 2.5% per year (*Time*, 2002). In developing countries, the primary source for fuel is wood or fossil fuels. Because of poorer systems, these sources often emit more carbon dioxide and greenhouse gases than countries with pollution-control systems. Cheaper sources of power such as hydroelectric plants have proven unfavorable with local residents because rivers and streams are dammed. Cleaner fuels such as ethanol have been developed from agricultural products. Cheaper and cleaner sources of energy, that utilize *renewable energy sources* (e.g., the sun and the wind), are being developed. The use of garbage or methane by-products as fuel to create energy (known as *green power*) is available in some communities with economic incentives for industries to use them. The key is matching the right energy source to the right users.

Global Collaboration

o one country has more of an obligation to preserve the environment and address environmental degradation than another.

Each country needs to cooperate with global efforts because these efforts eventually affect each member of society. This has not been an easy task considering the history between countries that has been going on for centuries. Even so, the 1970s provided the impetus for global collaboration addressing environmental concerns.

STOCKHOLM CONFERENCE (1972)

The first attempt to discuss global environmental issues was in 1972 when the United Nations met for 2 weeks in Stockholm, Sweden. Delegates from 113 countries met reporting the state of their national environments. Industrialized countries were concerned about preventing pollution, controlling overpopulation, and conserving natural resources. Developing nations were concerned with widespread hunger, disease, poverty, and the effects of growing industrialization. Delegates agreed that population growth needed to be controlled, natural resources needed to be conserved, and the human environment needed to be protected from the negative effects of industrialization in all countries. As a result, the United Nations Environment Program (UNEP) was established to monitor changes in the physical and biological resources of the Earth (Evans, 2003). The UNEP launched the Global Environmental Project in 1995, involving experts from over 100 countries (Yassi et al., 2001).

An outcome from the resolutions of this meeting and recommendations of the World Health Assembly was the establishment of the World Health Organization (WHO) Environmental Health Criteria Programme in 1973 (Figure 2-6). Objectives of the program included:

1. assessment of information on the relationship between exposure to environmental pollutants and human health and provide guidelines for setting exposure limits

2. identification of new or potential pollutants

3. identification of gaps in knowledge concerning the health effects of pollutants

4. promotion regarding the harmonization of toxicological and epidemiological methods for internationally comparable results

MONTEGO BAY (1982)

In 1982, many countries met in Montego Bay, Jamaica, to set up a comprehensive law establishing rules concerning pollution of the marine (sea and ocean) environment. The intent of the law was to prevent, reduce, and control pollution. There was discussion concerning the seabed, ocean floor, and sub-floor. Other issues concerned scientific research, the development and transfer of marine technology, and the settlement of disputes.

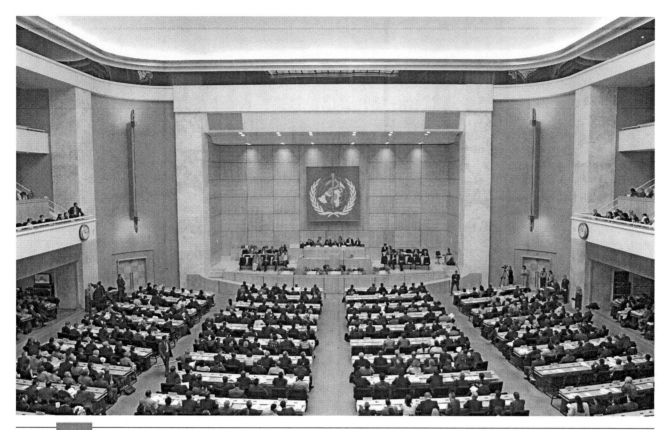

FIGURE 2-6 The purpose of the United Nations is to keep peace, promote respect for human rights, promote justice and respect for international laws and treaties, promote social progress, and strive for better standards of living throughout the world.

MONTREAL PROTOCOL (1987)

In 1985, 20 nations met in Vienna, Austria, regarding depletion of the ozone layer. Negotiators finalized the agreement to decrease CFC production by 50% by 2000 in 1987 in Montreal, Canada (United Nations Environment Programme, 1995). This was considered to be the most ambitious attempt ever to combat environmental degradation on a global scale and was a landmark in international environmental diplomacy. The resulting document was named the Montreal Protocol on Substances that Deplete the Ozone Layer and was signed by 24 nations. The intent of the protocol was to eliminate halon, carbon tetrachloride, methyl chloroform, and methyl bromide emissions into the environment. The agreement called for industrial nations to cut CFC emissions in half by 1998 and reduce halon emissions to 1986 levels by 1992. It called for the use of methylchloroform to be phased out by the year 2005. It has since been ratified by 175 countries. Developing countries were granted deferrals due to low-production levels.

THE HELSINKI DECLARATION (1989)

Following the signing of the Montreal Protocol in 1987, more information was shared regarding the hole in the ozone layer over Antarctica and thinning of the ozone layer over North America (International Institute for Sustainable Development, 1999). In May of 1989 another meeting in regard to the Montreal Protocol was held in Helsinki, Finland to create the Helsinki Declaration calling for the phaseout of CFC production by no later than the year 2000, the phaseout of halon production and other ozone-depleting substances (ODS), and calling for environmentally safe alternatives. The London amendment of 1990 added 10 more CFCs to the list, including carbon tetrachloride, which was to be phased out by 2000, and methyl chloroform, which was to be eliminated by 2005. The Copenhagen Amendment of 1992 added methylbromide, hydrobromofluorocarbons, and hydrochlorofluorocarbons (HCFCs) to the list with agreement to accelerate the ban by four years. The Montreal amendment of 1997 added a new licensing system for customs officials to monitor worldwide trade so that CFCs were not marketed illegally from one country to another. Meetings continued regarding the implementation of the Montreal Protocol after the Helsinki Declaration in Cairo (1998), Geneva (1999), and Beijing (1999).

EARTH SUMMIT (1992)

In 1992, the United Nations Conference on Environment and Development (UNCED) was held in Rio de Janeiro,

Brazil, to avoid a predicted **ecocatastrophe** (Swartzman, 1996) through uncontrolled development. It was the largest number of world leaders ever assembled for a single purpose—to solve global environmental problems through international collaboration. World leaders from 178 nations met for 12 days to address population growth problems, pollution, depletion of resources, destruction of land (deforestation), loss of biodiversity, climate change, and the eradication of poverty. It was the second time a world organization held a major international gathering to focus on environmental concerns. Common goals of the conference, known as the "Millennium Development Goals," included eradication of poverty and hunger, reduced child mortality/gender equality, and universal primary education.

The Earth Summit (also known as the Rio Summit) led leaders of the countries belonging to the United Nations to the adoption of Agenda 21, a wide-ranging blueprint for action to achieve **sustainable development** worldwide (Parson, Haas, and Levy, 1992). The plan was not without its problems. Many participants refused to discuss certain issues and others refused to agree to the proposition. In particular, the Vatican and Islamic nations were opposed to controlling population growth. U.S. delegates, under orders from President George Bush, refused to sign international agreements to protect endangered species, reduce carbon dioxide emissions, and to increase funding to Third World nations for development and pollution abatement programs.

There were, however, some notable outcomes, in spite of the differences among nations. A positive outcome was the formation of thousands of ecological groups around the world and official environmental agencies to confront problems of pollution and resource pollution in many nations.

COPENHAGEN (1996)

In 1992, 87 nations met in Copenhagen, Denmark, to stop the production of halon and advanced the deadline for halting the production of CFCs to January 1996. Leaders also attempted to eliminate HCFCs, temporary substitutes for CFCs. Recycled halon is still available today for fire protection, but only under EPA approval. The implementation has encountered problems with the Soviet Union in eliminating CFCs and countries such as Russia, China, and India undermining the phase out by selling CFCs through the black market (Dini, 2000).

THE KYOTO PROTOCOL (1997)

Global commitment to environmental concerns continued as global leaders held a meeting in Kyoto, Japan. Known as the United Nations Framework Convention on Climate Change (UNFCCC), the meeting addressed environmental causes of climactic change. Discussion centered around the production of six greenhouse gases (water vapor, carbon dioxide, nitrous oxide, methane, chlorofluorocarbons, and ozone) from the burning of fossil fuels. A treaty, known as the Kyoto Protocol, was signed by representatives from over 170 nations, including the United States, the European Union, Canada, and Japan. The Kyoto treaty was the first effort to combat concerns about global warming. Critics of the treaty said the focus was on restrictions for developed nations of the world and not on developing countries such as China, India, and Brazil. In 2001, President George W. Bush announced that the United States would withdraw from the Kyoto Protocol. U.S. representatives said the United States would combat global warming in other ways by encouraging energy-efficient technology, incentives to encourage industries to voluntarily reduce greenhouse gas emissions, and conservation programs that help sequester carbon in the soil.

At first this action was considered a major setback because the United States was responsible for about 25% of the 1990 carbon dioxide emissions. Experts predicted that without U.S. participation, the Kyoto Protocol would never be implemented. However, in 1994 the European Union, Japan, Canada, Russia, Australia, and 170 other nations reached an agreement to proceed with the treaty. In order to secure the support of highly industrialized nations, the European Union was forced to make substantial concessions. The targets for emissions reduction were reduced by two thirds from the original goals, and countries were given the option of planting carbon-absorbing forests to earn pollution credits, in lieu of reducing emissions. The European Union and other nations continued to encourage President George W. Bush to adopt the Kyoto Protocol, but he has refused in spite of the fact that the United States produces 36% of the world's greenhouse gases. In 2001 he proposed a reduction in greenhouse gases in the United States but continued to call the Kyoto Protocol unrealistic because it would hurt the U.S. economy. On November 5, 2004, Russian President Vladimir Putin signed the Kyoto Protocol. Russian emissions account for 17% of the world's greenhouse gases. Although Australia signed the Protocol in 1997, it continues to be the world's worst polluter in regard to greenhouse gas emissions per capita although it only accounts for 1.4% of the world's greenhouse gases (Roarty, 2002).

THE CONVENTION ON BIOLOGICAL DIVERSITY (1998)

The Convention on Biological Diversity was negotiated under the United Nations Environment Programme (UNEP) and opened a document for signature at the June 1992 United Nations Conference on Environment and Development. The document promoted conservation of biodiversity, sustainable use of its components, as well as fair and equitable sharing of benefits arising out of the utilization of genetic resources. The Subsidiary Body on Scientific Technical and Technological Advance (SBSTTA) met in Nassau, Bahamas (1995), Paris (1995), Jakarta, Indonesia (1995), Montreal (1996, 1997, and 1999), Buenos Aires (1996), and Bratislava, Slovakia (1998). By 2000 more than 176 countries had signed the document.

WORLD SUMMIT ON SUSTAINABLE DEVELOPMENT (2002)

In 2002, presidents, prime ministers, and other leaders convened at the World Summit on Sustainable Development in Johannesburg, South Africa, for the purpose of developing cooperative strategies aimed at improving uncontrolled pollutants and other hazardous practices. The goal was to get countries who favor growth to care about the environment. Officials emphasized that prosperity, while destroying the environment, was not prosperity at all, but a temporary reprieve from future disaster. They urged leaders to become interested in the concept of sustainability, integrating respect for the environment with development and economic initiatives. The call for political commitment was made. For more information about the World Summit, visit http://www.johannesburgsummit.org.

Countries Helping Other Countries

he United Nations has addressed population control issues in Third World countries. In 1994 in Cairo, Egypt, the United Nations hosted the International Conference on Population and Development (ICPD), the most comprehensive international meeting ever held regarding world population issues. Attendees from 180 different countries agreed that economic development, family planning, and the improved status of women were deemed essential for reducing population growth rates and set goals to achieve by 2015 (International Conference on Population Development, 2004). Initiatives such as the World Bank and the U.N. Fund for Population Activities (UNFPA) were created to help countries in need.

Most of the wilderness preservation issues are in developing countries that are being utilized by developed countries. Countries such as the United States have taken the initiative to help with forest and wildlife issues in other countries. Wildlife corridors are being established between countries so that large animals may roam and mate to maintain their population. Acres of land have been set aside as preservation areas and national parks to help preserve natural resources and land surface area. Some countries also took the initiative to establish marine reserves in coastal waters where fishing is prohibited and coral reefs are protected. A movement known as **ecotourism** has been experimented with in some countries with endan-

gered forest and species. This movement engineers low-impact tours for visitors to learn how to appreciate the fragile ecosystems, yet preserve them at the same time.

Predicting Global Advancements in Environmental Health Issues

n the book *Critical Issues in Global Health*, former President Jimmy Carter asked readers to study history in order to help shape the future. Major advances in the twentieth century in science have produced side effects of emerging health problems. C. Everett Koop, former U.S. surgeon general, reiterates these concerns. He also announced that health has a higher price tag than ever before. As the planet "shrinks" and nations grapple over resources, nations must work together to maintain the quality of life enjoyed today. Environmental issues are more important than ever before in preventing infectious disease, chronic diseases, injury, and premature death.

When it comes to global health concerns, according to Cartledge (1994), there are three "P's" of major concern: population, poverty, and pollution. As populations increase, there is a greater need for water, food, land, energy, education, employment, resources, and health care. In all countries, poverty contributes to famine, disease, crime, and violence. Pollution contributes to the spread of disease. It has been suggested that the three P's be replaced with the three "E's": consideration for economics, ethics, and ecology. An emphasis on macroeconomics compromises the environment and quality of life. Consideration for wealth and economic growth oftentimes supercedes ethical concerns. It makes sense to be conservative, erring on the side of nature, rather than greed, and leaving a wasteland behind for future generations.

Ecocatastrophe
Sudden, widespread disaster or calamity with extensive damage to the environment threatening quality of life and death. The term was first coined by Georgescu-Roegen in 1971 as he predicted a "heat death of the universe" due to economic activity. Some believe Earth will face an ecocatastrophe from overpopulation or a nuclear disaster.

Sustainable development
Development that meets the needs of the present without compromising the ability of future generations to meet their own needs.

Ecotourism
Travel such as hiking or camping that minimally impacts the natural environment and its wildlife, while providing economic benefits to local communities.

Since the 1992 Earth Summit, numerous domestic and international crises have occurred, lowering the priority of environmental stability for many national leaders, but the future may not be as grim as special interest group extremists would like to believe. Problems of population growth, food needs, and energy demands exist in every country, making environmental issues more important than ever. All countries must work on their own problems, enlist the aid of other countries, and above all, work together to maintain the standard of living enjoyed.

Summary

Problems concerning climate changes and environmental quality are affected by population growth and migration, increased energy needs, exploitation of natural resources, disasters, and careless waste management. Diseases, toxic substances, and pollution affect everyone. Experts push for population control, land preservation, water conservation, and new sources of energy. Global organizations have devoted efforts toward a united effort to preserve our planet by monitoring potentially endangered species, limiting greenhouse gas emissions, discouraging ocean pollution, and encouraging sustainable development. Many countries agree that current practices should be changed, but not all agree on the best methods for change or compliance deadlines. Globally, the three main problems concerning preservation of the plant are population, poverty, and pollution. Approaches to these problems, according to experts, are concern for economics, ethics, and ecology.

REFERENCES

Ashford, L. (2004). World population highlights—2004. Population Reference Bureau. Retrieved from http://www.prb.org/Template.cfm?Section=PRB&template=/ContentManagement/ContentDisplay.cfm&ContentID=11267.

Ashton, J., & Laura, R. (1999). *The perils of progress: The health and environment hazards of modern technology and what you can do about them*. New York: Zed Books Ltd.

Bertini, C. (2003). Educate girls: The 2003 World Food Prize Laureate Lecture. The United Nations Association of Minnesota. Retrieved November 5, 2004 from http://www.unamn.org/Catherine%20Bertini.htm.

Bhart, A. (1994). Rajkot chronic scarcity. *The Hindu Survey of the Environment*, May 31, 1994, 113–117.

Brown, L., Renner, M., & Flavin, C. (1998). *Vital signs 1998: The environmental trends that are shaping our future*. Worldwatch Institute. New York: W.W. Norton.

Camarota, S. (2001). Immigrants in the United States—2000: A snapshot of America's foreign-born population. Center for Immigration Studies. Retrieved November 6, 2004 from http://cis.org/articles/2001/back101.pdf.

Carnell, Brian. (2004). U.N. population fund holds forum on Europe's low fertility rates. Retrieved November 3, 2004 from http://www.overpopulation.com/articles/2004/000014.html.

Cartledge, B. (Ed.) (1994). *Health and the environment: The Linacre lectures 1992–1993*. Oxford, England: Oxford University Press.

Coker, R. J. (2000). *From chaos to coercion: Detention and the control of tuberculosis*. New York: St. Martin's Press.

Dini, J. (2000). CFC treaty fuels black market. The Heartland Institute. Retrieved November 5, 2004 from http://www.heartland.org/Article.cfm?artId=9614.

Evans, K. (2003). *The environment: A revolution in attitudes*. Detroit: Thomson Publishers.

Gleick, P. H., Cohen, M., Haasz, D., & Wolfe, G. (2002). Water: Facts, trends, threats, and solutions. Pacific Institute for Studies in Development, Environment, and Security Retrieved November 5, 2004 from http://www.pacinst.org/reports/water_fact_sheet/water_factsheet.pdf.

Haub, C. (2002). Has global population growth reached its peak? *Population Today*, August/September. Retrieved August 9, 2004 from http://www.prb.org/Template.cfm?Section=PRB&template=/Content/ContentGroups/PTarticle/July-Sep2002/Has_Global_Growth_Reached_Its_Peak_.htm.

Harrington, C. R. (Ed.) (1992). *The year without a summer: World climate in 1816*. Ottawa: Canadian Museum of Nature.

International Conference on Population and Development. (2004). Investing in people: national progress in implementing the ICPD Programme of Action 1994–2004, a summary report. Retrieved November 6, 2004 from http://www.unfpa.org/upload/lib_pub_file/278_filename_icpd04_summary.pdf.

International Institute for Sustainable Development. (1999). Summary of the 11th meeting of the parties to the Montreal Protocol and the fifth conference of the parties to the Vienna Convention: November 29–December 3, 1999. *Earth Negotiations Bulletin*, 19, 1–14. Retrieved November 5, 2004 from http://www.iisd.ca/download/pdf/enb1906e.pdf.

International Institute for Sustainable Development. (2000). Summary of the 5th session of the subsidiary body for scientific, technical, and technological advice of the convention on biological diversity: January 31–February 4, 2000. *Earth Negotiations Bulletin*, 9, February, 1–2. Retrieved November 6, 2004 from http://www.iisd.ca/download/pdf/enb09141e.pdf.

Kluger, J., & Dorfman, A. (2002). The challenges we face. Special report: How to save the Earth, *Time*, 160, August 26, A6–A12.

Koop, C. E., Pearson, C. E., & Schwarz, M. R. (2001). *Critical issues in global health*. San Francisco: Jossey-Bass.

Martin, P., & Midgley, E. (2003). Immigration: Shaping and reshaping America. *Population Bulletin*, 58.

National Environmental Health Association. (1998). New global health report warns about health risks of environmental degradation. *Journal of Environmental Health*, 61, 31–34.

National Research Council (1997). *Premature death in the new independent states*. Washington, DC: National Academy Press.

Parson, E. A., Haas, P. M. & Levy, M. A. (1992). A summary of major documents signed at the earth summit and the global forum. *Environment*, 34, 12–15, 34–36.

Population Reference Bureau. (2004). Human population growth: Fundamentals of population growth. Three patterns of population change. Retrieved November 2, 2004 from http://web.cocc.edu/lminorevans/soc303_hw1.htm.

Population Reference Bureau (2002). World population growth 1750–2150 in *Human population: Fundamentals of growth, population growth, and distribution.* http://www.prb.org/pdf/worldpopgrowth.pdf.

Roarty, M. (2002). The Kyoto Protocol—issues and developments through to conference of the parties (COP7). *E-Brief: Online Only,* 13 September 2002. Retrieved November 5, 2004 from http://www.aph.gov.au/library/intguide/SCI/kyoto.htm.

Schwartzman, D. (1996). Solar communism. *Science & Society, 60,* Fall, 307–331. Retrieved November 5, 2004 from http://www.dccofc.org/Documents/Solar%20Communism.doc.

Tobias, M. (1998). *A paradox of souls: China; World War III: Population and the biosphere at the end of the millennium.* New York: Continuum Publishing.

United Nations Development Programme. (2000). *World resources 2000–2001.* Washington, DC: World Resources Institute.

United Nations Environment Programme (1995). Report of the implementation committee under the non-compliance procedure—tenth meeting. Retrieved November 5, 2004 from http://www.unep.org/ozone/10impcom.shtml.

United States Census Bureau. (1999). Dynamic diversity: Projected changes in the U.S. race and ethnic composition 1995 to 2050. U.S. Department of Commerce. Retrieved November 3, 2004 from http://www.mbda.gov/documents/unpubtext.pdf.

WASH. (2004). Water Supply and Sanitation Collaborative Council. Retrieved November 4, 2004 from http://www.wsscc.org/home.cfm?CFID=595322&CFTOKEN=21122738.

World Commission on Environment and Development (1987). *Our common future.* Oxford: Oxford University Press, 43. (Often referred to as The Brundtland Report cited on http://sdgateway.net/introsd/definitions.htm.)

Yassi, A., Kjellstrom, T., de Kok, T., & Guidotti, T. (2001). *Basic environmental health.* New York: Oxford University Press.

ASSIGNMENTS

1. Find three articles to abstract about one of the following topics: global warming, acid rain, species endangerment, population growth, famine, poverty, war, natural disasters.

2. List four effects of global warming and how an individual can decrease the source.

3. Gather information on one of the global meetings held in Sweden, Brazil, Japan, or Canada.

4. Investigate an environmental problem in a country of your interest, such as atmospheric radiation in Russia, water pollution in Africa, and so forth.

5. As a class or as an individual, develop an environmental statement regarding the three "P's" and the three "E's" with resolutions on a particular global environmental problem.

6. Investigate political efforts in the United States to place effective controls on environmental concerns.

7. Select an international or national organization devoted to environmental concerns and research their mission and efforts to help.

8. Visit the library and select an international journal in which an interesting environmental article can be found. Bring it to class for discussion.

9. Learn more about one of the international collaboration efforts to help reduce environmental concerns that have a negative impact on health.

10. Select a journal article from one of the journals below and share the content and potential impact on global health with the class.

ENVIRONMENTAL LAW

1969 National Environmental Policy Act (NEPA) (42 USC 4321-4347)
The U.S. charter for protection of the environment establishing policy, goals, and means to carry out the policy.

PROFESSIONAL JOURNALS

Bulletin of the World Health Organization
Global Change and Human Health
International Family Planning Perspectives
International Journal of Global Health
International Journal of Infectious Diseases
International Journal of STD and AIDS
International Migration Review
Pan-American Journal of Public Health
Public Health Reports
Social Science and Medicine
WHO Bulletin
WHO Weekly Epidemiologic Record
World Health Forum
World Health Report
World Watch

ADDITIONAL READING

Ashton, J., & Laura, R. (1999). *The perils of progress: The health and environment hazards of modern technology and what you can do about them.* New York: Zed Books Ltd.

Conly, S. R., & Camp, S. L. (1992). *India's family planning challenge: From rhetoric to action.* Country Study Series #2, The Population Crisis Committee.

Lappe, F., & Lappe, A. (2003). *Hope's edge: The next diet for a small planet.* New York: The Putnam Publishing Group.

Lomborg, B. (2001). *The skeptical environmentalist: Measuring the real state of the world.* New York: Cambridge University Press.

World population projections to 2150. (1998). *Population Newsletter, 65,* June.

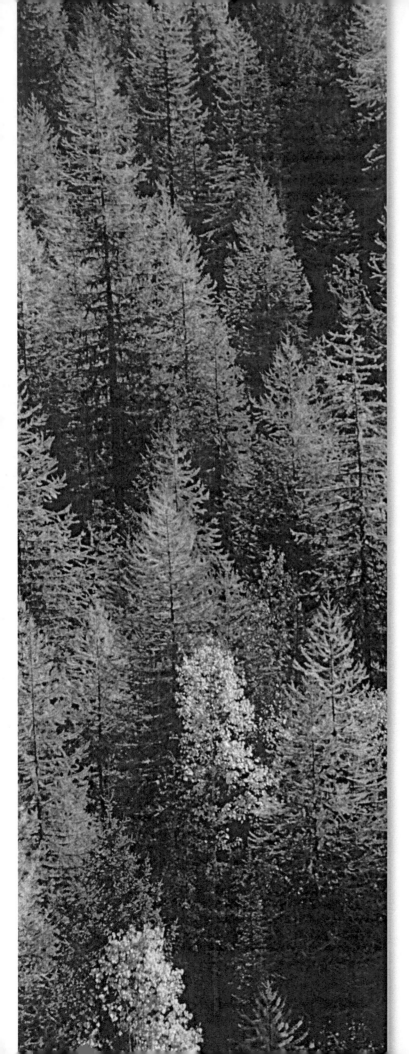

Effects of the Environment on Public Health

3

The first wealth, is health.

Ralph Waldo Emerson

OBJECTIVES

1. Briefly describe public health problems and practices in ancient cities.

2. Explain how the atomic theory of disease influenced the study and treatment of diseases.

3. Describe the main public health contribution of the Roman Empire.

4. Explain how the religious leaders influenced personal and public health practices during the Middle Ages.

5. Describe how the bubonic plague prompted the development of public health departments.

6. Give a brief historical account of events leading to the establishment of the U.S. Public Health Service during the "age of enlightenment."

7. Contrast post-Industrial Revolution public health efforts in England with those in the United States.

8. Differentiate public health advancements before and after the Great Depression.

9. Give a brief overview describing the development of the Healthy People Objectives 2010.

10. Examine the Healthy People Objectives 2010 for environmental health priorities and goals.

Introduction

The quality of air, water, food, shelter, and the climate of the environment has a dramatic effect on individual lives. The threat of destruction and disease has always been present. Wars have been waged, cities have been wiped out, and entire cities have been threatened by disease. Mass movements of people demand drinking water, food, goods, services, transportation, and solid waste disposal. As people migrated from rural areas to the cities, sanitation, public water systems, and public health services grew out of necessity. Scientific advancement exploded during the twentieth century and that growth will continue. An overview of problems from the past can provide a perspective on the importance of environmental issues.

Public Health Efforts in Ancient Cities

Ancient inscriptions indicate that in China and Egypt wells for drinking were dug, rainwater was collected, and sewage was processed. In India, bathrooms and drains were common; streets were paved and drained by covered sewers (Rosen, 1958). Minoans (3000–1430 B.C.) and Myceneans (1430–1150 B.C.) built drainage systems, toilets, and water systems (Pickett & Hanlon, 1990). About 1500 B.C., Hebrews advocated hygienic practices such as bodily cleanliness, protection against the spread of diseases, isolation of lepers, disinfection of dwellings after illness, sanitation of campsites, and disposal of excreta and refuse, as well as the protection of water and food supplies.

THE ATOMIC THEORY OF DISEASE

A famous Greek, Hippocrates (460–377 B.C.), developed a theory of disease causation believing that all things were composed of atoms. He hypothesized that there were only four kinds of atoms: earth, air, fire, and water. He believed the human body was made up of four "humours" or fluids (blood, phlegm, yellow bile, and black bile), which gave off vapors to the brain, and a person's physical, mental, and moral characteristics were explained by the state of threat to the humans. Each humour was made of one type of atom. Blood was made up of air, phlegm was made up of water, yellow bile was fire, and black bile was earth. Hippocrates believed that disease was the result of an imbalance of these four humours. He observed and recorded associations between diseases and geography, climate, diet, and living conditions. He has been credited as the first epidemiologist and is noted as the father of modern medicine. One of his contributions is the distinction between endemic and epidemic diseases (Duncan, 1988). He is credited with prescribing that rainwater be boiled and strained before drinking.

THE ROMAN EMPIRE: HYGIENE AND SANITATION (753 TO 509 B.C.)

The first sewers of Rome were built 500 years before the first aqueduct. The underground sewer systems emptied into the Tiber River, which is part of the sewer system of Rome still today. Roman aqueducts brought water from the Anio Valley to citizens for drinking and baths (Hansen, 2004). Attention was given to water purity. Water flowed through aqueducts along contours of the land utilizing gravity. At its peak development, aqueducts carried about 300 gallons of water for every citizen. Roman baths were emptied and filled at least once a day. By the fourth century A.D., Rome had 11 public baths, 1,352 public fountains and **cisterns**, and 856 private baths (Fox, 2004). The location of cities was determined according to the drainage of dwellings. The Romans regulated building construction and the destruction of decaying buildings, and prevented sewage accumulation in streets. Building regulations provided for ventilation and central heating. In addition to the aqueducts, there were paved streets with gutters and street cleaning.

THE MIDDLE AGES: SIN THEORY OF DISEASE (500 B.C. TO A.D. 1400)

The Middle Ages, also known as "the medieval era," had three periods: early, high, and late. The time known as the Early Middle Ages, extends from the collapse of the Roman Empire at about 500 B.C. to A.D. 1000. Germanic barbarians moved into Britain, destroying everything in their path. The curative powers of the Roman hot baths, already part of English legend by the sixth century, were lost when the last Romans fled Britain. Roman bathhouses became synonymous with debauchery, wild parties, and brothels when both sexes began to use them together. Most of the health standards established in ancient cultures were lost. Civilization and sanitation regressed to the most basic forms. There were almost no schools because education and cultural activities were ignored and almost forgotten. This is why the period is also known as the Dark Ages. The only civilizing force during the Middle Ages was the Catholic church. Church leaders became governmental officials and obtained large areas of land. The Roman Catholic church controlled religion, philosophy, morals, politics, art, and education. The church set up schools and some churches served as hospitals. Catholic leaders rejected most anything Roman, including the value of cleanliness. Diseases were thought to be acts of God attributed to sin with the only treatment being penitence.

The High Middle Ages (1000 to 1300) saw improvements in government and economics. From 1150 to 1200,

there was major climate warming throughout Europe. Diets improved and populations grew. The Crusades (1095 to 1204) encouraged trade with the Middle East. Lack of fresh water and sewage removal continued to be major problems in cities. Streets were unpaved, narrow, crooked, dark, and filthy and people threw garbage and rubbish into them, providing the opportunity for epidemics. More Crusaders were defeated by dysentery and other epidemics, than by their enemies. During the 1200s, some towns began to pave their streets and attempted sanitation improvements.

The "Little Ice Age" came through the area with a colder climate ending in 1351. Severe droughts and floods also brought death, disease, and famine. Crop yields reduced, the general health of people declined, and the pest population increased. Around 1330, the bubonic plague (also known as "The Black Death") infected the Orient and spread by trade routes established between the East and Europe. It was the most severe epidemic in human history, ravaging Europe from 1347 to 1351. Europe lost one quarter to one third of its entire population (Donan, 1898). It was first thought that lepers had deliberately spread the plague. Because of this, some were asked to leave their homes. Many areas of Europe were abandoned, food was in short supply, and crime was rampant.

THE RENAISSANCE PERIOD: THE RECOVERY (1400 TO 1700)

During this time, also known as the Late Middle Ages, basic hygiene was still discouraged. Water was not to be used for anything except drinking and cooking. Disposal of human waste was a problem (Gray, 1940). Disease continued to ravage Europe. Typhus fever was attributed to bad sanitation and putrid surroundings. In Russia, thousands of Napoleon's men were lost due to typhus. Then typhoid fever, a slightly different ailment than typhus, emerged. Sexually transmitted diseases were common, particularly in the royal courts.

As Europe started to recover from the major epidemics, physicians began to see differences in the diseases: bubonic plague, influenza, smallpox, tuberculosis,

Digging Deeper

The cause of epidemics was thought by medieval Europeans to have been caused by five factors: the wrath of God, the corruption of dead bodies, water and vapors formed in the Earth, unnatural hot and humid winds, and the conjunction of stars and planets (Winslow, 1974). A group of people,

known as "the order of flagellants," went from town to town whipping themselves with iron spikes. Many of them died of infections from the open wounds. They may have also carried the plague with them in their travels. A syphilis epidemic killed thousands of people in 1492 (McKenzie & Pinger,

1997). Citizens were afflicted with other diseases such as smallpox, diphtheria, measles, influenza, tuberculosis, anthrax, and trachoma. Unaware that microorganisms carried the disease, residents tried all types of methods (except hand washing and bathing) to eradicate the disease to no avail.

leprosy, impetigo, scabies, anthrax, and trachoma. As early as 1546, Fracastoro (1478–1553), a physician of Verona, theorized that microorganisms caused disease and that sexual intercourse transmitted syphilis also known as "the French disease" (Thyresson, 1995). Dr. Thomas Sydenham (1624–1689) believed that diseases such as scarlet fever, malaria, dysentery, and cholera, should be differentiated. He developed three levels or classes of fevers: continued, intermittent, and smallpox (Timmreck, 1998). Thanasius Kircher (1602–1680) examined the blood of plague victims using a crude microscope finding red blood corpuscles (Carr, 1997). Zacharias Janssen, a Dutch lens maker invented the first compound microscope with more than one lens in 1595. Anton van Leeuwenhoek developed a more powerful microscope in 1673 and proved there were very small organisms that he called "little animalcules", but it was not known that any of them caused disease. Various fields of science evolved, but the public received little benefit.

Between 1600 and 1665, Europe suffered three severe pandemics of bubonic plague that killed 23% of London residents (Duncan & Scott, 2004). The "Black Death" was so bad that some considered the Great Fire of London in 1666 as a blessing in disguise consuming the garbage, muck, and black rats. The fire essentially ended the plague.

The only public health actions were in times of epidemics. Primary methods included sanitation, which meant more tidy housekeeping, **quarantine**, and **isolation** of the sick. New initiatives were aimed at raising public sanitation and governmental regulations. In Italy, health boards (forerunners of today's health departments) were initiated to fight the plague; market foods, wine, and water; monitor sewage systems; regulate hospital activities; and oversee physicians and the sale of drugs (Cipolla, 1976).

In America, Europeans were developing colonies. Smallpox, measles, typhus, and scarlet fever were carried over with them. Smallpox eliminated nearly 50 to 90% of American Indian populations because they had no natural resistance to the disease (Robertson, 2001). By 1640, the Huron nation was reduced by half. Some of the early settlements were wiped out from disease. Major epidemics broke out in 1633 in the Massachusetts Bay colonies and New York (at that time named the "New Netherlands") in 1663.

AGE OF ENLIGHTENMENT: THE FILTH
THEORY OF DISEASE (1700–1800)

During this period of time, revolutions, industrialization, and urban growth were active but plagues and diseases continued to be problems. It was believed that disease was from filth and epidemics were caused by "miasmas," the Greek word for pollution or "bad air" (Tesh, 1995). The miasthma theory of disease was developed on the belief that inhaling noxious air or vapors from decaying animals and humans, vapors in the outdoor air at dusk, vapors from stagnant waters, and putrid odors from sewage or poor hygiene caused diseases. It was not known that contaminated water could cause diseases. Dr. James Lind (1716–1794), a Royal Navy surgeon, discovered that scurvy, characterized by a loosening of the teeth, could be controlled on long sea voyages by having sailors drink lime juice (BBC, 2004). Edward Jenner (1749–1823) noticed that cowpox, a disease that struck cattle, provided immunity against smallpox for the milkmaids who contracted cowpox while milking the infected cows. He produced a crude vaccination procedure against smallpox by scratching cowpox into the skin (Vetter, 1997).

Growing concern among shipping and mercantile businessmen resulted in the drafting of public health laws (Fox, 2001). In 1701, Massachusetts passed laws to isolate smallpox patients and to quarantine ships as needed (Institute of Medicine, 1989). By the end of the eighteenth century, Boston, Philadelphia, New York, and Baltimore established the enforcement of isolation and quarantine rules. In a 1721 Boston epidemic alone, 5,980 of the city's 11,000 residents caught the disease. Of those afflicted, 844 died (Aronson & Newman, 2002). In 1746, regulations were passed to prevent the pollution of Boston Harbor. In 1752, Boston experienced a major smallpox epidemic with only 174 people of the 15,684 population escaping the disease.

In 1780, the first local board of health was established in Petersburg, Virginia. In the United States, Philadelphia had the largest epidemic when in 1793 23,000 people out of a population of 37,000 contracted yellow fever. Over 4,000 died from the disease (Powell, 1993). Citizens rallied to set up regulations such as cleaning the sickrooms, providing hospital accommodations for the poor, keeping streets and wharves clean, encouraging hygienic measures, and having quick burials. People used vinegar and camphor on handkerchiefs to prevent infection and burned gunpowder in the streets (Unknown, 2004).

The first public health efforts in the United States were initiated in 1798 by President John Adams. He initiated programs for seamen who traveled extensively and were unable to seek medical care on a regular basis (NIH, 2004). The Marine Hospital Service (MHS) Act required

Cistern
Large receptacles for storing water, such as an underground tank.

Quarantine
A period of time when infected individuals are isolated from healthy individuals to prevent the spread of the disease; the term literally means "40 days."

Isolation
Separation; a place apart from others to prevent the spread of infection.

The mid-nineteenth century journalist and legislator, Lemuel Shattuck (1793–1859), recommended keeping vital statistics in the United States. He had an interest in sanitation and was appointed to prepare a report on the sanitation conditions with a plan for reform. The report, regarding the entire state of Massachusetts, was submitted in 1850. The *Report of the Sanitary Commission of Massachusetts* is known today as the *Shattuck Report.* The report included a detailed consideration of present and future public health needs of Massachusetts and the nation. At the time, there were no national or state public health programs. The report laid

out ideas and modes of action that formed the basis of public health practice. The report contained 50 recommendations including the creation of a state board of health; a public health program based on vital statistics; sanitary improvements; control of adulterated foods, beverages, and medicine; vaccination against smallpox and a maritime quarantine; intensive study of tuberculosis problems; promotion of infant and child health; protection of school children by providing sanitary school buildings, health education, and systematic studies of sickness; the establishment of institutions to educate nurses; mobilization of public support

for the public health program; and the distribution of educational information to everyone. Thirty-six of the recommendations are accepted

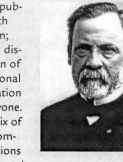

principles of public health practice (Goerke and Stebbins, 1968). Recommendations from the report, however, were not acted upon until 1869, 19 years later.

 During George Washington's lifetime, 90% of the people living after the age of 21 had smallpox and 25% of those died. The average life expectancy was age 29.

shipowners to pay 20 cents per month for each seaman they employed and was collected from shipmasters by the customs collectors in various U.S. ports. This was one of the first direct taxes enacted by the new republic and the first medical insurance program in the United States. The MHS was placed under the Revenue Marine Division of the treasury department. The money was used to build hospitals and provide medical services in all major seaports. The demand for medical services far exceeded the funds available so sailors with chronic or incurable conditions were excluded from the hospitals and a 4-month limit was placed on hospital care for the remainder. This was the beginning of what is now known as the U.S. Public Health Service. The first board of health was estab-

lished in Boston the year 1796 with Paul Revere as its first president (Public Health Museum, 2004).

INDUSTRIAL REVOLUTION: THE GREAT SANITARY AWAKENING (1800–1880)

The Industrial Revolution throughout Europe and America in the 1800s was known for the explosion of manufacturing industries for the production of goods. The steam engines that ran the machinery required fuels. Wood supplied much of it at first, then coal, then oil. As factories and mechanization grew, the demand for raw materials increased dramatically. Innovations in technology provided jobs in manufacturing plants, producing goods for increasing urban populations. As people migrated to the cities in search of jobs, cities became crowded with poverty and filth in tenements and slums, providing opportunities for the second and third pandemics of cholera. There was little or no provision for **cesspools** or fresh water supplies. Until the 1840s, a sewer was simply an elongated cesspool overflowing at one end. Street pumps provided the only source of water, running only a few minutes a day in poor districts. When sea merchants returned to Russia and Europe from India, the disease traveled with them from port to port. By 1827 cholera had become the most feared disease of the century. In the nineteenth century, it became the world's first truly global disease (Guynup, 2004).

In 1828, Edwin Chadwick, a London attorney, began his campaign for sanitary reform in England (UCLA, 2004). He expressed concerns about the health of London citizens due to industrialization and sanitation concerns. His report, *Sanitary Conditions of the Labouring Population,* was presented in 1842 to the British parliament. As a result,

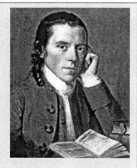 In 1800, Dr. Benjamin Waterhouse, a Harvard Medical School professor (1754–1846), introduced the idea of smallpox vaccinations in America based on results from the work of Dr. Edward Jenner in England, inoculating members of his household. He was the first American physician to establish inoculation as general practice.

Seven pandemics of cholera have occurred since the first one in 1817. The first major cholera pandemic began along the Ganges River, progressing to Calcutta, India, in 1817. It spread throughout Asia by 1823, sailing from port to port in contaminated kegs of water, in the excrement of infected victims, or infected travelers (Marks & Beatty, 1976). The second pandemic of cholera reached the British Isles in the 1830s and Canada in 1847 when Irish immigrants arrived. The third pandemic occurred from 1852 to 1859 and cholera became rampant in the United States. The fourth pandemic brought cholera to cities and towns along the Mississippi, Missouri, and Ohio rivers. The fifth pandemic affected South America with high mortality in Argentina, Chile, and Peru. It was during this time that Robert Koch isolated the cholera bacilli. The sixth pandemic occurred from 1899 to 1923, affecting the near and middle East and Balkan peninsula. Except for a large epidemic in Egypt in 1947, cholera remained confined to south and southeast Asia from the mid-1920s. The seventh pandemic began in Indonesia in 1961 and was the most extensive of the pandemics, spreading to the Philippines, Sabah, and Taiwan by the end of 1962. From 1963 to 1969 cholera spread to the Asian mainland, reaching the Middle East and West Africa in the early 1970s. It reached South America beginning in Peru in 1991, then to Ecuador, Columbia, and Chile, traveling along the Pacific coast to Central America. The seventh pandemic is ongoing and continues with seasonal outbreaks in many developing countries (Faruque, Albert, & Mekalanos, 1998).

England passed the national Public Health Act of 1848, which initiated the world's first public health department. The act also contained a code mandating toileting facilities in every home, whether it was a flushing toilet (invented in 1775), privy, or an ash pit. Cholera hit England through the town of Sunderland in 1831. Medical doctors believed that cholera was not contagious. Merchants found plenty of reasons to deny that they had cholera to avoid the 40-day quarantine in ports. Another pandemic of cholera spread throughout Asia, the Middle East, Europe, Britain, and North and South America in 1837. A third and a fourth cholera pandemic spread. Epidemics of smallpox, yellow fever, cholera, typhoid, and typhus persisted. Tuberculosis and malaria continued to be major problems. In another medical breakthrough, in 1844, a Viennese physician, Ignaz Semmelweis (1818–1865), advocated the washing of hands to prevent the transmission of "childbirth fever" (streptococcal infection) (CDC, 2000).

Once filth was identified as the cause of disease and transmission of diseases in 1923 by Charles Chapin, cleanliness was advocated. Sanitation theories changed the way the public thought about health. Illness was seen as an indicator of poverty as filthy conditions and the spread of disease among the working class became common. Industrialization had produced both a population that was more susceptible to disease and conditions in which disease was more easily transmitted. Sanitation efforts were accompanied by ideas that protecting the health of populations was a social responsibility. The rich quickly learned that the best way to protect themselves against getting a disease was to help the poor who were afflicted. The emphasis on isolation and quarantine changed to cleaning up and improving the environment. Public health agencies and institutions grew at local and state levels. Clean air, decent food and water, decent housing, vaccination programs, proper waste disposal, and knowledge of personal health needs and practices helped improve the health of communities.

About 1857, discussion concerning the prevention and control of typhus, cholera, and yellow fever convened in the United States with what was known as "quarantine conventions." These events resulted in the forming of a national sanitary association (Bernstein, 1972). State boards of health were established in Massachusetts (1869), Virginia (1870), and California (1870) (Institute of Medicine, 1988). In 1872, the American Public Health Association was founded in New Jersey with Dr. Stephen Smith as its first president. In 1879, Congress created the National Board of Health. The primary function of this board was to receive information on all matters related to public health. Grants were provided to state boards of health and universities on topics of health-related interest. The board was not popular, however, because some felt the research grant expendi-

Cesspools
Deep holes or pits in the ground, usually covered, receiving sewage from sinks, toilets, and other areas of the house.

 During the Crimean War (1854–1856) in Europe, Florence Nightingale (1820–1910) served as a military hospital nurse and advocated sanitary methods. She also kept statistics showing the reduction of preventable deaths due to these procedures.

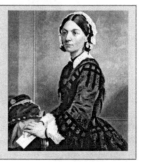

As Europeans settled in North America, the forests and grasslands provided new opportunities. The supply seemed without end. In the South, plantations diminished the fertility and texture of the soil with cotton and tobacco crops so erosion became a problem (McDonald, 1941). In the 1860s, railroads opened up the Great Plains, bringing about the slaughter of bison and pronghorns by the millions. Ranchers brought in cattle that overgrazed the land. The steel plow was invented by John Deere in 1837 and the rich, heavy soils and deep sod of the Midwest changed dramatically (Drake, 2004).

tures were extravagant. The board also was not popular with state health departments and the shipping industry because of quarantine practices. In 1882, the board's functions were transferred to the Marine Hospital Service, which carried on with quarantine functions, but the grants program was discontinued (USDHEW, 1976). There were gains in life expectancy from 34.5 years in 1789 to 42.5 years in 1890 (Indiana Historical Bureau, 2004).

The Age of Bacteriology (1864–1910)

In 1865, while the Civil War was going on, Joseph Lister (1827–1912) (Figure 3-1) began to use antiseptics to care for wounds and during surgery, used carbolic acid (Hallsal, 1998). The first book on public health, *Hygiene and Public Health,* was published by A. H. Buck in 1895. In Europe, Joseph Devaine (1812–1882) identified anthrax bacillus, often transferred from animals to humans by milk.

In 1864, Louis Pasteur (1822–1895) (Figure 3-2) developed a technique known as **pasteurization** that killed bacteria in food. After Pasteur published his book in 1878 regarding his germ theory of disease, the identification of pathogens began. Causes of malaria, anthrax, typhoid, pneumonia, tuberculosis, and diphtheria were identified. Pasteurization of milk was rec-

ommended, vaccines were developed, and vaccination programs by public health officials began.

In the United States, cities continued to grow and many people lived in poor conditions. The Federal Quarantine Act was passed in 1878 (NIH, 2004). Aware that a federal program could not meet local needs, states took matters into their own hands. State hygienic laboratories were developed in Massachusetts, Michigan, and Rhode Island to detect bacteria in water systems.

W. T. Sedgwick, a biologist and professor at the Massachusetts Institute of Technology, was one of the most famous scientists in sanitation and bacteriologic research (Sedgwick, 1891). In 1881, he identified fecal bacteria in water as the cause of typhoid fever and developed the first sewage treatment techniques. He investigated typhoid epidemics and was a spokesperson on the rules for handling and pasteurizing milk. J.W. Hyatt and I.S. Hyatt, developed a water filtration technique using chemical and coagulation filtration processes and patented it about 1884 (Zink, 2004). Theobald Smith (1859–1934), a pathologist from Massachusetts, developed vaccines, antitoxins, and diagnostic tests for smallpox, meningitis, tuberculosis, and typhoid (American Child Health Association, 2004). In 1887, a hygienic laboratory was established at the Marine Hospital Service on Staten Island, New York. Herman Biggs, a pathologist in New York, suggested the application of bacteriology to the detection and control of cholera. W.H. Park, a pathologist in New York, introduced bacteriological diagnosis of diphtheria and production of an antitoxin. It became clear that epidemiologists and their laboratories could lead the effort to reduce infectious diseases. Public health efforts were guided by engineers, chemists, biologists, and physicians.

In 1878, 20,000 people along the Mississippi River died of yellow fever (Ellis, 1992). In 1898, Henry Carter, a yellow fever expert employed by the Public Health Service (PHS) discovered that yellow fever virus was transmitted by mosquitoes. In 1893, the PHS required the documentation and publication of death and disease statistics and

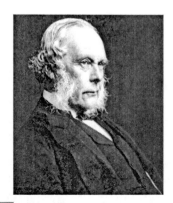

FIGURE 3-1 **Dr. Joseph Lister** A physician during the Civil War, he recognized the need for handwashing and sterilization to prevent infection.

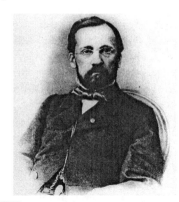

FIGURE 3-2 **Dr. Louis Pasteur** Known for his technique to eliminate and reduce food-borne pathogens to make food safer.

the *Morbidity and Mortality Weekly Report* has been published ever since.

The bubonic plague first struck the United States in San Francisco in 1900. The disease was carried by flea-infected rats to ground squirrels (Chase, 2003). Dr. Joseph Kinyoun, the director of the MHS hygienic laboratory set up a quarantine station, provoking criticism and violent protest from local residents. Dr. Rupert Blue (1867–1948) was assigned to the "plague laboratory" and the plague was proclaimed eradicated in 1905 after 121 cases and 113 deaths. It re-emerged in 1907 after the San Francisco earthquake. It re-emerged yet again in New Orleans in 1914. Rat trappers were hired and as many as 4,000 to 5,000 rats per day were caught, labeled according to the location where they were caught, and examined for signs of the disease.

The most common cause of death in 1900 was influenza accompanied by pneumonia (Ausubel & Meyer, 2001). By then there were 38 states with state boards of health. County health departments began to emerge as the need for local health departments was realized. The first county health department was set up in Jefferson County, Kentucky, in 1908 (University of Louisville, 2004). Public health efforts to control diseases, such as utilizing filtering water systems, were effective. Disease registries were set up; some states passed laws requiring that certain diseased individuals be reported.

In 1902, Congress renamed the Marine Hospital Service the Public Health and Marine Hospital Service and provided it with an organizational hierarchy under the direction of the surgeon general. Concerns about food **adulteration**, vendors misleading potential customers, and mislabeling of products led to the Pure Food and Drug Act which was enacted in 1906. Standard methods of water analysis were also adopted in 1906. The U.S. Department of Labor and the Bureau of Mines was created in 1910 to oversee conditions of mine workers in order to prevent black lung disease and to reduce hazards to miners (Wright, 1995). The first clinic for occupational diseases was also established. During World War I, public health service officials worked overseas using oil and kerosene in water where mosquitos would breed to prevent the spread of malaria (Soper et al., 1947).

HEALTH RESOURCES EXPANSION (1910 TO 1945)

In accordance with the Immigration Law of 1891, in 1910, public health service physicians began to exam immigrants entering the United States through Ellis Island, New York, and Angel Island, San Francisco (The History Channel, 2004 and National Museum of Health and Medicine, 1998). The main disease inspectors were looking for was trachoma, a chalmydia infection of the eye, leading to blindness endemic in Europe. In 1912, trachoma was found in rural Kentucky. Dr. John McMullen,

who had extensive experience working with immigrants on Ellis Island, was assigned to diagnose and treat the disease (Mabey & Bailey, 1999). Some of the first health education efforts were set up, encouraging basic hygiene practices such as handwashing in order to prevent its spread. Immigrants were also examined for insanity, heart disease, lameness, and scalp diseases.

In 1911, Yakima County, Washington, organized a full-time county health department in response to a typhoid epidemic. Pasteurization of milk continued to prove effective in controlling the spread of disease. In 1922 the first school of public health, the Harvard School of Public Health, was established. Dr. Charles Chapin (1880–1941) became well-known for his public health work related to such contagious diseases as diphtheria, scarlet fever, and typhoid (Salotto, 2001). His research showed that contagious diseases were not airborne, but were spread through contact. He emphasized a focus on finding living human germ carriers. As a result of his work, entire families were inoculated against typhoid fever.

In 1912, the Public Health and Marine Hospital Service became known as the U.S. Public Health Service. Congress enacted the Public Health Service Act of 1912. Under the direction of Dr. Rupert Blue, the U.S. Public Health Service became more active in research and public campaigns against disease initially to prevent outbreaks of typhoid fever from contaminated drinking water. The Act of 1912 authorized the investigation of water pollution as a cause of disease and guidelines were put into place for potable water and pasteurized milk. Campaigns were also extended to include the control of occupational and environmental threats (USDHHS, 2004). In 1913, a lab was opened in Cincinnati, Ohio, to study water pollution targeting the spread of cholera and typhoid from sewage and industrial waste.

The first health status assessment for Americans began in 1917 with the Selective Services Act. Medical examinations were given to classify men inducted into the armed services during World War I (1914–1918). The military rejected 30% of the young men because they were physically unfit for duty (Fee, 1987). The Chamberlain-Kahn Act of 1914 established a comprehensive venereal disease control program for the military and provided funding for the quarantine of infected civilians (Brandt, 1985). World War I greatly increased the demand for wheat. Wetlands were drained and ecosystems were disrupted.

Pasteurization
A method of destroying disease-producing bacteria by heating the liquid to a prescribed temperature for a specified period of time.

Adulteration
To make inferior, impure, by adding a harmful, less valuable, or prohibited substance.

By 1915, there were more than 500 tuberculosis clinics and 538 baby clinics in America, most of which were run by city health departments. The clinics provided medical care and health education to decrease morbidity and mortality from disease (Starr, 1982). In 1918, the Spanish flu came to the United States and killed 675,000 people, more than ten times the casualties of World War I (Billings, 1997). In the United States, 28% of the citizens were infected with the Spanish flu decreasing the life expectancy by 10 years. At least half of the soldiers who died in Europe died from the Spanish flu. The Spanish flu grew into a pandemic as outbreaks swept through North America, Europe, Asia, Africa, Brazil, and the South Pacific killing 20 to 40 million people worldwide. Sanitation programs continued, adding programs for draining swamps, spraying for mosquitoes, regulating sewage disposal and water supplies, and inspecting food sources and restaurants. C. E. A. Winslow, professor of public health at Yale University from 1915 to 1945, defined public health as "the science of not only preventing contagious disease, but also prolonging life and promoting physical health and efficiency" (1923).

During the 1920s, malaria was a major problem in the southern United States (Moore, 2004). Public health workers advised residents to drain swamps, put screens on their porches and windows, and quinine was shipped to treat malaria. Kerosene, crude oil, and DDT were used to reduce mosquito populations. In 1922, a laboratory was set up in Hamilton, Montana, to study Rocky Mountain spotted fever, a rickettsial disease transmitted by ticks (Multimedia Museum of Medicine, 2004). From that laboratory, a vaccine was developed, and between 1927 and 1940, half a million people in the Rocky Mountain area were vaccinated. Only 61 people developed the disease and only 3 died. Work began on other insect-transmitted diseases. Developing into three separate labs, they were known as the Rocky Mountain Laboratories.

As the nation suffered during the Great Depression in the 1930s, it became clear that the health needs of the people could not be met without government intervention. In 1933, President Franklin D. Roosevelt created the "New Deal" in order to help the disadvantaged. His plan created agencies and programs to provide public health services. Funds were available for the construction of municipal water and sewage systems, building of hospitals, and to control infectious diseases such as malaria. Public health officials began to make house-to-house inspections in rural areas regarding the disposal of human excrement in outdoor privies, assurance of safe water supplies, and the presence of disease-bearing insects, especially flies and mosquitoes, in the home. Efforts began at the state and local levels to continue with the inspections. Through these inspections, the incidence of typhoid fever and hookworm were dramatically reduced. Health education campaigns included the distribution of flyers to prevent the spread of disease. The Social Security Act of 1935 provided funds for state health departments and their programs to develop sanitary facilities and improve material and child health.

The Ransdell Act of 1930 (PL 71-251) changed the name of the Hygienic Laboratory to the National Institute of Health, now known as the National Institutes of Health. The primary function of this agency was to determining the cause, prevention, and cure of disease (USDHEW, 1976). The institutes are known as the most prestigious medical research facilities in the world.

After the 1930s, local, state, and federal responsibilities for public health continued to increase. The role of the federal government became more prominent in ensuring social welfare. Penicillin was introduced in 1943 and the U.S. government distributed it among military soldiers in an effort to control the spread of syphilis and gonorrhea.

THE AGE OF SOCIAL ENGINEERING (1945 TO 1975)

From 1945 to 1950, U.S. troops were used to combat malaria in the Philippines where as many as 4 to 5 million cases per year were reported (Ejercito, Hess, & Willard, 1954). The Communicable Disease Center (CDC) was organized in Atlanta, Georgia, on July 1, 1946. It is now known as the Centers for Disease Control and Prevention. The World Health Organization (WHO) was developed in 1947 to monitor the spread of infectious diseases worldwide. The outbreak of the Korean War in 1950 was the impetus for creating CDC's Epidemic Intelligence Service (EIS) as the threat of biological warfare became a concern (Ostroff, 2001). Medical discoveries and immunizations drastically reduced childhood diseases such as diphtheria, whooping cough, measles, and scarlet fever.

During the mid-1950s, poliomyelitis was a major health concern. In 1954, Jonas Salk developed a polio vaccine and children across the United States were immunized. Unfortunately there was some controversy when vaccines produced by Cutter Laboratories were found to have live viruses in California (Spector, 1980). In 1957, epidemiological surveillance traced the Asian influenza pandemic and national guidelines for the influenza vaccine were developed. In 1962, a smallpox surveillance unit was established.

> The Sheppard-Towner Act of 1922 established direct funding of personal health services, setting guidelines for public health programs. All states were to meet minimum guidelines for funding such as the provision of nursing, home care, health education, and obstetric care to mothers; a state agency to administer the program; and reports to the federal board. As a result, federal and state partnerships for health programs were developed, increasing the need for public health workers.

The 1960s saw the promotion of a "Great Society" under the Johnson administration. Several federal programs for the improvement of education and health were initiated. Under the Partnership in Health Act of 1966, the federal government funded state and county public health efforts. In 1967, the Comprehensive Health Planning Act (CHP) was passed establishing community health centers across the country. The National Health Service Corps Program assigned physicians to provide medical care in underserved areas. The amount of money spent on health care increased dramatically, making the containment of health care costs a national objective.

President Lyndon B. Johnson's vision for a Great Society also included the improvement of health and education with equal access for all and the responsibility for control of our environment. Medicaid and Medicare programs were established and environmental laws were developed. Johnson stated:

> The air we breathe, our water, our soil and wildlife, are being blighted by poisons and chemicals which are the by-products of technology and industry. The society that receives the rewards of technology, must, as a cooperating whole, take responsibility for [their] control. To deal with these new problems will require a new conservation. We must not only protect the countryside and save it from destruction, we must restore what has been destroyed and salvage the beauty and charm of our cities.
> Our conservation must be not just the classic conservation of protection and development, but a creative conservation of restoration and innovation. (Califano, 1999)

President Johnson provided the rationale for laws creating the Environmental Protection Agency (EPA) and the Superfund Act extracting financial payments from industrial polluters. Laws inspired by the quest for a Great Society included the Clean Air Act (enacted in 1970), Clean Water Act (1972), the Solid Waste Disposal Act (1965), the Motor Vehicle Air Pollution Control Act (1965), and the Aircraft Noise Abatement Act (1968). Efforts to conserve untouched environments included the Wild and Scenic Rivers Act (1968) protecting 155 river segments in 37 states and the National Trail System Act (1968) establishing more than 800 recreational, scenic, and historic trails covering 40,000 miles.

Efforts to collect information about health practices among citizens began in 1971. A major health survey, known as the National Health And Nutrition Examination Survey (NHANES) was conducted by the National Center for Health Statistics of the Centers for Disease Control. This survey provides useful information about health, nutritional status, health knowledge, and health behaviors, enabling public health workers to determine needs and measure outcomes. The NHANES II was conducted from 1988 to 1994. The NHANES III (1999 to 2004) included a physical exam, dental exam, body measurements, as well as hearing, allergy, lung capacity, electrocardiogram (ECG), and bone density tests. The Health Maintenance Act of 1973 promoted organizations that provided less costly health care services.

In July of 1976, public health officials identified the bacterium causing Legionnaire's disease. Since then, more than 20 different species have been identified. In 1981, the acquired immunodeficiency syndrome (AIDS) was first mentioned in an issue of the *Morbidity and Mortality Weekly Report,* published by CDC, identifying the HIV-I retrovirus as the cause.

HEALTH PROMOTION PERIOD (1974 TO PRESENT)

During this era, national initiatives in Canada and the United States for childhood immunization, adolescent pregnancy, smoking, and nutrition were announced. In 1974, the Canadian Ministry of Health and Welfare published a report titled *A New Perspective on the Health of Canadians,* presenting epidemiological evidence of environmental and lifestyle factors responsible for disease and calling for health promotion strategies to encourage Canadians to be more responsible for their health. In 1979, the U.S. Public Health Service produced *The Healthy People* report, emphasizing the need to shift away from the traditional medical model of health care (emphasizing treatment approaches to disease) to a preventive approach. In 1980, the first *Promoting Health/Preventing Disease: Objectives for the Nation* report was generated by the Centers for Disease Control and Prevention. Its purpose was to improve preventative health measures directed by governmental agencies and services for the public. The aim was to set national disease prevention and health promotion objectives to be achieved by 1990. The report contained 226 objectives in 15 priority areas for the United States providing the framework for public health efforts (USDHHS, 1980).

In 1990, the report, *Healthy People 2000: National Health Promotion and Disease Prevention Objectives,* was released. This time 332 objectives were written in 22 priority areas to be achieved over a 10-year period. Soon it became apparent to public health leaders that change was difficult without considering social, political, and economic factors impacting the individual (Cottrell, Girvan, & McKenzie, 1999). As a result, *Healthy People 2010* was developed to continue the collaborative efforts among federal, state, and territorial governments, as well as private, public, and nonprofit organizations throughout the nation. Environmental health was one of the 10 priority areas with 30 objectives.

The goal and 30 objectives pertinent to environmental health include the following:

Goal: Promote health for all through a healthy environment.

Outdoor Air Quality
8-1 Harmful air pollutants
8-2 Alternative modes of transportation
8-3 Cleaner alternative fuels
8-4 Airborne toxins

Water Quality
8-5 Safe drinking water
8-6 Waterborne disease outbreaks
8-7 Water conservation
8-8 Surface water health risks
8-9 Beach closings
8-10 Toxic chemicals

Toxics and Waste
8-11 Elevated blood lead levels in children
8-12 Risks posed by hazardous sites
8-13 Pesticide exposures
8-14 Toxic pollutants
8-15 Recycle solid waste

Healthy Homes and Healthy Communities
8-16 Indoor allergens
8-17 Office building air quality
8-18 Homes tested for radon
8-19 Radon-resistant new home construction

8-20 School policies to protect against environmental hazards
8-21 Disaster preparedness plans and protocols
8-22 Lead-based paint testing
8-23 Substandard housing

Infrastructure and Surveillance
8-24 Exposure to pesticides
8-25 Exposure to heavy metals and other toxic chemicals
8-25 Information systems used for environmental health
8-27 Monitoring environmentally related diseases
8-28 Local agencies using surveillance data for vector control

Global Environmental Health
8-29 Global burden of disease
8-30 Water quality in the U.S.–Mexico border region

Food Safety
10-7 Reduce human exposure to organophosphate pesticides from food

Oral Health
21-9 Increase the proportion of the U.S. population served by community water systems with optimally fluoridated water

Physical Activity and Fitness
Increase the proportion of trips made by walking
Increase the proportion of trips made by bicycling

Tobacco Use
27-9 Reduce the proportion of children who are regularly exposed to tobacco smoke at home
27-10 Reduce the proportion of nonsmokers exposed to environmental tobacco smoke
27-11 Increase smoke-free and tobacco-free environments in schools, including all school facilities, property, vehicles, and school events
27-12 Increase the proportion of worksites with formal smoking policies that prohibit smoking or limit it to separately ventilated areas
27-13 Establish laws on smoke-free indoor air that prohibit smoking or limit it to separately ventilated areas in public places and worksites

Environmental Health: An Important Component of Public Health Efforts

Two factors have shaped public health efforts globally, nationally, and locally: (1) advancements in scientific knowledge and (2) the acceptance that disease control is a public health responsibility. The average life span for U.S. citizens has increased by 30 years from 47 years of age in 1900 to 76 years of age in 1990. Twenty-seven of those years of gain are due to the control of infectious diseases and environmental threats (MMWR, 2003; Research to Prevention, 2004). In the United States, less than 4% of improvements in life expectancy are credited to modern medicine. Environmental concerns such as clean water, decent housing, vaccination programs, proper waste disposal, knowledge of health needs and practices, un-contaminated food, and breathable air have had more impact on human health than any other effort.

Public health officials have worked collaboratively with epidemiologists, environmental scientists, engineers, businesspeople, and many others to determine the potential, scope, and means of correcting environmental problems affecting the health of the public. The assessment of potential environmental health **risks** analyzes the **impact** of the environmental concern, the **source** of the problem, **etiology**, the effects in terms of **exposure** and **dosage**, and whether controls can be applied. The source of the problem is sometimes difficult to determine and may come from several sources or over a prolonged period of time. When environmental concerns adversely affect human health, the **severity** and **scope** of the problem are important considerations. Problems can diminish or increase with time. When control measures are not possible, acceptable limits of exposure are established. This process is often referred to as **risk management** (see Chapter 6).

Future Public and Environmental Health Concerns

The environment is important to longevity and quality of life. Issues regarding nuclear power, pesticides, climate changes, and the balance between humans and nature are public health issues. Szreter (2003) predicts that the third millennium will have rapid and unregulated economic growth with massive disruptions in the environment and public health. He says:

> . . . we have become ever more intimately interdependent on ourselves, on the consequences of our collective actions, and on the enormous, complex network of relationships that we call "the market . . . However, far more insidious threats to our collective security and health are posed by the continuous and accumulating social inequality and environmental degradation produced by unregulated free market growth; these may, in the long run, be even more devastating to global population health. (p. 429)

These ideas forecast the continued importance of environmental effects on human health for generations to come.

Risk
The possibility of injury, disease, or death.

Impact
To have an effect; the power of an event to produce change.

Source
The starting point, person, place, or thing by which something develops; the point by which something begins.

Etiology
The science of causes or origins of a disease.

Exposure
Contact by swallowing, breathing, or direct contact (such as through the skin or eyes). Exposure may be either short term (acute) or long term (chronic).

Severity
The harshness or intensity of an event.

Scope
The range of extent of an action.

Risk management
The process of deciding how and to what extent to reduce or eliminate risk factors by considering the risk assessment, engineering factors, social, economic, and political concerns.

Digging Deeper — U.S. PUBLIC HEALTH CHRONOLOGY HIGHLIGHTS

1798 The Marine Hospital Service (MHS) Act was created by President John Adams designating responsibility for diagnosing infectious diseases from incoming ship seamen and passengers.

1836 The Library of the Army Surgeon General's Office was founded. It is now known as the National Library of Medicine. After the Civil War, it became the leading medical library in the United States.

1862 The library was moved on to the mall in Washington, D.C., sharing quarters with the Army Medical Museum.

1870 Because additional funds were requested from Congress to maintain the MHS, Congress reorganized a network of locally controlled hospitals to a centrally controlled national agency with its own administrative staff, administration, and headquarters in Washington. The MHS became a separate bureau of the U.S. Treasury Department under the supervision of the supervising surgeon, who was appointed by the secretary of the U.S. treasury. Additional money to fund the reorganized service was appropriated by raising the hospital tax on seamen from 20 to 40 cents per month. The money collected was deposited in a separate MHS fund. The 1870 reorganization also changed the general character of the service. It became national in scope and military in outlook and organization. Medical officers, called surgeons, were required to pass entrance examinations and wear uniforms.

1875 The title of the central administrator was changed to Supervising Surgeon General. It was changed again in 1902 to Surgeon General.

1884 Taxing seamen to fund the MHS was abolished. From 1884 to 1906, the cost of maintaining the marine hospitals was paid from the proceeds of a tonnage tax on vessels entering the United States, and from 1906 to 1981 when the Public Health Service hospitals were closed, by direct appropriations from Congress.

1887 The Hygienic Laboratory was established in the basement of a medical hospital on Staten Island to apply findings in bacteriology for the control of epidemic diseases. Diseases such as cholera, yellow fever, smallpox, and the plague were studied. Water was tested, various disinfectants were tried, and fumigants were developed in the lab.

1891 The Hygienic Laboratory moved to Washington, D.C.

1902 The 1902 Biologics Control Act gave the lab authority to inspect the production of vaccines and grant licenses to assure cleanliness and purity. This expanded the scientific research work at the Hygienic Laboratory and gave it a definite budget. The bill also required the surgeon general to organize annual conferences to coordinate better state and national public health activities. The name of the MHS was changed to the Public Health and Marine Hospital Services (PHMHS) to reflect its broader scope.

1912 The Public Health and Marine Hospital Service was renamed the U.S. Public Health Service (PHS).

1918 The Chamberlain-Kahn Act established the U.S. Interdepartmental Social Hygiene Board, a venereal disease control program for the military. It provided funding for the quarantine of infected civilians.

1921 The Sheppard-Towner Act established the Federal Board of Maternity and Infant Hygiene, administrative funds for the Children's Bureau, and funding for states to establish programs in maternal and child health.

1930 The Ransdell Act of 1930 officially changed the name of the Hygienic Laboratory to the National Institute of Health. The primary function of this agency was to determine the cause, prevention, and cure of disease. It is known as one of the most prestigious medical research facilities in the world. The National Institute of Health was moved to Bethesda, Maryland, in 1938. After World War II, federal support was given to expand research to include the study of chronic diseases, human biology, immunology, genetics, and DNA. Because of the expansion, the Institute became the National Institutes of Health (NIH).

1935 The Social Security Act was passed establishing and maintaining public health services for training public health personnel.

1936 The library collections were transferred from the Department of Defense to the U. S. Public Health Service and named the National Library of Medicine (NLM).

1939 The PHS was transferred by President Franklin D. Roosevelt to the newly created Federal Security Agency (FSA), which combined a number of New Deal government agencies and services related to health, education, and welfare. Over 140 years of association between the PHS and the treasury department came to an end.

1944 For the first time, the Public Health Services Act consolidated all the laws affecting the functions of the services.

1953 President Eisenhower submitted a reorganization plan to Congress that called for the dissolution of the FSA and the transfer of all its responsibilities to a newly created Department of Health, Education, and Welfare (HEW). A major objective of this reorganization was to ensure that the important areas of health, education, and social security be represented in the president's cabinet.

1962 The National Library of Medicine was moved to the NIH campus in Bethesda, Maryland.

1979 HEW's educational tasks were transferred to the new Department of Education and the remaining divisions of HEW were reorganized as the Department of Health and Human Services (HHS). The duties and functions of the PHS were expanded to include disease control and prevention, biomedical research, regulation of food and drugs, mental health and drug abuse, health care delivery, and international health.

1966 The National Institute of Environmental Health Sciences (NIEHS) was established in the Research Triangle Park in North Carolina. The purpose of NIEHS was to provide a scientific base for protecting the health of Americans by preventing environmentally related diseases. The Division of Extramural Research and Training provides grants to colleges, universities, and research foundations. Environmental Health Sciences Centers were established at universities throughout the country. Marine and Freshwater Biomedical Sciences Centers were also established. Research Manpower Development Programs support pre- and postdoctoral training in toxicology, pathology, mutagenesis, epidemiology, and biostatistics as they pertain to the environment.

1966 The Partnership in Health Act established a "block grant" approach for a variety of programs, providing federal funding of state and county activities for public health, tuberculosis control, dental health, home health, mental health, and so forth.

1966 The Comprehensive Health Planning Act was passed to establish a nationwide system of health planning agencies and develop community health centers across the United States.

1972 The first edition of the journal *Environmental Health Perspectives*, a NIEHS publication, was issued.

1973 The Health Maintenance Act promoted health maintenance organizations as a means of providing less costly health care.

1978 The National Toxicology Program, headquartered at NIEHS, was established.

1997 The Environmental Genome Project was initiated to explore gene variations that influence susceptibility to environmental exposures.

1998 The Children's Environmental Health Research Center was established.

1998 First National Allergen Survey was conducted.

REFERENCES

(1999). Achievements in public health, 1900–1999: Changes in the public health system. *MMWR, 58,* 1141–1147.

(2001). A history of public health. *New Internationalist, 331,* 30–32.

American Child Health Association (2004). Retrieved November 11, 2004 from http://www.ecommcode2.com/hoover/research/hooverpapers/hoover/commerce/acha5.htm.

(2004). Charles Edward Armory Winslow. Retrieved November 11, 2004 from http://ourworld.compuserve.com/homepages/CarolASThompson/Winslow.htm.

Aronson, W. M., & Newman, L. (2002). God have mercy on this house: Being a brief chronicle of smallpox in colonial New England. Part of an exhibition entitled Smallpox in the Americas 1492 to 1815: Contagion and Controversy. Retrieved November 11, 2004 from Brown University News Service at http://www.brown.edu/Administration/News_Bureau/2002-03/02-017t.html.

Ausubel, J. H., & Meyer, P. S. (2001). Death and the human environment: The United States in the twentieth century. *Technology in Society, 23*(2):131–146.

Author Unknown. (2004). Theobald Smith. 1999–2004 Today in Science History. Retrieved November 11, 2004 from http://www.todayinsci.com/cgi-bin/indexpage.pl?http://www.todayinsci.com/7/7_31.htm.

BBC. (2004). Historic figures: James Lind. Retrieved November 7, 2004 from http://www.bbc.co.uk/history/historic_figures/lind_james.shtml.

Berstein, N. (1972). *APHA: The first one hundred years.* Washington, DC: American Public Health Association.

Billings, M. (1997). The influenza pandemic of 1918. Stanford University. Retrieved November 11, 2004 from http://www.stanford.edu/group/virus/uda/.

Califano, J. (1999). What was really great about the Great Society: The truth behind the conservative myths. *Washington Monthly,* October. Retrieved November 11, 2004 from http://www.washingtonmonthly.com/features/1999/9910.califano.html.

Carr, I. (1997). Nature of disease: The nineteenth century medical revolution. Retrieved November 11, 2004 from Hippocrates on the Web at http://www.umanitoba.ca/faculties/medicine/history/histories/path.html.

Centers for Disease Control. (2000). Why is handwashing important? Press release issued from the Division of Media Relations. Retrieved November 11, 2004 from http://www.cdc.gov/od/oc/media/pressrel/r2k0306c.htm.

Chase, M. (2003). *The Barbary plague: The black death in victorian San Francisco.* New York: Random House.

Cipolla, C. (1976). *Public health and the medical profession in the Renaissance.* Cambridge, England: Cambridge University Press.

Cottrell, R., Girvan, J., & McKenzie, J. (1999). The history of health and health education, pp. 32–69. *Principles and foundations of health promotion and education.* Boston: Allyn & Bacon.

Donan, C. (1898). *The Dark Ages 476–918.* London: Rivingtons.

Drake, H. M. (2004). The impact of John Deere's plow. Retrieved November 8, 2004 from http://www.lib.niu.edu/ipo/iht810102.html.

Duncan, C. & Scott, S. (2004). The history of the Black Death. Retrieved November 7, 2004 from http://www.firstscience.com/site/articles/history-of-the-black-death.asp.

Ellis, J. H. (1992). *Yellow fever and public health in the New South.* Lexington, KY: The University Press of Kentucky.

Ejercito, A., Hess, A. D., & Willard. A. (1954). The six-year Philippine-American malaria control program. *American Journal of Tropical Medicine and Hygiene, 3,* 971–980.

Faruque, S. M., Albert, J. M., & Mekalanos, J. J. (1998). Epidemiology, genetics, and ecology of toxigenic vibrio cholerae. *Microbiology & Molecular Biology Reviews, 62,* 1301–1314.

Fee, E. (1987). *Disease and discovery: A history of the Johns Hopkins School of Hygiene and Public Health 1916–1939.* Baltimore, MD: Johns Hopkins University Press.

Fox, D. (2001). The professions of public health. *American Journal of Public Health, 91,* 1362–1364.

Fox & Co. (2004). The history of plumbing. Retrieved November 7, 2004 from http://www.muswell-hill.com/foxandco/pages/history.htm.

Gray, H. Farth. (1940). Sewerage in ancient and medieval times. *Sewage Works Journal, 12,* 939–946. Retrieved November 7, 2004 from http://www.sewerhistory.org/articles/whregion/1940_as201/article1.pdf.

Guynup, S. (2004). Cholera: Tracking the first truly global disease. *National Geographic News.* Retrieved November 7, 2004 from http://news.nationalgeographic.com/news/2004/06/0614_040614_tvcholera.html.

Hallsal, P. (1998). Modern History Sourcebook: Joseph Lister (1827–1912) Antiseptic principle of the practice of surgery, 1867. Retrieved November 8, 2004 from http://www.fordham.edu/halsall/mod/1867lister.html.

Hansen, R. (2004). Water and wastewater systems in Imperial Rome. Retrieved November 7, 2004 from http://www.waterhistory.org/histories/rome/rome.pdf.

History Channel. (2004). What happened on Ellis Island? Retrieved November 11, 2004 http://www.historychannel.com/ellisisland/gateway/inspectorstory.html.

Indiana Historical Bureau. (2004). Public health in Indiana. Timeline in an issue of the Indiana Historian. Retrieved November 8, 2004 from http://www.statelib.lib.in.us/www/ihb/publications/tlph.html.

Institute of Medicine. (1988). A history of the public health system. In *The future of public health,* pp. 56–72. Washington, DC: National Academy of Sciences, National Academies Press.

Institute of Medicine. (1989). A history of the public health system. In *The future of public health.* Washington, DC: National Academy Press.

Mabey, D., & Bailey, R. (1999). Eradication of trachoma worldwide. *British Journal of Opthalmology, 83,* 1261–1263.

Marks, G., & Beatty, W. (1976). *Epidemics.* New York: Charles Scribner & Sons.

McDonald, A. (1941). Early American soil conservationists. Miscellaneous Publication No. 449. Retrieved November 8, 2004 from http://www.soilandhealth.org/01aglibrary/010107earlyam/010107earlyamsoil.html.

McKenzie, J., & Pinger, R. (1997). *An introduction to community health.* Boston: Jones and Bartlett.

Moore, T. G. (2004). In sickness and in health: The Kyoto protocol versus global warming. Essays in Public Policy, Hoover

Institution. Retrieved November 11, 2004 from http://www.hoover.stanford.edu/publications/epp/104/104b.html.

Morbidity and Morality Weekly Report. (2003). Trends in aging—United States and worldwife. *MMWR, 14,* 101–104, 106.

Multimedia Museum of Medicine on the World Wide Web. (2004). Biomedical research. Retrieved November 11, 2004 from http://www.etg.nlm.nih.gov/project/m3w3/phs_history/phs_history_69.html.

National Institutes of Health. (2004). NIH almanac: Legislative chronology. Retrieved November 8, 2004 from http://www.nih.gov/about/almanac/historical/legislative_chronology.htm.

National Museum of Health and Medicine. (1998). Doctors at the gate: The U.S. Public Health Service at Ellis Island. Retrieved November 11, 2004 from http://ublib.buffalo.edu/libraries/e-resources/ebooks/records/7150.html.

Ostroff, S. M. (2001). The Epidemic Intelligence Service in the United States. *European Surveillance, 6,* 34–365.

Pickett, G., & Hanlon, J. (1990). *Public health administration and practice, 9th ed.* St. Louis: Times Mirror/Mosby.

Public Health Museum. (2004). Pioneers of public health in Massachusetts. Retrieved November 11, 2004 from http://www.publichealthmuseum.org/exhibits-pioneers.html.

Research to Prevention. (2004). Rationale for increased investment in prevention. Retrieved November 11, 2004 from http://www.researchtoprevention.org/html/aboutus.html.

Rosen, G. (1958). *A history of public health.* New York: MD Publications.

Salotto, L. (2001). Charles V. Chapin papers. Rhode Island Historical Society. Retrieved November 11, 2004 from http://www.rihs.org/mssinv/Mss343.htm.

Sedgwick. W. T. (1891). An epidemic of typhoid fever in Lowell, Massachusetts. *Boston Medical & Surgical Journal, 124,* (April 23), 397–402.

Soper, F. L., Knipe, F. W., Casini, G., Riehl, L. A., & Rubino, A. (1947) Reduction of *Anopheles* density effected by the pre-season spraying of building interiors with DDT in kerosene, at Castel Volturno, Italy, in 1944–45 and in the Tiber Delta in 1945. *American Journal of Tropical Medicine, 27,* 177–200.

Spector, B. (1980). The great Salk vaccine mess. *Antioch Review, 38,* 291–303.

Starr, P. (1982). *The social transformation of American medicine.* New York: Basic Books, Inc.

Swazey, J. P., & Reeds, K. (1978). Louis Pasteur: Science and applications of science. In *Today's medicine, tomorrow's science: Essays on paths of discovery in the biomedical sciences.* DHEW Publication No. (NIH) 78-244. Retrieved November 11, 2004 from http://newman.baruch.cuny.edu/digital/2001/swazey_reeds_1978/default.htm.

Szreter, S. (2003). The population health approach in historical perspective. *American Journal of Public Health, 93,* 421–431.

Tesh, S. N. (1995). Miasma and "social factors" in disease causality: Lessons from the nineteenth century. *Journal of Health Politics, Policy and Law, 20,* 1001–1024.

Thyresson, N. (1995). Girolamo Fracastoro and syphilis. *International Journal of Dermatology, 34,* 735–739.

Timmreck, T. (1998). *An introduction to epidemiology, 2nd ed.,* pg. 73. Boston: Jones & Bartlett Publishers.

Unknown. (2004). Yellow fever along the Gulf Coast. Retrieved November 11, 2004 from http://plantpathology.tamu.edu/kbgs/yellowfever.htm.

University of Louisville. (2004). List of history and manuscript collections. Kornhauser Health Sciences Library. Retrieved November 22, 2004 from http://library.louisville.edu/kornhauser/info/manuscript.html#C.

University of Southern California School of Public Health. (2004). Brief history during the Snow Era (1813–58). Retrieved November 11, 2004 from http://www.ph.ucla.edu/epi/snow/1859map/chadwick_edwin_a2.html.

U. S. Department of Health, Education, and Welfare. (1976). *Health in America 1776–1976.* Publication No. (HRA) 76-616. Washington, D.C.: U.S. Government Printing Office. DHEW.

U. S. Department of Health and Human Services (USDHHS). (1980). *Promoting health/preventing disease: Objectives for the nation.* Washington, DC: U.S. Government Printing Office.

U. S. Department of Health and Human Services. (2004). *Surgeon General Biography: Rupert Blue (1912–1919).* Retrieved November 11, 2004 from http://www.surgeongeneral.gov/library/history/bioblue.htm.

Vetter, R. T. (1997). Vaccines and the power of immunity: Teaching the body to fight back. *Postgraduate Medicine, 101,* 154–156, 159.

Wild, R. (2004). The Black Death. The History Magazine, Retrieved November 7, 2004 from http://www.history-magazine.com/black.html.

Winslow, C. (1923). The evolution and significance of the modern public health campaign. *Journal of Public Health Policy.* South Burlington, Vermont.

Wright, J. (1995). Statement of Secretary of the Interior Bruce Babbitt on the closure of the U.S. Bureau of Mines. U.S. Department of Interior. Retrieved November 11, 2004 http://www.doi.gov/news/archives/pr28m.html.

Zink, C. W. (2004). The Hackensack Water Works: Sparkling history, cloudy future. New Jersey Reporter. Retrieved November 11, 2004 from http://www.njreporter.org/NJH200204/njr_waterworks1.html.

ASSIGNMENTS

1. Write a five-paragraph essay expressing the importance of the environment on human health. Provide historical evidence for support.

2. Investigate the background and career of Herman Biggs.

3. Select one of the previous references and visit the Web site to learn more about the function of that agency, its goals, and current programs.

4. Visit the library and find an article regarding a current environmental health concern from the list of the following professional journals.

5. Read one of the following books and write a book report.

6. Provide an overview of the history of the American Public Health Association.

7. Present a debate expressing both sides of the argument concerning the importance of economic growth and environmental health concerns.

8. Select one of the following laws and provide a historical account of its development and impact.

9. Review the Healthy People 2010 objectives as related to environmental health.

10. Develop a short paper on how the Sheppard-Towner Act was developed and implemented.

SELECTED ENVIRONMENTAL LAWS

1878 *Federal Quarantine Act (20 Stat. L. 37)*
Legislation that permitted confinement of individuals carrying a contagious disease; for the purpose of preventing an epidemic. In 1892, the federal government issued requirements for quarantine and in 1893 the federal government assumed responsibility for quarantine inspections. As a result, quarantine facilities were built. By 1921, all quarantine facilities were under federal control.

1918 *Chamberlain-Kahn Act (40 Stat. L. 886)*
Provided for the study of veneral diseases by the Public Health Services.

1921 *Sheppard-Towner Act (PL 67-97)*
Increased funding for the federal government to reduce infant mortality via prenatal and child health.

1930 *Ransdell Act (PL. 71-251, 46 Stat. L. 379)*
Reorganization, expansion, and redesignation of the Hygienic Laboratory at the National Institute of Health. The construction of two buildings and fellowships were authorized.

1935 *Social Security Act (PL. 74-271, 49 Stat. L. 634)*
This act authorized health grants to states to improve public health programs for the control of diseases.

1944 *Public Health Services Act (PL. 78-410, 58 Stat. L. 682)*
This act consolidated the Public Health Service, dividing it into the Office of the Surgeon General, Bureau of Medical Services, Bureau of State Services, and the National Institute of Health.

1966 *Comprehensive Health Planning Act (PL 89-749)*
Offered grant money to states to establish public health services to move to comprehensive health coverage.

1973 *Health Maintenance Act (PL 93-222)*
An attempt at organized medicine to provide an alternative method of financing and delivery of health care services with an emphasis on screening and prevention.

PROFESSIONAL JOURNALS

American Journal of Public Health
Emerging Infectious Diseases
Morbidity and Mortality Weekly Report

ADDITIONAL READINGS

Bess, C. (1982). *Story for a Black Night.* Oakland, CA: Parnassas Press.

Colborn, T., Dumanowski, D., & Peterson Myers, J. (1996). *Our stolen future: Are we threatening our fertility, intelligence, and survival?* New York: Penguin Books.

Hopkins, D. R. (2002). *The greatest killer: Smallpox in history.* Chicago, IL: University of Chicago Press.

Hudson, J. (1989). *Sweetgrass.* New York: Philomel Books. (A 19th century, 15-year-old Blackfoot Indian girl saves her family from a smallpox epidemic).

Melosi, M. (2000). *The sanitary city.* Baltimore, MD: Johns Hopkins University Press.

Melosi, M. (2001). *Effluent America: Cities, industry, energy, and the environment.* Pittsburgh, PA: University of Pittsburgh Press.

Robertson, D. R. G. (2001). *Rotting face: Smallpox and the American indian.* Calwell, ID: Caxton Press.

Wilslow, O. E. (1974). *A destroying angel: The conquest of smallpox in colonial Boston.* Boston: Houghton Mifflin.

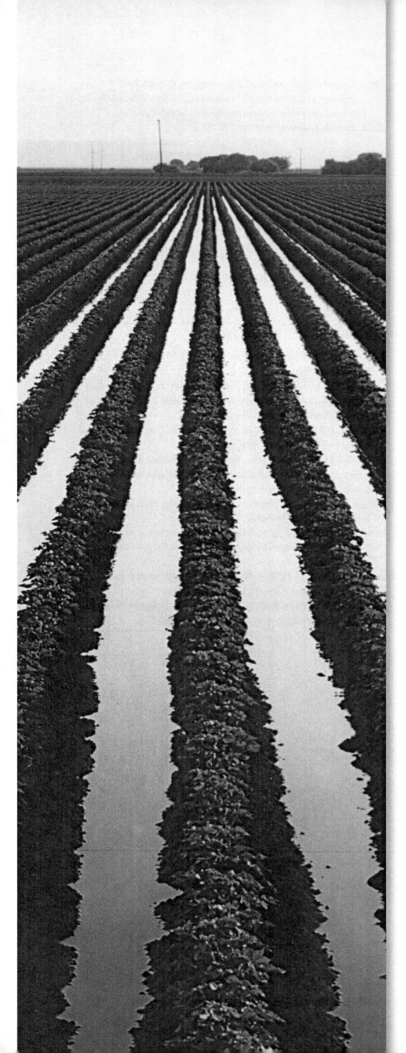

Epidemiology and Environmental Diseases

4

Extreme remedies are very appropriate for extreme diseases.

Hippocrates (460–370 B.C.)

OBJECTIVES

1. Define the term emerging diseases and give five examples.

2. Give accounts of how bioterrorism has been used as an offensive tactic in wars.

3. List and describe three types of agents known to cause environmentally related diseases.

4. Describe natural immunity, active immunity, and passive immunity.

5. Explain how genetic mutation can influence disease transmission.

6. Tell who is most vulnerable to environmental factors resulting in disease states.

7. Explain how an allergen or a pathogen influences the body.

8. Describe six ways diseases can be transmitted.

9. Differentiate diseases caused by bacteria, viruses, prions, fungus, or protozoan.

10. List ways to protect against exposure to and transmission of diseases.

Introduction

This chapter provides information about current environmental concerns important to the spread of disease, disease agents, immunity, susceptibility, **infection, epidemiology**, and specific disease-producing **pathogens**.

The Relationship of Environmental Health and Disease Prevention

Global warming affects weather patterns that can affect health by changing disease patterns. Warm winters and hot, dry summers that increase **vector**-borne infectious diseases and what were once tropical diseases now are found in more temperate zones. Increased rainfall and flooding in some areas provides a suitable climate for mosquitoes that carry disease. Malaria, the West Nile virus, and encephalitis are common to warm areas of the United States, as they are in other parts of the world. Flooding infiltrates sewer systems spreading waterborne illnesses in many places. Storm water runoff increases the incidence of diseases such as typhoid and cholera. Drought lowers water levels and creates stagnant water opportunities for laying eggs. There has been an increase in allergies and hay fever believed to be caused by the increase in pollen produced by higher carbon dioxide levels associated with global warming. Plants that grow in an enriched carbon dioxide atmosphere usually grow faster and larger, producing pollen as much as 61% higher than normal levels (Wayne, Foster, Bazzaz, & Epstein, 2002; Weber, 2002).

International travel has increased dramatically in recent years, making disease prevention a global concern because diseases can easily move from one continent to another with the traveling public, by invaders from another country, migration, or immigration (Bayer, 2004). In 430 B.C., 200,000 people migrated to Athens as they fled from the Spartans. One third of the population died from an infection from an unidentified agent, ending the Golden Age of Athens. In A.D. 166, a plague (possibly smallpox, bubonic plague, or measles) was brought to Rome when Roman troops returned from Syria. The Antoine plague was brought from India by the Huns. Estimates are that the Antoine plague killed 4 to 7 million people throughout Europe resulting in the collapse of the Roman Empire. As early as A.D. 160 the bubonic plague, known as Barbarian boils, carried to China from northern invaders, caused the collapse of the Han Empire. In the Middle Ages, multitudes of people in Asia, the Middle East, and Europe died. The bubonic plague became pan-

demic starting from China through South Russia to Crimera in 1346 to 1350 killing nearly one third of the population of Europe. When Columbus traveled to the Carribean in 1492, 8 million residents of Hispanola died when they were infected by diseases the explorers brought with them such as influenza, smallpox, tuberculosis, and gonorrhea. As slaves were brought to the Caribbean and Americas, infectious diseases from Africa (malaria and yellow fever) killed many European settlers. In addition to malaria and yellow fever, travelers to Africa encountered dysentery and worm infestations, calling Africa "the white man's grave." The bubonic plague, starting in Egypt and spreading throughout Europe in 1542, killed 40% of the population of Constaninople. In the sixteenth century, diseases were spread in Central and South America by Spanish invaders, decreasing the population by 33% in 10 years and by 95% in 75 years. European sailors brought tuberculosis and venereal disease to the Pacific Islands killing 9% of the population. Major **epidemics** have occurred since colonial days when malaria caused the death of Jamestown colonists. In 1724, nearly one third of the population of Williamsburg died of typhoid fever. During the seventeenth and eighteenth centuries, smallpox was the deadliest disease in America. Smallpox epidemics have killed people all over the world. During the Industrial Revolution, cholera swept entire conti-

2010 HEALTHY PEOPLE OBJECTIVES
14-3   Reduce hepatitis B
14-28   Increase hepatitis B vaccine coverage among high-risk groups
8-28   Local agencies using surveillance data for vector control

Infection
The invasion of pathogens in the body of sufficient toxicity to cause illness.

Epidemiology
The science of the occurrence, causes, frequencies, and distribution of diseases in a human population.

Pathogens
Microorganisms that cause diseases such as bacteria, viruses, fungi, protozoa, and richettsiae.

Vector
An insect or animal, usually an invertebrate (insect, tick, or snail) that transmits a disease-producing organism from a host to an uninfected individual; usually through a bite or environmental or food contamination.

Epidemic
Any excessive and related incidence of a particular disease transmitted by an infectious agent in excess of what is normally observed or expected in a region during a particular time period.

A newly emerged disease is one that is (Lederberg et al., 1992):
- a newly described disease or syndrome recognized within the past few decades
- an expanded distribution of a familiar disease into a new region or habitat
- increased local **incidence** of a disease
- increased severity or duration of a disease or increased resistance to treatment

nents. In 1952, 200,000 Americans contracted polio. In the 1980s, human immunodeficiency virus syndrome (HIV/AIDS), genital herpes, and chlamydia moved from Central and South Africa to the United States. Influenza viruses migrate from Asia to all parts of the country each year. Cooperation with international agencies such as the Pan American Health Organization (PAHO), World Health Organization (WHO), and the World Trade Organization (WTO) monitor and provide services for the containment and prevention of epidemics and pandemics.

Emerging Diseases

ew diseases and diseases that were once thought to be controlled are spreading across the globe (Figure 4-1). The emergence of new disease in a geographical area occurs when the agent is introduced in a new **host** population and is transmitted to another host population. Most emerging diseases are thought to be caused by pathogens that existed in the environment previously but were given an opportunity to infect new host populations under altered conditions. These might include global warming, agricultural or economical development, human migration, microbial adaptation, or the breakdown of public health measures (Morse, 1995). Hemorrhagic fevers, for example, are connected to the clearing of land; eliminating of snakes, owls, and jaguars that normally ate the rodents; and the development of grain economics where rodents thrive. Clearing away tropical rainforests leaves behind tropical slums, providing the perfect breeding ground for the *Aedes aegypti* mosquitoes that carry dengue and yellow fever. Some of the new infections are transferred from animals to humans. Examples of **emerging diseases** recognized in the United States since 1947 include Legionnaire disease, Lyme disease, Cryptosporidiosis, acquired immunodeficiency syndrome (AIDS), *Escherichia coli* 0157:H7, hantavirus pulmonary syndrome (HPS), and West Nile disease.

Diseases found in one part of the globe that quickly moved to other areas include Argentine hemorrhagic fever, Bolivian hemorrhagic fever, Chagas disease (American Trypanosomiasis), Ebola hemorrhagic fever (Figure 4-2), Lassa fever, Venezuelan hemorrhagic fever, human granulocytic ehrlichiosis (HGE), dengue hemorrhagic fever, bubonic plague, bovine spongiform encephalopathy (BSE), paratyphoid, malaria, yellow fever, and tuberculosis. With continued population growth, international travel, climate changes, poverty, and urban migration, the time may never come when infectious diseases will be eradicated.

The Threat of Biological Warfare

ar between nations has been a problem since the beginning of time. **Biological warfare** has been noted

FIGURE 4-1 **Emerging Infectious Disease Journal** A good source of information for accurate and timely information about new and re-emerging diseases. (Source: Courtesy of Centers for Disease Control (PHIL).)

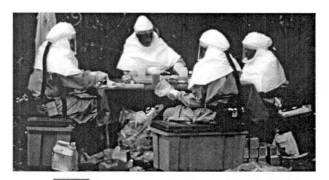

FIGURE 4-2 **Ebola Testing** The U.S. Public Health Service was actively involved in identifying and isolating the virus to prevent its spread.

throughout history. In the fifth century B.C., Romans contaminated water sources with animal carcasses. Around 400 B.C., Scythian archers dipped their arrowheads in feces and cadavers. Hannibal was said to have launched pottery with poisonous snakes onto enemy ships in 190 B.C. During the fourteenth century, Mongols catapulted plague-infected cadavers into Kaffa, a city in the Ukraine.

The first documented use of biological warfare in the United States was during the French and Indian Wars (1754–1767). British soldiers, under orders by Lord Jeffrey Amherst, were said to have taken blankets from a local sanitarium where smallpox was being treated and given the blankets to the Indians. This was in hopes of initiating an outbreak of smallpox in the tribes. It was not known at the time that the disease was caused by contact or inhalation of the disease-causing agent, but the intent was still the same.

During the U.S. Civil War, a Confederate surgeon imported clothes infected with yellow fever. During World War I, Germany used anthrax (*Bacillus anthracis*) and glanders (*B. mallei*) to infect livestock and animal feed exported to Allies. During World War II, Japan conducted research on anthrax, meningitis, shigella, cholera, and the plague as potential military weapons. Germany infected Nazi prisoners with diseases such as hepatitis A to learn more about vaccinations and drugs to treat them. Nazi secret agent Reinhardt Heydrich was assassinated with botulinium toxin. In 1942, Britain developed strategic amounts of anthrax. At the same time, the United States filled as many as 5,000 bombs with anthrax. During the Korean War, U.S. efforts in biological warfare were expanded. In 1955, human experiments were conducted using rabbit fever (*F. tularensis*) and Q fever (*C. burnetti*). From 1949–1968, a stimulant organism was released off the coast of San Francisco and in the New York City subway system. Only in 1969 did the United States terminate offensive biological weapons programs.

Today the threat of **bioterrorism** is as real as it has been ever been. By 1995, it was suspected that 17 countries had biological weapons. Key elements of biological weapons include the low cost of using pathogens as military weapons and the ability to disperse them in a multitude of ways. In addition, they are invisible, odorless, and tasteless making them difficult to detect.

Environmental Disease Agents

here are several determinants of environmentally induced diseases. Biological hazards include pathogens that cause diseases or infec-

tions and are discussed in this chapter. Chemical hazards include toxic substances and will be discussed in Chapter 5. Physical hazards include environmental conditions that permit repeated exposure to situations that impact negatively on health. Physical hazards include noise, heat, humidity, and equipment that cause health problems (see Chapter 16).

Explaining Immunity

he immune system consists of the skin, the lymphatic system composed of glands, and cells within the body that ward off or act upon foreign substances in the body (Figure 4-3). The primary defense against infection is the skin, the largest organ of the body. The skin provides protection unless there is an opening where foreign substances can enter the body. It is for this reason that hand washing and personal **hygiene** are so important. Bone marrow, the thymus gland, spleen, and lymph nodes are also important to the body's defense system. Cells acting upon foreign substances include leukocytes, phagocytes, inflammatory agents, and natural killer cells. Leukocytes, also known as *white blood cells,* indicate that an infection is present. Phagocytes attempt to destroy infected cells. Natural killer cells include B-cells that are produced in the bone marrow of the body and T-cells that are also produced by bone marrow but require action from the thymus gland

Incidence
The number of *new* cases of a disease that occur within a defined population over an established period of time; given as a rate of cases per 100,000 population.

Host
An animal or plant that provides an environment conducive to growth of an infectious agent.

Emerging diseases
Diseases of infectious origin with an incidence that has increased in human populations or threatens to increase in the near future.

Biological warfare
The use of biological agents, or pathogens, to inoculate populations with a disease capable of killing large numbers of people.

Bioterrorism
The use of biological or chemical agents to harm or destroy large populations of people associated with acts of terrorism.

Hygiene
The practice of cleanliness; sanitary practices; hand washing and bathing.

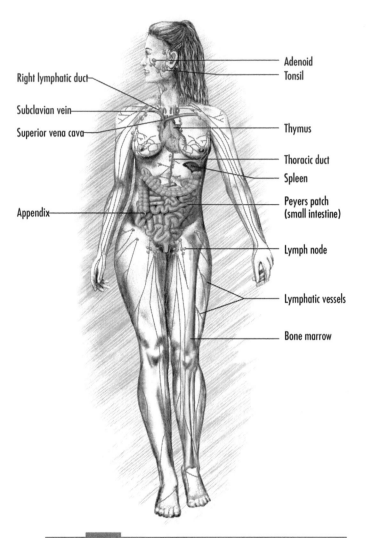

Right lymphatic duct

Subclavian vein

Superior vena cava

Appendix

Adenoid

Tonsil

Thymus

Thoracic duct

Spleen

Peyers patch
(small intestine)

Lymph node

Lymphatic vessels

Bone marrow

FIGURE 4-3 **Immune System** The immune system provides cells and pathways for the body to fight infection when it invades the body.

to mature. The body responds to infection by reacting to **antigens** produced by the foreign agent.

Immune system functioning is important to ward off contagious illnesses from contact with pathogens and sensitivity to **allergens**. Immunity to diseases is aided by the skin, circulatory system, respiratory system, digestive system, and lymphatic system. Proper housing, sanitation, nutrition, and decreased exposure to environmental agents that cause disease are especially important. Immunity can be active or passive or naturally or artificially acquired. **Active immunity** occurs when the human body produces antibodies in response to an antigen. This can take several days. **Passive immunity** provides antibodies through other means. **Naturally acquired immunity** can be active or passive. **Naturally acquired active immunity** occurs when the body encounters an antigen and produces antibodies. **Naturally acquired**

passive immunity occurs when an infant receives antibodies through the placenta or breast milk. **Artificially acquired immunity** usually takes place actively with immunizations or passively by other medical intervention. **Artificially acquired active immunity** is induced when **attenuated** (live or killed) **vaccine**, fragmented, or a DNA–altered agent is injected into the body (Harper, Fukuda, Cox, & Bridges, 2003). The body responds to the antigens by producing antibodies. **Artificially acquired passive immunity** occurs when an **antibody**-containing serum or immunoglobin from another person or animal is transferred to an infected or poisoned person, or a person with severe immunodeficiency, but the effect is short-lasting and may cause anaphylaxis or a blood-borne illness such as HIV or hepatitis (Ghaffar, 2004). **Herd immunity** refers to the resistance within a population to a particular infection (Wilson, 2001). The more people in a population that are immune to a particular pathogen, the less likely the infection will persist or spread. Herd immunity can increase either because an infectious disease spreads or because large numbers of people are vaccinated. Environmental changes can alter herd immunity.

Evolution of Immunity

Individual susceptibility to disease is determined by hereditary predisposition. Some individuals are naturally more susceptible to diseases than others. Weak immune systems can be transferred from parents to offspring. Genes and DNA can be altered in response to environmental influences.

The two most important mechanisms of evolution are **natural selection** and **genetic drift**. Natural selection is known as "survival of the fittest," a phenomenon observed by Darwin. When populations are struck by epidemics, disasters, or war, victims are killed unselectively. The result is a genetic pool of survivors who pass their characteristics on to their offspring. As humans (plants and animals) adapt to a new or stressful environment in order to survive, the resulting genes are then passed on to future generations, known as genetic drift. The process of altering genetic material is known as **mutation**. During the lifetime of an individual, approximately 30 mutations take place. Mutations occur two different ways: genetically and somatically.

Genetic mutations occur in sperm or egg sex cells that unite during reproduction and are passed on to the next generation. Some mutations are minor (such as color blindness), some are beneficial (strengthening survival mechanisms), and some cause diseases that pass on to the next generation. Genetic diseases are linked to either dominant or recessive genes. A dominant gene may be passed to a child from one parent while recessive genes may go unnoticed unless both parents have the same recessive gene. Genetic mutations can occur in response to environmental influences, such as in the case of sickle cell anemia and Tay-Sachs disease.

Sickle cell anemia (SCA) is an inherited blood disorder consisting of crescent or sickle-shaped red blood cells that are difficult to circulate through the small blood vessels. Individuals with SCA experience anemia, pain, and destruction of tissues that lack circulation. The disease occurs primarily among African Americans, Arabs, Greeks, Italians, Latin Americans, and those from India, zones of high malaria incidence. SCA is a recessive disease associated with a protective factor against malaria.

Tay-Sachs disease is a genetic neurological disorder that results in fatty accumulations of nerve cells in the brain resulting in blindness, deafness, paralysis, and death in children by the age of five. Researchers at the Stanford University Medical Center discovered that Ashkenazi Jews have an unusually high risk of several genetic diseases that have been passed on for the past 150 generations (Risch, Tang, Katzenstein, & Ekstein, 2003). This particular population comprises 90 percent of the Jewish population and is known for its high incidence of lysosomal storage disease. Researchers estimate mutations occurred 50 generations ago when Jewish people formed a distinct population in the Middle East. Because Ashkenazi Jews tend to marry within their own population, those mutations remain common today.

Somatic mutations occur in the genes of cells (other than sex cells) as a result of mistakes made during DNA copying or cell division. Exposure to harmful environmental factors will increase susceptibility of cancer and other diseases. It is known that approximately 15% of cancer is due to inherited cancer-disposing genes. An example of this would be exposure of a fair-skinned person to ultraviolet light and the development of a melanoma gene. Predisposition to breast, ovarian, and colorectal cancer are other examples (Venne, Cronister, Greene, Mullineaux, & Klein, 1999).

Antigens
Substances that can trigger an immune response, resulting in production of an antibody as part of the body's defense against infection and disease. Many antigens are foreign proteins (those not found naturally in the body). An allergen is a special type of antigen that causes an IgE antibody response.

Allergens
Substances that trigger an immune response, producing an IgE antibody.

Active immunity
Immunity occurring when the human body produces antibodies in response to an antigen.

Passive Immunity
Immunity provided for the body.

Naturally acquired immunity
Immunity that develops when the body, either actively or passively) encounters an antigen and produces antibodies.

Naturally acquired active immunity
Immunity acquired when the body encounters an antigen and produces antibodies.

Naturally acquired passive immunity
Immunity acquired when an infant receives antibodies from the mother through the placenta or breast milk.

Artificially acquired immunity
Immunity provided by the production of antibodies from immunizations or medical intervention.

Artificially acquired active immunity
Immunity from a vaccine (**attenuated** live, killed, fragmented, or DNA-altered agent) injected into the body results in the production of antibodies so the recipient has mild or no symptoms.

Attenuated vaccine
A vaccine prepared from a microorganism to produce an immune response. A killed attenuated vaccine can no longer reproduce. A live attenuated vaccine is made from living, reproducing microorganisms selected to produce milder effects than the natural (wild) strain; for example, cowpox used to increase immunity to smallpox.

Artificially acquired passive immunity
Immunity induced when an antibody-containing serum or immunoglobin is transferred from another person or animal.

Antibody
A protein (also called an immunoglobulin) manufactured by lymphocytes (a type of white blood cell) to neutralize an antigen or foreign protein; a protein found in blood and tissue fluids produced by B-lymphocytes, binding to antigen-carrying cells to destroy them and provoking an inflammatory response.

Herd immunity
The resistance of a population to an infectious agent.

Natural selection
A complex mechanism by which the genetic structure of a population changes over time because of survival of particular members of that population in different environments.

Genetic drift
Accidental random events that influence genetic codes (alleles) found in DNA of cells passed from one generation to another; usually evidence in small and isolated populations.

Mutation
An inheritable change in a cell's genetic material (DNA).

Individuals Susceptible to Disease

omen are more susceptible to diseases because of their multiple roles. Women must work, bear children, and tend to household duties. This exposes them to many pathogens and chemical agents. Children are more susceptible to disease because they may be exposed to hazards beyond their control. Day cares and schools provide breeding grounds for pathogens, particularly because children are less likely to wash their hands and prevent the spread of disease. Women and children are equally exposed during pregnancy when agents cross the placental barrier from mother to fetus. Disabled and elderly persons are susceptible to diseases when they do not have good nutrition and physical activity habits. More than any other population, poor people are more susceptible to disease. Poverty creates many undesirable conditions and less access to preventative care.

Disease Control Efforts

iseases, such as the plague, malaria, typhoid, smallpox, yellow fever, cholera, and influenza have had devastating effects across the world. They have killed many people, disabled others, spread panic and fear, disrupted communities, and caused government officials to change priorities in order to stop their importation and spread. Disease prevention practices began when Edward Jenner (1749–1823) observed that individuals who had cowpox were less likely to get sick from smallpox than other residents. Biological agents were first discovered when Dr. Robert Koch of Germany (1843–1910), "the father of microbiology," discovered that **microorganisms** caused diseases such as anthrax, tuberculosis, and cholera. When the cause of communicable disease was identified, scientists including Louis Pasteur (1822–1895) developed preventive techniques such as pasteurization of foods and vaccinations. Joseph Lister (1827–1912) advocated the use of **antiseptics** and **sterilization** of medical equipment to reduce deaths from bacterial infections.

Digging Deeper — ADVANCES IN DISEASE EPIDEMIOLOGY CHRONOLOGY

1878 Louis Pasteur publishes *The Germ Theory and Its Applications to Medicine and Surgery.*
Robert Koch publishes *Investigations into the Etiology of Traumatic Infectious Diseases.*

1880 Alphonse Laveran identifies parasites that cause malaria.
Louis Pasteur develops vaccines for chicken cholera and anthrax with attenuated bacilli.
Carl Eberth identifies the typhoid bacillus.

1881 Pneumococcus bacilli are identified as a cause of pneumonia by Louis Pasteur.

1882 Robert Koch announces the discovery of the tuberculosis bacteria.

1883 Diphtheria bacillus is discovered by Edwin Klebs and Fredrich Loeffler.

1885 Pasteur develops the rabies vaccine and it is first used on a 9-year-old boy bitten by a rabid dog.

1886 Pasteurization of milk is first recommended by Franz Soxhet.

1887 Diphtheria and tetanus antitoxins were developed as well as steam-disinfecting techniques.

1890 Shibasaburo Kitsato and Emil Behring develop tetanus and diphtheria toxin vaccines and antitoxins for treatment.

1896 Amroth Wright develops vaccine for typhoid using heat-killed bacilli.

1897 Malaria transmission through the *Anopheles* mosquitoes is proven.

1901 Dr. Walter Reed and colleagues implicate the *Aedes aegypti* mosquito as a carrier of yellow fever.

1918 Worldwide Spanish influenza epidemic kills 20 million people.

1929 Alexander Fleming discovers penicillin. It was first used on humans in 1941. It was recommended for the treatment of bacterial infections in 1943.

1936 Yellow fever vaccine is developed.

1947 The World Health Organization is established to monitor the spread of infectious diseases worldwide.

1955 The Salk polio vaccine is distributed through a nationwide immunization campaign.
The World Health Organization launches a global malaria eradication program, relying on DDT spraying.

1956 The Asian influenza (H2N2) pandemic emerges.

1963 Measles vaccine is developed.

1968 Mumps vaccine is developed.

1969 Hong Kong (H3N2) influenza pandemic emerges.

1976 First Legionnaire's disease outbreak occurs.
First case of human infection with cryptosporidium is discovered.
Swine flu outbreak prompts a federal vaccination program.

1977 Lyme disease is reported in three Connecticut communities.

1979 Hepatitis B vaccine is developed.

1982 *E. coli* 157:H7 is recognized as a pathogen.

1983 HIV-I retrovirus is identified as the cause of AIDS.
H. pylori bacteria identified as a cause for gastric ulcers.

1987 Toxic shock syndrome is identified.

1989 Hepatitis C is identified.

1993 Hanta virus outbreaks in the Four Corners region of the United States.

1999 The West Nile virus first makes its appearance in the United States.

Epidemics have raged through communities, destroying large numbers of people. In fact, epidemics are responsible for more deaths than war. There are two different types of epidemics: common source epidemics and host-to-host epidemics. Common source epidemics are due to **contamination** of water and food from human excretion. Bacteria, viruses, and protozoan are the agents of common source epidemics such as anthrax, dysentery, botulism, brucellosis, cholera, giardiasis, hepatitis, and typhoid fever. Host-to-host epidemics are transmitted from one host to another. In order to produce an epidemic, offending microbes must be transmitted to new hosts. Examples of host-to-host infections include respiratory diseases (e.g., hantavirus pulmonary syndrome, meningococcal meningitis, pneumococcal pneumonia, and tuberculosis), sexually transmitted diseases, other diseases (e.g., typhus, Lyme disease, malaria, plague, and Rocky Mountain spotted fever), and direct-contact diseases (rabies and tularemia).

Epidemiology

The field of epidemiology developed out of necessity to determine the origin, route of transmission, and measures to control the spread of disease. Epidemiology studies populations and groups measuring disease, injury, and disability patterns. The objective of epidemiologists is to find the etiologies of diseases and patterns of transmission or distribution. This enables other health professionals to locate points of intervention before people get sick or injured. Epidemiological information consists of statistical facts such as **morbidity** and **mortality rates**. Epidemiologists found that the transmission of diseases could be airborne, waterborne, foodborne, or transmitted by a vector. This information is vital when planning to interrupt the transmission of diseases through isolation, quarantine, pest control, water purification, food protection, immunization, or solid waste disposal. Epidemiologists also help determine the relative risk of a population for disease, injury, disability, and death. Relative risk is calculated by the following method:

$$\text{Relative risk} = \frac{\text{incidence among those exposed}}{\text{incidence among those not exposed}}$$

The epidemiological approach to disease prevention includes interactions of host, agent, and environment.

Microorganisms
A plant, animal, or pathogen visible only with a microscope.

Antiseptics
Substances that inhibit the action of microorganisms, preventing infection or decay.

Sterilization
Removing microorganisms incapable of reproduction by using heat or chemicals.

Contamination
The presence of toxins or pathogens on inanimate objects such as clothing, furnishings, food, water, soil, eating utensils, or needles.

Morbidity
Any departure, subjective or objective, from a state of physiological or psychological well-being; illness.

Morbidity rate
Also known as the sickness rate; a rate of incidence of sickness to the number of well people in a given group of people over a specified period of time; usually expressed as number of cases per 100,000 people.

Mortality rates
Ratio of the number of deaths during a defined time period to the number of persons at risk of dying during the period; usually expressed in terms of the incidence in a population of 100,000.

Digging Deeper — FATHER OF EPIDEMIOLOGY

In 1845, a cholera outbreak in London occurred. John Snow (1813–1858) studied the incidence of cholera where residents received water supplies from two different companies. He determined the source of the epidemic to be the Broad Street pump and removed the pump handle, putting an end to the outbreak. Although this discovery was his most famous, his work concerning the spread of cholera through water pollution was even more significant. The Southwark Company provided sewage-polluted water from the Thames River. The Lambeth Company provided water from the Thames that was upstream from the pollution. Snow examined cholera deaths and found that homes served by the Lambeth Company had a much lower incidence of cholera. His study of the disease provided a springboard for the study of epidemiology. In 1859, a "manual of hygiene" was developed by E. A. Parks, a professor of military hygiene.

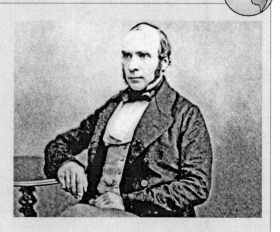

The **disease host** refers to the person in whom the disease resides. The **disease agent** refers to that which carries the disease to the person. Epidemiology views the environment as a means to control disease-causing agents in water, air, food, and waste products.

Biological Agents

iological agents include all forms of life that cause illness and disease including allergens, pathogens, plants, insects, animals, and other humans. Disease may also result from toxins and other nonliving aspects of the biological agent, rather than the agents themselves. Allergens produce antibody reactions, pathogens may produce toxins, plants produce oils, insects produce feces, animals have dander, and humans wear chemicals that may be noxious to other individuals.

Allergens are foreign substances introduced to the body that cause the immune system to produce an antibody reaction to it. This is known as an *allergy*. Pollen (Figure 4-4), molds, dust, peanuts, milk, shellfish, sulfa drugs, penicillin, wheat, and bee sting venom are allergens that produce an allergic reaction in sensitive individuals. When an individual is exposed to an allergen, an antigen or antibody response occurs. Bacteria, viruses, and other microorganisms commonly contain many antigens. Although many types of antibodies are protective, inappropriate or excessive formation of antibodies may lead to illness. When the body forms a type of antibody called IgE (immunoglobulin E), allergic rhinitis, **asthma**, or eczema may result when the patient is again exposed to the substance that caused IgE–antibody formation (allergen). IgE antibodies on basophile cells and mast cells produce a **histamine** reaction and a broncho-constriction effect may occur. This

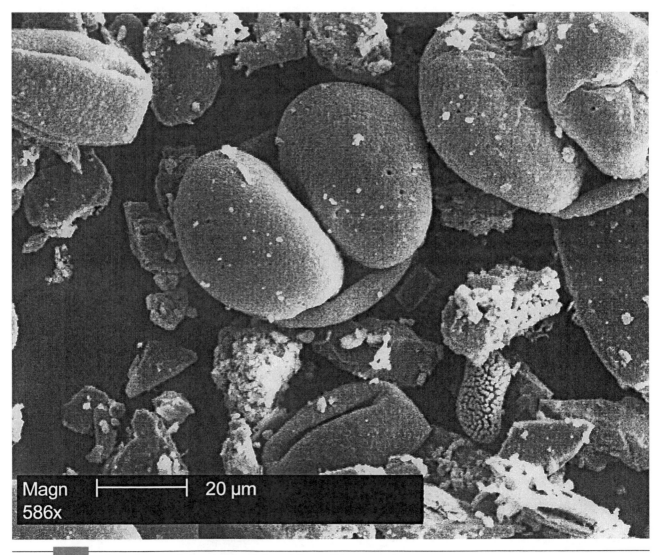

FIGURE 4-4 **Pollen** Microscopic image of pollen on Atlanta, GA campus.

may manifest itself as a rash, hives, or severe itching. In extreme cases, anaphylactic shock can occur. This occurs because of swelling of the respiratory passages, resulting in an extreme emergency. Individuals most likely to have allergic reactions usually have a family history of hay fever, allergies, or asthma. Asthma is a reactive airway disease that occurs as a result of exposure to allergens. It is a chronic condition that requires surveillance and some medications to control acute reactions to an allergen.

The incidence and **prevalence** of allergies and respiratory disease is ever-increasing. This incidence is attributed, in part, to the effects of global warming. Environments with higher-than-normal atmospheric carbon dioxide produce plants much quicker. Warmer temperatures also enable some plants to pollinate quicker and live longer. Warmer climates produce drought conditions that make the reproduction of disease-carrying insects easier. Warmer seasons also mean longer seasonal exposure to plants, insects, and mold.

Allergy tests consist of skin and blood tests. The skin tests are conducted by injecting the agent into the skin. Several agents can be injected using a grid indicating which type of agent was used. The allergist checks the site for redness, itching, or raised bumps or welts. A Radio-AllergoSorbent Test (RAST) is a blood test, using blood from a vein and testing for allergen-specific antibodies. The RAST test is not considered to be as sensitive as the scratch skin test.

Allergy treatments consist of shots and medication to manage allergic symptoms. In the case of asthma, bronchodilators are administered with inhalers. There is not much that can be done to prevent allergies because exposure to allergens is the problem. After an allergen has been identified, it is best to avoid it or to prevent contact with it. Certain foods, plants, animals, smoke, and chemicals can be avoided. Keeping a clean house or office reduces exposure to dust, molds, and chemicals. More information on the indoor environment is provided in Chapter 15.

PATHOGENS

Biological pathogens include bacteria, viruses, prions, fungi, protozoa, rickettsiae, and worms. Disease occurrence depends on exposure to a pathogen and other factors. Biological pathogens need the proper air, moisture, pH, and temperature to grow. Inside the human body, microorganisms flourish. Some can grow without detection, but others multiply to the point of infection. This is when disease symptoms are noticed. An infection spread from one person to another is called **contagious** or **communicable**. These infections are **acute**, with a sudden onset and severe effects, but lasting for a short period of time. Many infections are **chronic**, developing gradually and lasting a long time.

Pathogens may be spread through the air, water, food, by contact with others, by insects and vermin (known

as vectors), and by contaminated objects (known as **vehicles**). Pathogens may be spread in the form of droplets from coughing, sneezing, sputum, or a runny nose. They may enter the body by inhalation, ingestion, injection, or absorption. Pathogens can be found in air, food, and in water. Pathogens may enter the body through inhalation, breaks in the skin, ingestion, direct contact with an infected person, or from handling contaminated objects. Pathogens may be restricted to a specific site or they can be systemic, spreading to various parts of the body. Pathogens may also generate toxins that damage organs and systems of the body.

The five major infectious killers in the world are acute respiratory infections, diarrhea, HIV, tuberculosis, malaria, and measles. Public health officials (Figure 4-5) are

Disease host
The animal or person in which the disease agent resides.

Disease agent
The biological agent or pathogen causing a disease.

Biological agents
Forms of life that cause illness and disease including allergens, pathogens, plants, insects, animals, and other humans.

Asthma
A chronic, inflammatory lung disease characterized by recurrent breathing problems.

Histamine
A chemical released during an allergic reaction; responsible for inflammation, runny nose, sneezing, itching, and bronchial constriction.

Prevalence
The number of diseased individuals at any one time (point prevalence) or over a given period (period prevalence); given as a rate of cases per 100,000 population.

Prevalence rate
Ratio of the total number of individuals who have a disease at a particular time relative to the population at risk of having the disease at that point in time.

Contagious
A disease spread from person to person, caused by direct or indirect contact.

Communicable
A disease that can be transmitted or spread.

Chronic disease
A disease lasting a long time or recurring often.

Acute infection
An infection or illness having sudden onset with severe effects lasting for a short period of time.

Vehicle
An object used to carry a pathogen or transmit an infection from one person to another.

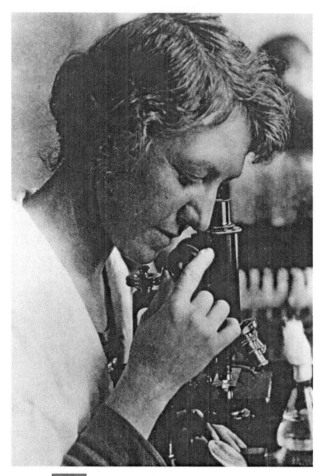

FIGURE 4-5 **Ida Bengston** A bacteriologist for the U.S. Public Health Service.

event during the winter months when most people are inside longer. Legionnaire's disease, the Norwalk virus, anthrax, smallpox (Figure 4-6), influenza, and tuberculosis are diseases that threaten large numbers of people because they can spread very quickly and can be lethal. The severe acute respiratory distress syndrome (SARS) virus created a stir in Asia, North America, and Europe with an epidemic in 2003 (Centers for Disease Control, et al., 2003).

WATERBORNE ILLNESSES

Waterborne illnesses are designated as such because they are transferred from one individual or animal to another from either contaminated drinking water, swimming in contaminated water, eating sewage-contaminated food, consuming fish contaminated by unclean waters, or improper hand washing. Examples of waterborne illnesses include typhoid, cholera, campylobacteriosis, and shigellosis.

ZOONOSES

Diseases may be transmitted from animals to humans. An example would be tetanus, a common intestinal bacteria transmitted from an animal bite. Anthrax can be transmitted from goats, sheep, and cattle to humans by handling contaminated hides and wool. Rabies is carried by wild animals such as skunks, bats, and squirrels to domestic animals and their owners. Giardia is often called "beaver fever," because its most common source is drinking water from streams. Histoplasmosis may be transferred from pigeon feces to humans. The hantavirus is spread by field mice. It was thought that the Ebola virus is present in animals but can be transferred to humans. Bovine spongiform encephalitis was transmitted to humans by consuming the meat from infected cattle. Other diseases transmitted from animals to humans include the plague from fleas carried by rats; tetanus from horses; tuberculosis from cattle; trichinosis from swine; psittacosis from parrots and parakeets; rabies from rodents, dogs, and bats; toxoplasmosis from cats; schistosomiasis from snails; and tularemia from rodents.

concerned about new diseases resulting from changes in the environment (Lake, Bock, & Acrill, 1993; Roizman, 1995).

Transmission of Diseases

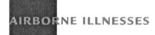
AIRBORNE ILLNESSES

In any area inhabited by humans, bacteria and viruses are easily spread. When an individual coughs, it is thought to spread microbes as far as 20 to 30 feet in diameter. When an individual sneezes, the microbes may be sprayed as far as 40 to 50 feet away. Indoors, this means that anyone in the immediate vicinity is automatically exposed to contagious respiratory diseases. If there are a large number of people in the building, eventually each person is exposed. The incubation times vary from disease to disease and by person to person, depending on their immunity. An increased incidence of colds and flu is often a common

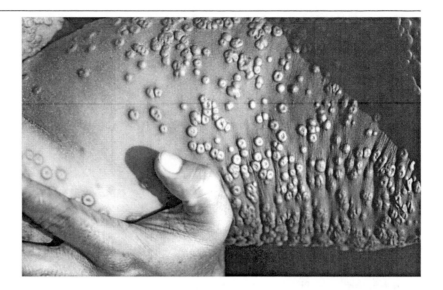

FIGURE 4-6 **Smallpox Victim** The size and proliferation of the nodules are quite frightening and can cause deformity.

VECTOR-TRANSMITTED ILLNESSES

Vectors are animals or insects that transmit pathogens to humans (see Chapter 6). Some animals carry insects that transmit diseases; this includes the flea-carrying rats responsible for the bubonic plague. Arthropods such as mosquitoes and flies transmit illnesses by biting or blood sucking. Malaria, dengue fever, yellow fever, encephalitis, and the West Nile virus are examples of mosquito-transmitted diseases. Rocky Mountain spotted fever is carried by wood or dog ticks. Lyme disease is an infection transmitted by a bacteria-infected deer tick.

SOIL

Soil may harbor hookworm, tetanus, anthrax, and botulism. Some diseases are obtained when an individual eats a food with soil on it, does not wear shoes and socks, or does not wash their hands.

FOMITE

A **fomite** is an inanimate object other than air, water, milk, food, or soil that is a vehicle of disease. Often called vehicles, contaminated objects such as discarded tissues, needles, and other items could spread disease organisms from one person to another. Additional fomites include handrails, door knobs, grocery carts, clothing, bed linens, and toys.

NOSOCOMIAL INFECTIONS

Nosocomial infections are transferred from a health care worker to patients, patients to health care workers, and patient to patients after a hospitalization or period of infirmity. The most common of nosocomial infection is *staphylococcal* infection (Figure 4-7). In the 1990s,

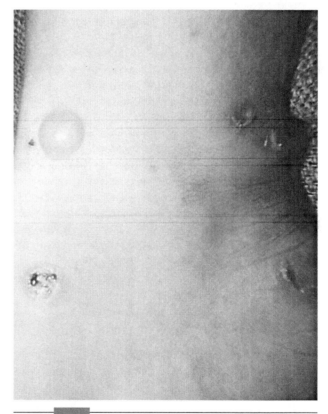

FIGURE 4-7 **Staph Infection** Common acne, impetigo, and other skin lesions are considered staph infections.

Fomite
An object, such as a comb, pencil, toothbrush, or anything that might transmit pathogens, that is infected by an individual.

Nosocomial infections
Infectious diseases contracted while in a medical facility.

between 100,000 to 150,000 patients died from infections they contracted inside a U.S. hospital (Koplan & Fleming, 2000). Even in air-conditioned rooms, conditions are right for certain pathogens.

Pathogens

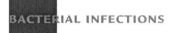

BACTERIAL INFECTIONS

Anthrax

Anthrax is an acute infectious disease caused by the spore-forming bacterium *Bacillus anthracis*. The spores are stable and may remain viable for many years in soil and water. They will resist sunlight for varying periods. Anthrax is a zoonotic disease that can be transferred from animals to humans. The animal most commonly affected are goats, sheep, and cattle. It is not transmitted from human to human. In order to be infected, the organism must be rubbed into abraded skin, swallowed, or inhaled as a fine, aerosol mist.

The skin form of the infection (known as cutaneous anthrax, Figure 4-8) occurs most frequently on the hands and forearms of persons working with infected livestock or contaminated animal products and represents 95% of cases of human anthrax (U.S. FDA, 2004). It is initially characterized by a small solid elevation of the skin, which progresses to a fluid-filled blister with swelling at the site of infection. The scab that typically forms over the lesion can be black. With treatment, the case fatality rate is less than 1% among people who get the skin form of the disease. Left untreated, the illness can progress rapidly to respiratory distress and shock in 2 to 4 days followed by a range of more severe symptoms, including breathing difficulty and death.

The swallowed form of the disease comes from eating insufficiently cooked infected meat or ingesting food with hands contaminated with anthrax spores. Symptoms include nausea, loss of appetite, vomiting, fever, followed by abdominal pain, vomiting blood, and severe diarrhea. Intestinal anthrax results in death of 25% to 60% of cases (CDC, 2004a).

Cases of inhaled anthrax were associated with bioterrorism activity in the United States in 2001. Spores were sent through the mail and postal workers became infected as they inhaled the bacteria while sorting the mail. The inhaled form is gradual with symptoms resembling a cold or flu without the runny nose. After several days, breathing problems and shock develop. The current mortality for inhaled anthrax in the United States is 80% to 90% (Bartlett, Inglesby, & Borio, 2004).

Botulism

Botulism is a serious illness caused by a toxin produced by the rod-shaped bacterium *Clostridium botulism*, commonly found in soil. Food-borne botulism is caused by eating foods that contain the botulism toxin (e.g., home-canned foods with low acid content such as green beans, asparagus, beets, and corn; home-canned or fermented fish; chopped garlic in oil; chili peppers; tomatoes; improperly handled baked potatoes wrapped in aluminum foil; and honey). Wound botulism is caused by a toxin produced from a wound infected with *Clostridium botulinum*. Infant botulism is caused by consuming the spores of the botulinum bacteria, which then grow in the intestines and release toxin (Figure 4-9). All forms of botulism can be fatal and are considered medical emergencies. The classic symptoms of botulism include double vision, blurred vision, drooping eyelids, slurred speech, difficulty swallowing, dry mouth, and muscle weakness. Respira-

---

FIGURE 4-8 **Cutaneous Anthrax Victim**
The black spots on the skin are found in cutaneous anthrax, but not the respiratory type.

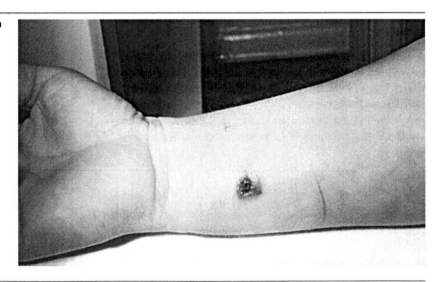

tory failure and paralysis occurs with severe botulism may require a breathing machine (ventilator) for weeks and intensive medical care.

Brucellosis

Brucellosis is caused by the bacteria *Brucella* that affects sheep, goats, cattle, deer, elk, moose, wild pigs, dogs, and other animals. Humans are infected by eating or drinking something that is contaminated with *Brucella* (e.g., wild game or unpasteurized milk or cheeses), inhaling the organism, or through skin wounds and contact with infected animals. Those most at risk are persons working in slaughterhouses or meatpacking plants, veterinarians, and hunters. Symptoms are flu-like but more severe infections of the central nervous system and heart can develop. Most cases of brucellosis are in countries that do not have effective public health and animal disease control programs such as the Mediterranean Basin (Portugal, Spain, southern France, Italy, Greece, Turkey, and North Africa), South and Central America, Eastern Europe, Asia, Africa, the Caribbean, and the Middle East (CDC, 2004b). In the U.S., cases have been reported in California, Florida, Texas, and Virginia. Mortality is less than 2%, usually due to cardiac complications. Treatment consists of several antibiotics and preventing secondary infections.

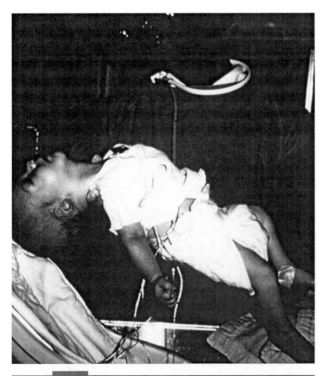

FIGURE 4-9 **Six-week Old Botulism Victim** Public health officials have warned that honey may contain botulism and is not to be given to a child less than 2 years of age.

Campylobacteriosis

Campylobacteriosis (*Campylobacter jejuni*) is the most common cause of bacterial diarrhea in the United States. Many cases go unreported. The bacteria is a spiral shape and is most often found in raw poultry, unpasteurized milk, contaminated water, or contact with the feces of an infected animal. Forty to 60% of the raw poultry produced in the United States has campylobacter bacteria on it (Hingley, 1999). Symptoms include diarrhea, cramping, abdominal pain, nausea, vomiting, and fever within 2 to 5 days after consumption. The illness usually is short-lived, but some individuals develop arthritis or Guillian-Barre syndrome afterward. Most cases of campylobacteriosis could have been prevented by handwashing, careful handling of poultry while preparing, and cooking poultry meat completely.

Clostridium Tetani

Clostridium tetani is a bacterium that causes *tetanus* (also known as *lockjaw*) in humans. The rod-shaped bacteria is found in soil and animal feces. The bacteria forms spores that multiply and produce toxins that affect the nervous and muscular system. Tetanus is preventable with immunization. In the United States, immunizations begin with four shots in the first two years of birth, with a booster shot every 10 years.

Cholera

Cholera (*Vibrio cholerae*) is an enteric bacterium present in sewage-contaminated food or water. It is a normal inhabitant of surface water growing in association with plankton. Symptoms of cholera include watery diarrhea and vomiting, leading to dehydration and death. During the last 170 years, cholera has occurred as a **pandemic** disease (Huq, Sack, & Colwell, 2001). Originally found in Asia, it has been in Africa and South America for almost 100 years. Since 1975, there have been sporadic cases of cholera along the Gulf Coast of the United States.

V. cholerae is the most common type of cholera found in the United States today. The *V. cholerae* is a rod-shaped bacteria that secretes an enterotoxin. Vibrio bacteria are common in surface waters, both ocean and freshwater habitats. Transmission to humans is usually through water or seafood (mostly crabs and oysters) during warm summer months. The first symptom is a sudden onset of watery diarrhea. This loss of fluid leads to dehydration, acidosis, and shock. Untreated cholera frequently results

Pandemic
An epidemic extending beyond the confines of a wide area, typically a continent, such as HIV/AIDS; a widespread problem.

in high (50% to 60%) mortality rates. Most antibiotics do not cure the disease, but may shorten the duration.

E. coli

E. coli (Escherichia coli) is commonly found in the intestines of healthy humans and animals. It is a common cause of diarrhea, particularly traveler's diarrhea. It is transferred by the oral-fecal route, when human and animal feces is in water or food. During rainfalls, snow melts, or other types of precipitation, E. coli may be washed into creeks, rivers, streams, lakes, or groundwater. Agricultural and food-processing companies have also been known to reuse wastewater. When these waters are used as sources of drinking water and the water is not treated or inadequately treated, E. coli may end up in drinking water. E-coli can also contaminate meat during slaughter. It has been found on cattle udders and equipment used for milking. It has also been found in swimming pools and unpasteurized juices as well as alfalfa sprouts. E. coli can be transmitted person-to-person in families, child care centers, and nursing homes. Officials warn that the chance of infection increases dramatically during the summer months.

One strain, E. coli 0157:H7, is particularly harmful. This strain produces a powerful toxin and can cause severe illness. Infection often causes hemorrhagic colitis, characterized by severe bloody diarrhea and abdominal cramps, or severe nonbloody diarrhea. Frequently, no fever is present and occasionally vomiting will occur. Symptoms usually appear within 2 to 4 days, but can take up to 8 days. Diagnosis is based on detection of bacterium in the stool and is indicated for anyone with bloody stool. Most people recover without antibiotics or other specific treatment in 5 to 10 days. In some people, particularly children under 5 years of age and the elderly, the infection can also cause a complication called hemolytic uremic syndrome (HUS), in which the red blood cells are destroyed and the kidneys fail. HUS is the principal cause of acute kidney failure in children. About 8% of persons with HUS have lifelong complications such as high blood pressure, seizures, blindness, paralysis, and long-term kidney damage (CDC, 2001). Prevention of E. coli transmission includes the washing of hands after using the bathroom.

Lyme Disease

Lyme disease is caused by the Borrelia burgdorferi bacteria. It is spread to humans by the bite of ticks in the Ixodes family such as the deer tick and the black-legged tick. The ticks feed on deer, lay their eggs, and the eggs develop from larvae to nymphs, which infect an unsuspecting host. The disease was first reported in 1975 near Lyme, Connecticut. The disease occurs primarily in coastal regions of the northeastern United States, but is reported in California, Nevada, Oregon, and many Midwestern states. A circular red rash appears 3 to 30 days after the tick bite on humans (Figure 4-10). Lyme disease can be treated with antibiotics. Untreated, it can result in death, but this is rare.

Meningitis

Meningitis is caused by either bacteria or a virus in humans. Meningitis is an infection of the spinal cord and brain fluid, sometimes referred to as spinal meningitis. Symptoms of the disease include high fever, headache, and a stiff neck. The illness progresses very quickly and can be fatal. It is important to know which type of meningitis is present to prevent spreading the infection. Viral meningitis is less severe and resolves without specific treatment. Bacterial meningitis can be quite severe and may result in brain damage, hearing loss, or learning disability. Haemophilus influenzae type b (Hib) was the lead-

---

Digging Deeper   E. COLI AND FOOD-BORNE ILLNESSES

In the summer of 1997, 100 people reported E. coli in Michigan and Virginia after consuming alfalfa sprouts. It was later traced back to a food producer in which animal feces had contaminated the seeds where they had been harvested (Breuer et al., 2001).

An outbreak occurred during a fair in Albany, New York, in 1999. Nine hundred and twenty-one people reported diarrhea. It was later determined that the water supply used to make ice and beverages was contaminated with runoff from a cattle barn (CDC, 1999). Stool cultures confirmed 116 persons had the disease and 65 required hospitalization. Eleven children developed hemolytic uremic syndrome (HUS) and two people died. Another case occurred in 1999 in Vancouver, Washington when thirty-two people were infected with E. coli after swimming in a lake. It was unclear whether the source was human or from the ducks inhabiting the area. Three young children required dialysis (Rojas-Burke, 1999). In 1998, 13 children were diagnosed with E. coli after visiting a kiddie pool near Atlanta, Georgia. Five were hospitalized with HUS. In Illinois, 5,400 people became ill from a milder form of E. coli by eating contaminated potato salad (CNN, 1998). E. coli in apple cider was also detected in 1999. Since 1999, ground beef has been recalled after finding evidence of E. coli by the Food Safety and Inspection Service during routine monitoring.

---

ing cause of bacterial meningitis, but a **vaccine** is given to children to reduce the occurrence. *Streptococcus pneumoniae* and *Neisseria meningitidis* are the leading causes of bacterial meningitis.

Rocky Mountain Spotted Fever

Rocky Mountain spotted fever (*Ricettsia rickettsii*) is the most severe and most frequently reported rickettsial bacteria illness in the United States. The disease is spread to humans by dog and wood ticks. Rocky Mountain spotted fever was first recognized in 1896 in the Snake River Valley of Idaho and was originally called "black measles" because of the characteristic rash (CDC, 2000). The name Rocky Mountain spotted fever is somewhat of a misnomer. Beginning in the 1930s, it became clear that this disease occurred in many areas of the United States other than the Rocky Mountain region. Initial symptoms of the disease include sudden onset of fever, headache, and muscle pain, followed by the development of a rash. The disease can be difficult to diagnose in the early stages, and without prompt and appropriate treatment it can be fatal. Rocky Mountain spotted fever can be a severe illness and patients often require hospitalization. Because *R. rickettsii* infects the cells lining blood vessels throughout the body, respiratory system, central nervous system, gastrointestinal system, or renal system complications can occur. Long-term health problems include partial paralysis of the lower extremities; gangrene requiring amputation of fingers, toes, arms, or legs; hearing loss; loss of bowel or bladder control; movement disorders; and language disorders.

Shigellosis

Shigellosis (dysentery) is caused by a group of bacteria called *Shigella*. Infected individuals develop stomach cramps, diarrhea, and fever a day or two after they are exposed. The illness usually resolves itself in 5 to 7 days. Shigella is contracted through the fecal-oral route of infection or from eating food contaminated by infected food handlers, sewage-contaminated vegetables, flies, drinking contaminated water, swimming in contaminated water, or diaper changing. Shigella dysenteriae type 1 (Sd1) is the most virulent type of Shigella, causing epidemic dysentery. *Dysentery* is defined as diarrhea containing blood. This form of Shigella is antimicrobial resistant, making treatment difficult. Complications can develop including seizures, renal failure, and HUS. It may require hospitalization of children and elderly adults.

Staph Infections

Staph infections are caused by *Staphylococcus aureus* bacteria. *Staphylococcus aureus* normally occur in the nasal passage, mouth, and rectum and is relatively harmless. It is also found in acne and boils on the skin. *S. aureus* is the leading cause of soft tissue infections and a major cause of hospital-acquired infections of surgical wounds. An uncontrolled staph infection may cause permanent damage

---

Vaccine
Biological preparation administered to a person to induce immunity against an infectious agent.

FIGURE 4-10 **Lyme Disease Rash** The circular rash after a deer tick bite is the most distinguishing sign of Lyme disease.

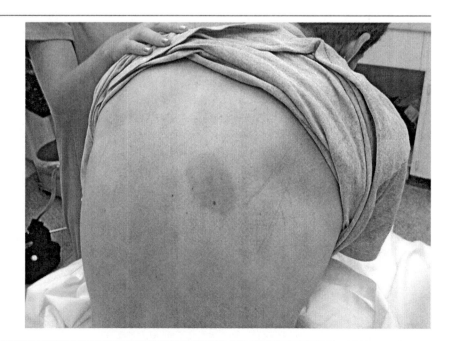

to the heart and lead to pneumonia. The infections are difficult to treat because it is resistant to some antibiotics. It is also the agent in pneumonia, meningitis, boils, arthritis, and toxic shock syndrome (TSS). Staph infections can be found in food. After consuming contaminated food, symptoms occur quickly with cramps and severe vomiting.

Typhoid Fever

Typhoid fever is caused by the bacterium *Salmonella typhi*. It is a life-threatening illness. *Salmonella typhi* lives only in humans. Infected individuals carry the bacteria in their bloodstream and intestinal tract. Carriers of the disease may show no symptoms but can infect others when they shed the bacteria in their feces. Another person can become infected with typhoid fever by eating food or drinking beverages handled by an infected person who has not practiced correct hygiene. A famous carrier known as Typhoid Mary is featured in Chapter 13.

Another source of typhoid is sewage-contaminated drinking water. Typhoid is found in developing countries. Individuals from the United States primarily are infected when they travel internationally. Persons with typhoid fever usually have a high fever, stomach pains, headache, and loss of appetite. Persons traveling internationally are usually advised to obtain the vaccine, drink bottled water, and avoid ice in their drinks.

Tuberculosis

Tuberculosis is a chronic infectious disease of the lower respiratory tract caused by *Mycobacterium tuberculosis* bacteria (Figure 4-11). The disease is passed from one person to another by inhaling airborne droplets from the coughing of infected individuals. Tubercle bacilli form in the lungs and can be active or dormant. It is the most deadly infectious disease worldwide because it is so widespread. Efforts to control tuberculosis have been difficult because drug-resistant strains are developing. The drug-resistant strains have developed as a result of noncompliance with antibiotic therapy among patients who stop taking it after they feel better. In the United States, tuber-

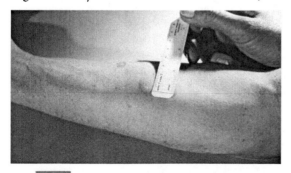

FIGURE **4-11** **Tuberculosis** Tuberculosis reaction to Mantoux test.

culosis patients have been ordered to take their medicine under supervision for 6 months and be tested regularly. Some patients in New York City have been placed in detention facilities until they are well (Coker, 2000).

Tularemia

Tularemia is a disease caused by a bacteria, *Francisella tularemsis* and is being considered as a bioterrorism weapon. Known as "rabbit fever," the disease can affect humans and animals and is most often associated with rabbits, although it can be carried by rodents, ticks, and deerflies. Exposure to the tularemia bacteria can be from contact with the skin, mucous membranes, blood, or tissue of infected animals or a bite from infected ticks or flies. Less common means of contracting the disease include drinking contaminated water, inhaling dust from contaminated soil, or handling pelts of infected animals. The most common symptoms are a skin lesion and swollen glands. Antibiotics are effective in treating tularemia.

VIRAL INFECTIONS

Dengue fever

Dengue fever is considered an "urban tropical disease" because it is distributed in cities in tropical areas globally with cases reported in Taiwan, China, Pakistan, the Pacific Islands, Africa, and along the Mexican border. The illness is carried by the *Aedes* mosquito moving from one area to another by sailing ships. There are four virus serotypes that cause dengue and dengue hemorrhagic fever (DHF): *DEN-1, DEN-2, DEN-3,* and *DEN-4*. Having the disease does not give immunity from the same infection or another type. Initial symptoms are flu-like. When an infected individual begins to feel better, blood vessels leak, and untreated individuals go into shock and die.

Epidemics were reported in Asia, Africa, and North America from 1779 to 1780. A pandemic occurred in the 1950s after World War II; by 1975 it was the leading cause of hospitalization and death in Southeast Asia (CDC, 2003a). In the 1980s dengue fever expanded to Sri Lanka, India, the Maldive Islands, the People's Republic of China, and Taiwan. An epidemic of dengue fever was reported in Pakistan in 1994. Dengue fever has spread to the Americas and remains the most dangerous of mosquito-borne illnesses.

Ebola Virus

Ebola virus is feared because of the high fatality rate. The **filovirus** was first discovered in 1976 in Zaire, Africa. It is spread from bodily fluids and secretions. Flu-like symp-

 Navajo medicine lore says mice are the bearers of an ancient illness and are to be avoided.

toms occur 4 to 16 days after infection, followed by rashes, bleeding, and kidney or liver failure. Infected individuals become extremely ill with massive internal hemorrhaging, causing death.

Encephalitis

Encephalitis is inflammation of the brain, caused by a viral infection. The most common type of encephalitis in the United States is St. Louis encephalitis (SLE), where the first cases were recognized in 1933. The virus is thought to live in birds and other animals and is transferred to humans by the *Culex* mosquito. Most people who are infected do not show symptoms. Those who do have symptoms begin with flu-like symptoms. Severe cases include seizures, paralysis, and death. Antibiotics are not effective and there is no vaccine.

Hanta Virus Pulmonary Syndrome

Hanta virus pulmonary syndrome (HPS, *sin nombre virus*) received national attention when it was identified in 1993 when Navajo residents living in the Four Corners region of the southwest (New Mexico, Arizona, Colorado, and Utah) were infected. The spread of the disease was attributed to global warming. After six years of drought, an extensive rainfall produced an abundance of pinion nuts and field mice migrated in search of food. Humans contracted the disease by inhaling virus particles from rodent feces or by being bitten by an infected rodent. Initial symptoms are flu-like but within a short time the lungs fill with fluids causing severe respiratory distress.

Retroactive studies found the hanta virus as far back as 1959. As of February 2000, 238 cases of hantavirus pulmonary syndrome had been reported in the United States with 42% resulting in death (Ellis, 2003). As of June 2002, 318 cases of HPS were identified in 31 states, with a case fatality of 37% (Mills, Corneli, Young, Garrison, Khan, & Ksiazek, 2002).

Hepatitis

Hepatitis is inflammation of the liver. There are five types of hepatitis: hepatitis A, hepatitis B, hepatitis C, hepatitis D, and hepatitis E. *Hepatitis A* (HAV) can occur as an isolated case or a widespread epidemic. The infection is acute and there is a vaccine for it. The symptoms are nausea, diarrhea, and fever accompanied by jaundice. The HAV virus is spread by the fecal-oral route. *Hepatitis B* (HBV) and *Hepatitis C* (HCV) are more serious with long-term effects, causing cirrhosis of the liver, liver cancer, liver failure, and death. Approximately 30% of those infected with HBV have no symptoms and approximately 80% of those with HCV have no symptoms. Both HBV and HCV are transmitted by shared needles and sexual intercourse. There is a vaccine for HBV, but there is no vaccine for HCV. The HCV virus is the most common cause of chronic liver disease in the United States. More than 2.7 million persons in the United States (or 1.3% of the population) are infected with HCV. Many of these will develop end-stage liver disease (Heintges & Wands, 1997; Alter, Kruszon-Moran, Nainan et al, 1999). *Hepatitis D* (HDV) infection can be acquired either as a coinfection with HBV or as a **superinfection** of persons with chronic HBV infection (CDC, 1990). *Hepatitis E* (HEV) is commonly recognized in large outbreaks. HEV is transmitted primarily by the fecal-oral route and fecally contaminated drinking water. Unlike hepatitis A virus, which is also transmitted by the fecal-oral route, person-to-person transmission of HEV appears to be uncommon. However, nosocomial transmission, presumably by person-to-person contact, has been reported to occur. Virtually all cases of acute hepatitis E in the United States have been reported among travelers returning from high HEV-**endemic** areas.

Human Immunodeficiency Virus

Human immunodeficiency virus (HIV) is caused by a retrovirus that attacks white blood cells, essential to a healthy immune system. The virus attaches to the T cell and transfers genetic information to the cell. The genetic information then is reproduced. HIV is transmitted by contact with blood, body fluids, and from mother to fetus. Infected individuals will not manifest symptoms for months or years after acquiring the infection. HIV antibodies can be detected by the Enzyme-Linked Immunosorbent Assay (ELISA) and Western Blot tests, but it may take as much as 6 months to be detected after an infection. HIV may progress to acquired immunodeficiency syndrome (AIDS). When the immune system breaks down, many different infections can occur. The most common and frequently fatal infection is *Pneumocystic carinii pneumonia*. AIDS patients may also develop Kaposi's sarcoma or lymphomas. Worldwide, it is estimated that 1 in every 100 sexually active adults is HIV-infected, including children under the age of 15. Since the epidemic began in 1970, it is responsible for about 20% of

---

Filovirus
A virus with the appearance of long threads or filaments, causes hemorrhagic fevers in humans and primates.

Superinfection
Reinfection with an altered type of the same infection; difficult to treat.

Endemic
A relatively stable transmission of an infectious agent in a human population; any disease with a low to moderate normal base level incidence rate in the population, but not necessarily constant; e.g., the common cold is endemic.

all deaths (UNAIDS and WHO, 1997; Centers for Disease Control and Prevention, 1997).

Influenza

Influenza was first described by Hippocrates in 412 B.C. Epidemics of certain viruses have been reported worldwide. In 1918, the Spanish flu (Type A HINI) caused an estimated 500,000 deaths in the United States and 20 million deaths worldwide (Moore, 2002). In 1957, the Asian flu (Type A H2H2) caused 70,000 deaths in the United States. The Hong Kong flu (Type A H3N2) caused 34,000 deaths worldwide in 1968 and remains the most destructive of viruses currently circulating.

Influenza is commonly referred to as the flu, but there are three basic types. Influenza C causes a mild respiratory illness and is not thought to cause epidemics. The flu shot does not protect against Influenza C. Two basic types, type A and type B, have spanned the globe. Both types of influenza viruses have mutated so that immune cells do not recognize the new strains of the viruses. Flu viruses spread from November through March. Symptoms can be very mild with a fever, cough, sore throat, stuffy nose, muscle aches, and extreme fatigue. Usually the illness lasts 1 to 2 weeks. Influenza A causes the worst symptoms and the most complications. Death can occur among those who are young, debilitated, or elderly.

Norwalk Viruses

Norwalk viruses (*Noroviruses*) are a class of viruses that cause acute **gastroenteritis**. Symptoms of norovirus illness include nausea, vomiting, diarrhea, and some stomach cramping. The illness begins suddenly and the infected person may feel very sick. The illness is usually brief, with symptoms lasting only about 1 or 2 days. Noroviruses are very contagious and can spread easily from person to person. The most common cause of a Norwalk-like virus is eating food contaminated by a food handler. Persons who are infected with norovirus should not prepare food while they have symptoms and for 3 days after they recover from the illness.

Rabies

Rabies (*Mononegavirales*) is a viral infection transmitted from animals to humans because of contact with saliva, either from a bite or droplet spread (Figure 4-12). The virus causes acute encephalitis and the outcome is almost always fatal. Although all warm-blooded animals are susceptible, only a few species are **reservoirs** for the disease. In the United States, rabies is associated with bats, raccoons, skunks, foxes, and coyotes. The first symptoms of rabies are flu-like, which may last for days. Within days, symptoms of cerebral dysfunction, anxiety, confusion, and agitation progress to delirium, abnormal behavior, hallucinations, and insomnia lasting 2 to 10 days. A vaccine for animals is available to prevent the spread of this disease.

Severe Acute Respiratory Syndrome

Severe acute respiratory syndrome (SARS) is a respiratory illness reported in Asia, North America, and Europe. SARS is caused by a corona virus, a common cause of upper respiratory viruses, which is resistant to normal **disinfection** techniques (Figure 4-13). SARS is spread by close person-to-person contact, contaminated objects, or droplet spread from coughing and sneezing. Symptoms begin with a fever, headache, and body aches. Some people also experience mild respiratory symptoms. After 2 to 7 days, SARS patients may develop a dry cough and have trouble breathing. Approximately 8% of cases are fatal.

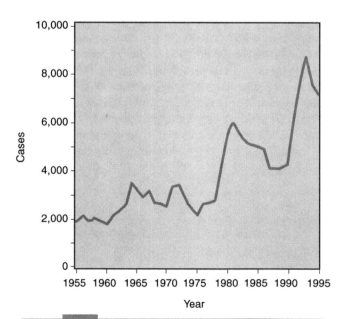

FIGURE 4-12 **Animal Rabies, United States, 1955 to 1995** Because of the wide dispersion of the rabies virus animal vaccinations are required in all states. (Source: Courtesy of Centers for Disease Control (PHIL).)

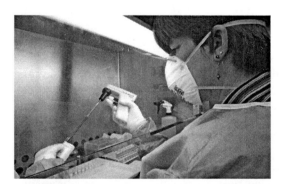

FIGURE 4-13 **SARS Prevention** Concern over the rapid spread of SARS created worldwide panic in 2003.

West Nile Fever

West Nile Fever is caused by transmission of the virus from birds to horses and humans by mosquitoes (Figure 4-14). The bird species *Corvidae* (crows, blue jays) provide the reservoir. Transmission of the virus from one person to another has not been documented. Birds and horses have died from the illness and usually indicate that the virus is in a particular geographical area. Most human cases have no signs or symptoms. In the elderly, the very young, and those with depressed immune systems, the disease can cause inflammation and encephalitis.

PRION INFECTIONS

A **prion** is a disease-producing protein particle related to a number of illnesses such as *bovine spongiform encephalitis* (BSE, or "mad cow disease") and chronic wasting disease in animals, as well as Cruetzfeldt-Jakob disease in humans. Prions convert the protein from normal cells into prions. Prions enter the central nervous system (brain and spinal cord) through the immune system and leukocytes (Aguzzi, Montrasio, & Kaeser, 2001). Prions enter brain cells and they eventually misfire, function poorly, or do not function at all. Prions eventually move over to healthy brain cells and destroy them, resulting in a "spongy" appearance with holes. The transmission of prions to humans comes from eating animal meat.

FUNGAL INFECTIONS

Histoplasmosis

Histoplasmosis (*Histoplasma capsulatum*) is a disease caused by inhaling the spores of the fungus found in soil with a high nitrogen content. The disease can be carried by wild birds and bats, and transferred to other areas by their droppings. Histoplasmosis primarily affects a person's lungs and a great majority of infected individuals do not have symptoms. If symptoms occur, they are mild and flu-like. A chest X-ray can reveal distinct markings on

Gastroenteritis
Inflammation of the gastrointestinal system evidenced by nausea, diarrhea, bloating, gas, and other symptoms.

Reservoir
The host or substance in which a parasitic organism normally resides that is essential for parasitic replication or development.

Disinfection
Killing or removing pathogens capable of causing infection using chemicals or radiation; decontamination.

Prion
A disease-producing protein particle related to bovine spongiform encephalitis, chronic wasting disease, and Cruetzfeldt-Jakob disease.

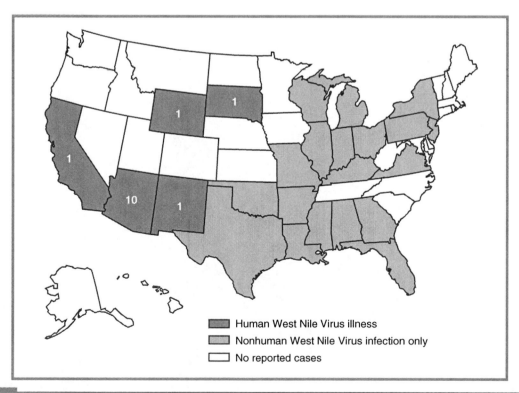

Human West Nile Virus illness
Nonhuman West Nile Virus infection only
No reported cases

FIGURE 4-14 **West Nile Virus Activity, United States, 2004** Considered an invasive species, the West Nile virus has spread to many areas of the United States. (Source: Courtesy of Centers for Disease Control. Available: http://www.cdc.gov/mmwr/preview/mmwrhtml/mm5323a6.htm.)

an infected person's lungs. Chronic lung disease due to histoplasmosis resembles tuberculosis and can worsen over months or years. The best way to prevent exposure to *H. capsulatum* spores is to avoid situations contaminated with bird droppings that can become aerosolized and subsequently inhaled.

PROTOZOAN INFECTIONS

Cryptosporidium Parvumis

Cryptosporidium parvum is a protozoan transmitted in the intestines of animals and humans. It is found in feces, soil, drinking water, recreational water, food, unwashed hands, and contaminated surfaces. The parasite is highly infectious and widely distributed because it is resistant to chlorine disinfection and is hard to filter out of water supplies. Individuals drinking contaminated water swallow the cysts that protect the protozoan. Infected individuals develop watery diarrhea, stomach cramps, nausea, and a slight fever. Symptoms last 2 weeks or less except in individuals with weakened immune systems. In 1993, 400,000 people were infected with *Cryptosporidium* by contaminated drinking water in Milwaukee. Other outbreaks have been reported from recreational waters, unpasteurized apple cider and through day care centers and hospitals. The illness is usually **self-limiting**.

Giardiasis

Giardiasis is the most common cause of waterborne illness in the United States. It is a diarrheal illness caused by *Giardia intestinalis* (also known as *Giardia lamblia*) (Figure 4-15). *Giardia* may be found in soil, food, water, or surfaces that have been contaminated with the feces from infected humans or animals. The most common source is swallowing recreational water or untreated water from shallow wells, lakes, rivers, springs, ponds, and streams. Symptoms occur 1 to 2 weeks after exposure and include diarrhea, loose or watery stool, stomach cramps, and upset stomach. These symptoms may lead to weight loss and dehydration. Some people have no symptoms.

Malaria

Malaria is caused by the *Plasmodium* parasites. The protozoan are transmitted from human to human by the *Anopheles* mosquito. The mosquitoes become infected when they feed on an infected person. Sporozoites develop in the stomach of the mosquito and are transferred from the salivary glands. After entering a human, the sporozoites enter the liver and cells begin to split, producing merozoites. The merozoites attach to red blood cells, convert hemoglobin to hemozoin, and symptoms of malaria develop such as bouts of chills and fever for sev-

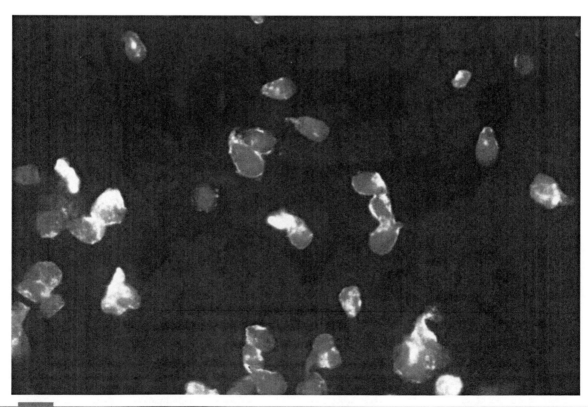

FIGURE 4-15 **Giardia** A parasite common in areas where campers drink water that has not been chlorinated or boiled.

eral hours every 3 to 4 days. Waves of parasitemia develop, producing a fever. Certain strains of the parasite can cause cerebral malaria and death. Most malaria cases are in the tropical and subtropical regions (Figure 4-16). It is estimated that malaria kills two million people per year, but debilitation from malaria is the most significant effect of the disease. Malaria has occurred in the United States in California, Texas, and Florida in individuals who traveled or lived overseas.

National and Local Precautions

fforts to prepare for possible mass epidemics of deadly diseases have been initiated by the federal government. Public health departments in all 50 states were issued a mandate to have a bioterrorism disaster preparedness plan in effect. All public health workers were to receive training and create mechanisms to issue immediate communications should an alert occur. Health care facilities and clinics, including dental and veterinarian services, are required to notify state laboratories about unusual occurrences of certain diseases. Military and public service workers are prepared to handle emergencies requiring protective clothing, mass immunization, and temporary housing for affected populations. U.S. residents have also been instructed to keep emergency food supplies, water, medicines, and other essentials in the event of isolation or evacuation. Some programs have given advice to providing airtight residences should a bioterrorism emergency occur.

Medical Precautions

he most important thing in the treatment of diseases is early detection and treatment. Physicians, pathologists, and other health care workers need to be updated on new pathogens and diseases so they can recognize them when they are presented in clinical areas. The next most important thing is proper treatment. Bacterial and parasite infections can be slowed down or killed by antibiotics. Although a healthy person may be able to recover without antibiotics, the use of drugs has made recovery much faster. When an individual is sick, the drugs may save a person's life. However, not all pathogens respond to antibiotics and other drugs. Increasingly, pathogens are becoming antibiotic resistant as individuals do not take antibiotics as directed at specific intervals until it is gone. Antibiotics cannot be applied to viral infections. New diseases and the re-emergence of

Self-limiting
A disease that resolves on its own.

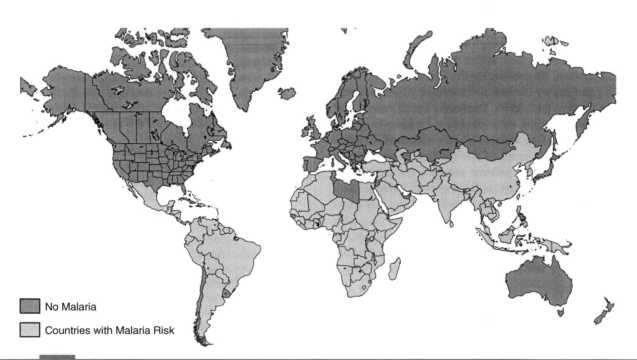

□ No Malaria

□ Countries with Malaria Risk

FIGURE **4-16** **Malaria Endemic Countries, 2003** It is apparent that malaria is a problem in many areas of the world where there are mosquito populations. Note: This map shows countries with endemic malaria. In most of these countries, malaria risk is limited to certain areas. (Source: Centers for Disease Control.)

diseases thought to be eradicated continuously challenge the medical profession and scientists.

The primary means of controlling contagious diseases has always been sanitation, control of vectors, and isolation.

Summary

The spread of disease is as much a problem now as it has ever been. Individuals, families, communities, and entire populations of people can be affected. Sanitation, vaccines, and good personal health practices are the best defenses against contact with disease-causing pathogens. Treatment has advanced, but it is dependent upon early detection by knowledgeable health care providers and compliance with medical treatment by patients. Not all of the medical innovations or technologies can help prevent some of the devastating effects of disease. In fact, technologies thought to help humankind may actually be sabotaging it. The best strategy is to be personally accountable by complying with mandatory immunizations, proper hygienic practices, avoiding others presenting disease symptoms, and taking responsibility by not spreading diseases to anyone else.

REFERENCES

Aguzzi, A., Montrasio, F., & Kaeser, P. (2001). Prions: Health scare and biological challenge. *Nature Reviews Molecular Cell Biology, 2,* 118–126.

Alter, M., Kruszon-Moran, D., Nainan, O., et al. (1999). The prevalence of hepatitis C virus infection in the United States, 1988 through 1994. *New England Journal of Medicine, 341,* 556–662.

American Cancer Society (2003). Cancer facts and figures: 2003. Retrieved May 3, 2003 from http://www.cancer.org/downloads/STT/CAFF2003PWSecured.pdf.

Aron, J., & Patz, J. (2001). *Ecosystem change and public health: A global perspective.* Baltimore, MD: The Johns Hopkins University Press.

Bartlett, J. G., Inglesby, T., & Borio, L. (2004). Anthrax for the pulmonary physician. From the Web site of the American College of Chest Physicians. Retrieved November 7, 2004 from http://www.chestnet.org/education/online/pccu/vol16/lessons1_2/lesson01.php.

Bayer Pharmaceutical Corporation. (2004). A brief history of infectious disease: Epidemics. Retrieved November 7, 2004 from http://www.bayermhc.com/healthcare/hc0102.asp.

Benensen, A. (1990). *Control of communicable diseases in man.* Washington, DC: American Public Health Association Publications.

Blostein, J. (1991) Shigellosis from swimming in a park pond in Michigan. *Public Health Reports, 106,* 3317–3322.

Breuer, T., Benkel, D., Shapiro, R., Hall, W., Winnet, M., Linn, M., Neiman, J., Barrett, T., Dietrich, S., Downes, F., Toney, D., Pearson, J., Rolka, H., Slutsker, L., Griffin, P., and the investigation team. (2001). A multistate outbreak of Escherichia coli 0157:H7 infections linked to alfalfa sprouts grown from contaminated seeds. *Emerging Infectious Diseases, 7.* Retrieved November 7, 2004 from http://www.cdc.gov/ncidod/eid/vol7no6/breuer.htm.

Centers for Disease Control and the Council of State and Territorial Epidemiologists (CSTE). (2003). Revised U.S. surveillance case definition for Severe Acute Respiratory Syndrome and update on SARS cases—United States and worldwide, December 2003. *MMWR, 52,* 1202–1206.

Centers for Disease Control and Prevention. (2004a). Questions and answers about anthrax. Retrieved November 7, 2004 from http://www.bt.cdc.gov/agent/anthrax/faq/index.asp.

Centers for Disease Control and Prevention. (2004b). Brucellosis. Retrieved November 7, 2004 from http://www.cdc.gov/ncidod/dbmd/diseaseinfo/brucellosis_t.htm.

Centers for Disease Control and Prevention. (2003a). Dengue fever. Retrieved November 7, 2004 from http://www.cdc.gov/ncidod/dvbid/dengue/.

Centers for Disease Control and Prevention. (2003). Retrieved from http://www.bt.cdc.gov/Agent/Anthrax/Anthrax.asp.

Centers for Disease Control and Prevention. (2001). Diagnosis and management of food-borne illnesses: A primer for physicians. *MMWR, 50.* Retrieved November 7, 2004 from http://www.cdc.gov/mmwr/PDF/rr/rr5002.PDF.

Centers for Disease Control and Prevention. (2000). Rocky mountain spotted fever: Introduction. Retrieved November 7, 2004 from http://www.cdc.gov/ncidod/dvrd/rmsf/.

Centers for Disease Control. (1999). Escherichia coli 0157:H7:H7 and campylobacter among attendees of Washington County Fair. Retrieved March 20, 2002 from http://www.cdc.gov/ep/mmwr/.

Centers for Disease Control and Prevention. (1997). Update: Trends in AIDS incidence, deaths, and prevalence, United States, 1996. *MMWR, 46,* 165.

Centers for Disease Control and Prevention. (1990). Protection against viral hepatitis recommendations of the Immunization Practices Advisory Committee. *MMWR, 39,* RR-2, 1–26.

CNN. (1998). Food poisoning outbreaks hit hard nationwide, July 10. Retrieved November 7, 2004 from http://www.cnn.com/HEALTH/9807/10/summer.bad.food/.

Coker, R. J. (2000). *From chaos to coercion: Detention and the control of tuberculosis.* New York: St. Martin's Press.

Ellis, S. (2003) Hantavirus pulmonary syndrome. Retrieved June 24, 2003 from http://www.austin.cc.tx.us/microbio/2704f/hanta.htm.

Ghaffar, A. (2004). Microbiology and immunology on-line. University of South Carolina School of Medicine. Retrieved November 7, 2004 from http://www.med.sc.edu:85/ghaffar/immunization.htm.

Harper, S. A., Fukuda, K., Cox, N. J., & Bridges, C. B. (2003). Using live, attenuated influenza vaccine for prevention and control of influenza. Supplemental recommendations of the Advisory Committee on Immunization Practices (ACIP). *MMWR, 52,* September 26, 1–8.

Heintges, T., & Wands, J. (1997). Hepatitis C virus: Epidemiology and transmission. *Hepatology, 26,* 521–526.

Hingley, A. (1999). Campylobacter: Low-profile bug is food poisoning leader. *FDA Consumer, 33.* Retrieved November 7, 2004 from http://www.fda.gov/fdac/features/1999/599_bug.html.

History of Epidemics and Plagues. (2001). Retrieved May 2003 from http://uhavax.hartford.edu/bugl/histepi.htm.

Huq, A., Sack, R., & Colwell, R. (2001). Cholera and global ecosystems. In Aron, J., & Patz, J. *Ecosystem change and public health: A global perspective,* pp. 347–352.

Koplan, J., & Fleming, D. (2000). Current and future public health challenges. *JAMA, 284,* 1696.

Lake, J., Bock, G., & Acrill, E. (Eds.). (1993). *Environmental change and human health.* New York: J. Wiley & Sons.

Mills, J., Corneli, A., Young, J., Garrison, L., Khan, A., & Ksiazek, T. (2002). Hantavirus pulmonary syndrome—U. S.—Updated recommendations for risk reduction. *MMWR, 51,* 1–12.

Moore, G. (2002). *Living with the earth: Concepts in environmental health science,* 2nd ed. Boca Raton: Lewis Publishers.

Morse, S. (1995). Perspectives: Factors in the emergence of infectious diseases. *Emerging Infectious Diseases, 1.*

Risch, N., Tang, H., Katzenstein, H., & Ekstein, J. (2003). Geographic distribution of disease mutations in the Ashkenazi Jewish population supports genetic drift over selection. *The American Journal of Human Genetics, 72,* 812–822.

Rojas-Burke, J. (1999). Investigation confirms lake as source of E. coli cases. The Oregonia, September 15. Retrieved March 7, 2000 from http://www.oregonlive.com/news/99.

Roizman, B. (Ed.). (1995). *Infectious diseases in an age of change: The impact of human ecology and behavior on disease transmission.* Washington, DC: National Academy Press.

UNAIDS and WHO. (1997). Report on the global HIV/AIDS epidemic. Available from http://www.unaids.org/unaids/document/epidemio/report97.html.

U. S. Food and Drug Administration. (2004). Anthrax. Retrieved November 7, 2004 from http://www.fda.gov/cber/vaccine/anthrax.htm.

Venne, V., Cronister, A., Greene, M., Mullineaux, L., & Klein, C. (1999). Genetic and cancer syndromes, *Genetic Drift, 17.* Retrieved May 1, 2003 from http://www.mostgene.org/gd/gdlist.htm.

Wayne, P., Foster, S., Connolly, J., Bazzaz, F., & Epstein, P. (2002). Production of allergenic pollen by ragweed is increased in CO2-enriched atmospheres. *Annals of Allergy and Asthma Immunology, 88,* 279–282.

Weber, R. (2002). Mother nature strikes back: Global warming, homeostasis, and implications for allergy. *Annals of Allergy, Asthma, & Immunology, 88,* 251–252.

Wilson, M., (2001). Ecology and infectious disease. In Aron, J., & Patz, J. *Ecosystem change and public health: A global perspective,* pp. 283–324.

ASSIGNMENTS

1. Select one of the newly emerging diseases mentioned in this chapter or in recent newspaper or magazine articles and learn the symptoms, how it is transmitted, the incubation period, how it is treated, the predicted prognosis or recovery, and residual effects. Suggestions include Argentine hemorrhagic fever, Bolivian hemorrhagic fever, Chagas disease (American Trypanosomiasis), Ebola hemorrhagic fever, Lassa fever, Venezuelan hemorrhagic fever, human granulocytic ehrlichiosis (HGE), dengue hemorrhagic fever, bubonic plague, bovine spongiform encephalopathy (BSE), malaria, yellow fever, and tuberculosis.

2. Search the Internet pages of the Centers for Disease Control and Prevention (http://www.cdc.gov/) and two other resources listed in the following resources and learn more about public health programs. Select Web pages from at least three different areas of interest to learn what types of information are provided.

3. Invite an epidemiologist to class to discuss current diseases threatening local populations.

4. Go to the National Library of Medicine or other reputable source for historical information related to the use of prevention and management of diseases in the United States.

5. Read the book *The Tipping Point* and discuss how diseases and ideas spread.

6. Find the *Morbidity and Mortality Week Report* Web site and locate information about a particular disease that is monitored by vital statistics and governmental agencies.

7. Compose a list of diseases transmitted by contaminated food and water that one might encounter and how they can be prevented.

8. Discuss reasons why military and health care personnel refused mandatory smallpox vaccinations by federal bioterrorism training programs.

9. Research the efficacy of vaccinations by selecting a specific disease and follow past national immunization programs.

10. Learn your personal immunization history and your compliance with health recommendations.

SELECTED ENVIRONMENTAL LAWS

1984 Health Promotion and Disease Prevention Amendments (P 98-551)
Amended the Public Health Service Act to extend provisions related to health promotion and disease prevention and establish research and demonstration centers.

2002 Public Health Security and Bioterrorism Response Act (PL 107-188)
Addressed the need to combat threats to public health, providing funds to every state to assess needs, develop a health alert network (HAN), and to prepare for emergencies.

SELECTED PROFESSIONAL JOURNALS

American Journal of Epidemiology
American Journal of Infection Control
American Journal of Preventive Medicine
American Journal of Public Health
American Journal of Tropical Medicine and Hygiene
Applied and Environmental Microbiology
Emerging Infectious Diseases
Environmental Health Perspectives
Epidemiology
Infection Control and Hospital Epidemiology
Journal of Community Health
Journal of Community Health Nursing
Journal of Environmental Medicine
Journal of Epidemiology and Community Health
Journal of Genetic Counseling
Journal of Hospital Infection
Journal of Immigrant Health

Journal of Infectious Disease
Journal of Parasitology
Journal of Public Health Medicine
Morbidity and Mortality Weekly Report
Occupational and Environmental Medicine
Vector-Borne and Zoonotic Diseases
Weekly Epidemiological Record
World Health Report

ADDITIONAL READING

Cipolla, C. (1992). *Miasmas and Disease: Public Health and the Environment in the Pre-Industrial Age.* New Haven, CT: Yale University Press.

Gladwell, M. (2002). *The Tipping Point: How Little Things Can Make a Big Difference.* New York: Little, Brown and Company.

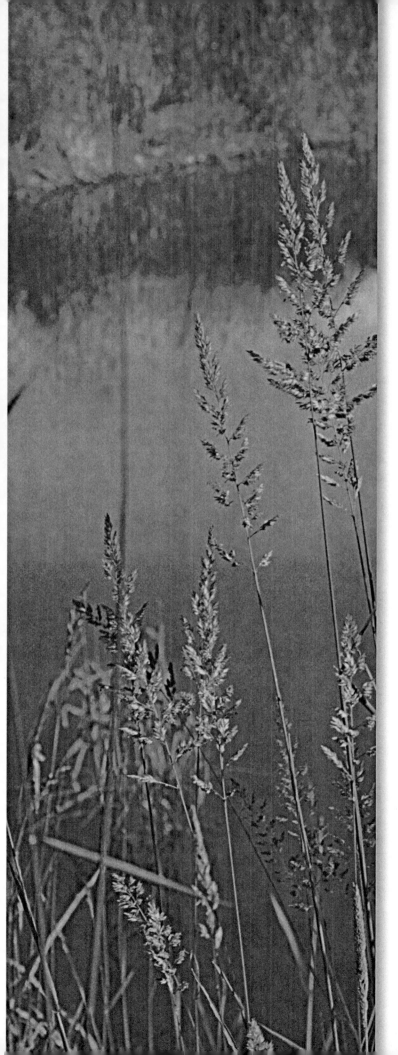

Environmental Toxins and Toxicology

5

We've got to start looking at exposure from conception to birth.

Theo Colborn (1927–)

The dose makes the poison.

Paracelsus (1493–1541)

OBJECTIVES

1. Define the terms ambient, teratogen, toxic, hazardous, poisonous, contamination, and corrosive.

2. Explain what toxicologists do.

3. Define what is meant by the term MRL and how it is derived.

4. List the 10 most hazardous materials in the environment.

5. Give examples of heavy metals.

6. List the harmful effects of asbestos, acetone, benzene, carbon disulfide, cyanide, dioxin, formaldehyde, styrene, vinyl acetate, and vinyl chloride and where they can be found.

7. Give examples of organophosphates and PCBs.

8. Describe why DDT is no longer recommended for use as a pesticide today.

9. Explain what is meant by the term endocrine disrupter and give an example.

10. Describe how toxicologists and government officials determine the "risk" associated with environmental toxins.

Introduction

Environmental health hazards consist of natural and human hazards, including biological (Chapter 4), chemical, and physical hazards. Chemical hazards include **toxic** substances found in gas, liquid, and solid form, often referred to as **pollutants**, and are discussed in this chapter. Physical hazards include conditions likely to cause harm such as radiation (Chapter 12), unhealthy food (Chapter 13), poor sanitation practices (Chapter 14), unfavorable housing conditions (Chapter 15), and machinery, traffic, and noise (Chapter 17). Health hazards can be found everywhere from the home, school, or work environment; public buildings; dump sites; and in recreational areas. When health risks due to infectious diseases are reduced, exposure to **hazardous** chemicals becomes even more important.

Contamination of the air, water, or soil with toxins can frequently lead to serious health problems. A **toxin** is a substance that **poisons** or harms a living organism. Toxins can cause immediate harm or may accumulate in the tissues after long-term exposure. Irritation to the eyes and respiratory system, cancer, endocrine disruption, birth defects, methemoglobinemia, suppressed immune systems, and mutations are just some of the effects documented to date.

The most controversial topic regarding environmental hazards is the association with cancer. There is some evidence that exposure to some environmental toxins may be associated with some types of cancer. Known environmental **carcinogens** include arsenic, nickel, asbestos,

---

Toxic
A chemical, poison, or something contaminated by a poisonous or harmful substance that provokes an adverse systemic effect on living organisms.

Pollutants
Harmful chemicals or waste material discharged into land, water, or the atmosphere.

Hazardous
The capacity to do harm; risky, danger; a substance is one that an organism is likely to come into contact with and has the capacity to do harm to the organism.

Toxin
A poisonous compound produced by pathogens or chemicals that cause illness.

Poison
An agent that kills, injures, or impairs a living thing; very small doses are needed.

Carcinogen
Substances with cancer-causing properties.

According to Paracelsus (1593–1541), a Swiss physician, alchemist, the "father of modern toxicology:" *"All substances are poisons; there is none which is not a poison. The right dose differentiates a poison and a remedy."* Paracelsus determined that specific chemicals were responsible for the toxicity of a poison. He documented the body's response to chemicals according to the dose, revealing that small doses could be harmless or beneficial, while larger doses could be toxic. This is now known as the *dose-response relationship*.

A Spanish physician, Orfila, is often referred to as the founder of toxicology. Orfila was the first to prepare a systematic correlation between the chemical and biological properties of poisons of his time. He demonstrated effects of poisons on specific organs by autopsying tissues for damage.

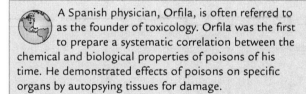

Digging Deeper | 2010 HEALTHY PEOPLE OBJECTIVES

8-11 Eliminate elevated blood lead levels in children.

8-14 Reduce the amount of toxic pollutants released, disposed of, treated, or used for energy recovery.

8-25 Reduce exposure of the population to pesticides, heavy metals, and other toxic chemicals, as measured by blood and urine concentrations of the substances or their metabolites (Heavy metals = arsenic, cadmium, lead, manganese, mercury), (Pesticides = 2, 4,-D, o-phenylphenol, permethrins, diazinon), (Persistent chemicals = polychlorinated biphenyls, dioxins, furans), (Organochlorine compounds = chlordane, dieldrin, DDT, lindane).

8-26 Improve quality, utility, awareness, and use of existing information systems for environmental health.

8-27 Increase or maintain the number of territories, tribes, and states and the District of Columbia that monitor diseases or conditions that can be caused by exposure to environmental hazards (lead poisoning, pesticide poisoning, mercury poisoning, arsenic poisoning, cadmium poisoning, methemoglobinemia, acute chemical poisoning, carbon monoxide poisoning, hyperthermia, hypothermia, skin cancer, malignant melanoma, other skin cancer, birth defects).

ultraviolet radiation, methylene chloride, and some viruses (e.g., *hepatitis* B, *human papilloma,* and *Epstein-Barr*). Studies by the Department of Veterans Affairs (1999) revealed an association with DDT and various types of cancer including soft-tissue sarcomas, non-Hodgkin's lymphoma, Hodgkin's disease, chloracne, respiratory cancers, prostate cancer, and multiple myeloma. Higher levels of PCB and DDE have also been found in the tissue of women with breast cancer.

Another controversy is the potential harm from **endocrine disrupters.** Endocrine disrupters may disrupt a biological process by binding to hormone receptors, thereby blocking the function of the natural hormone when it is needed. On the other hand, an endocrine disrupter might activate a biological process when it should otherwise be dormant. Blocking normal hormone function when it is needed, or turning on a process when it is not necessary, can have profound effects on the development and maintenance of organisms. Indeed a substantial body of research has linked endocrine disrupters to human cancer and developmental anomalies in wildlife. Examples of endocrine disrupters are some **pesticides**, PCBs, nonphenyls, components of epoxsies (bisphenol A), and plasticizers such as the phthalates. **Heavy metals** such as arsenic are also suspected of endocrine disrupting activity.

A **teratogen** produces malformation or defective development in a fetus. Although not toxic to adults, some substances can have teratogenic effects on the unborn. Examples include alcohol, rubella or fifth disease, X-rays, and chemical wastes such as lead, methyl mercury, PCBs, dioxin, and other pollutants. Only 23% of chemicals are tested for teratogenic effects. No safe levels are known for the pregnant mother and her developing fetus. Toxic effects of alcohol include Fetal Alcohol Syndrome (FAS), a permanent congenital disorder.

Toxicology

oxicology is a science that determines harmful effects of toxic agents (substances or chemicals). A **toxic agent** is anything chemical, physical, or biological that can produce an adverse biological effect. **Toxicity** is primarily determined in three ways:

1. Observing people during normal use of a substance or from accidental exposure

2. Experimental studies using animals

3. Cellular studies

Definitions of Toxic Substances

t is important to know the difference between hazardous materials, toxins, and poisons. A toxic substance is one that can damage or disrupt living tissue. Toxicity is often indicated by the terms *hazardous* and *poisonous*.

1. Hazardous. For a substance to be hazardous, it depends on its inherent ability to do harm and on the likeliness of that substance coming into contact with humans. A hazardous chemical would be one that is potentially dangerous in either large or small amounts. Hazardous substances must be labeled. Some of the labels include statements such as:
   "May be fatal if swallowed."
   "Harmful if swallowed."
   "Causes severe burns."
   "Extremely flammable liquid and vapor; vapor may cause fire."
   "Flammable solid."
   "Strong oxidizer. Contact with other materials may cause fire."

2. Poison. This term refers to a chemical that can cause illness or death at a very low dose of exposure. A highly toxic substance can be lethal and is usually called a poison. A very small amount of a poison (about ¾ teaspoon for an adult and ⅛ teaspoon for a toddler) will cause illness, injury, or death. The effects are immediate and acute. A poisonous chemical is one

Digging Deeper	THE TOP 20 ENVIRONMENTAL HAZARDOUS MATERIALS

1. Arsenic	8. Polycyclic aromatic hydrocarbons (PAHs)	14. Arochlor 1260
2. Lead	9. Benzo(a)pyrene	15. Cibenozo(a,h)anthracene
3. Mercury	10. Benzo(b)fluoranthene	16. Trichloroethylene
4. Vinyl chloride	11. Chloroform	17. Chromium, hexavalent
5. Polychlorinated biphenyls (PCBs)	12. DDT, P,P'	18. Dieldrin
6. Benzene	13. Arochlor 1254	19. Phosphorus, white
7. Cadmium		20. Chlordane
		Source: CERCLA, 2003.

that causes severe illness, disability, or death with a small dose. In addition to the dose, the manner in which the hazardous substance enters the body is important. Poisons can enter the body through the skin, respiratory system, or the gastrointestinal system. The faster the poison is absorbed, the more dangerous the poison. For example, an inhaled poison takes approximately 7 seconds to reach the brain. When the poison is ingested, it may take 15 minutes to 2 hours, depending upon the contents of the stomach. A poison can be absorbed through the skin through injection (as in a bee sting) or through a crack in the skin surface. When the poison is injected, it is absorbed faster than if it passes over several layers of skin. The time by which the toxic reaction occurs is related to the sensitivity of the individual. Poisons are absorbed more readily by infants, the elderly, and those who have an immune deficiency.

Acute toxicity occurs when one is exposed to a large amount of the substance in a short period of time, resulting in severe effects. It may result with a single exposure. Chronic toxicity occurs when one is exposed to low concentrations of a substance over a long period of time. **Bioaccumulation** occurs when a person is exposed to a

Endocrine disrupters
Chemical substances that mimic the effects of the hormone estrogen; sometimes called environmental estrogens.

Inorganic pesticides
Chemicals used to prevent or destroy pest infestations that contaminate the environment and are passed from animal to animal through the food chain.

Heavy metals
Natural elements such as lead, mercury, cadmium, and nickel.

Teratogen
An agent (pathogen or chemical) that causes malformation of a fetus.

Toxicology
The science of poisons; the study of the adverse effects of chemicals or physical agents on living organisms.

Toxic agent (toxic substance)
A substance (pathogen or chemical) that causes harm from exposure.

Toxicity
The degree of danger posed by a toxic or poisonous substance to animal or plant life; harmful effects of a chemical on a target organ.

Acute toxicity
A sudden and serious illness developed from exposure to a toxic substance.

Bioaccumulation
The accumulation of toxic substances in living tissue over time.

 HOW MUCH IS HARMFUL?
If you are exposed to hazardous chemicals, several factors will determine whether harmful health effects will occur and what the type and severity of those health effects will be. These factors include:

- The dose (how much)
- The duration (how long)
- The route or pathway by which you are exposed (breathing, eating, drinking, or skin contact)
- The other chemicals to which you are exposed
- Characteristics such as age and susceptibility (via gender, nutritional status, family traits, lifestyle, immune system, and state of health)

Consider the Cost · TO DETOXIFY OR NOT TO DETOXIFY, THAT IS THE QUESTION . . .

Detoxification is known as a process of reducing or eliminating toxic impurities in the body. The rationale is that the incidence and prevalence of cancer, multiple chemical sensitivity, attention deficit hyperactivity disorder (ADHD), chronic fatigue immune deficiency syndrome (CFIDS), autoimmune diseases (rheumatoid arthritis, fibromyalgia, multiple sclerosis) are increasing, possibly due to environmental toxins. We are involuntarily exposed to food additives, pesticides, heavy metals, and air pollutants. In addition to these, we voluntarily pollute our own bodies with carbonated beverages (phosphoric acid), caffeine, alcohol, tobacco, refined and processed foods, hormones (steroids and estrogens), and other drugs. The result is decreased energy, joint pain, headaches, dental caries, increased anxiety and irritability, respiratory problems, gastrointestinal problems, and a depressed immune system.

Common detoxification methods include breathing exercises, specific diets, herbs, supplements, sauna, and massage. Advocates of detoxification also ascribe to "cleansings" that include strict dietary restriction and enemas. This procedure can be quite harsh and can wipe out important bacteria in the gastrointestinal system. A more prudent approach would be to limit exposure to toxins, eat a healthy diet with whole grains, eliminate the use of stimulants (sodas, coffee, tea, and tobacco), and practice relaxation strategies daily.

substance over a period of time, accumulating higher levels of the substance in the body. **Biomagnification** occurs when organisms low on the food chain are consumed by organisms higher on the food chain, increasing levels of the toxic agent in the predator as a result of concentration in the prey. **Subchronic toxicity** is the ability of the substance to cause effects for more than 1 year but less than the lifetime of the exposed organism.

Environmental Toxins

Toxic substances occur naturally and are also by-products of industry, transportation, and other human activities (Table 5-1). The most common toxins include heavy metals (lead, cadmium, aluminum, mercury, and manganese), chlorine, organic chemicals (pesticides and herbicides), and radiation. Toxic metals include cadmium, chromium, copper, lead, manganese, mercury, nickel, and arsenic. When referring to toxic metals, it must be understood that these metals cause damage, primarily because they are stored in fat and bone tissues of the body for extended periods of time. They can persist in the environment for years.

TABLE 5-1 Natural vs. Toxic Substances

Naturally Occurring Toxic Substances	Manufactured Toxic Chemicals
Cadmium	Acetone
Chromium	Benzene
Copper	Carbon disulfide
Lead	Chlorinated hydrocarbons Organochlorines
Manganese	Cyanide
Mercury	Dieldrin
Radon	DDT
Silver	Dioxins
	Formaldehyde
	Methyl chloride
	Nitrites
	PCBs
	Pentachlorophenol
	PBBs and PBDES
	Polycyclic aromatic hydrocarbons
	Phthalates
	Sodium hypochlorite
	Styrene
	Vinyl acetate
	Vinyl chloride

Harmful chemical toxins include DDT, dioxin, polychlorinated biphenyls (PCBs), furans, and some plastics. Of the thousands of chemicals produced in the United States, many have not been tested for their harmful effects. It is important to know where a toxic substance comes from and when it was first released to the environment. The movement of a toxic substance through the environment is influenced by its chemical properties. Major forces that influence movement and accumulation of toxic agents in ecosystems are important. Wind, rain, and leaching through soils are all possible means of contamination.

Natural Elements

ARSENIC

Arsenic occurs naturally in soils, rocks, water, air, plants, and animals. Arsenic in its purest form is a gray, brittle, crystalline, semimetallic solid. As much as 100,000 tons of arsenic is produced worldwide, mostly as a by-product of smelting copper, lead, cobalt, and gold ores (Calvert, 2004). Approximately 90% of all arsenic in the United States is used for preserving wood. Smaller quantities are used to produce insecticides, herbicides, algaecides, growth stimulants for plants and animals, the production of glass and nonferrous alloys, and in electronic semiconductors. Pure arsenic is used to make light-emitting diodes (LEDs), solar cells, infrared devices, and lasers.

Adverse health effects from arsenic include skin, bladder, and lung cancer. Most arsenic exposure in the United States comes from drinking water (Natural Resources Defense Council, 2001). Drinking water can be contaminated from naturally occurring arsenic, resulting from iron oxides. Other sources of arsenic include geothermal waters and sulfide minerals. Geothermal springs in Yellowstone National Park often have arsenic concentrations exceeding 1,000 **ppb** (Welch et al., 2000). The Environmental Protection Agency (EPA) has established a maximum contaminant level (MCL) for arsenic in drinking water of 10 ppb. Arsenic concentrations exceeding 10 ppb have been found in the western United States, the Great Plains, and New England areas.

CADMIUM

Cadmium is a natural element in the Earth's crust found in all soils and rocks. It is extracted from the Earth like zinc, lead, and copper. It does not corrode easily and has many uses; it is used in batteries, paint pigments, metal coatings, and plastics. Cadmium stays in the body an extremely long time and can build up from many years of exposure. Breathing high levels of cadmium in the workplace severely damages the lungs and can cause death.

Long-term exposure to lower levels of cadmium in air, food, or water leads to a buildup of cadmium in the kidneys and possible kidney disease. Many substances like cadmium accumulate in the body (liver and fat stores) over time. Other effects are long-term lung damage and fragile bones (Bellinger et al., 2004). Cadmium and cadmium compounds may be carcinogenic. Exposure to cadmium is most likely in the workplace where cadmium products are made.

CHROMIUM

Chromium is a naturally occurring element found in rocks, animals, plants, soil, and in volcanic dust and gases. It is present in the environment in several different forms, the most common of which are chromium, chromium III, and chromium VI. Chromium is used for making steel. Chromium III and VI are used for chrome plating, dyes/pigments, leather tanning, and wood preserving. Chromium III occurs naturally in the environment and is an essential nutrient. Chromium VI is produced by industrial processes. The toxicity of chromium compounds depends on the oxidation state of the metal (Agency for Toxic Substances and Disease Registry [ATSDR], 2000; Pesticide Action Network [PAN], 2004). Chromium is considered to be hazardous if inhaled, with a possible link to lung cancer.

The EPA has set a limit of 100 μg chromium (III) and chromium (VI) per liter of drinking water (100 μg/L). The Occupational Safety and Health Administration (OSHA) has set limits of 500 μg water soluble chromium (III) compounds per cubic meter of workplace air (500 μg/m³), 1,000 μg/m³ for metallic chromium (0) and insoluble chromium compounds, and 52 μg/m³ for chromium (VI) compounds for 8-hour work shifts and 40-hour work weeks.

COPPER

Copper occurs naturally in rocks, soil, water, air, plants, and animals. Copper compounds are commonly used in agriculture to treat plant diseases such as mildew, for water treatment, and as preservatives for wood, leather, and fabrics. Older homes may have copper plumbing. The copper is carried in the water and can be ingested. Copper cups and plates should not be used, particularly if the drinks or foods are acidic. The U.S. **maximum contaminant level goal (MCLG)** for copper in water is 1.3 mg/L (Copper Development Association, 2005). Acute copper poisoning is rare, usually from accidental spills of copper nitrate or copper sulfate. Symptoms include nausea, vomiting, abdominal pain, and jaundice. Normally the effects of copper poisoning are short lived, as the victim usually vomits or the liver excretes it.

LEAD

Lead is found in small amounts in the earth's crust but can be found in many areas due to the burning of fossil fuels, mining, and manufacturing. Lead has been mined in the United States since 1621 for bullets, pipes, and paint (Lewis, 1985). Lead was also added to gasoline to reduce the "knocking" sound and increase power and efficiency in car engines. It is used in the production of batteries (Figure 5-1), ammunition, metal products (solder and pipes), paint, plumbing, and devices to shield X-rays. Lead is also used in brass coverings, television tubes, cosmetics, crayons, pottery, and cables. Lead poisoning is a continuing problem in the United States. It is highly toxic, causing harm to the brain, kidneys, bone marrow, and central nervous system. It can be inhaled or ingested. It can move through the body and expelled, but some is deposited into the bones where it can stay for many years. Lead accumulates in the body so that high levels can develop.

Lead-based paint remains the most common high-dose source of lead exposure for preschool children (CDC, 2004). The EPA has estimated that up to 20% of a child's lead exposure can potentially be attributed to lead-contaminated water. The most likely source of

> At the conclusion of World War II, residents along the Jinzu River Basin near Toyama, Japan displayed symptoms of pain, kidney damage, and loss of bone strength. By 1968 the cause was determined to be from chronic cadmium poisoning, traced to effluent from the Mitsui Mining and Smelting Company. The cadmium poisoning was from discharges from the Kamiska Mine into river water used to irrigate rice fields. By 1991, 129 people were diagnosed with the condition and 116 of them died (Nogawa et al., 2004).

Biomagnification
Otherwise known as biological magnification; the tendency of toxic agents to become concentrated in organisms higher on the food chain by consuming animals lower on the food chain.

Subchronic toxicity
A type of illness occurring with less intensity and for less duration than chronic toxicity.

Ppb
Parts per billion.

Maximum contaminant level goal (MCLG)
A goal set for contaminants in drinking water that may post a threat to public health. The goal is set at a level below which there is no known or expected health risk, allowing for a margin of safety.

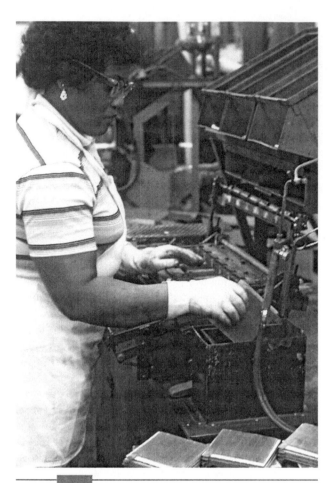

FIGURE 5-1 **Lead Exposure in Battery Factory** One of the many cases that have created the need for occupational health and safety practices.

lead in drinking water is from corroded pipes in older homes. Most health professionals are aware of the threat of lead (Pb) toxicity, particularly its long-term impact on children in the form of cognitive and developmental deficits, which are often cumulative and subtle. The effects of lead poisoning continue into adulthood. Lead toxicity may alternatively be present as acute illness. Signs and symptoms in children may include irritability, abdominal pain, emesis, marked ataxia, and seizures or loss of consciousness. In adults, diffuse complaints—including headache, nausea, anorexia (and weight loss), constipation, fatigue, personality changes, and hearing loss—coupled with exposure opportunity may lead to suspicion of lead poisoning. Lead inhibits heme synthesis. The standard screening method is investigation of blood lead (PbB) levels that reveal recent exposure to lead. If sufficiently high PbB levels are confirmed, chelation therapy may be indicated. Suspected low-level lead contamination cannot be accurately identified by an erythrocyte protoporphyrin (EP) finger-stick test, but requires blood lead analysis.

Lead poisoning via ingestion has been most widely publicized, stressing hazards from nibbling of flaking paint by infants and toddlers and by the use of lead-containing food ware (glass and soldered metal-ceramic ware) by adults. Lead levels in paints for interior use have been increasingly restricted since the 1950s, and many paints are now virtually lead-free. However, older housing and furniture may still be coated with leaded paint, sometimes surfacing only after layers of later, non-lead paint have flaked away or have been stripped away in the course of restoration or renovation. In these circumstances, lead dust and fumes can permeate the air breathed by both adults and children. Additional sources of airborne lead include art and craft materials, from which lead is not banned. However, the U.S. Consumer Product Safety Commission (CPSC) requires its presence to be declared on the product label if it is present in toxic amounts. Significant quantities are found in many paints and glazes and stained glass, as well as in some solder.

Airborne lead, however, is also a worrisome source of toxicity. Lead dust flaking or "chalking" off of lead-painted walls is a major concern indoors. Airborne lead outdoors, originating chiefly from gasoline additives, has been effectively controlled since the 1980s through regulation at the federal level. Between 1976 and 1980, blood levels of lead declined over 30% due to the phase out of leaded gasoline and paint (Annest et al., 1983). Lead is still found in enormous levels in the environment due to illegal dumping and residues left in soil, water, old dishes, and the air. Much of this lead remains in the soil near heavily trafficked highways and in urban areas and can become airborne at times. It may enter dwellings via windows and doors, and contaminated soil can also be tracked inside. Hazardous levels of atmospheric lead have been found at police and civilian firing ranges. Repair and cleaning of automobile radiators in inadequately ventilated premises can expose workers to perilous levels of airborne lead. The use of treated or painted wood in fireplaces or improperly vented wood-burning stoves may release a variety of substances, including lead and other heavy metals, into the air.

MANGANESE

Manganese is a naturally occurring trace element found in many types of rocks. Exposure can occur from breathing air where manganese is used in manufacturing or from drinking water and food contaminated with manganese. Iron, steel, and power plants and mining operations can emit manganese. It can enter the water and soil from natural deposits and it exists naturally in rivers, lakes, and underground water. Manganese exposure is relatively common in welders who work in confined spaces because it is a component of all steel and welding materials. A recent study found 40% of welders showed signs of the disorder. Symptoms of manganese poisoning include tremors, loss of balance, delayed movements, walking problems, slurred speech, impotency, extreme drowsiness, and nighttime leg cramps (Electronic Library of Construction Occupational Safety and Health [ELCOSH], 2003). At high levels, manganese can cause damage to the brain, liver, kidneys, and the developing fetus. There is no human cancer data available for manganese.

MERCURY

Mercury occurs naturally in the environment and exists in several forms. There are two types of mercury: inorganic and organic. Inorganic mercury is metallic and is harmful when inhaled, but not swallowed. It is a shiny, silver-white, slightly volatile metal liquid at room temperature and is used in thermometers and sphygmomanometers. At room temperature, some of the metallic mercury will evaporate and form mercury vapors. Metallic mercury has been found at 714 hazardous waste sites nationwide (ATSDR, 1999). It is used in the production of chlorine gas, fungicides, and metal extraction. It is also used for electroplating, making paper, making plastics, in fluorescent light bulbs, and in medicines. Mercury binds with proteins and once it enters the body, it is distributed to many organs, doing the most damage to the brain and kidneys. Symptoms of mercury poisoning include headache, rapid heart beat, intermittent fever, and muscle cramps or tremors. Young children exposed to mercury can develop "pink disease," characterized by a rash, itching, excess sweating, hypotonia, and photophobia. In the United States, mercury exposures were reported from latex paint. It has been banned since 1990 (Agocs et al., 1990).

Organic mercury is discharged into waterways by industries and found in fish or shellfish (these should be eaten in moderation). In 1950, those in the fishing industry and other citizens in Minamata City, Japan, were exposed to mercury discharged from a chemical plant into waters where seafood was caught for food (Ellis, 1989). Other exposures to mercury were reported when seed grain treated with fungicide preparations of methyl mercury were consumed in Iraq, Guatemala, Ghana, and Pakistan (Elhassani, 1983).

NICKEL

Pure nickel is a hard, silvery-white metal with properties desirable for making alloys. Nickel compounds dissolve easily in water and have a green color (ATSDR, 2003). There is no characteristic odor or taste. It can be mixed with iron, copper, chromium, and zinc to make metal coins, jewelry, valves, and heat exchangers. Most nickel is used to make stainless steel. It is also used for nickel plating, to color ceramics, and to make batteries. It is found in all soil and is emitted from volcanoes. It is also found in meteorites and is released into the atmosphere during nickel mining and industries. Nickel can be discharged in industrial waste water by oil-burning power plants, coal-burning power plants, and trash incinerators. Most of the U.S. nickel is from Russia, Canada, and Japan. There was one mine in Riddle, Oregon but it closed in 1998 (Naro, 2001).

Nickel particles can leave the lungs with mucus and can get into the bloodstream and travel to all the organs, especially the kidneys. The most common adverse health effect of nickel is an allergic reaction by sensitive individuals. Wearing nickel earrings may sensitize people and once sensitized, further contact with the metal will produce a reaction. Eczema and asthma attacks can be attributed to nickel. The most serious effects of nickel, cancer of the lung and nasal sinus, have occurred in people who have breathed nickel dust from refineries or processing plants.

RADON

Radon is a naturally occurring, odorless, and colorless gas produced when uranium in soil, rock, and water breaks down. The gas can enter buildings through cracks in the foundation and other openings. The radon decays into

---

DOES YOUR HOUSE HAVE MERCURY-BASED PAINT?

A report detailed elevated levels of mercury in persons exposed to interior latex (water-based) paint containing phenyl mercuric acetate (PMA) (Agocs et al., 1990). PMA was a biocide that was used to kill bacteria and fungus. Initial action by the U.S. Environmental Protection Agency resulted in the elimination of mercury compounds from indoor latex paints at the point of manufacture as of August 1990, with the requirement that paints containing mercury, including existing stocks originally designed for indoor use, be labeled or relabeled "For Exterior Use Only." As of September 1991, phenyl mercuric acetate is forbidden in the manufacture of exterior latex paints as well. Latex paints containing hazardous levels of mercury may still remain on store shelves or in homes where they were left over after initial use, however.

In 1908, a fertilizer plant was established near Minamata, a coastal town in Japan with 12,000 people. The plant eventually became one of Japan's largest manufacturers of chemicals. By the 1920s, damage to fisheries were noted. By 1956, patients with a severe neurological disease were observed. It was not until 1968 that the disease was associated with ingestion of seafood containing high concentrations of methylmercury, a by-product of acetaldehyde discharged into Minamata Bay near Shiranui Sea. By 1991, 2,248 people were identified with Minamata disease and received compensation from the Chisso Corporation. Unfortunately 1,004 died.

radioactive solids that attach to dust particles in the air and can be inhaled. The inhalation of radon particles has been linked to lung cancer (National Institute of Environmental Health Sciences [NIEHS], 2004). Unfortunately there are no early symptoms of radon poisoning.

Radon gas can be found in drinking water, although the **risk** of that is extremely small. Surface waters such as rivers, lakes, or reservoirs usually do not carry radon because it evaporates before it reaches municipal water supplies. There is no federally enforced drinking water standard for radon, but maximum contaminate levels have been recommended. Homeowners whose water supply is from a private well could reduce radon content in their drinking water by installing a carbon filter or device that bubbles air through the water and is diverted through an exhaust fan.

SILVER

Silver is an element found naturally in the environment with other elements such as sulfide, chloride, and nitrate. It is often found as a by-product during the retrieval of copper, lead, zinc, and gold ores. It is used to make jewelry, flatware, electronic equipment, and dental fillings. It is also used to make photographs, in alloys and solders, to disinfect drinking water and water in swimming pools, and as an antibacterial agent. It has been used in lozenges and chewing gum to help people stop smoking. At very high levels, it may cause argyria, a blue-gray discoloration of the skin and other organs. Lower-level exposures may cause silver to be deposited in the skin and other parts of the body; however this is not known to be harmful. Skin contact with silver can cause mild allergic reactions such as rash, swelling, and inflammation in some people.

Manufactured (Chemical) Substances

oxic agents are found in chemicals, which are all toxic to some degree. What once amounted to a few chemicals listed as harmful has become an extremely long list. In 1976, the United Nations Environment Program (UNEP) established the International Registry of Potentially Toxic Chemicals (see http://irptc.unep.ch/irptc/databank.html) listing hundreds of chemicals and how to handle them. Chemicals are continually being evaluated regarding toxic effects, but the number of chemicals produced each year exceeds the ability to measure all the short- and long-term effects they might have. The risk to chemicals is determined by the toxicity of the substance and exposure to it.

Chemicals may be distinguished by their chemical structure. Organic chemicals have a carbon structure de-

rived from living organisms. **Inorganic** chemicals contain few carbon atoms and are derived from mineral sources having a consistent and distinctive set of physical properties. Inorganic chemicals include halogens, **corrosives**, metals, and many other substances. Halogens include fluorine, chlorine, bromine, and iodine in either gas or liquid form. Corrosive materials consist of alkaline compounds such as ammonia, calcium hydroxide (caustic soda), calcium oxide (lime), potassium hydroxide (caustic potash), sodium carbonate (soda ash), sodium hydroxide (lye), and acid materials such as sulfuric acid and chromic acid. Air pollutants such as ozone and nitrogen oxides are also corrosive. Corrosive substances irritate sensitive tissues such as skin, eyes, respiratory tract, and digestive tract. Inorganic compounds are extremely stable and tend to persist over time. They are sometimes referred to as **persistent organic pollutants (POPs)**.

ACETONE

Acetone (dimethyl formaldehyde) is a manufactured chemical found naturally in the environment. It is a colorless liquid with a distinct smell and taste and is used to make plastic, fibers, drugs, and other chemicals. It is also used as a solvent in paints, inks, adhesives, degreasers, and varnishes. It occurs naturally in plants, trees, volcanic gases, and forest fires. It can be found in second-hand tobacco smoke, vehicle exhaust, and landfill sites. A large percentage of acetone is released during its manufacture in the air. It doesn't bind to soil but rather can move into groundwater from spills or landfills. Exposure is mostly from breathing air, drinking water, or coming in contact with products or soil that contain acetone. Exposure to moderate-to-high amounts can irritate the eyes and respiratory system. Very high exposure may cause unconsciousness. Acetone can be measured in the breath, blood, and urine.

BENZENE

Benzene is a colorless liquid with a sweet odor. It evaporates quickly into the air and dissolves slightly in water. It is highly flammable and is formed from both natural processes and human activities. Benzene is widely used in the United States; it ranks in the top 20 chemicals for production volume (ATSDR, 1997). Some industries use benzene to make other chemicals that are used to make plastics, resins, and nylon and synthetic fibers. Benzene is also used to make some types of rubbers, lubricants, dyes, detergents, drugs, and pesticides. Natural sources of benzene include volcanoes and forest fires. Benzene is also a natural part of crude oil, gasoline, and cigarette smoke. Breathing extremely high levels of benzene can result in death, while high levels can cause drowsiness, dizziness, rapid heart rate, headaches, tremors, confusion, and unconsciousness. Eating or drinking foods containing high levels of benzene can cause vomiting, irritation of the

HOW TO SELECT THE LEAST TOXIC SUBSTANCE

The front label of potentially harmful products must include a "signal word" warning and description of the hazard. *Caution* indicates the lowest level of toxicity, meaning that 1 pint of the product would be considered poisonous if it were swallowed. *Warning* means that 1 teaspoon or more of the product would be considered poisonous. The word *Danger* indicates the highest level of toxicity because less than 1 teaspoon would be poisonous if consumed. *Poison* might be another word on a label. Labels should also have a list of ingredients and an EPA registration number.

- Read the labels of cleaners and buy the least harmful product. The word *nontoxic* has no governmental definition and can be used as the manufacturer wants to market the product. It does not mean it is not hazardous.

- Check the label for a list of ingredients and instructions for safe use. If there is no list of ingredients or instructions on safe use, then it is best to buy another product.

- If you must purchase solvents, corrosives, poisons, or other toxic substances, buy only what you need and use it up in a short period of time.

STORING HAZARDOUS PRODUCTS IN THE HOME

There is always a danger when hazardous products are stored and used by more than one person.

- Always store chemicals in locked cabinets and in areas where children cannot get to them.

- The storage area should also be in a place where temperatures remain constant or at normal room temperature. Make sure containers will be kept dry to prevent rusting.

- Store volatile products (with vapors and fumes) in well-ventilated areas such as a storage shed.

- Make sure the lids and caps are tightly sealed.

- Put cleaning rags in sealed, marked containers when disposing or keeping them for reuse.

- Do not put hazardous materials in unmarked containers so an unsuspecting person would not know what they are using.

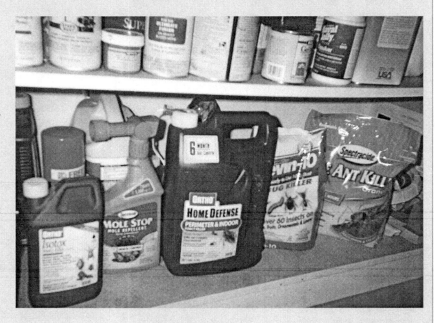

stomach, dizziness, sleepiness, convulsions, rapid heart rate, and death. It is a common source of methemoglobinemia.

The major effect of benzene from long-term (1 year or longer) exposure is on the blood. Benzene causes harmful effects on the bone marrow and can cause a decrease in red blood cells, leading to anemia. It can also cause excessive bleeding and can affect the immune system, increasing the chance for infection. Some women who breathed high levels of benzene for many months had irregular menstrual periods and a decrease in the size of their ovaries. It is not known whether benzene exposure affects the developing fetus in pregnant women or fertility in men. The U.S. Department of Health and Human Services (2002) has determined that benzene is a known human carcinogen. Long-term exposure to high levels of benzene in the air can cause leukemia, cancer of the blood-forming organs.

Risk
Vulnerability; likelihood that an event will occur with an unfavorable outcome.

Inorganic
A type of matter that is not animal or vegetable or from a living thing; a substance that does not contain carbon and may be found from mineral sources.

Corrosives
Substances that gnaw, eat, wear away, or cause another substance to deteriorate.

Persistent organic pollutants (POPs)
A set of toxic chemicals that persist in the environment for a long period of time and biomagnify as they move up the food chain; they have been linked to cancer, damage to the nervous system, reproductive disorders, and disruption of the immune system in humans and animals.

CARBON DISULFIDE

Carbon disulfide is a colorless liquid with a pleasant, sweet odor. It evaporates at room temperature and easily explodes or catches fire. It is used to make things such as rayon, cellophane, and carbon tetrachloride. It is also used to dissolve rubber to make tires and pesticides. Most carbon disulfide in the air and surface water is from manufacturing and processing activities, however, it is found naturally in coastal and ocean waters. It can enter the body by breathing, drinking, or eating substances that contain it. There is no information on the health effects of people who eat or drink it. Skin contact can lead to burns.

CHLORINATED HYDROCARBONS

Chlorinated hydrocarbons contain carbon, hydrogen, and chlorine and are often called **organochlorines.** The use of chlorinated hydrocarbons has harmful effects for humans and wildlife because of disruption of the endocrine system. The endocrine system regulates blood sugar, reproduction, metabolism, and the central nervous system development from birth to death. Endocrine disruptors such as organochlorines can cause genetic, reproductive, and behavioral abnormalities in humans and wildlife. Cancer, birth defects, and nervous system disorders have also been found. Endocrine disrupters can be found in rain, surface water, groundwater, and food. Examples of organochlorines that are endocrine disruptors include dichloro-diphenyl-trichloroethane (DDT) and polychlorinated biphenyls (PCBs). DDT was used as a pesticide. PCBs are fire retardant and used in many products. Endocrine disrupters used as pesticides, herbicides, and industrial-cleaning compounds are banned in the United States today but still remain in the environment and are used in other countries.

CHLORINE

Chlorine was used as a poisonous gas in World War I (Smart, 2004). Used to purify water since the early 1900s, it is the world's most used water disinfectant. It has sup-

Most of the pesticides used in the 1960s have been replaced by other types of pesticides, such as pyrethroids. Dieldrin and chlordane have also been restricted because they persist in the environment. PCBs and DDE have been found in cancerous breast tissues. Some of the newer pesticides are designed to be less persistent in the environment. Natural methods such as crop cover, crop rotation, mechanical tilling, the introduction of pest predators, and other means can be used to control pests. Consumers have indicated a desire for more organically grown foods to avoid pesticide residues found on fresh produce.

pressed typhoid fever, cholera, and dysentery across the world. The EPA recommends that drinking water contain no more than 4 mg of chlorine per liter of water (4 mg/L) (ATSDR, 2002). When chlorine is added to water with organic matter, it produces trihalomethanes, known to cause cancer (Environmental Research Foundation, 1998). Most experts believe that if chlorine were not used, the public health risks would be worse than the effects of the by-products. The use of ozone and ultraviolet radiation are alternatives, but they are either too costly or less effective against viruses, cysts, and worms found in water. They must also be used in combination with chlorine to be used as disinfectants.

CYANIDE

Cyanide is used to make paper, textiles, plastics, and photographs. It is released naturally from some foods and is found in cigarette smoke. It has been used to exterminate pests and vermin. Hydrogen cyanide (Zyklon B) was used by the German Nazis as a genocidal agent in World War II. It may have been used in subsequent wars (CDC, 2004). Cyanide is rapidly absorbed through inhalation and is distributed by the blood throughout the body. Acute inhalation exposure to high levels leads quickly to death preceded by dyspnea, convulsions, and central nervous system depression. In lesser amounts, it can produce peripheral vision loss. It inhibits the use of oxygen by cells.

DIELDRIN AND ALDRIN

Dieldrin and aldrin are insecticides, but aldrin quickly breaks down to dieldrin in the body and in the environment. From the 1950 to 1970s, aldrin and dieldrin were widely used pesticides for crops such as corn and cotton and insects such as termites. Both have been banned by the EPA since 1987. These insecticides bind tightly to the soil and break down slowly so they are still in the environment. Humans can consume either chemical by eating fish or shellfish from contaminated lakes or streams, contaminated root crops, contaminated dairy products or meats, or living in a home that was once treated with aldrin or dieldrin to control termites. There is no evidence that either causes cancer but nervous system disorders have been reported.

DICHLORO-DIPHENYL-TRICHLOROETHANE

These pesticides are used to kill or control insects in agriculture. Pesticide use grew during the 1960s and 1970s. Popular pesticides included DDT and toxaphene. DDT is a white, crystalline solid with no odor or taste and can be found in surface water, groundwater, and rainfall. It was banned in 1974 because of damage to wildlife but is still used in some countries. Although DDT has not been found to cause cancer or birth defects, the effects on wildlife and the central nervous system of humans is a concern. Eggshells of bald eagles and peregrine falcons became fragile, endangering the species because chick embryos could not hatch. Exposure to large amounts of DDT has been linked to several different types of cancer, acute peripheral neuropathy, and spina bifida in children of veterans (Figure 5-2). In the natural environment, human exposure is due to consumption of contaminated foods such as root and leafy vegetables, fatty meat, fish, and poultry. Infants may be exposed to it from breast milk. A major concern with pesticide use is that it stays in the environment for an extended time and accumulates in fatty tissues of humans and animals. Due to bioaccumulation, pesticide exposure moves up the food chain to toxic levels.

DIOXINS

Dioxin is the common name used to refer to the chemical 2,3,7,8-tetrachlorodibenzo-p-dioxin (2,3,7,8-TCDD). Dioxin is one of the most toxic chemicals known. During the Vietnam War, Agent Orange, which contained dioxin, was used as a defoliant. Dioxin is highly toxic to humans and persists in the environment. In September 1994, the EPA described dioxin as a "serious public health threat" (APHA, 1996). Dioxins are carcinogens, highly toxic to many cells of the body and can cause death. Dioxin accu-

mulates in fat cells in the body. It takes approximately 7 years to remove half of the dioxin levels in the body.

Dioxins are chemical **contaminants** formed during combustion processes, such as waste incineration, forest fires, and backyard trash burning and during manufacturing processes such as herbicide manufacture and paper manufacture. The Food and Drug Administration is concerned about the general population exposed to low levels of dioxins as environmental contaminants in coffee filters, milk cartons, and paper plates. It has received a great deal of attention since the Vietnam War when it was used in **Agent Orange**.

In laboratory animals, dioxins are highly toxic, cause cancer, and alter reproductive, developmental, and immune function. The effects of dioxin on humans have been observed in populations that were highly exposed. A well-known health effect in humans is **chloracne**. Studies of chemical workers found a higher incidence of cancer in workers who had chloracne (Bertazzi et al., 2001; Sweeney, 2002).

In addition to dioxin itself there are other compounds, such as the polychlorinated dibenzodioxins (PCDDs), polychlorinated dibenzofurans (PCDFs), and some polychlorinated biphenyls (PCBs), that have similar structures and activity as dioxin.

FORMALDEHYDE

At room temperature, formaldehyde is a colorless, flammable gas. It has a pungent, distinct odor and may cause burning to the eyes, nose, and lungs at high concentrations. It is also known as methanol, methylene oxide, oxymethylene, methylaldehyde, and oxomethane. It can react with other chemicals and will break down into methanol (wood alcohol) and carbon monoxide at very high temperatures. A major source of formaldehyde is smog in the lower atmosphere. Automobile exhaust from cars without catalytic converters emit formaldehyde. However, the most common place to be exposed to

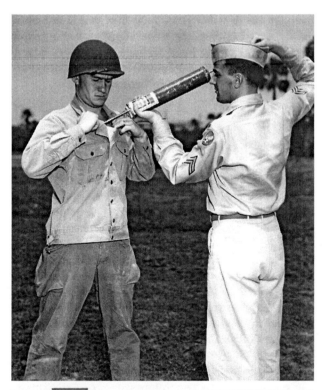

FIGURE 5-2 **DDT Spraying in WWII** Soldiers received instruction on how to protect against pests causing diseases.

Organochlorines
A class of organic chemical compounds containing chlorinated hydrocarbons, such as dioxins, PCBs, CFCs, and DDT.

Contaminant
A compound that pollutes, making the original substance impure or unusable.

Agent Orange
A herbicide and defoliant used during the Vietnam War to which several servicemen were exposed.

Chloracne
A severe skin disease characterized by follicular hyperkeratosis with or without cysts and pustules associated with chronic exposure to high levels of dioxin.

Consider the Cost   DIOXIN IN TAMPONS?

Dioxin is a by-product of the chlorine bleaching process used to whiten paper products such as diapers, sanitary pads, and tampons. About 70% of American women use tampons. It is estimated that a woman may use as many as 11,400 in a lifetime. Manufacturers believe that humans already consume dioxin, so a little more will not hurt. Tampons also include elements such as aluminum, copper, waxes, surfactants, alcohols, and acids. The effect of these substances is unknown. In addition to dioxin concerns, tampons are made from cotton. The type of cotton is important because 10% of the world's pesticides are used on cotton.

Dioxin exposure has been associated with increased risk for toxic shock syndrome, endometriosis, immune system depression, increased pelvic inflammatory disease, decreased fertility, cervical cancer, bladder cancer, and ovarian cancers. When questions about dioxin arose a number of years ago, FDA asked tampon manufacturers to provide information about their pulp purification processes and the potential for dioxin contamination. Manufacturers have provided FDA with test results of studies conducted at independent laboratories, using the most sensitive test methods available. The detectable limit of this assay is currently approximately 0.1 to 1 parts per trillion of dioxin, much less than found in the environment. It appears that while tampons do generate dioxins, it is at extremely low levels.

The EPA has been working with paper manufacturing companies for non-dioxin methods of bleaching paper. The Robin Danielson Act (HR 360) directs the CDC to collect and report on toxic shock syndrome and the National Institute of Health to conduct research determining the extent to which dioxin and other tampon additives pose a health risk to women.

Sources:

Nassar, S. (2003). Tampon safety. National Center for Policy Research. Retrieved March 3, 2003 from http://www.cpr4womenandfamilies.org.

U.S. Food and Drug Administration. Tampons and Asbestos, Dioxin, & Toxic Shock Syndrome. http://www.fda.gov/cdrh/consumer/tamponsabs.html.

---

formaldehyde is indoors. At home, formaldehyde can be produced by tobacco products, gas cookers, and open fireplaces. It is also used as a preservative in some foods such as cheeses, dried foods, and fish. It is found in many products such as antiseptics, medicines, cosmetics, dishwashing liquids, fabric softeners, shoe care agents, carpet cleaners, adhesives, lacquers, paper, plastics, and some wood products. People living in new mobile homes may be exposed to higher levels of formaldehyde from the manufactured wood products used in these homes. It is used in many industries for the production of latex, leather tanning, wood preser-

vation, and photographic film production. It is combined with methanol and other substances to make embalming fluid and it is used to preserve tissue specimens in laboratories and hospitals. The most common exposure to formaldehyde is in the air. It can be found in water but does not last a long time and is not commonly found in drinking water supplies. Some people are more sensitive to formaldehyde than others. Severe pain, vomiting, coma, and possible death can occur after ingesting large amounts of formaldehyde.

NITRITES

Nitrates and nitrites are nitrogen-oxygen chemical units that combine with various organic and inorganic compounds. Once taken into the body, nitrates are converted into nitrites. The greatest use of nitrates is as a fertilizer. Inorganic nitrates used for fertilizer, such as potassium nitrate and ammonium nitrate, may contaminate drinking water. Excessive levels of nitrates in drinking water have caused serious illness and sometimes death. This is a serious illness in infants due to the conversion of nitrate to nitrite by the body, which can interfere with the oxygen-carrying capacity of the child's blood. This can be an acute condition in which health deteriorates rapidly over a period of days. Symptoms include shortness of breath and blueness of the skin, often leading it to be called blue baby syndrome. Lifetime exposure of nitrates and nitrites may produce diuresis, increased starchy deposits, and hemorrhaging of the spleen. Farmers and chemical manufacturing workers are most likely to have

Estrogens are steroid hormones for men and women that are important to human reproduction and secondary sex characteristics. To develop and function normally, hormonal levels must be regulated. Regulation can be disturbed when exposed to environmental chemicals. Xenoestrogens are found in phytoestrogens metabolized and excreted in the urine after consuming plant foods (such as soybeans). Other xenestrogens are toxic, such as polychlorinated biphenyl (PCB), dioxin, and furans. PCB affects sperm motility and density. Other xenoestrogens have been linked to fibrocystic breast disease and breast cancer. A synthetic hormone, diethylstilbestrol (DES) used in pregnant women, resulted in increased risk and incidence of cancer in female offspring. Because xenoestrogens have nearly the same chemical structure as estradiol and DDT, the effect on humans is not well known. Xenoestrogens are another substance found in foods heated with plastic wrap.

lifetime exposure. The MCLG for nitrates in drinking water has been set at 10 parts per million (ppm) and at 1 ppm for nitrites.

POLYCHLORINATED BIPHENYLS

PCBs are a class of chlorinated organic compounds manufactured during the 1930s to late 1970s. They were widely used throughout the world for their heat resistance and electrical characteristics. They were also used as an additive in transformer and hydraulic fluids and continue to be used in a variety of applications. PCBs enter the body via the gastrointestinal tract through the fish, meats, and milk consumed. They can remain in the body for several years in fatty tissue. PCBs are widespread, do not break down easily in the environment, and can accumulate. Human studies provide evidence that PCBs are carcinogenic, affecting the liver, biliary tract, intestines, and skin. Exposure in occupational settings may result in chloracne, hyperpigmentation of the nails and skin, and skin irritation.

METHYLENE CHLORIDE

Methylene chloride is known to cause cancer in animals and is known to convert to carbon monoxide in the body of humans. Poisoning symptoms include drowsiness, nausea, and unconsciousness leading to death. Consumer products that contain methylene chloride include paint strippers, adhesive removers, and aerosol spray paints. Carefully read the labels containing health hazard information and cautions on the proper use of these products. Use products that contain methylene chloride outdoors when possible; use indoors only if the area is well ventilated.

PENTACHLOROPHENOL

Pentachlorophenol (PCP) is used as a pesticide and wood preservative. Since 1984, the purchase and use of PCP has been restricted to certified applicators, and is no longer available to the general public. Used industrially as a wood preservative for utility poles, railroad ties, and wharf pilings, pentachlorophenol can be found in the air, water, and soil. It enters the environment through evaporation from treated wood surfaces, industrial spills, and disposal at uncontrolled hazardous waste sites. It can be broken down by sunlight, other chemicals, and microorganisms within a couple of days to several months. PCP is found in fish and other foods, but tissue levels are usually low. Exposure to high levels of pentachlorophenol can cause the cells in the body to produce excess heat (ATSDR, 2001). When this occurs, a person may experience a high fever, profuse sweating, and difficulty in breathing. In addition, the body temperature can rise to dangerous levels. Damage to the liver and immune system

has also been observed in individuals who are exposed to high levels of PCP for an extended time. The EPA and International Agency for Cancer Research (IARC) have determined that pentachlorophenol is a probable human carcinogen.

POLYBROMINATED BIPHENYLS AND POLYBROMINATED DIPHENYL ETHERS

Polybrominated biphenyls (PBBs) and polybrominated diphenyl ethers (PBDEs) are manufactured chemicals found in plastics used in computer monitors, televisions, textiles, plastic foams, and other consumer products. During their manufacture and use, PBBs and PBDEs find their way into air, water, and soil. Most of what is known about the health effects of PBBs in people comes from studies of people in Michigan who, for several months from 1973 to 1974, ate PBB-contaminated animal products. Some residents complained of nausea, abdominal pain, loss of appetite, joint pain, fatigue, and weakness, but it was not established that PBBs were the cause of these problems. There is stronger evidence that PBBs may have caused skin problems, such as acne, in some people who ate contaminated food, breathed in, or had skin contact with PBBs. The manufacture of PBBs was discontinued in the United States in 1976.

POLYCYCLIC AROMATIC HYDROCARBONS

Polycyclic aromatic hydrocarbons (PAHs) are a group of over 100 different chemicals that are formed during the incomplete burning of coal, oil and gas, garbage, or other organic substances like tobacco or charbroiled meat. Exposure to PAHs usually occurs by breathing air contaminated by wild fires or coal tar or by eating foods that have been grilled. Respiratory problems occur due to exposure. The Department of Health and Human Services (DHHS) has determined that some PAHs may reasonably be expected to be carcinogens. Some people who have breathed or touched mixtures of PAHs and other chemicals for extended periods of time have developed cancer of the skin, lung, and stomach.

PHTHALATES

Known as plasticizers, phthalates are used to make plastics flexible without sacrificing strength or durability. It is used to make polyvinyl chloride (PVC) plastic flexible enough to make toys and other flexible plastic products. Mono-ethyl phthalates are used as solvents in paint, nail polish, perfume, hand lotion, soaps, shampoo, and deodorant. Mono-butyl phthalates are used in cosmetics, printing ink, coating on pharmaceuticals, and insecticides. Benzylbutyl phthalate is used in adhesives for vinyl flooring, sealants, and car care products. Other phthalates include mono-cyclohexyl phthalate, mono-2-ethylhexyl phthalate, mono-n-octyl phthalate, and mono-isononyl phthalate. Nearly everyone has phthalates in their body. The Centers for Disease Control maintains, however, that simply because people have this in their system does not mean it is harmful.

SODIUM HYPOCHLORITE

Sodium hypochlorite is found in household products such as bleaching agents, cleaning products, or disinfectants. Sodium hypochlorite solutions are clear or greenish to yellow liquids with an odor of chlorine. They are found in drinking water, waste water purification systems, and swimming pools. The toxic effects are due to the corrosive properties. Inhaled chlorine gas from concentrated hypochlorite solutions may cause nasal irritation, sore throat, and coughing. Contact with the skin may cause burning pain, inflammation, and blisters. Ingestion of sodium hypochlorite will cause severe corrosive injuries to the mouth, throat, esophagus, and stomach with bleeding, perforation, and death. Permanent scars and narrowing of the esophagus may occur in survivors. It can cause irritation of the eyes, skin, respiratory, and gastrointestinal tract. Exposure to high levels can result in severe corrosive damage to the eyes, skin, and respiratory and gastrointestinal tissues and can be fatal.

STYRENE

Pure styrene is a colorless liquid that evaporates easily and has a sweet smell. It is used to make rubber and plastics for packaging, insulation, fiberglass, pipes, automobile parts, drinking cups, and carpet backing. Styrene is also present in cigarette smoke and automobile exhaust. It can be found in the air, soil, and water, but it is quickly broken down in the air within 1 to 2 days. Styrene is usually not found in drinking water unless it is discharged from factories, coal gasification plants, and hazardous waste sites. It can be a natural part of foods such as fruits, vegetables, nuts, beverages, and meat. It can also be transferred to food from polystyrene packing materials. Styrene enters the body quickly if it is inhaled or ingested. For those who work in manufacturing plants producing styrene, large amounts can cause depression, concentration problems, muscle weakness, tiredness, and nausea. Styrene may also cause lower birth weight and has an increased risk of spontaneous abortion. It can be found in blood, urine, and body tissues for a short time following exposure to moderate-to-high levels.

VINYL ACETATE

Vinyl acetate is an industrial chemical used to make other industrial chemicals: glues, paints, textiles, paper, plastic films for packaging, and as a modifier of food starch. It is a clear, colorless liquid with a sweet, fruity smell. It is flammable and may be ignited by heat, sparks, or flames. It enters the environment from industries that make, use, or process it. It breaks down readily in the environment; about 6 hours in the air, 7 days in water, and it is not known how long it stays in the soil. The major effects of breathing high levels of vinyl acetate for a short time are irritated eyes, nose, and throat. It can cause skin irritation and blisters if spilled on the skin.

VINYL CHLORIDE

Exposure to vinyl chloride occurs mainly in the workplace. At normal room temperatures, vinyl chloride is a colorless, flammable gas with a mild, sweet odor. It is used to make polyvinyl chloride for piping, wire and cable coatings, furniture, and automobile upholstery. It also results from the breakdown of other substances such as trichloroethane, tricholorethylene, and tetrachloroethylene. Liquid vinyl chloride evaporates easily into the air and can break down within a few days. Breathing high levels of vinyl chloride can cause dizziness or drowsiness. At very high levels, it can cause unconsciousness and death. Breathing vinyl chloride for extended periods of time can result in permanent liver damage, immune reactions, nerve damage, and liver cancer. It is a known carcinogen.

The Role of Environmental Scientists

Environmental science is concerned with the identification and control of factors that affect health (Table 5-2). Environmental scientists work with epidemiologists and toxicologists to assess risk and develop strategies to manage or reduce risk from exposure to toxins. Environmental risk assessment includes a four-step process, developed by the National Research Council, to determine risk to human health:

1. Hazard identification. Identification of potential health effects that may occur.

2. **Dose-response.** The amount of substance to which the person is exposed.

3. **Exposure.** The substance may be inhaled, ingested, absorbed, or injected.

4. Risk. Consideration of the substance, dose-response, and exposure to determine the overall risk (risk = toxicity $\times$ exposure) (Griffith, Aldrich, & Drane, 2002).

TABLE 5-2 Toxic Substances and Their Impact

Toxic Substances	Effects on Health
Acid rain	Lowers soil fertility, damages vegetation and buildings
Carbon monoxide	Prevents RBCs from carrying oxygen, produces fatigue, nausea, vomiting, unconsciousness, and death
Cigarette smoke	Contains 43 toxic substances, including benzene, which cause cancer
Fertilizers	Pollute water and kill fish
Herbicides	Cause brain and nerve disorders, birth defects, cancer, and reproductive and endocrine disorders
Mercury and lead	Cause brain damage, mental retardation, nerve disorders, kidney disorders, paralysis, and loss of vision
Noise	Causes permanent hearing loss
Pesticides	Cause lymphoma, prostate cancer, endocrine disruption, birth defects, low birth weight, and breast cancer
Radon	Causes lung cancer, particularly among smokers and women
Sewage	Cause transfer of pathogens that cause illness, such as hepatitis, cholera, typhoid fever, and E. coli
Smog and other gases	Causes or worsens respiratory illnesses such as asthma and chronic obstructive pulmonary disease
UV radiation	Causes sunburn, cataracts, and cancer

Substances can be rated according to risk using the following scale:

1 = cause irritation but only minor residual injury

2 = temporary incapacitation or possible residual injury

3 = cause serious temporary or residual injury

4 = major residual injury and could cause death

The minimal risk level (MRL) for hazardous substances is also assessed. It is an estimate of the daily human exposure to a hazardous substance without appreciable risk of adverse non-cancer health. MRLs are determined using animal studies, assuming that humans are more sensitive to effects over a specified duration of exposure. Public health officials utilize the MRL estimate to identify hazardous waste. MRLs for many substances are provided on the Agency for Toxic Substances and Disease Registry (ATSDR) Web site at http://www.atsdr.cdc.gov/atsdrhome.html.

Laboratory studies of the carcinogenicity of environmental and industrial chemicals are conducted by the National Toxicology Program (NTP). The NTP is a cooperative effort to coordinate toxicology research and testing activities within the Department of Health and Human Services. The NTP receives funds for conducting its studies from the National Institute of Environmental Health Sciences (NIEHS), the National Institute for Occupational Safety and Health, and the National Center for Toxicological Research.

The National Report on Human Exposure to Environmental Chemicals was first released in 2001. The aim of the report was to provide information to scientists, physicians, and health officials to help prevent disease resulting from exposure to environmental chemicals. The report measured lead, mercury, cadmium, dialkyl phosphate, organophosphate pesticides, cotinine, and phthalates. The second report was released in 2003 and added information about polycyclic aromatic hydrocarbons, dioxins, furans, PCBs, phytoestrogens, organophosphate pesticides, organochlorine pesticides, carbamate pesticides, herbicides, pest repellents, and disinfectants.

Scope of Environmental Toxin Problems

xamples of environmental poisoning include the cases of the Hudson River, Shenandoah River, Chattahoochee River, Ohio River, and

Dose-response
The type of response to a toxic agent in response to a particular dose.

Exposure
Contact with or proximity to a toxic agent that may have harmful consequences.

Mississippi River (particularly in the Louisiana delta region). The pollution of the Hudson River started in 1929 when Monsanto Company began to manufacture PCBs. In 1947 General Electric began to manufacture PCBs, contributing to more pollution. In 1973, a dam was built, moving water from the upper Hudson River to the lower Hudson River, increasing pollution levels. When high PCB levels were found in fish in 1974, the effects were studied and the production of PCBs were eventually banned. In the 1970s, mercury pollution in the South River and South Fork of the Shenandoah River was discovered from a synthetic fibers plant. More recently, increasing levels of PCBs are causing concern for local residents. Pollution is a concern for the Chattahooche River, the Mississippi River, and the Missouri River as dams are built and new construction along the rivers contribute to pollution from urban runoff. As a result, Congress passed the Emergency Planning and Community Right-to-Know Act of 1986 (PL 99-499). The act established a database called the Toxics Release Inventory (TRI), regarding 650 chemicals released by manufacturing, mining, power plants, chemical distributors, petroleum companies, storage facilities, and hazardous water treatment facilities (Figure 5-3). The greatest number of chemical emissions were from the mining industry (47%), followed by manufacturing companies (32%), and electric facilities (16%).

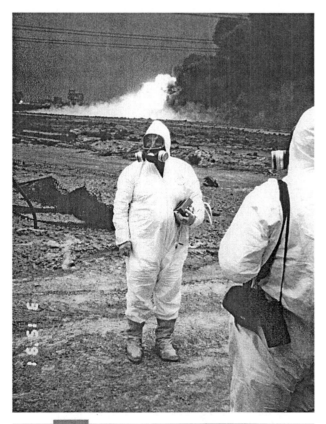

FIGURE 5-3 **Hazardous Materials** The identification and containment of hazardous materials is an important role for environmental health specialists.

Summary

The environment has a dramatic impact on how long humans live and how healthy their lives will be. The environment provides the air, the water, the food, the shelter, and the climate needed to exist. Environmental quality then, determines the quality of life each shall have. Air quality, water quality, and food quality are major concerns today, in part because of the way in which human interactions affect the spread of contagious and chronic diseases. Less obvious are concerns regarding natural resources, preservation of the land, respect for other living creatures, and the need for safe outdoor areas.

Scientific advancements have exploded during the twentieth century and similar growth is predicted for the future. Advancements in science have beneficial as well as harmful effects that must be weighed. Chlorination of drinking water reduced waterborne illnesses, but the interaction of chlorine and organic matter produces trihalomethanes, a harmful substance. Automobiles made it possible for individuals to get to work and school but contribute to smog and acid rain. Smog contributes to respiratory diseases and acid rain destroys vegetation and buildings. Chlorofluorocarbons used for refrigeration made it possible to store food and vaccines longer, but reduce the protective ozone layer. Pesticides and herbicides boost food production, but remain in the environment for long periods of time, accumulating in fatty tissues of animals and humans, causing reproductive problems and cancer.

In an effort to improve the quality of life, humans create new problems. In turn, individuals with a sense of moral responsibility can organize resources, develop environmentally friendly technology, push local officials to regulate sources of pollution, and control their own behavior. Environmentalists can help by educating the public and government officials about environmental problems and possible solutions. Conservationists can encourage the wise use of land and water for the production of food and sustainable development. Physicians and government officials have set up public health agencies to determine disease-causing agents to protect citizens. Federal agencies required the testing of new products and their effect on human health. Scientific studies are scrutinized for potential harm to human subjects. The ultimate goal for all of these efforts is to sustain the environment and quality of life enjoyed today.

Toxic substances are abundant in the environment today, largely in an effort to increase farm production, store radioactive materials used for energy, control disease-carrying vectors, and technology. Many of the toxic substances occur naturally, but exposure from mining, development, manufacturing new items, and wars increases the risk substantially. Risks include DNA mutations, cancer, autoimmune deficiencies, illnesses, and burns. Many toxic substances are regulated and their management is regulated by laws. In order to decrease the number of toxic

Consider the Cost HOW TO REDUCE TOXIC ACCIDENTS

Many instances of accidental contact with toxins can be prevented by two simple steps:

- Before using, read the label to know how to use the product safely and what to do if the products splashes or is spilled on you.
- Keep containers of hazardous products closed while using them to prevent fumes and toxic spills.

SAFE USE OF HAZARDOUS PRODUCTS

- Pregnant individuals should avoid using toxic substances as much as possible because many products have not been tested for effects on unborn children.
- Do not wear soft contact lenses when using solvents or pesticides

because they can trap chemicals on the eyes so you cannot wash them out.

- Use hazardous materials outdoors or open the windows to be sure there is enough ventilation. Use an exhaust fan and do not stay in the area for more than a few minutes. Take frequent "fresh air" breaks.
- Do not eat, drink, or smoke while using hazardous products. You may inadvertently swallow them, which can be more harmful than absorbing them on the skin.
- Use eyeglasses or goggles to prevent chemicals from getting into the eyes.
- Have fresh water and a towel or rag nearby in the event you spill chemicals on your skin.

- Wear protective gloves and wash your hands immediately after using.
- *NEVER combine ammonia and bleach products together.* The reaction causes toxic fumes that can harm human and animal health or require evacuation from a building.
- Wash with detergent (soap leaves a residue-trapping chemical on the skin) and water after wiping up spills.
- Throw away your clothes if acid is spilled on them. Battery acid will continually eat through clothing with repeated washings. Dispose of clothing as if they were hazardous materials (as indeed they are).

Consider the Cost WHAT TO DO IN THE EVENT OF AN EMERGENCY

When using hazardous materials, pay attention to the type of substance used, the time that has passed since exposure occurred, and the amount before starting the job. Keep a telephone close by or have another person nearby whom you can call for help, in the event you need assistance.

- Call the Poison Control Center number (1-800-922-1117 or 800-222-1222) for directions if an emergency occurs.

- If another person absorbs or swallows a hazardous substance, estimate what has been ingested or absorbed, the amount, and the approximate time the chemical was ingested.
- Refer to the container to determine the exact type of substance. There may be a hazardous product number (EPA registration number) that emergency personnel will need to determine the appropriate antidote or treatment.

- Be prepared to dilute the poison, absorb the poison (with activated charcoal and water), or induce vomiting (with syrup of ipecac, followed by a glass of water) if it has been swallowed.
- Never induce vomiting if a petroleum or corrosive product has been swallowed because the esophagus can be re-injured.

substances in the environment, the demand for convenience and technology could be decreased.

REFERENCES

Agocs, M., Etzel, R., Parrish, R., Paschal, D., Campagna, P., Cohen, D., Kilbourne, E., & Hesse, J. (1990). Mercury exposure from interior latex paint. *New England Journal of Medicine, 323,* 1096–1101.

Agency for Toxic Substances and Disease Registry (ATSDR). (2003). CERCLA Priority list of hazardous substances. Retrieved November 12, 2004 from http://www.atsdr.cdc.gov/clist.html.

Agency for Toxic Substances and Disease Registry (ATSDR). (1997). ToxFAQs for benzene. CAS# 71-43-2. Retrieved November 12, 2004 from http://www.atsdr.cdc.gov/tfacts3.html.

Agency for Toxic Substances and Disease Registry (ATSDR). (2001). ToxFAQs for pentachlorophenol. CAS# 87-86-5. Retrieved November 12, 2004 from http://www.atsdr.cdc.gov/tfacts51.html.

Agency for Toxic Substances and Disease Registry (ATSDR). (2004). Proceedings of the expert panel workshop to evaluate the public health implications for the treatment and disposal of polychlorinated biphenyls—Contaminated waste. Chapter 2—Expert Panel Report, Health Effects Panel. Retrieved November 12, 2004 from http://www. atsdr.cdc.gov/HAC/PCB/b_pcb_c2b.html.

Agency for Toxic Substances and Disease Registry (ATSDR). (1999). Public health statement for mercury. CAS# 7439-97-6. Retrieved November 12, 2004 from http://www.atsdr. cdc.gov/toxprofiles/phs46.html.

Agency for Toxic Substances and Disease Registry (ATSDR). (2000). Case studies in environmental medicine: Chromium toxicity. ATSDR Publication No.: ATSDR-HE-CS-2001-0005. Retrieved November 12, 2004 from http://www. atsdr.cdc.gov/HEC/CSEM/chromium/.

Agency for Toxic Substances and Disease Registry (ATSDR). (2002). ToxFAQs for Chlorine. CAS# 7782-50-5. Retrieved November 12, 2004 from http://www.atsdr.cdc.gov/ tfacts172.html.

Agency for Toxic Substances and Disease Registry (ATSDR). (2003). ToxFAQs for Nickel. Retrieved November 12, 2004 from http://atsdr1.atsdr.cdc.gov/tfacts15.html.

American Public Health Association. (1996). Prevention of dioxin generation from PVC plastic use by health care facilities. Retrieved November 12, 2004 from http://www.apha. org/legislative/policy/policysearch/index.cfm?fuseaction= view&id=125.

Annest, J. L., Pirkle, J. L., Makuc, D., Neese, J. W., Bayse, D. D., & Kovar, M. G. (1983). Chronological trend in blood lead levels between 1976 and 1980. *New England Journal of Medicine, 308,* 1373–1377.

Bellinger, D., Bolger, M., Goyer, R., Barraj, L., & Baines, J. (2004). WHO food additives Series 46: Cadmium. Retrieved November 12, 2004 from http://www.inchem.org/ documents/jecfa/jecmono/v46je11.htm#_46112210a.

Bertazzi, P., Consonni, D., Bachetti, S., Rubagotti, M., Baccarelli, A., Zocchetti, C., & Pesatori, A. (2001). Health effects of dioxin exposure: A 20-year mortality study. *American Journal of Epidemiology, 153,* 1031–1044.

Calvert, J. B. (2004). Arsenic. Retrieved November 12, 2004 by http://www.du.edu/~jcalvert/phys/arsenic.htm.

Centers for Disease Control. (2004). Facts about cyanide. Retrieved November 12, 2004 from http://www.bt.cdc.gov/ agent/cyanide/basics/facts.asp.

Centers for Disease Control. (2003). Lead and drinking water from private wells. Retrieved November 12, 2004 from http://www.cdc.gov/ncidod/dpd/healthywater/factsheets/ lead.htm.

Centers for Disease Control. (2004). Preventing lead poisoning in young children. Retrieved November 12, 2004 from http://www.cdc.gov/nceh/lead/publications/books/plpyc/ chapter3.htm#Introduction.

Copper Development Association. (2005). www.copper.org. Retrieved April 1, 2005.

Department of Veterans Affairs. (1999). Review of the literature on herbicides, including phenoxy herbicides and associated dioxins. III. Health effects of phenoxy herbicides and contaminants. *Environmental Health, 15,* 12. Retrieved November 12, 2004 from http://infoventures. com/e-hlth/orange/phd-he2.html.

Electronic Library of Construction Occupational Safety and Health (ELCOSH). (2003). Welding and manganese poisoning. *International Brotherhood of Electrical Workers Journal,* July/August issue. Retrieved November 12, 2004 from http://www.cdc.gov/elcosh/docs/d0500/d000595/ d000595.html.

Elhassani, S. (1983). The many faces of methyl mercury poisoning. *Journal of Toxicology. Clinical Toxicology,* 19, 875–906.

Ellis, D. (1989). *Environments at Risk.* Berlin: Springer-Verlag Publishers.

Environmental Research Foundation. (1998). Dangers of chlorine in water. Rachel's Environment and Health Weekly #599, May 21. Retrieved November 12, 2004 from http:// www.monitor.net/rachel/r599.html.

Griffith, J., Aldrich, T., & Drane, W. (2002). Risk assessment. In *Environmental epidemiology and risk assessment,* pg. 215. Hoboken, NJ: John Wiley & Sons, Inc.

Hesse, J. (1990). Mercury exposure from interior latex paint. *New England Journal of Medicine, 323,* 1096–1101.

Lewis, J. (1985). Lead poisoning: A historical perspective. *EPA Journal,* May, 11. Retrieved November 12, 2004 from http://www.epa.gov/history/topics/perspect/lead.htm.

Naro, K. (2001). Nickel. *Ductile Iron News, 1.* Retrieved November 12, 2004 from http://www.ductile.org/magazine/2001.

National Institute of Environmental Health Sciences (NIEHS). (2004). Radon testing. Retrieved November 12, 2004 from http://www.niehs.nih.gov/external/faq/radon.htm

National Institute of Environmental Health Sciences (NIEHS). (2001). Dioxin Research at the National Institute of Environmental Health Sciences. Retrieved April, 2003 from http://www.niehs.nih.gov/oc/factsheets/dioxin.htm.

Natural Resources Defense Council. (2001). Arsenic in drinking water. International Programme on Chemical Safety Retrieved November 12, 2004 from http://www.nrdc.org/ water/drinking/qarsenic.asp#health.

Niemeyer, S., Heiden, K., & Wolt, W. (1994). Handling wastes: Household paints and paint related products. Nebraska Cooperative Extension Service document NF94-194.

Nogawa, K., Kobayashi, E., Okubo, Y., Suwanzono, Y. (2004). Environmental cadmium exposure, adverse effects and preventive measures in Japan. *BioMetals,* 17, 581–587.

Nordenberg, T. (2000). Cell phones and cancer: No clear connection. *FDA Consumer, 34,* 19–21, 23.

Pesticide Action Network (PAN). (2004). Chromium III compounds. Retrieved November 12, 2004 from http://www. pesticideinfo.org/Detail_Chemical.jsp?Rec_Id=PC40088.

Smart, J. K. (2004). History of chemical and biological warfare: An American perspective. Textbook of military medicine: Medical aspects of chemical and biological warfare, Chapter 2. Retrieved November 12, 2004 from http://www.vnh. org/MedAspChemBioWar/chapters/chapter_2.htm.

Sweeney, M. H. (2002). Cancer in humans related to exposure to Agent Orange and other chemicals contaminated with 2, 3, 7, 8-TCDD. Retrieved November 12, 2004 from http:// www.niehs.nih.gov/external/usvcrp/conf2002/abs_pdf/ diox-049.pdf.

U.S. Department of Health and Human Services (USDHHS). (2002). Report on Carcinogens, 10th edition. U.S. Public Health Service, National Toxicology Program, December. Retrieved November 12, 2004 from http://ehp.niehs.nih.gov/roc/toc10.html.

U.S. Environmental Protection Agency. (1996). Radiation: Risks and realities. Retrieved 3/27/2000 from http://www.epa.gov/radiation/rrpage/rrpage1.html.

Weiss, B., & Elsner, J. (1996). The intersection of risk assessment and neurobehavioral toxicity. *Environmental Health Perspectives, 104* (Supplement 2), 173–177.

Welch, A. H., Westjohn, D. B., Helsel, D. R., & Wanty, R. B. (2000). Arsenic in ground water of the United States—occurrence and geochemistry: *Ground Water, 38,* 589–604.

Yassi, A., Kjellstrom, T., de Kok, T., & Guidotti, T. (2001). Nature of environmental health hazards, pgs. 52–103. *Basic Environmental Health.* Oxford, NY: World Health Organization.

ASSIGNMENTS

1. Select a toxic substance described in this chapter and learn more about it by using the Web site for the Agency for Toxic Substances and Disease Registry Division of Toxicology (http://www.atsdr.cdc.gov/toxfaq.html).

2. Find RADNET on the Internet and report on interesting information you discover.

3. Look up information about other toxic substances (such as acetone, nickel, vinyl acetate, silver, phosphoric acid, styrene, cyanide, carbon disulfide, DDT, sodium hypochlorite, and manganese) and consider sources of exposure in your environment.

4. Look up four alternative medicine techniques that people claim "detoxify" the body to determine whether they are effective and determine their effectiveness.

5. Discuss ethical concerns related to pesticide use.

6. Ask a pest control expert to speak to the class about requirements for pesticide training.

7. Research the effects of Agent Orange on Vietnam veterans and citizens and compensation from the U.S. government.

8. Read *Silent Spring* and write a book report.

9. Perform additional research on the harmful effects of PCBs, nonphenyls, components of epoxies (bisphenol A), and phthalates to determine the potential risk to you and your family.

10. Search your home and garage for pesticides and read the labels to determine toxicity and the best means of disposal.

SELECTED ENVIRONMENTAL LAWS

1976 Toxic Substances Control Act (TSCA) (PL 96-469)
Requirements for EPA notification on use, testing, and restriction of certain chemical substances on human health and the environment (all chemicals produced in or imported into the United States).

1990 Pollution Prevention Act (42 U.S.C. 13101 and 13102)
Requirements for prevention, reduction, or treatment of pollution at its source, recycled or treated, and disposed of or released only as a last resort.

1992 Residential Lead-Based Paint Hazard Reduction Act (PL 102-550)
Issued to stop the use of lead-based paint and remove old paint in federal buildings. It was later amended to establish funds for lead abatement training.

2001 Comprehensive Environmental Response, Compensation and Liability Act (CERCLA, U.S.C. 9604)
As amended by the Superfund Amendments and Reauthorization Act (SARA, PL 99-499) requires that the Agency for Toxic Substances and Disease Registry (ATSDR) with the EPA develop, in order, a list of hazardous substances most commonly found at facilities on the Superfund national priorities list.

SELECTED PROFESSIONAL JOURNALS

Archives of Environmental Contamination and Toxicology
Archives of Toxicology
Bulletin of Environmental Contamination and Toxicology
Ecotoxicology and Environmental Safety
Environmental Research
Environmental Toxicology and Chemistry
EPA Journal
Experimental Lung Research
Health Physics
Journal of American College of Toxicology
Journal of Analytical Toxicology
Journal of Environmental Pathology, Toxicology and Oncology
Journal of Exposure Analysis and Environmental Epidemiology
Journal of Toxicology and Environmental Health
Nature
Toxicology
Toxicology and Applied Pharmacology

ADDITIONAL READING

Carson, R. (1962, 1994, 2002). *Silent Spring.* Boston, MA: Houghton Mifflin.

Colborn, T., Dumanowski, D., & Peterson Myers, J. (1996). *Our Stolen Future: Are We Threatening our Fertility, Intelligence, and Survival?* New York: Penguin Books.

Fagin, D., Lavelle, M., & Center for Public Integrity Staff (1999). *Toxic Deception: How the Chemical Industry Manipulates Science, Bends the Law, and Endangers Your Health.* Monroe, ME: Common Courage Press.

Krimsky, S. (2002). *Hormonal Chaos: The Scientific and Social Origins of the Environmental Endocrine Hypothesis.* Baltimore, MD: Johns Hopkins Press.

Steingraber, S. (1998). *Living Downstream: A Scientist's Personal Investigation of Cancer and the Environment.* New York: Knopf Publishing Group.

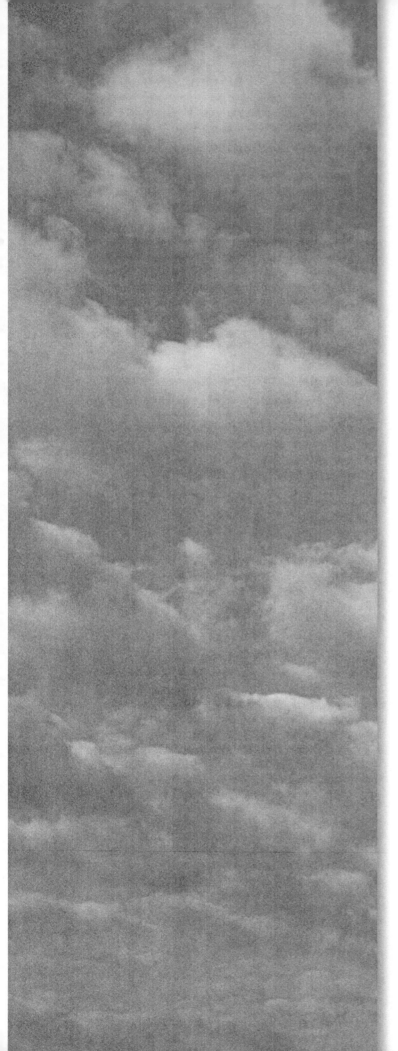

Environmental Health Risk Assessment and Intervention

First weigh the considerations, then take the risks.
Helmuth von Moltke (1800–1891)
What you risk reveals what you value.
Jeanette Winterson (1959–)

OBJECTIVES

1. Identify four federal agencies with the mandate of monitoring health risks for citizens.

2. Explain why public laws are needed for any action on the part of government officials, business leaders, and citizens.

3. Differentiate between a standard, code, regulation, guideline, and policy.

4. Describe two models used to assess environmental health risks.

5. List the four aspects of risk analysis to be considered.

6. Identify ways in which epidemiological methods contribute to risk identification.

7. Name four types of studies used to assess environmental health risks.

8. Explain how uncertainty affects the environmental health risk determination of acceptable risks.

9. Explain how the precautionary principle is applied to risk management and guides risk monitoring.

10. Describe three different types of risk control strategies by giving examples.

Introduction

The methods used in risk assessment, management, control, and communication are important in achieving the desired outcome. Several federal agencies have been issued the duty and authority for monitoring harmful products, substances, and practices in order to **mitigate** illness, disability, and death. They include:

Consumer Product Safety Commission (CPSC)

Environmental Protection Agency (EPA)

Food and Drug Administration (FDA)

National Institute of Environmental Health Sciences (NIEHS)

National Institute for Occupational Safety and Health (NIOSH)

Occupational Safety and Health Administration (OSHA)

The authority and duties of these agencies are dictated by public laws already identified in chapters of this text. State agencies are also given the mandate for adhering to federal regulations and standards. In some areas, local laws are developed to deal with problems specific to an area or community. The federal, state, and county agencies employ epidemiologists, toxicologists, safety personnel, industrial hygienists, and other environmental health specialists to carry out the intent of the law, sometimes aided by law enforcement officials.

The Determination of Risk

A **health risk** is a deviation in normal functioning of the body due to exposure or a series of exposures that can have a damaging effect ranging from a mild affliction to premature death (RAIS, 2005). Environmental health risks are unavoidable but must be managed and reduced where feasible. The risk can be preventable or unavoidable. The unavoidable risks are considered a "fact of life" or "fate," something one has little control over. It is the avoidable risks with which physicians, attorneys, public health officials, and citizens are concerned. No one wants to suffer or die unnecessarily. For centuries, researchers, environmentalists, and educators have studied the effects of the environment on human and other life. It is only recently that the effects of humans on the environment have been seriously considered. It seems an insurmountable task to identify potential risks to human health and to get people to change their behaviors in order to protect others.

Risk Assessment

Risk assessment is the characterization of potential adverse health effects of human exposure to environmental hazards (Griffith, Aldrich, & Dane, 2002). **Risk assessment** considers the risk of a particular exposure event or scenario and estimates its impact to human health. In some cases, there is an acceptable risk or the type of risk understood to be natural or expected. Some environmental hazards or substances occur naturally in the environment and exposure cannot be avoided if one happens to live there. Some would argue that if the risk is known, then citizens should be warned so they can relocate to a safer area. Others would say that there is no reason to create alarm by alerting citizens to health risks that have not caused significant health impacts in a population. Sensitive and vulnerable individuals will always be at greater risk but are not the sole basis for changes in risk management policy or action. On the other hand, would-be parents who have lost a child due to a miscarriage that is suspected to have been caused by radioactive contamination in drinking water supplies would disagree. Parents who watch their children die of leukemia or anemia would also unanimously agree that if someone had told them of the health risks, their child might still be alive and would not have had to suffer. Risk assessment is applied to populations; estimating the probability and magnitude of an event.

Risk Assessment Models

Models are used to construct a framework for examining a problem and finding solutions to combat the problem. There are two models from the sciences that can be applied to environmental problems; the epidemiologic model and the exposure-disease models.

Mitigate
To make less harmful or severe.

Health risk
Anything having a negative effect on health status, from mild affliction to premature death. The likelihood that a given exposure or series of exposures may have or will damage the health of individuals.

Risk assessment
The determination of adverse health effects attributed to exposure to environmental hazards; the combination of risk identification and risk estimation.

EPIDEMIOLOGIC MODEL

The epidemiologic model, also known as the "epidemiologic triad," is considered to be the traditional model of disease causation (Last, 1996). The model suggests that disease occurs when three components are brought together:

1. a susceptible host, vulnerable to the disease

2. an agent that can infect or cause symptoms in the susceptible host

3. an environment that supports growth of the agent, exposure to the agent, and circumstances that transport the agent to many individuals (Figure 6-1).

This model presupposes that if one of the components of the model is missing or an intervention is applied to one of the components, then the risk of the disease is lessened or removed. An example would be that the *Aedes* mosquito that carries the West Nile virus (agent). During the summer months, the *Aedes* population is likely to proliferate due to warmer temperatures and a wetter climate. In the evenings or in shaded areas, humans, chickens, and horses are susceptible to being bitten by the *Aedes* mosquito. Interventions to reduce the risk of West Nile virus can occur at any of the three levels. If there were less areas with standing or stagnant water, there would be less breeding grounds for *Aedes* mosquitoes and less mosquitoes. If citizens and animals were inoculated with a mosquito deterrent or if they were kept inside during normal biting times, then they would be less likely to be bitten and contract the West Nile virus.

THE EXPOSURE-DISEASE MODEL

In the case of health problems presumed to be related to toxic substances or hazardous materials (Figure 6-2), this model can be applied with its four elements:

1. exposure to the substance

2. dosage absorbed

3. biological effects from the absorbed dose

4. resulting clinical illness or disease

The exposure-disease model provides a useful way to consider the effects of toxic substances on people, but involves considerably more time to make a determination. For example, persons can inadvertently be exposed to a substance and the degree to which the substance is harmful may be unknown until an illness or disease is discovered in a relatively unique sample. Once the disease and contributing factors are noted, the amount of the substance that is absorbed and the biological effect of the absorbed dose must be recorded. This can take years of observation. When cause and effect cannot be established, a precautionary principle can be applied.

Risk Assessment Methods

In order to assess risk, estimates of exposure, dose, and effect are needed. In order to achieve these estimates, epidemiological and toxicological studies are needed. The challenge to risk assessment is that information needed for analysis is often absent or missing. Risk can be determined in several ways; some more powerful than others. The usual process is to look for historical data from a past problem to compare with current data and look for trends. Sometimes knowledge about similar substances is used. When neither of these techniques provides the information needed, others such as epidemiological studies, clinical studies, animal studies, in vitro tests, and comparative studies are used.

HISTORICAL DATA

Risk determined from historical data is the easiest to understand. If records kept showing the number of motor vehicle accidents (MVAs) in a particular area at one point in time are compared to the number of MVAs 5 years later and the number of MVAs has increased three-fold, then it can be assumed that the risk needs to be examined further to see why more accidents are occurring. If cars are made

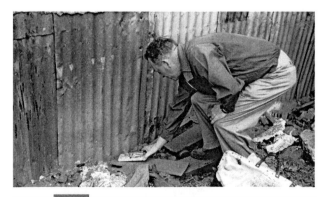

FIGURE 6-1 **Public Health Worker Trapping Rats in Louisiana** Sanitary engineers sometimes have to trap vectors that transmit disease to prevent an epidemic.

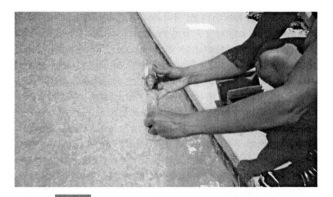

FIGURE 6-2 **Water Sampling** Pool owners test the water regularly for chlorine, pH, and turbidity so the water is safe for swimmers.

better, intersections are more visible, and laws pertaining to obtaining a license are more stringent, then the need to understand driver factors could account for the increase in accidents. Perhaps more drivers are using cellular phones than they did 5 years ago. Perhaps a new fast food restaurant has been added, increasing the amount of traffic and driving problems due to the location.

KNOWLEDGE OF COMPARATIVE RISKS

Sometimes experiences with certain substances in the past provide information about similar substances. An example of this would be exposure to radiation from iridescent dials made from radioactive substances. In a Westinghouse plant in 1930, workers exposed to the paint used to illuminate the dials suffered severe illness and skin damage. Because the paint was radioactive, the effects of X-rays on X-ray technicians could be estimated to be similar to those of the plant workers. After radiation exposure from Chernobyl, experts could now recognize the risk to citizens living within a similar distance to a nuclear power plant should an accident or natural disaster threaten.

CLINICAL AND EPIDEMIOLOGICAL STUDIES

The most direct means of determining risks to human health from exposure to hazardous substances are clinical and epidemiological studies. These studies are used to analyze populations who were accidentally exposed to a chemical or agent, often in conjunction with their employment. Medical and veterinary clinics, hospitals, and laboratories provide information about specific types of cases identified. Sometimes medical centers receive grant funds for research regarding a particular health problem. When patients cannot be identified for the study, newspaper ads or other methods are used to recruit subjects with problems investigated by researchers. Epidemiological studies are supervised by public health officials for reportable diseases and injuries.

LONGITUDINAL STUDIES

In the event of long-term exposure or delayed effects, **longitudinal studies** are often necessary. Longitudinal studies take years and are costly. When subjects who have been exposed to a harmful substance can be identified and followed over time, long-term effects can be determined. If these subjects are continually exposed to low levels of a substance, cumulative effects can also be studied.

LABORATORY STUDIES

When there is no other study to compare the effects a substance has on a person or animal, laboratory studies are used. The advantage to laboratory studies is that they can be accomplished in a much shorter time period than clinical, epidemiological, or longitudinal studies. This hastens conclusions about risk so that a product is not released to the public or is recalled due to unforeseen problems. In most cases, animals are used for laboratory studies. Critics of laboratory studies argue that animals are different from humans and the effects of toxic agents are different. In addition, laboratory animals are often exposed to higher doses and may give a **false negative** result. Researchers compensate for this procedure by subjecting the animal to lower levels of a toxin, thereby providing a better estimate for humans. The risk to the animal is then estimated by mathematical means to predict risk for humans.

Another type of laboratory study is an **in vitro** study. An in vitro study involves growing cells outside the body in a test tube or Petri dish for observation. Sometimes cells are kept alive in order to study the effect of cells when inoculated with a substance to determine its toxicity or ability to change DNA.

Calculating or Estimating Risk

Risk estimation is accomplished by the use of three mathematic models (McCally, 2002). The **tolerance distribution model** assumes that each individual in a population has a threshold level and tolerance levels are different from individual to individual. The **mechanistic model** is based on the assumption that cancer originates from one cell and cell growth is estimated mathematically. The **time-to-tumor model** is used when the time between initial exposure and development of a tumor are known.

Most risk assessments have focused on the risk of birth defects and cancer risk. It is generally recognized that a

---

Longitudinal studies
Observations made over a long period of time.

False negative
A negative result from a test that has the possibility of being in error.

In vitro
Outside the living organisms, in a test tube or Petri dish.

Tolerance distribution model
The assumption that each individual has a threshold and tolerance level different from another individual regarding risk of harm from environmental hazards.

Mechanistic model
A mathematical model used to estimate the potential exponential growth of cancer cells.

Time-to-tumor model
A model of risk estimation used when the time an individual is exposed to an environmental hazard is known as well as the development of a tumor.

high enough dose of any agent at a crucial time in development time will have an adverse effect on fetal development. A major problem with using birth defects as a determinant of risk is the fact that many fetuses die in utero and the abnormality goes unnoticed. Models are being applied so that the risk for children and other vulnerable population subgroups can gain attention. Carcinogens can be identified but cancer risk determinations are tricky because developmental growth and processes differ in individuals from one point to another. Although done less often, more emphasis is being placed on immune suppression and neurological problems today.

Systematic Risk Analysis

The National Research Council (NRC) defined risk assessment for potential neurotoxicity from environmental toxins as having four components:

1. **hazard** identification (chemical properties and the ability to cause disease)

2. exposure assessment (estimating exposure from contact with the hazardous agent)

3. dose-response assessment (the potential of a substance to cause disease as a result of contact)

4. risk characterization (toxicity, routes of exposure, and probable effect on a population)

This established guidelines for the EPA to follow (NRC, 1983).

HAZARD IDENTIFICATION

Experts such as biologists, chemists, and toxicologists use available data to determine the risk a potential hazard might have. Hazards include chemical agents (lead, asbestos, dioxin, and benzene), physical agent (radiation, noise, and accidents), and biological agents (pathogens and allergens). Toxicity is the level to which harmful effects are determined for a particular substance or agent. Toxicity is determined by the use of blood samples and is measured in units of micrograms per deciliter (mg/dL).

Toxicity can be determined through research designs used by epidemiologists. Three designs used include descriptive studies, analytical studies, and experimental studies (Commission on Life Sciences, 2001). **Descriptive studies** address the occurrence of disease or health-related problems in specific populations or representative samples of a population. There is no control group. Descriptive studies provide information from **case studies**, cross-sectional sampling, and the state of ecological factors. They do not test a hypotheses, they generate a hypothesis. Analytical studies assess associations or they may test hypotheses about risk factors and health. Analytical studies include the comparison of case studies to control groups or the examination of a phenomenon in **cohort studies**. Experimental studies compare the effects of a toxin in an experimental group compared to a control group. Members of the experimental and control groups are randomly assigned. The appropriate design is determined when research questions and goals are identified.

EXPOSURE

Exposure refers to the intensity and duration of contact with a substance (such as pesticides or particulate matter) or an agent (pathogens or radiation). Exposure occurs through four possible routes of exposure:

1. inhalation

2. skin absorption

3. ingestion

4. injection

Exposure assessment often utilizes hydrologists, meteorologists, and chemists. Epidemiologists and industrial hygienists help identify hazards by determining cause-and-effect relationships and human studies. Exposure assessment occurs with the help of environmental monitoring. Environmental health professionals measure air pollution and the components discharged; for example, from a steel mill or paper company. Water samples are taken to assure that contaminant levels do not exceed the safety margin. **Dosimeters** worn by employees at a nuclear plant or radiologists are monitored by health physicists to make sure that accidental exposure has not occurred. Exposure assessment also includes the effects of hazardous substances on environmental degradation, cumulative effects, deposition rates, and **biomagnification**.

DOSE-RESPONSE

How much a person actually absorbs from exposure is considered the **dose**. The dose is determined according to the type of substance, the concentration or intensity of the agent, the amount, the route, and the duration of exposure. The type of substance is usually assessed in terms of its toxicity. Toxicity is often determined according to the concentration or intensity of the agent. Once the toxicity is determined, the amount absorbed must be determined or estimated. The absorbed dose is generally greater if exposure level is high or for a prolonged length of time. Exposure levels are also considered to be high if the chemical is highly soluble in fat. The response to the dose is particularly important. Dose-response relationships require collaboration between statisticians, pathologists, and epidemiologists.

Digging Deeper | BIOMAGNIFICATION

Biomagnification occurs when organisms at the bottom of the food chain (e.g., insects) transfer a toxic substance (e.g., DDT) to the organism above it (e.g., fish). Following this example, note that the fish will consume large amounts of insects containing DDT. When the smaller fish that ate the insects is eaten by a larger fish, the DDT from the insects is stored in the fatty tissues of the larger fish after it consumed the smaller fish. When a human eats several of the larger fish with the DDT in its fatty tissues, levels in the body become much higher. In order for a pollutant to biomagnify, the following conditions must be met:

1. The pollutant must be long-lived.

2. The pollutant must be concentrated by the producers.

3. The pollutant must be fat-soluble.

Fortunately water-soluble substances cannot biomagnify because they are excreted in the waste products of animals and humans.

BIOLOGICAL EFFECT

The biological effect of an environmental toxin or infectious agent depends upon the substance's chemistry or a physical agent's type, the dose, and the person's **susceptibility** to disease. Individuals may have different **thresholds** for experiencing an effect from a biological, chemical, or physical hazard. This means that some people can be exposed longer to a harmful substance with minimal effect while others subjected to a small amount can have an acute reaction.

Determination of Risk

Risk from exposure to a hazard is communicated in terms of individual lifetime risk, annual population risk, the percentage of increase in risk, and loss of life expectancy. An example of how risk was communicated was based on years of life lost to young adults from the use of or exposure to cigarette smoke. For a long time, many companies, government officials, and individuals denied that a substantial risk existed because not every smoker acquired lung cancer. Their argument was further supported by the fact that nonsmokers could get lung cancer. Although researchers estimated that smokers were 10 to 15 times more likely than nonsmokers to get lung cancer, the concept was not accepted. Researchers tried again to convince others that the dangers from smoking were high, particularly for vulnerable individuals such as infants, the elderly, and individuals with suppressed immunity. In 1982 U.S. Surgeon General C. Everett Koop addressed "the most important public health issue of our time" and called for a "smokeless society" by the year 2000. He emphasized risks associated with smoking and cancer, pressing legislation for warning labels on each package. As a result, smokers who incurred damage as the result of tobacco use have filed claims against the tobacco industry and won. Even so, smoking is still a prevalent habit and adopted by new people every day.

Studies regarding the potential of harm for those using sugar substitutes such as saccharin also met opposi-

Acute exposure usually refers to a potent dose in a short period of time.
Chronic exposure usually refers to a low dose over a long period of time.

Hazard
Sources of potential harm; a substance, hazard, or microorganism that could lead to harm.

Descriptive studies
Studies designed to assess "what is"; often used to assess needs.

Case studies
Studies that examine dynamics of one subject or the group as a whole.

Case study
A study that gathers information about specific health conditions and past exposures.

Cohort studies
The use of subjects with similar characteristics; used in longitudinal and comparative designs.

Dosimeter
An instrument used for measuring ionizing doses of radioactivity.

Biomagnification
Otherwise known as *biological magnification;* the tendency of toxic agents to become concentrated in organisms higher on the food chain by consuming animals lower on the food chain.

Dose
The amount of a toxin absorbed by the body.

Susceptibility
The tendency toward a particular problem; vulnerability.

Thresholds
Points at which a substance causes problems; the beginning of symptoms showing that there is a problem.

Acute exposure
Exposure to a large or potent dose in a short period of time.

Chronic exposure
Exposure to a low dose over a long period of time.

tion. Laboratory animals were fed large amounts of saccharin and developed bladder cancer, but individuals refused to consider the potential harm to human health. When the product was taken off the market, many consumers became upset. A few years later the product was back, largely due to consumer demand.

In another example, the use of the drug Tamoxifen for breast cancer still continues in spite of the risks of ovarian cancer.

No one would argue that automobiles themselves do not cause accidents. The risk of having an accident depends on the training and status of the driver, condition of the automobile, road conditions, and probability of encountering another driver who will make an error. Actuarial studies are conducted by insurance companies in order to establish risk based upon the age of the driver, gender, previous driving record, and other public offenses to determine the cost to the company based on driver risk. Because no one can be perfectly free of risk, many choose to drive, knowing there are major risks involved.

THE ACCEPTANCE OF RISK

From experience, society has learned that:

- Not every person exposed to a potential hazard will have an adverse response.

- The occurrence or magnitude of an adverse response depends on the type of exposure to the hazard and the threshold of an individual.

- Individuals have different responses to the same dose or exposure to a hazardous agent according to age, gender, prior exposure, concurrent exposure with other substances, and the level of detoxifying enzymes in the body.

- The data used to assess risk in humans is inadequate or absent.

- A certain amount of risk is acceptable, particularly if it is voluntary, if the risk is to an individual or small group of people, if the risk is outweighed by convenience, or if compensation can be received for damages.

RISK EQUATIONS

In spite of the difficulties of risk assessment, standard equations are used to determine if a population is at increased risk or if there is an increased number of cases compared to the normal population. Epidemiologists have used measures of incidence and prevalence for quite some time.

Disease rate =

$$\frac{\text{Number of cases of illness in the population at risk}}{\text{Number of persons in the population at risk}}$$

The disease rate is expressed in terms of per 1,000 or 10,000 cases. For example, if a factory employing 1,000 workers had 13 workers with skin cancer, the disease rate would be 13/1000 or 130/10,000.

Risk ratio =

$$\frac{\text{Rate of illness in a population with the risk factor}}{\text{Rate of disease in a population without the risk factor}}$$

The risk ratio for the at-risk population would be expressed as N times greater than the population not at risk. If there was a disease rate of 13/1000 at an industrial plant using benzene and a disease rate of 5/1000 at an industrial plant not using benzene, then the risk ratio for the at-risk population would be 2.6 times greater (13/1000 divided by 5/1000) for the workers at the plant using benzene.

It must be remembered, however, that risk does not imply cause. Only a scientifically controlled study could determine that. It may be that benzene is only associated with the risk for skin cancer. The real reason could be another chemical was used in conjunction with benzene, the benzene plant had more Caucasian workers, or a greater exposure to the sun during lunchtime due to the location of the plant.

In some cases, the risk is unavoidable or economically disadvantageous and acceptable daily limits are established. In these cases, the EPA determines acceptable daily intake (ADI) or tolerable daily intake (TDI) levels based on **no observed adverse effect level (NOAEL)** or **lowest observed adverse effect level (LOAEL)** determinations divided by **uncertainty factors (UF)**.

$$\text{ADI} = \frac{\text{NOAEL or LOAEL}}{\text{UF}}$$

The uncertainty factors, also known as *safety factors,* include vulnerability of individuals, physiological diversity within a population, measurement errors, undetectable effects, and measures that are impossible to acquire. The uncertainty of the measurements reflects the degree of uncertainty that must be taken into account when using incomplete information. *The less that is known, the higher the uncertainty factor.*

Many organizations and agencies have what are known as quality assurance measures to monitor daily activities and reduce the number of errors that result in injuries or illnesses. Measurement tools are calibrated, human errors are detected, and training occurs.

Risk Management

The goal for studying relationships between hazardous substances and health is to mitigate or eliminate the potential for harm. This is the foundation of risk management. The management of risk integrates risk assessment with cost-benefit analysis for the purpose of developing strategies to regulate and control risk. The management of risk for a widely used material or widely dispersed agent can require many hours of highly trained experts and cost millions of dollars.

When risk is determined, **margins of safety** are also determined. Using previous data, scientists look at the highest dose or exposure that has produced no effect in humans or animals and the lowest dose that did produce an adverse effect. The factors are used to set an exposure limit of one-one thousandth of the highest dose known to not cause problems. Another estimate uses a statistical regression model to estimate doses associated with specific responses. Either method is based on assumptions.

SETTING STANDARDS

For recognized environmental health risks, efforts to control the amount of hazardous or toxic materials include the issuance of federal or state standards and regulations. **Regulations** are usually set by government officials in accordance with laws. In fact, *laws* usually provide directives for federal and state agencies to provide programs in an effort to regulate programs and services. If there were not a law or legal directive, the regulations could not be issued or enforced. **Codes** are rules that explicitly state how standards are achieved. When building or remodeling a structure, the structure must adhere to specific codes. For example, in areas where hurricanes occur with regularity, roofs must have hurricane clips to tie the roof down more securely.

Standards are expectations of conduct, services, or facilities usually set with the health of citizens in mind. Standards are set for the good of all and agencies or businesses are expected to strive to achieve those standards. An example of a standard would be that all restaurants must have dishwashers that heat water to a certain temperature for a period of time to sanitize dishes. Standards send a message that if the rules or laws are not followed, citizens may be at risk for health problems due to negligence or carelessness. Standards are taken seriously by those who enforce them.

SETTING GUIDELINES

There are some situations in which standards are not set, either because the hazards and risks have not been identified and confirmed, or when there is strong objection to proposed standards. When hazards and their accompanied risks have not been substantiated by experts but it seems logical that there is a serious risk involved, guidelines are issued to protect the public. Guidelines are not enforced by law.

Guidelines are suggestions, often developed by researchers or associations interested in protecting the environment while recognizing that economic issues are at stake. Sometimes guidelines raise the standard already identified and imposed. When researchers suggest guide-

lines, they may go above federal or state requirements to decrease the risk even further. When associations suggest guidelines, they may be making a political statement that protects the interests of their membership for liability and economic reasons. Those who follow guidelines are

UNCERTAINTY
There are three types of uncertainty: model uncertainty, statistical uncertainty, and fundamental uncertainty. **Model uncertainty** refers to the way in which cause and effect is determined. There are few times when a direct cause-effect relationship can be determined. In most cases, there are multiple causes or a complex set of conditions that make it hard to say any one factor is more responsible than another. **Statistical uncertainty** refers to the inability to measure or quantify the level of certainty with any precision. **Fundamental uncertainty** refers to the fact that nothing in life is certain and not everything is predictable.

No observed adverse effect level (NOAEL)
The point on a dose-effect curve at which a threshold is reached with no symptoms or problems.

Lowest observed adverse effect level (LOAEL)
The lowest level at which some symptoms and problems are found.

Uncertainty factors (UF)
Sometimes called "safety factors." Mathematical adjustments used when knowledge is incomplete; used to account for variations in people's sensitivity, differences between animals and humans, and differences between a LOAEL and a NOAEL to decide whether an exposure will cause harm to people.

Margins of safety
Confidence that exposure to a toxin will not produce an adverse effect.

Regulations
Rules, ordinances, or laws that must be enforced.

Codes
Laws organized for easy reference for a nation or a city.

Standards
A measure, gauge, yardstick, or criterion used to establish that which is acceptable, optimal, or ideal.

Guidelines
A standard or principle used to make a judgment, formulate a policy, or follow a course of action.

Model uncertainty
The manner in which cause and effect is determined when a direct cause-effect relationship cannot be determined.

Statistical uncertainty
The inability to measure or quantify the level of certainty with any precision.

Fundamental uncertainty
A premise that nothing in life is certain and not everything is predictable.

exercising professional courtesy, extending good citizenship, and making an effort to convince their communities that the welfare of citizens is important to them.

An example of a guideline would be a statement that women who are pregnant should not consume alcohol. A pregnant woman who drinks alcohol is not arrested or incarcerated, but it is generally known that the possibility of fetal alcohol syndrome (FAS) increases if she does. A prudent woman would not consume alcohol, but there are no legal consequences if she does.

DEVELOPING POLICIES

When there are regulations, standards, and guidelines, sometimes a business may provide additional measures known as policies. **Policies** are specific measures (otherwise known as standard procedures) within an organization that state exactly how a problem is to be managed. Sometimes there is a specific **protocol** to be followed, according to the situation. An example would be the steps taken to correct a problem once an employee recognizes one. The employee may be required to report the problem to his or her immediate supervisor. The supervisor must then take some type of action to correct the problem and if that action is not effective, report it to the next person in the chain of command. Another example would be the documentation of a problem. If an employee were to become injured because of an environmental hazard, the date of the incidence, circumstances involved, and measures taken to help the individual must be recorded. Policies are helpful when actions taken to prevent or correct problems are questioned. When it is determined that the business or organization ignored the problem or that there was some **liability** involved, policy and procedures manuals are reviewed to see if potential problems were anticipated and efforts were made to plan what to do in the event a problem occurred.

Control Strategies

here are several solutions to environmental problems affecting human health. The best solutions include primary prevention and secondary prevention. Primary prevention includes efforts to prevent a problem. Secondary prevention occurs when a problem is detected early and treated.

PRIMARY PREVENTION

Primary prevention employs three techniques known as:

1. control at the source
2. control along the path
3. control at the level of the person

Control at the source means to prevent exposure altogether. Use of the substance may be eliminated entirely by using a less-harmful substitute. Exposure may also be minimized by providing ventilation to move large amounts of air and decreasing the concentration of the substance that might cause health problems. Sometimes product, process, or emissions standards are set. When product standards are established, sometimes the product can be redesigned to minimize the amount of substance required. An example would be to use alkaline batteries instead of cadmium batteries. Process standards may set limits of harmful by-products such as mercury or dioxin by providing tax incentives to businesses to find ways of diverting or recycling them. Emission standards for pollutants can be set and monitored so when conditions become hazardous, immediate interventions can contain risks to the public. An example would be to monitor smog levels and alert citizens that levels are such that individuals with asthma, emphysema, or other breathing problems should remain inside or limit outdoor activities. In the situation where an accident has spilled hazardous materials over public roads or on private property, the clean-up can take place immediately, diverting traffic and halting or moving other activities where citizens may be unnecessarily exposed while cleanup crews work on the area.

When control at the source is not possible or if it is not the sole means of controlling potential exposure, **control along the path** is used. In situations where the transport of hazardous materials is unavoidable, standards can be established for packaging, handling, transportation, storage, and disposal procedures. If potential exposure is at a work site, provide ventilation, protective barriers, and other measures so that exposure is reduced or eliminated. An example would be to keep workers away from excessive noise, installing acoustic barriers on walls or ceiling, or providing frequent breaks from the noise. An example of this type of control was when miners used canaries underground with them to detect harmful gases. If the small birds showed effects of the gas, the miners could escape before they were overcome.

If neither of these measures are feasible, **control at the level of the person** is used by providing protective equipment, quality control, immunization, safety training, and other preventive measures to provide some assurance that the individual handling the material has minimal risk. Examples of this type of control would be the training of personnel to wear face masks, self-contained breathing devices, reflective clothing, badges, gloves, rubber boots, safety goggles, hard hats, and/or ear plugs. When chemicals are used, showers are installed nearby so if the chemical are inadvertently splashed on a person, they can be immediately washed off before damage occurs. In health care settings, workers are required to have tuberculosis screening and hepatitis B vaccinations for their own safety.

Secondary prevention consists of **early detection** when exposure is determined and remedial efforts are used to treat the individual or other contaminated area. Health physicists may determine ion exposure and require hazard management procedures to dispose of contaminated material and decontamination procedures. If the individual has suffered injuries as a result of the contamination, they may require medical treatment or hospitalization.

When an emergency spill has occurred, the material must be controlled or contained, the extent of the damage must be determined, affected individuals must be identified, and survivors should be monitored. The protection and treatment of emergency care workers is also very important.

Special procedures are necessary and need to be rehearsed using "mock situations" and "trial runs" so that personnel can respond quickly and appropriately if an emergency should occur.

TERTIARY PREVENTION

A third type of prevention, not always considered as prevention, is the application of occupational and environmental medicine. Once an exposed individual is identified, evaluated, and treated, the prevention of a chronic ailment or disorder becomes the goal. A physician with this type of expertise must first be able to diagnose the problem and distinguish it as an environmental disease rather than another type of diagnosis. Physicians may know that wrist problems related to repetitive work could be the cause of carpal tunnel syndrome. Although the treatment or rehabilitation for an environmental disease may be the same as one with a different etiology, the physician may be called upon to identify a disability that reduces the worker's capacity to work or prevents them from working at all. Evaluation of worker's compensation claims is an important part of an occupational and environmental medical professional.

RISK MANAGEMENT STRATEGIES

Risk management utilizes risk assessment information and determinations in a way that aids economic, social, political, and legal entities in making decisions about the best course of action. The problem may be prevented or an existing problem may need to be solved. Risk management strategies include:

- developing policies
- establishing priorities
- enacting statutes
- processing regulations and standards

- surveillance
- inspection
- issuing permits
- conducting epidemiological investigations
- holding public hearings
- providing public information
- fostering community support
- issuing administrative orders
- implementing embargoes
- issuing court orders or mandates
- charging offenders with citations
- imposing court or administrative penalties

Communication of Risk

he way information is disseminated or exchanged about the existence of a hazard, the nature of the substance, the severity of the risk, and acceptability of risk factors must be carefully considered. The communication of risk among scientists is handled differently than the way special interest groups and government officials communicate the risk to citizens. Scientists may appear to "sound the alarm" in a way that may sound like a doomsday prediction if nothing is done about it. After a risk has been confirmed by scientists, national organizations already aware of the issue

Policies
Principles, plans, or course of action for wise conduct or management.

Protocol
A formal set of rules and procedures to be followed during a particular research experiment, course of treatment, or situation.

Liability
The legal obligation or responsibility implied.

Control at the source
To prevent exposure from the point of origination.

Control along the path
Measures taken to minimize exposure when transporting the material.

Control at the level of the person
Equipment and training to provide minimal risk to the person handling the agent.

Early detection
To detect exposure before harm is done.

may magnify the problem to create public concern and, for instance, to draw in contributions to fund special projects. When information is given to those who have the power and authority to make decisions, information must be objective so that community leaders are not swayed or biased. When government officials plan risk communication for the public, it can become a delicate matter. Sometimes the media can distort facts and misquote representatives, creating public outrage. If this is a possibility, officials may issue a press release using their own words. The primary reason why risk communication can be a delicate matter is that individuals and groups may react differently when the same information is received. The possible ways information can be interpreted and acted upon include:

denying that there is a problem so it will not be exaggerated by the media

suppressing the information because it is too difficult to think consider

redefining the problem so positive effects are told first to diminish the negative impact on citizens (a good news, bad news scenario)

stating information in a way that sounds acceptable because there is nothing that can be done about it

amplifying concerns because of stressors and other factors making the problem seem larger than it is by itself

The communication of risks or potential risks can be done through various types of media, such as television spots, public service announcements (PSAs), billboards, local meetings, and educational programs. When federal, state, or county agencies are involved, the messages usually must be approved by public relations representatives before statements are released. If the reason for the communication is to encourage action by the individual, tailored messages must be used to promote behavior change. Different approaches must be used according to the needs, interests, attitudes, and skills of various types of individuals, groups, or communities.

Risk Monitoring

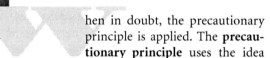

hen hazards have been identified, risks have been communicated, messages encouraging behavior changes have been distributed, and skills have been taught, the effectiveness of these techniques must be monitored. One example to monitor changes that have occurred is to regularly check emissions levels to see if atmospheric concentrations have decreased once control measures were implemented. This is known as checking the **air quality index**. Water samples can also be checked regularly to be certain that bacterial contamination and chlorine levels are satisfactory. Other monitoring includes regular inspections of restaurants and food service units, animal control, meat inspection, pesticide regulation, and radiation protection.

Another epidemiological study may be conducted to see if the incidence of new cases has decreased. The problem with epidemiological studies is that they require a great deal of time. Sometimes surveillance studies can be used by drawing blood samples and comparing them to baseline measures to see if the risks have increased, stayed the same, or decreased.

Increasingly, geographic information systems (GISs), remote sensing, and other related technologies are being used to study disease patterns and their geographical environments. The GIS applications have described the source, geographic distribution, and regions where people may be exposed to toxic and pathological agents. GISs are also being used to monitor water supplies, emissions, pollutant levels, and land uses.

Protecting the Public

hen in doubt, the precautionary principle is applied. The **precautionary principle** uses the idea that when threats of significant harm are evident, even in the face of scientific uncertainty, precautions should be taken to protect the public health and the environment. The precautionary principle urges the need for better ways of determining health risks due to environmental factors so that actions can be taken. The precautionary principle is based on:

■ Threat of potential harm. Harm can occur at the cellular level, for one individual, for a community or population, or an entire ecosystem.

■ Scientific uncertainty. The ability to predict harm requires the use of current knowledge, scientific measures, and methods available to reduce the potential for harm.

■ Precautionary action. Measures can be taken to reduce known and unknown risks.

The precautionary principle emphasizes anticipation and avoidance of damages from environmental hazards before they occur or to detect them early.

The term originates from the German environmental policies calling for *vorsorge* ("prior care, foresight, forward planning") for cleaner air in the 1970s (Boehmer-Christiansen, 1994). During the Rio Conference in 1992,

United Nations representatives further developed the precautionary principle to include any type of environmental hazard posing a risk to human health (Pugh, 1997). In 1998, the Wingspread Conference was held in Wisconsin inviting scientists, governmental researchers, environmentalists, and labor representatives from the United States, Canada, and Europe to discuss ways of implementing the precautionary principle (see "Interpretations and Intent of the Precautionary Principle"). Since then, the precautionary principle has been applied to public policy decisions about the protection of freshway, land development, genetic engineering, and food safety.

The precautionary principle has ethical underpinnings. **Ethics** involve a sense of what is right from what is wrong, based upon underlying values. Ethical issues prompt the responsibility for preserving what society has now and what will be available in the future. Not everyone shares the same values. Even those with the same values do not share the same philosophical approaches to managing the problem. Although each one can recognize that ecosystems are important and that natural resources should be sustained, not everyone will take action to protect them. Some believe in the right to individual freedoms, which often violate the rights of others, rationalizing that scientific gains will come about to address current problems. Others may believe that the problem is too big and on such a large scale, that only a Higher Power is able to resolve the problems.

Major limitations to the precautionary principle is the fact that scientific proof is difficult to achieve, that science sometimes is in conflict with human values, and that sometimes problems take care of themselves with no action. Even when programs are developed to address problems and successfully implemented, it is difficult to say whether problem reduction was due entirely to the intervention or other forces. Environmental health professionals argue that "something is better than nothing" and being "proactive is better than being reactive." Key issues are whether citizens, government officials, and businesses

---

Ethics
Moral standards, in this instance, as ascribed to by a professional group.

Deny
Declare untrue; refuse to accept as correct.

Suppressing
Keeping information from becoming known.

Air quality index
A guide used to show the amount of outdoor air pollution and health effects.

Precautionary principle
The identification of environmental risks so appropriate action can be taken.

Digging Deeper — INTERPRETATIONS AND INTENT OF THE PRECAUTIONARY PRINCIPLE

The precautionary principle, as stated at the Rio Declaration of 1992:

> When there are threats of serious or irreversible damage, lack of full scientific certainty shall not be used as a reason for postponing cost-effective measures to prevent environmental degradation.

The precautionary principle, as stated at the Wingspread Conference of 1998:

> When an activity raises threats of harm to human health or the environment, precautionary measures should be taken even if some cause-and-effect relationships are not fully established scientifically.

The precautionary principle means more than "foresight planning." It addresses an ethical obligation for mankind to maintain the integrity of natural systems particularly when there is a lack of human understanding concerning the risks due to uncertainty factors. This principle is important because there are economic incentives for delaying action regarding environmental harm or risk. If we intend to sustain our environment, we cannot argue that human innovation, ingenuity, imagination, and adaptation will eventually curtail environmental damage or loss of resources.

Six basic concepts considered in the precautionary principle are:

1. Anticipation that further delay will ultimately prove more costly to nature and society of future generations.

2. Safeguarding ecology rather than widen the margins of tolerance to environmental degradation.

3. Comparison of the risk to future generations when the risk could have been avoided without excessive cost.

4. Duty to change environmental damage with emphasis on the liability of offenders and obligation to correct the situation.

5. Ethical regard for the rights of all to a clean and healthy environment.

6. Regard for the responsibility of all who coexist in the environment with the burden of cost-sharing from the most grievous offenders.

The precautionary principle encourages prudent actions when there is sufficient evidence and the precautions to be taken can be justified; particularly when there is potential irreversibility or harm to future generations (O'Riordan, T., & Cameron, J., 1994).

Environmental Impact Studies

strategy that places some of the responsibility for protecting and preserving the environment is the requirement of environmental impact studies. This measure mandates that government officials and developers share some of the burden in determining how destruction or a change in the ecosystem affects and/or enhances the quality of life for residents and other life. When projects or activities are planned, the results of environmental impact studies are presented before the project can proceed. The studies include the identification and assessment of environmental and health effects of development projects before they are approved. Environmental impact assessments are only estimated guesses based upon findings from similar projects. The impact (or harm) can be physical, ecological, social, cultural, economical, or political. Costs and risks are weighed in regard to economic development as well as human health. Sometimes an alternative design is warranted before the project is approved. Unfortunately, some projects are still approved when it is clear that the environment will be significantly changed because trade-offs are acceptable. For example, when a developer wants to put in a large shopping mall on a wetlands area, the developer can "donate" other land close by to absorb runoff and excessive rainfall so the environmental impact of the mall will be less.

Summary

he difficulty of determining risk associated with exposure to hazardous materials or agents is difficult and not without controversy. In some cases, toxicity can be determined, the biological response can be explained by toxicological investigations, longitudinal studies, and other historical information. Risk can be reduced by creating laws, setting standards, and enforcing compliance with the law. In many cases, the extent to which an agent is established as the primary cause of a health problem is still under speculation and only estimates or educated guesses can be applied. In those instances, the precautionary principle is applied to reduce risk by erring on the side of being too cautious rather than not cautious enough. Oftentimes the risk is weighed according to the costs and benefits involved in reducing the risk for specific health problems. In nearly all cases, there are economical and political issues at odds with personal safety issues. Because the science of de-

termining environmental health risks is still fairly new, the best that can be done is to adhere to the scientific method of inquiry, also known as **experimental design**, to establish cause-and-effect relationships. When this is not possible, **quasi-experimental methods** can be used to determine potential risks for the prediction of problems similar to those already identified. When neither is possible, some degree of risk is accepted. The management of risk includes the communication of risk to public officials and citizens. It calls for surveillance, protective equipment or gear, and containment of a problem to limit the damage likely to occur. In an ideal world, the identification and management of risk would be voluntary. In the world we live in, those who are concerned about the risks and potential risks are needed to sound the alarm, even to the point of being extremist, so that others do not become complacent.

REFERENCES

Agency for Toxic Substances and Disease Registry (ASTDR). (2001). Exposure-disease model. Case studies in environmental medicine: Pediatric environmental health. In: A primer on health risk communication principles and practices. Retrieved January 14, 2005 from http://www.atsdr.cdc.gov/HEC/primer.html.

Boehmer-Christiansen, S. (1994). The precautionary principle in Germany—Enabling government. In O'Riordan, T., & Cameron, J. (Eds). *Interpreting the Precautionary Principle*. London: Earthscan.

Commission on Life Sciences. (2001). Evaluating chemical and other agent exposures for reproductive and developmental toxicity, pg. 198. Washington, DC: National Academies Press.

Ewing, G. (1986). The Surgeon General C. Everett Koop. *Corporate Monthly*, February, pg. 21. Retrieved January 14, 2005 from http://www.surgeongeneral.gov/.

Griffith, J., Aldrich, T., & Dane, W. (2002). Risk assessment, pgs. 212–239. *Environmental Epidemiology and Risk Assessment*. Hoboken, NY: John Wiley & Sons, Inc.

Last, J. M. (Ed.). (1996). A *Dictionary of Epidemiology*. International Epidemiological Association and Oxford University Press. As cited on http://www.cdc.gov/excite/library/glossary.htm\.

McCally, M. (2002). Environment, health, and risk. In McCally, M. (Ed.). *Life support: The Environment and Human Health*. Cambridge, MA: The MIT Press.

Experimental design
The design of a research study that utilizes subjects randomly assigned to either an experimental or a control group for comparison. The experimental group experiences a treatment while the control group experiences no special treatment.

Quasi-experimental method
An experimental method that does not have random assignment into a control group or an experimental group; less controlled than experimental design.

National Research Council (NRC). (1983) Risk assessment in the federal government. Managing the process. Washington, DC: National Academy of Sciences. Retrieved January 14, 2005 from http://www.epa.gov/fedrgstr/EPA-TOX/1998/May/Day-14/t12303.htm.

O'Riordan, T., & Cameron, J. (1994). Interpreting the precautionary principal. Earthscan Publications, Ltd. Retrieved January 14, 2005 from http://dieoff.org/page31.htm.

Pugh, D. (1997). The precautionary principle and science-based limits in regulatory toxicology: the human experience, individual protection. *Archives of Toxicology, Supplement, 18,* 147–154.

RAIS. (2005). Glossary of useful terms found in risk assessment, EMBAM, health physics, and waste management reports. Retrieved January 14, 2005 from http://rais.ornl.gov/homepage/glossary.shtml.

Wingspread Statement. (1998). The precautionary principle. Accomplishments from the 1998 conference, January 23–25, 1998, Racine, Wisconsin. Retrieved January 14, 2005 http://www.johnsonfdn.org/miscellaneous.html.

ASSIGNMENTS

1. Find four Web sites of governmental agencies that have the mandate to regulate environmental hazards to investigate current issues and print the pages for reference.

2. Locate public laws and federal regulations on the Internet for a particular environmental issue of concern in your area and write down the web addresses.

3. Go to the GATHER Web site and find environmental hazard sites in your area, then discuss how further action can be taken by citizens.

4. Copy a GIS map showing distribution of a disease in the United States to show where the highest density of cases are located.

5. Attend a local government meeting (town council or county council) or public hearing to explore current issues of concern between residents, government officials, and business leaders.

6. Debate an environmental issue with another group in your class to see what conflicts arise and how they can be resolved.

7. Develop your own philosophical statement about the certainties of life regarding man, progress, economics, and the environment.

8. Give an example of an environmental health risk and the political environment governing how the risk is communicated to the public.

9. Give an example of how geographic information systems might be used to monitor environmental risks.

10. Provide an example when an environmental impact assessment might be necessary.

SELECTED ENVIRONMENTAL LAWS

1969 *National Environmental Policy Act (PL 91-190)*
Protection of the environment by declaration of a national environmental policy and establishing a Council on Environmental Quality.

1986 *Emergency Planning and Community Right-To-Know Act (EPCRA) (Title III of PL 99-499)*
Help local communities protect public health and the environment from chemical hazards.

SELECTED PROFESSIONAL JOURNALS

Environmental Impact Assessment Review
Health, Risk, and Society
Human and Ecological Risk Assessment Journal
Journal of the National Cancer Institute
Risk Analysis: An International Journal
Risk: Health, Safety, and Environment
Toxicological Sciences

ADDITIONAL READING

Allan, S., Adam, B., & Carter, C. (2000). *Environmental Risks and the Media.* Routledge Publishing.

Bailar, J., & Bailer, A. (2001).The science of risk assessment. In McCally, M. (Ed.). *Life Support: The Environment and Human Health.* Cambridge, MA: The MIT Press.

Cromley, E. (2003). GIS and disease. *Annual Reviews in Public Health, 24,* 7–24.

Hassi, A., Kjellstrom, T., de Kok, T., & Guidotti, T. (2001). Risk assessment. In *Basic Environmental Health.* New York: Oxford University Press.

Ropeik, D., & Gray, G. (2002). *Risk: A Practical Guide for Deciding What's Really Safe and What's Really Dangerous in the World Around You.* Boston: Houghton Mifflin.

Shettler, T., Barrett, K., & Raffensperger, C. (2002). The precautionary principle: A guide for protecting public health and the environment. In McCally, M. (Ed.). *Life Support: The Environment and Human Health.* Cambridge, MA: The MIT Press.

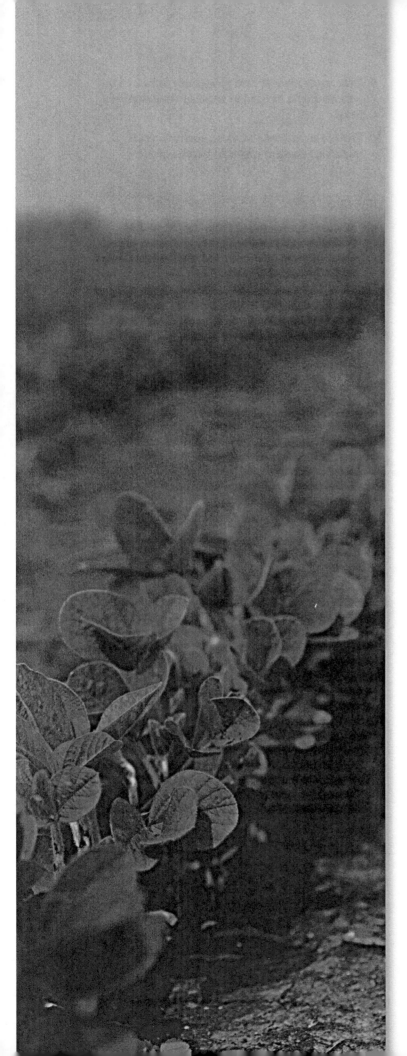

Pests and Pesticides

7

Man has lost the capacity to foresee and to forestall. He will end by destroying the earth.

Rachel Carson, marine biologist (1907–1964)

OBJECTIVES

1. Describe why it is necessary to reduce or eliminate pests in the environment, given what is known about ecosystems.

2. Explain the reason why garbage should be picked up at least twice per week to control fly populations.

3. Provide facts about the control of mosquito populations to prevent diseases.

4. Differentiate the three different types of cockroaches described in the chapter.

5. Explain how fleas and lice are transmitted among animals and humans.

6. Differentiate a deer tick from a dog tick or wood tick.

7. List various diseases associated with rats and mice.

8. Describe health problems associated with stinging insects.

9. Develop a table listing various rodenticides, insecticides, fungicides, and herbicides.

10. Discuss the problems of pesticide-resistant organisms.

Introduction

a **pest** is defined as an unwanted plant or animal. Pests negatively affect human interests such as causing

- loss of agricultural crops, food, and property
- damage to lawns and garden
- disease
- annoyance and discomfort

Unwanted plants are usually known as **weeds**. Some weeds have an oily substance that causes irritation to the skin. Some infectious diseases are transmitted by pests known as vectors (insects and vermin). Some individuals are sensitive to bites, stings, and contact with certain pests and plants.

The control of vector-borne diseases depends upon reducing the number of vectors. The most common type of vectors are arthropods and rodents. Flies, mosquitoes, cockroaches, fleas, body lice, ticks, mice, and rats all need to be controlled to prevent the spread of disease. Where there are human and animal activities, there are pests. Poverty and overpopulation has led to poor sanitation with greater opportunity for vectors. In order to live, pests require water, food, and breeding grounds. Unsanitary conditions provide what they need. Global warming and resistance to insecticides makes the control of disease-carrying insects difficult.

Arthropods

a **rthropods** have jointed appendages, an exoskeleton, and segmented bodies and include insects and arachnids.

INSECTS

Insects include ants, bees, wasps, termites, flies, mosquitoes, cockroaches, fleas, lice, bedbugs, and kissing bugs. Insects have three segments consisting of a head, thorax,

---

Pest
An unwanted insect, plant, or animal causing discomfort, disease, or damage.

Weeds
A plant that invades domesticated land that is usually not wanted; may be a native species.

Arthropods
Insects that have jointed appendages, an exoskeleton, and segmented bodies.

2010 HEALTHY PEOPLE OBJECTIVES

8-13 Reduce pesticide exposures that result in visits to a health care facility.

8-24 Reduce exposure to pesticides as measured by urine concentrations of metabolites [1-napthol (carbaryl), paranitrophenol (methyl parathion and parathions), 3, 5, 6-trichloro-2-pyridinal (chlorpyrifos), isopropoxyphenol (propoxur)].

Digging Deeper

Rachel Carson was a marine biologist, trained at Johns Hopkins University, and a writer. Born in Pennsylvania in 1907, Carson taught zoology at the University of Maryland and eventually took a job with the U.S. Fish and Wildlife Service. After her retirement, she began to write, and in 1952 she published *The Sea Around Us,* a bestseller. *The Edge of the Sea* was published in 1956. She published *Silent Spring* in 1962, describing how pesticides were affecting the air, water, and land to the extent that they were doing more harm than good. *Silent Spring* illuminated the harmful effects on lakes, rivers, oceans, and humans, of DDT

and other chemicals used to increase agricultural productivity. *Silent Spring* was pronounced the most influential book of its time. Carson testified in front of the U.S. Congress calling for new policies to protect human health. Rachel Carson and *Silent Spring* are often credited with the establishment of the U.S. Environmental Protection Agency and introduction of the term *ecosystem* to the general public.

Source: www.rachelcarson.org, a Web site devoted to the life and legacy of Rachel Carson.

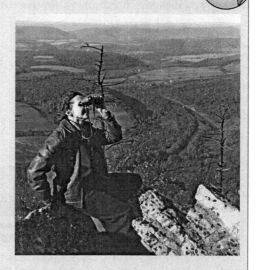

and abdomen. The head has a mouth, antennae, and eyes. Houseflies regurgitate fluids onto solid foods, liquefy them, and suck them up. They can carry pathogens on the body or in the digestive tract. Mosquitoes and fleas pierce the skin. Pathogens are inoculated into the bloodstream of their human victim while the insect feeds on the blood.

Most insects pass through a complete or incomplete metamorphosis. Insects such as roaches and lice go through three stages: egg, nymph, and adult. Mosquitoes and flies go through four stages of metamorphosis: egg, larvae, pupa, and adult (Figure 7-1). As insects develop, they molt by shedding their exoskeleton, forming a new skeleton underneath.

Flies

There are thousands of species of flies, several of which carry diseases. Flies can be categorized as nonbiting and biting. Nonbiting flies include the housefly or blow fly and absorb their food. Houseflies have spongy mouth parts. Houseflies "test" the food, excrete saliva or vomitus dissolving the food, and leave a light brown spot. The housefly is an important vector carrying food-borne illnesses. Houseflies travel several miles in 1 day feeding upon waste materials transporting pathogens on their bodies and in their feces. Nonbiting flies can carry salmonellosis, cholera, dystentery, typhoid, hookworm, pinworm, and whipworm.

Biting flies include black flies, deer flies, sand flies, horse flies, and stable flies and require a blood meal. The biting flies have rasping or sucking mouth parts. Because they bite or suck blood, they have the potential to carry bloodborne diseases. Biting flies can carry diseases such as onchocerciasis, African sleeping sickness, deerfly fever, and African eye worm disease. If an individual is bitten several times, they may have an anaphylactic reaction that begins with large blotchy, red-and-white hives, intense itching, and difficulty breathing as airways swell.

Flies breed rapidly laying several batches of 75 to 150 eggs on organic materials such as garbage and manure. Some species lay their eggs in wounds, hatching into larvae within hours (known as **maggots**), invading living tissue. The larval stage lasts approximately 4 to 7 days, entering into a pupa stage of 3 days to several weeks, depending on the temperature. Maturing very quickly, flies reach the adult stage within 1 to 2 weeks and begin to lay eggs of their own.

Because they multiply and grow rapidly, the control of flies through the handling of garbage, manure, and dead animals need to be managed by covering open containers, hauling trash away frequently, and either burying or incinerating waste materials. This is the reason why garbage needs to be kept in a covered trash can and removed at least twice each week. Additional measures should be used to protect food and humans from flies. The best way to keep flies out of buildings is to have screened areas around entrances. Fly strips with chemicals to attract them to the sticky surfaces can also be used.

Mosquitoes

Mosquitoes transmit all types of diseases including malaria, dengue fever, yellow fever, encephalitis, and West Nile fever. There are 3,000 species of mosquitoes worldwide (Clements, 1999, as cited in Crans, 2004). The species of most interest to public health officials are the *Culex, Aedes* (Figure 7-2), and *Anopheles* mosquitoes. The *Culex* species, known as house mosquitoes, carry encephalitis. *Aedes aegypti* carry the yellow fever virus. *Aedes albopictus* (known as the Asian Tiger mosquito) carries dengue fever, encephalitis, yellow fever, and the West Nile fever (Figure 7-3). *Anopheles* mosquitoes carry malaria. *Anopheles* mosquitoes transmit the malarial parasite *Plasmodium* while feeding on a blood meal. The parasites destroy red blood cells within 36 to 72 hours after the person has been bitten.

FIGURE 7-1 **House Fly Cycle**
This cycle occurs over the course of a few days. Source: Clemson University. Reprinted with permission.

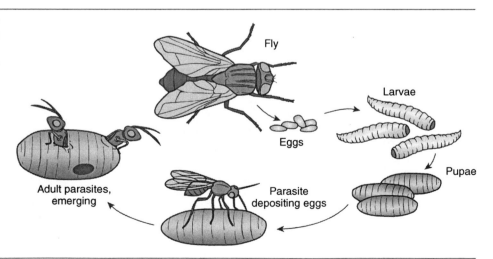

Fly

Eggs

Larvae

Pupae

Parasite depositing eggs

Adult parasites, emerging

Mosquitoes breed in stagnant water and produce larvae. All mosquitoes need water during their early life stages. Flood water, standing water, and ponds or lakes are where most mosquitoes lay their eggs. Mosquitoes lay several batches of 50 to 200 eggs, depending on the species (Clemson Extension Home & Garden Information Center, 2004). Mosquitoes go through four stages in the water. Eggs hatch into larvae or "wrigglers" that change into pupae or "tumblers" and then adults. It only takes about 5 days for a mosquito to change from an egg to an adult in hot, humid weather. Adults leave the water and seek vegetation to dry out. After they feed on bits of organic matter and mate, the female searches for a blood meal. The female mosquitoes are the ones that bite because they need the protein in blood to develop their

> The Asian Tiger Mosquito (*Aedes albopictus*) is an aggressive mosquito that has been spreading through the United States since its importation in 1985 in a load of used truck tires shipped from Japan to Texas.

eggs. The female mosquito has an elongated proboscis used for piercing and sucking. While the mosquito is feeding on its host, it injects saliva into the skin. The saliva prevents clotting and causes itching. The female lives from a few days to a few weeks, depending on the temperature. Mosquitoes can travel several miles to feed on humans, cattle, horses, domestic pets, and wildlife.

Control of mosquitoes can be done at the larvae or adult stage. Larvae may be controlled by chemicals, biological controls, or mechanical means. The most effective way is to eliminate standing or stagnant water in tin cans, flower pots, discarded tires, wading pools, bird baths, pet dishes, clogged gutters, refuse, ditches, and so forth. Modifying water flow in irrigation systems so water does not stagnate is also helpful. The addition of oil or pesticides to surface water has been effective, but present other environmental concerns. Adult mosquitoes can be temporarily controlled by area spraying with carbaryl or malathion. Mosquito traps can also be used to collect mature adults and larvae. Mosquito pesticides, often referred to as *dunks,* are placed into the water where mosquitoes accumulate, killing mosquitoes and their larvae (Rose, 2001). Homeowners can use screens or mosquito netting. Repellents such as DEET and Ind-

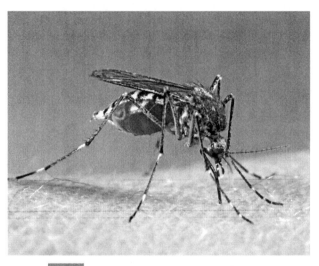

FIGURE 7-2 **Aedes Mosquito** The vector responsible for carrying the West Nile virus.

Maggots
The larvae stage of the fly life cycle lasting 4 to 7 days.

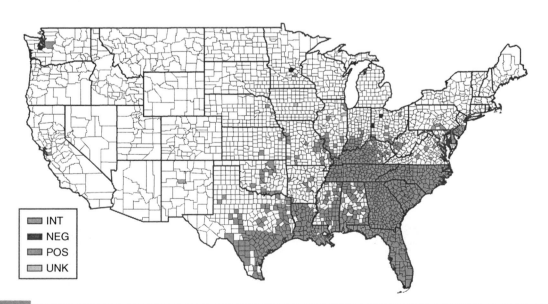

INT
NEG
POS
UNK

FIGURE 7-3 **Distribution of Aedes Albopictus, 2000.** Source: CDC.

alone offer some protection, but vary in effectiveness, depending on the species.

Mosquitoes are attracted to people by perfume, hair spray, deodorant, skin odors, and carbon dioxide from breath. Mosquitoes are most likely to swarm and bite when the sun is beginning to rise (dawn) or set (dusk) or in shady areas. Some species bite any time of the day; others prefer to bite after sunset. When outdoors, find an open, sunny spot away from trees, bushes, or high grass. Avoid going out unprotected at night or on cool or overcast days. Wearing long-sleeved shirts and pants in areas known for their mosquito populations (marshes, near standing water, or by roadside ditches) is always a good idea.

Screens and netting are also effective to keep mosquitoes from entering the home or biting. Some people spray their yards, light cigarettes or cigars, burn citronella candles, or plug in "bug zappers" to discourage mosquitoes, but these methods will not keep mosquitoes from biting. Foggers and yard sprays contain permethrin, a pesticide that kills and repels mosquitoes for several hours. Yard sprays should be sprayed around the perimeter of an outdoor area. A problem with foggers is that a slight breeze will carry it away from the desired site and they do not last long. Tobacco smoke may eliminate a few extra bites, but is not an effective mosquito repellent or insecticide (Ware & Whitacre, 2004). Citronella candles or torches filled with citronella oil and burned can be effective deterrents, but some individuals are sensitive to the smoke from citronella candles. Bug zappers are more likely to kill other insects, such as moths. Bug zappers work by luring insects into an area with ultraviolet light. New devices, known as "mosquito trappers," convert propane to carbon dioxide by attracting female mosquitoes. The best biological defense against mosquitoes are bats and birds. All of these methods, however, are not effective in controlling or repelling mosquitoes (Crans, 2004).

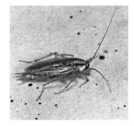

FIGURE 7-4 American Cockroach

The Centers for Disease Control and Prevention recommend that people use skin repellent when working, playing, eating, or resting in outdoor environments. The most effective mosquito repellent is N, N diethyl-m-toluamide (DEET) because it works the longest. A product containing 23.8% DEET will provide about 5 hours of protection; 20% for about 4 hours; and 6.65% for about 2 hours. Do not apply to eyes, lips, and mucous membranes or on skin that is cut, has an abrasion, or a rash. Open areas on the skin make it easier to absorb toxic amounts of DEET. The American Academy of Pediatrics recommends using low concentrations of DEET (10% or less) on children ages 2 to 12 years of age. Because children rub their eyes and often do not wash before they eat, it is a good idea not to put DEET on the hands of children. Bracelets do not provide full coverage. Insect repellents lose their effectiveness over a few hours or they may be washed away by sweating, swimming, or rain. Repellents also can harm certain fabrics. People with suspected metabolic disorders should check with their physician before using DEET.

Cockroaches

There are several species of roaches such as the American cockroach (*Periplaneta Americana*) (Figure 7-4), the German cockroach (*Blattella germanica*) (Figure 7-5), and the Oriental cockroach (*Blatte orientales*) (Figure 7-6). The American cockroach is the largest, growing up to two inches long. They are also known as water bugs and Palmetto bugs, depending on which area of the country they are found. Adults are brown to reddish brown in color. The German cockroach is pale yellowish-brown with two dark brown stripes on the head. The Oriental cockroach can be dark brown or black and are often referred to as sewer roaches.

Roaches carry their eggs in a capsule and attach them to an object out of sight. Cockroaches have a three-stage life cycle: egg, nymph, and adult. Nymphs hatch in 2 to 3 months and molt several times before reading the adult stage approximately 600 days later (Bell & Adiyodi, 1981). Cockroaches prefer dark, moist environments. They may also live in old bags or cartons carried home from the grocery store. They can hide in any crack or crevice. Roaches feed on manure, decayed food, glue, and any other accessible food. Diseases may be carried on the body or in the in-

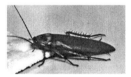

FIGURE 7-5 German Cockroach

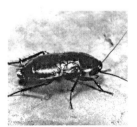

FIGURE 7-6 Oriental Cockroach

testines. When they eat, they regurgitate, transferring any pathogens they may be carrying onto food. No specific disease has been identified with the roach, but they have been known to aggravate allergies in infants and young children. To prevent cockroach infestations, the best methods are to keep food in covered storage containers, wipe up crumbs, keep kitchen and bathroom areas dry, and seal cracks. Dusting with borax powder is helpful. Organophosphate poisons such as malathion are also effective.

Fleas

Fleas (Figure 7-7) carry pathogens and usually access humans through pets or vermin. They feed on the blood of warm-blooded animals. Several species have the capacity to bite humans including the dog and cat flea (*Ctenocephalides*), the human flea (*Pulex irritans*), and the rat flea (*Xenopsylla cheopis*). After the female flea consumes a blood meal, she mates and lays her eggs. The eggs progress to an adult stage within 3 to 4 weeks (Robinson & Meola, 1997). Fleas are notorious for carrying the plague, typhus, tularemia, and salmonellosis. The rat flea carried the plague (*Yersinia pestis*) and typhus (*Rickettsia typhi*) from rat to rat and rat to human during the fourteenth century in Europe. The plague is still seen in India today. The plague is found in prairie dogs, chipmunks, and squirrels in the southwestern United States. Fleas are difficult to control in warm climate areas. The best way to prevent them is to treat infested animals and areas with a pesticide dust (flea powder).

Lice

Lice (Figure 7-8) have the capacity to bite and inject saliva into the bite, causing itching. Lice lay their eggs (or "nits") on hair and skin, depending on the species. The nits hatch

as nymph in 6 to 10 days and become adults in 10 days. Adult lice live on human hosts for about 30 days (CDC, 2003). There are three kinds of lice: the head louse (*Pediculis humanis capitis*), the body louse (*Pediculis humanis corporis*), and the crab louse (*Pthirius pubis*). Head lice is very common in preschool and elementary children and their families. Body lice can carry typhus (*Rickettsia prowazekii*), trench fever (*Rickettsia quintana*), and relapsing fever (*Borrelia spirochetes*). The disease is usually found in crowded and unsanitary conditions. Lice are transmitted by infected clothing, hair brushes, or direct contact with a person carrying the lice. The most common transmission of pubic lice, also known as "the crabs," is sexual intercourse.

Bedbugs

There are about seven species of bedbugs (Figure 7-9). The most common species in the United States is *Cimex lectularis*. Bedbugs come out at night to feed on humans and warm-blooded animals. Bedbugs do not carry diseases because infectious agents do not reproduce in them, however, a bite from a bedbug will make an itchy welt. Bedbug infestations in a home are difficult to control without the use of pesticides because they can live for a year without a blood feeding. Bedbugs hide in bedsprings, mattresses, and cracks in the wall.

Kissing Bugs

The kissing bug (*Triatoma*) (Figure 7-10) is found primarily in Mexico, Central America, South America, and in the southern United States (Vetter, 2001). They are carried by rodents, armadillos, and opossums. The bug lives in the crevices and cracks of stone or mud huts with

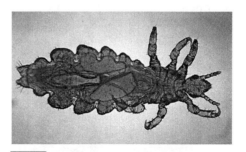

FIGURE 7-8 **Female Head Lice**

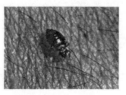

FIGURE 7-9 **Bed Bug**

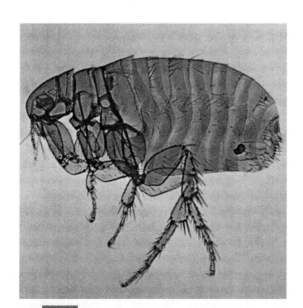

FIGURE 7-7 **Flea**

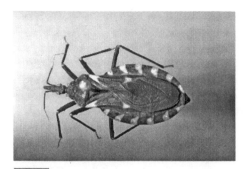

FIGURE 7-10 **Kissing Bug**

thatched roofs. It is distinguished from the bedbug by its well-defined wings. The bug appears at night and bites its victim near the lips, hence its name. It carries the protozoan parasite *Trypanosoma cruizi,* which is in the feces of the kissing bug. When a person scratches their skin, they may rub the kissing bug and its feces into an open bite wound. The disease causes severe inflammation, paralysis, and death in 10% of those affected.

Fire Ants

Most ants pose little problems unless they enter the house and get into food supplies. Fire ants are particularly harmful to humans because of their painful sting, ranging from an annoying burning sensation to anaphylactic shock and death. Between 30 to 60% of the population in infested areas are stung each year (Figure 7-11), especially children (Solley, Verderwoude, & Knight, 2002). The fire ant stings multiple times in a circular fashion with its abdominal stinger. The venom causes a welt within 30 to 60 minutes that becomes a pustule within 24 hours. The sting can be treated with anesthetic creams and oral antihistamines. Approximately 4% of those stung by fire ants

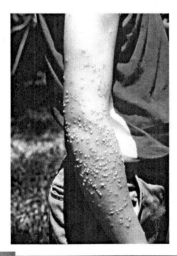

FIGURE 7-11 **Fire Ant Sting Victim**

> ### BIOINVASION: FIRE ANTS
> Red fire ants are an example of **bioinvasion**. They arrived from Paraguay and Brazil on shiploads of lumber to Mobile, Alabama, in the 1957. They have spread through the southern states (Schmidt, 1995; Texas Parks and Wildlife, 2001). They are very aggressive and adapt easily to most environments. However, they are not able to survive in areas where soil temperatures drop to near freezing temperatures for more than 2 to 3 weeks. Fire ants burrow underground to maintain tolerable temperatures. They damage gardens, yards, homes, and other structures in search of water. They can also invade the food supplies (insects, seeds, and young plants) for animals leading to starvation and hydration (Core, 1999). Finally, they severely damage crops and electrical equipment. Damage and control costs are estimated to be more than $6.5 billion each year (Core, 1999).

develop an allergic reaction. Reactions range from rapid flushing to hives; swelling of the face, eyes, or throat; chest pains; nausea; severe sweating; breathing difficulties; and faintness (Solley et al., 2002).

There are four species of fire ants: the red imported fire ant (*Solenopsis invicta*), the black imported fire ant (*Solenopsis richteri*), Southern fire ant (*Solenopsis xyloni*), and Tropical fire ant (*Solenopsis germinate*) (Tvedten, 2004). The black fire ant is similar to the red imported fire ant. It is found in northern Mississippi and Alabama. The Southern fire ant is found from North Carolina to northern Florida, along the Gulf Coast, and west to California. The Tropical fire ant is found from South Carolina to Florida and west to Texas.

These ants live in large colonies in dome-shaped mounts in sunny, open areas along highways, open fields, and yards. Spring and summer is mating season for fire ants. After mating, the females become queens and they burrow underground to lay their eggs and begin a new colony. Killing the queen is essential to eliminating the entire colony. Fire ant mounds can be very large and include as many as 200,000 ants. The queen may live up to 7 years of age. Fire ants travel up to 100 yards from their mound for food.

Control of fire ants is difficult because they reproduce rapidly. From the 1950s through the 1970s, helptachlor and mirex was used and was somewhat successful. Because the poisons killed wildlife as well, this practice was halted (Rigatuso, Bertoluzzo, Quattrin, & Bertoluzzo, 2000). The best way to eliminate fire ants is to apply a fire ant bait or granular insecticide. Baits are insecticides mixed with ant attractants. Baits are safer to use because they break down quickly when they get wet or are left in full sun. The best time to use fire ant bait is when ants are foraging for food, during 70 to 80°F temperatures. Worker ants carry it into the mound and break the bait into a liquid, feeding it back to the workers and queen. Granular insecticides can be applied directly to the mound or spread around the area. Granular, or contact, insecticides are faster acting. However, some granular insecticides last over 1 year and should be used with caution. A natural alternative to insecticides is to pour boiling water on the mound.

Most recently, scientists are trying a parasitic fly, known as the **phorid fly**, which is attracted to swarming fire ants. The fly hovers over the ants, looking for a victim. It then attacks the ant and lays its eggs in the fire ant's body, leaving the ant partly paralyzed and disoriented. The injected egg develops in the ant's thorax. Ten days later, the ant dies as the larva moves into its head. The head falls off and the larva develops inside the ant's body. Because of this process, the phorid fly is sometimes referred to as the decapitating fly. Adult flies emerge from pupae about 45 days after the original attack. This practice is still in the experimental process.

Bees and Wasps

Bees, yellow jackets, hornets, and wasps do not carry diseases, but they sting and some people are allergic to the venom. These flying insects live in nests and the best way to eliminate them is to get rid of the nest. Attempts to kill the insects in a nest should be done if the insects are a threat to people. Application of insecticides should be done at night when most insects are in or on the nest. Wear protective clothing including a hat, long pants, long-sleeved shirt, jacket, and netting over the head. Do not use a flashlight because it may attract the insects.

Termites

Termites (Figure 7-12) are small insects that cause severe destruction to wood. This is a problem unless the wood is intended to be recycled. They create tunnels making the wood porous, therefore collapsing utility poles, homes, and other structures. Termite colonies have a king, a queen, soldiers, and workers. Termites go through three stages: egg, nymph, and adult. Most species of termites have protozoa in their intestines that convert the wood into food for the colony (Lewis, 2001).

Signs of termite damage include "mud tubes" on the inside and outside surfaces of wood or damaged wood hollowed along the grain of the wood, lined with bits of mud or soil. To prevent termite infestations in the home:

1. Have a termite inspection (usually required by law) before purchasing a house.

2. Use decorative wood chips and mulch sparingly.

3. Never store firewood, lumber, or other wood debris against the foundation or inside the crawl space of the house.

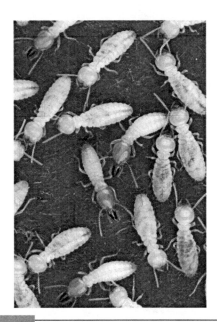

FIGURE 7-12 **Formosan Termite**

4. Don't allow moisture to accumulate near the foundation.

5. Eliminate wood contact with the ground.

ARACHNIDS

Arachnids include spiders, tarantulas, ticks, mites, and scorpions, and are carnivores. They have only one or two main segments: a **cephalothorax** and an abdomen. There are no antennae or wings. They have eight legs, multiple eyes, and use **booklungs** to breathe. The **pedipalp** is used by spiders to feel, and scorpions use them to grab. Their jaws are called **chelicerae** and have sharp fangs to burrow

---

Bioinvasion
The transfer of a species to another ecosystem that results in an overgrowth of the species.

Phorid fly
A type of fly that attacks and kills fire ants.

Cephalothorax
The head (cephalo) and thorax; one segment of the two arachnid body segments.

Booklungs
Lungs of an arachnid that expand with several layers.

Pedipalp
A set of appendages near the mouth of an arachnid used for feeling, hunting, and reproduction; carry the chelae of a scorpion.

Chelicerae
The fangs or claws of an arachnid used for grasping or piercing.

into the ground, inject venom into their prey (which breaks down the tissues), and suck their food.

Spiders and Tarantulas

There are many species of spiders. A tarantula is a large spider. Most species of spiders are harmless and content to live outdoors. The two species of health concern are the brown recluse spiders (Figure 7-13) and the black widow spiders (Figure 7-14).

The brown recluse spider (*Loxosceles recluse*) is not aggressive and may be found in clothing or bedding in the mid-United States (Jones, 2004) (Figure 7-15). It is most active at night, when it searches for food. A brown recluse spider bite is usually uneventful. In some people, however, it can be **cytotoxic**. When this happens, a bluish sinking patch with ragged edges and a surrounding redness appears within 24 to 72 hours, known as the "red, white, and blue sign." There is sometimes a blister. The spider venom has an enzyme that destroys cells in the wound area. Affected tissue gradually sloughs away, exposing underlying tissues. Within 24 hours, the bite site can erupt into a *volcano lesion* (a hole in the flesh due to damaged, gangrenous tissue). The wound becomes **necrotic**, but is treatable.

The black widow spider is more likely to be found outdoors. The venom of a black widow spider is more powerful than snake venom, but the amount of venom in a bite is very small. The reaction to a black widow spider bite depends on the area of the body bitten and sensitivity to the venom (Jones, 2004a). There is usually no swelling, but there will be two faint red puncture spots. There may be a short stabbing pain that progresses to the abdomen and back. Some people experience nausea, perspiration, labored breathing, restlessness, increased blood pressure, tremors, and fever. Symptoms may last one to several days. Fatalities from this spider bite are rare.

Both types of spiders like old rotting wood, such as wood stored outdoors for curing before it is burned in the fireplace. All spiders like damp areas where they can get water and food. Most, however, are considered beneficial because they eat insects. Spiders move into homes with insects so this is another reason to control the insect population.

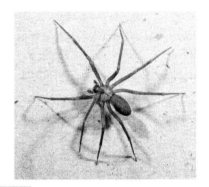

FIGURE 7-13 Brown Recluse Spider

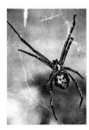

FIGURE 7-14 Black Widow Spider

FIGURE 7-15 **Distribution of Brown Recluse Spider, United States** Source: Rick Vetter, spiders.ucr.edu, http://spiders.ucr.edu/images/colorloxmap.gif. Reprinted with permission.

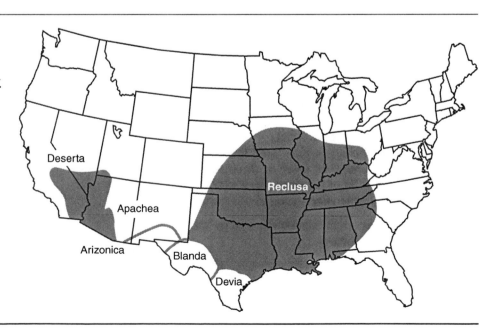

Ticks

Ticks feed on warm-blooded animals by the use of barbed feeding organs that pierce the skin and anchor the tick.

There are hard ticks (*Ixodidae*) and soft ticks (*Argasidae*). Hard ticks include the Brown dog tick (*Rhipecephalus sanguineus*), American dog tick (*Dermacentor variabillis*) (Figure 7-16), and Rocky Mountain wood tick (*Dermacentor andersoni Stiles*). There are three visible components of hard tick mouthparts: palps, chelicerae, and hypostome. The hypostome is a rod-shaped structure that is plunged into the host. A glue-like substance is used to hold it in place while the tick feeds. The tick may feed from several days to weeks while the tick grows from 200 to 600 times their unfed body weight (Vredevoe, 2004). A hard tick known as the deer tick (*Ixodes scapularis*) (Figure 7-17) can carry Lyme disease by transferring the spirochete *Borrelia burdorferi*. Deer ticks are about the size of a pin head, much smaller than the dog tick. The female tick feeds on a deer, mates, lays eggs, and the larvae fall to the ground where they are picked up by grass, leaves, rodents, and other animals. The nymphs cling to humans or animals that brush by them. Ticks can also transmit tularemia, Q fever, and Rocky Mountain spotted fever.

Hard ticks have four distinct life stages: egg, larvae with six legs, nymph with eight legs, and adult with eight legs. The female tick lays one batch of thousands of eggs, then dies. The time to completion of the entire life cycle may vary from less than a year in tropical regions to more than three years in cold climates. Ticks are known for transmitting the widest variety of pathogens including bacteria, rickettsiae, protozoa, and viruses.

Soft ticks include the common fowl tick (*Argas radiatus Raillet*) and the relapsing fever tick (*Ornithodorus turicata*). The life stages and mouthparts of soft ticks are not as distinguishable. The outside surface, or cuticle, expands from 5 to 10 times their unfed body weight.

Ticks like grassy and wooded areas. To prevent tick populations from breeding, it is best to keep grass cut short. When hiking or camping, wear long-sleeved shirts and long pants with the legs tucked into boots. Tie long hair back. Pets should be inspected often for ticks using a fine-toothed tick comb and flea and tick collars are helpful. When finding a tick, remove it with a pair of tweezers by the head. Clean the bite wound with soap and water. Despite urban tales, do not apply kerosene or Vaseline or use a hot match or a cigarette butt to remove the tick.

Mites

Mites (Figure 7-18) are extremely small and may not be easily seen. They develop from eggs into larvae, nymphs, and adults within 2 to 3 weeks. Mites live in

Cytotoxic
Toxic to cells; causes cells to die; destroys tissue cells.

Necrotic
The death of cells due to an infection or disruption of the blood supply.

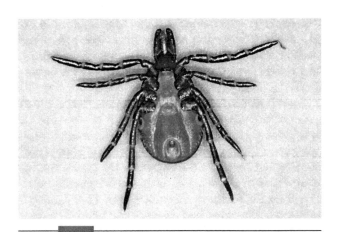

FIGURE 7-17 **Deer Tick**

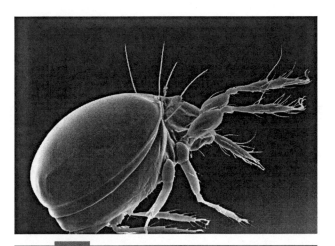

FIGURE 7-18 **Dust Mite**

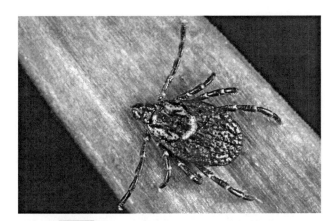

FIGURE 7-16 **American Dog Tick**

areas where human body cells are shed and body oils accumulate such as mattresses, couches, and beds. The scabies mite (*Scarcoptes scabiei*) burrows under the skin to lay its eggs. This causes intense itching, rashes, and redness on the skin. Mites are transmitted by direct contact with a person or an animal with mange. Mites can be carried by birds and rodents. A mite known as a chigger or redbug is the larvae of mites. They attach to the skin, inject saliva, and cause a welt to form. Mites can be vectors for scrub typhus, rickettsial pox, hemorrhagic fever, and encephalitis. Mites can be kept out of the house by keeping things cleaned and vacuumed.

Scorpions

Scorpions are found nearly everywhere, not just in desert areas (Figure 7-19). They are venomous creatures, but only one species presents a serious harm to humans. The world's most dangerous scorpions live in North Africa and the Middle East (species of *Androctonus, Buthus, Hottentotta, Leiurus*), South America (*Tityus*), India (*Mesobuthus*), and Mexico (*Centruoides*). The species most commonly found in the United States (*Centruroides exilicauda*) is found in the Southwest. The venom may produce severe pain and swelling, difficulties in breathing, muscle twitching, and convulsions. Death is rare if treatment is immediate.

Scorpions produce 25 to 35 embryos in the female ovariuterus. When they are born, they live on the mother's back for about a week, until they molt. Scorpions have a long gestation period, varying from several months to 18 months during which the young develop as embryos in the female's ovariuterus, gaining nutrients from the mother's digestive gland. They can live 3 to 5 years. Scorpions feed on pests and build their nests in mulch and woodpiles. Removing these items from the yard is a good way to control them.

Rodents

Rodents are mammals with teeth and jaws for gnawing. Without frequent gnawing their teeth can grow 5 to 6 inches long in 1 year. The destruction from gnawing is the most common problem associated with the animals.

Rodents are most active at night. Feces, nesting materials, holes gnawed into walls, or seeing a rodent during the day is an indication of infestation. Rats and mice usually go where there is food. Grain or pet food should be kept in a large metal container with a tight lid. There are two ways of getting rid of rats and mice: trapping or poison (Public Health Seattle and King County, 2004). For mice, traps may be successful. Discard the trap along with the mouse. Rats are harder to trap.

The house mouse (*Mus musculus*) (Figure 7-20) thrives wherever people live. It takes 19 to 29 days after impregnation for a mouse to have a litter (Timm, 2000). They can produce up to 5 to 10 litters per year with 5 to 6 young, and live indoors or outdoors. The deer mouse (*Peromyscus maniculatis*), known to carry the hantavirus, normally lives in the forest and meadows and feeds on nuts, fruits, and insects.

There are two main species of rats in the United States: the roof rat (*Rattus rattus*), also known as the black rat (Figure 7-21), and the Norway rat (*Rattus norvegicus*), also known as the brown rat (Figure 7-22). The female rat bears offspring 22 days after impregnation. Rats can have 4 to 6 litters per year with 6 to 8 offspring per litter. Rats reach sexual maturity 3 to 5 months after they are born. The roof rat prefers to live in attics, barns, and warehouses. The Norway rat arrived in the United States on boats during the 1600s and tends to burrow under foundations, along river banks, under garbage, and in lumber piles. They live in sewers and in the walls. Rats can pass through a hole the size of a quarter, climb vertically up a wall, jump over obstacles three feet high, walk on wires,

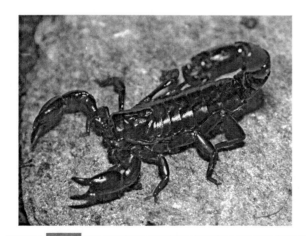

FIGURE 7-19 **Scorpion**

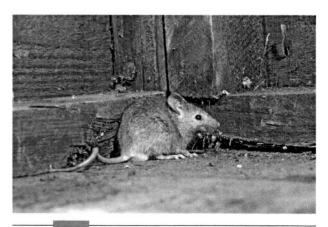

FIGURE 7-20 **House Mouse**

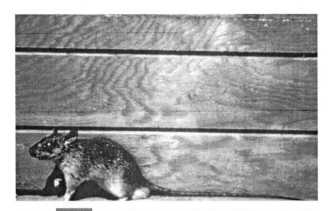

FIGURE 7-21 Roof Rat

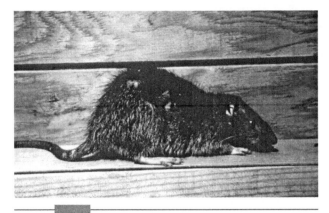

FIGURE 7-22 Norway Rat

and swim in the water. Rats damage food stores, contaminate food, and damage materials. They gnaw their way through walls and doors and can eat the coating from electrical wires, causing fires. Rats thrive in areas of poverty where there is garbage and poor sanitation. Rats can carry the plague, rickettsial pox, murine typhus, rat bite fever, lassa fever, salmonellosis, and trichinosis.

OTHER PESTS

There are other pests that cause property damage, can bite or sting, scare, or annoy people. Bees and wasps can sting. Snakes known as vipers bite and can damage skin, cause neurological problems, and left untreated, result in death. Wildlife such as bats, squirrels, skunks, deer, armadillos, racoons, bear, and feral cats can damage vegetation and lawns, and transmit diseases.

Pest Control and Elimination Methods

Pesticides control insects, fungus, weeds, worms, and rodents that destroy crops, buildings, and ornamental vegetation. Pesticides include insecticide, fungicide, herbicide, ascaricide, and rodenticide. Pesticide use is common in the United States to boost crop yield in agriculture. The goal of this first "green revolution" was to produce more crop yield in an effort to reduce world hunger.

The use of chemical pesticides began in the 1930s and became widespread after World War II (Table 7-1). There are five principal classes of pesticides: organochlorines, organophosphates, carbamates, pyrethroids, and phenoxy herbicides. Organochlorines, organophosphates, carbamates, and pyrethroids are used as insecticides. The organochlorines, developed in 1939 and used in 1942, were the first to be used extensively for agri-

culture and forestry. Some organochlorines, such as DDT (dichlorodiphenyltrichloroethane), were eventually banned because they persisted in the environment (CDC, 2004). Organophosphates were then developed but were highly toxic to humans. Carbamates were developed and became popular because they were not persistent in the environment, but still toxic to birds and fish. Synthetic pyrethroids were developed in the 1940s but not introduced until the 1970s and were found to be more stable to light, stronger than other chemical pesticides, and not harmful to birds or mammals, but still toxic to aquatic species. Phenoxy pesticides were developed in the 1940s.

Pesticides have become controversial because of their harmful effects on birds, fish, animals, and humans. The problem with pesticide use is that the pesticides may have harmful long-term effects on those who work in plants that manufacture the pesticides; those who use pesticides such as farm workers, aerial crop dusting pilots, or professional pest control workers; and vulnerable individuals, particularly children.

Pesticides
Substances used to kill insects, rodents, plants, and fungus; also includes insect and animal repellants, antimicrobial and cleaning products, wood and material preservatives, and insect and rodent traps.

Insecticide
A pesticide that kills insects.

Fungicide
A pesticide that kills fungus.

Herbicide
A substance, such as a defoliant, intended to kill weeds or other unwanted plants.

Ascaricide
A pesticide that kills worms.

Rodenticide
A pesticide that kills rodents (mice and rats).

TABLE 7-1 Chemical Pesticides and Their Effects

Class of Chemical Pesticides	First Used	Types	Type of Pesticide	Effects	Current Status
Organochlorines	1940	Dichlorophenylethanes (DDT, methoxychlor, dicofol) Hexachlorocyclohexanes (Lindane) Chlorinated cyclodine (Chlordane, Aldrin, Dieldrin, Endosulfan, Heptachlor) Other (Kepone, Mirex)	Insecticides and fungicides	Persist in the environment, bioaccumulative, endocrine disrupters	DDT banned in the 1960s
Organophosphates	1940s	Most toxic: Phosdrin, Parathion, Dichlorovos, TEPP Moderately toxic: DDVP, Dimethoate, Baytex, Diazinon Less toxic: Ronnel, Gardona, Abate, Malathion	Insecticide, ascaricide	Not persistent in the environment Toxic to humans, cholinesterase-inhibiting	Schradan was discontinued in 1964 with a move toward less toxic groups
Phenoxy	1946	2,4-D 2,4,5-T (Agent Orange)	Herbicide	Selective effects on humans and animals are not well known; potential cause of cancer in laboratory animals; 2,4,5-T is a source of dioxin	2,4-D is widely used 2,4,5-T has been banned in the U.S. and Canada but still used in other parts of the world
Carbamates	1950s	Carbaryl, Methomyl, Propoxur, Baygon	Fungicide, insecticide, ascaricide	Not persistent in the environment Cholinesterase-inhibiting Toxic to birds and fish	Aldicarb was discontinued in 1964
Pyrethroids	1980	Allethrin, Cyfluthrin, Resmethrin, Fenvalerate	Insecticide	Contact poisons, target-specific, toxic to aquatic species	

While some pesticides are highly toxic, others become toxic over time due to **bioaccumulation** or **biomagnification**. DDT was the first most controversial pesticide. It was used during World War II to kill mosquitoes, body lice, and other vectors carrying disease. High levels of DDT interfered with reproductive functions of birds and fish. It received widespread publicity for making the osprey and bald eagle endangered species when it was attributed to soft egg shells that could not develop properly and hatch. Agent Orange (2,4,5-T) was the second most controversial pesticide. It was used during the Vietnam War as a defoliant. The most harmful element of Agent Orange was dioxin. The effects of dioxin include birth defects, neurological and metabolic disorders, and cancer. DDT and Agent Orange have been found in human breast milk.

INSECTICIDES

Insecticides kill insects in different ways. Different types of insecticides include organochlorines, organophosphates, carbamates, and botanical insecticides. Organophosphates,

Possibly one of the worst cases of pesticide misuse was reported in Pascagoula, Mississippi, in 1996. Over 800 residents called the Mississippi Department of Health when they learned their homes were treated with methyl parathion. Methyl parathion, a powerful poison, is intended for outdoor use. Two men were charged with applying the chemicals indoors in homes, businesses, and schools to eradicate cockroaches and ants. Residents alerted the EPA and the Mississippi Department of Health after two infants suffered symptoms of pesticide poisoning. A call was also received from a church inquiring about a yellow stain on walls and carpets and a foul odor after the church had been sprayed. The EPA evacuated 47 homes sprayed by the two men. Six day-care centers voluntarily closed, three others were tested. Two motels were also sampled, and one closed voluntarily. Carol Kemker of the Atlanta regional EPA office said this case "could be one of the worst cases of pesticide misuse" in U.S. history. The men were suspected of having misapplied the pesticide between 5 to 15 years in Alabama, Mississippi, and Louisiana, according to health department officials.

As many as 2,600 homes and 100 businesses, including a day care, in Pascagoula and Hattiesburg were found to be contaminated with methyl parathion. At least two children had died. According to the CDC, similar incidences were reported in Alabama, Arkansas, Illinois, Louisiana, Michigan, Tennessee, and Texas. As of June 1998, 1,863 persons from 478 homes in the U.S. had been relocated until the pesticide could be cleaned up.

Source: CNN.com. Homeowners Worried After Pesticide Misuse. November 18, 1996. http://www.cnn.com/EARTH/9611/18/pesticide.abuse/.

---

organochlorines, and carbamates kill by acting on the nervous system of insects. Insecticides can be contact poisons, stomach poisons, fumigants, or desiccants. Contact poisons penetrate the exoskeleton. Stomach poisons enter the digestive system of biting or chewing insects. Fumigants enter through the respiratory system. A **desiccant** (such as nicotine) removes moisture from insects.

Organochlorines

These insecticides are contact poisons that attach the central nervous. They can kill many different types of insects, but exist in the environment for a long period of time. They are fat-soluble and accumulate in the body system of insects.

Organophosphates

Originally designed as nerve gases for wartime, organophosphates are responsible for more toxic exposures than any other group of pesticides. They vary dramatically in toxicity. One drop of the highly toxic organophosphates can be fatal. This class of pesticides causes more deaths and poisonings than any other category of pesticides.

Carbamates

Carbamates are contact poisons varying in toxicity. They are used as fungicides and insecticides. Some are toxic to fish and birds.

Synthetic Pyrethoids

Synthetic pyrethoids are contact poisons widely used in pest control for home and garden use. They can be used indoors.

Resistance to Pesticides

Insects, being the adaptable creatures they are, can become resistant to pesticides from one generation to another. These "super bugs" develop when all but a few insects survive. The survivors have a selective advantage by having a resistant gene to the pesticide. When these pesticide-resistant insects reproduce, their offspring are also resistant to the pesticide. More than 500 species of insects and mites are resistant to common pesticides, more than twice the number that was resistant just a few decades ago. According to the World Health Organization, 64 species of mosquitoes are pesticide resistant. Because of this, the incidence of malaria is on the rise (Brogdon & McAllister, 1998).

Botanical and Biological Insecticides and Alternatives

There have always been natural means of preventing and eliminating insect invasions. The chrysanthemum plant can be planted in areas where insects can do potential

---

Bioaccumulation
The accumulation of toxic substances in the body over time.

Biomagnification
The concentration of toxins in an organism high on the food chain that accumulates all the toxins present in its prey, possibly reaching lethal doses.

Desiccant
A substance that promotes drying by absorbing and removing moisture.

harm. The plant produces a natural alkaloid (pyrethrum) that kills insects but is not toxic to animals. This same chemical is used in synthetic pyrethroid insecticides. Gardeners can also use a solution of four teaspoons of dishwashing soap and one-quarter cup of water to deter small insects such as asphids, mealybugs, and spidermites. Boric acid is effective in deterring ants, cockroaches, and crickets.

Alternatives to pesticides also include the integration of natural predators. To kill mosquitoes, fish that eat mosquitoes (also known as "mosquitofish" or *Gambusia holbrooki*) can be introduced to water supplies. A protozoan parasite (*Thelohania solenopsae*) can be introduced in a fire ant colony, killing the colony within 9 to 18 months. Use of the phorid fly to kill fire ants is in the experimental stage.

Integrated pest management (IPM) is "the coordinated use of environmental and pest information with available pest control methods to prevent unacceptable levels of pest damage with the most economical and least hazardous means" (EPA, 2004). IPM methods include the introduction of natural predators, pathogens, sex attractants (pheromones), or insect growth regulators. Techniques such as manual trapping, sterilization, host plant resistance, and sanitation are also effective, but take more time. Farmers can use techniques such as crop rotation to control pests, minimizing the use of synthetic pesticide products that linger and accumulate in the environment. Bioengineered bacteria (*Bacillus thurengensis*) produces a protein (Bt toxin) that kills insects that eat it. Bioengineered seeds for soybeans and cotton have been developed.

Poison ivy (*Toxicodendron radicans*) is a plant that most people would not like to see. The plant is identified by its three oval-shaped leaflets with the middle leaflet usually longer than the other two. The leaves may be between 2 to 4 inches in length. Some plants are glossy and others are a dull green. It can be a woody vine, an upright shrub, or trailing plants. The vine is often seen growing on trees for support. The burning, blistery rash of poison ivy is caused by an oil toxicant called **urushiol**, found in all parts of the plant. Some people are more sensitive to urushiol than others. Irritation may begin immediately or take a few days to develop. The rash is followed by blisters that may break and ooze. When coming in contact with poison ivy, wash the area immediately with soap and cool water. Hot water may cause the poison to penetrate the skin faster. Isopropanol alcohol may be used to remove the resin and prevent irritation if it is applied soon enough. Methods for controlling poison ivy is to hand pull small plants with gloves or use an herbicide. Wear protective clothing and wash contaminated clothing separately before washing with other clothes.

Source: Conservation Commission of Missouri (2004).

FUNGICIDES

Fungicides are used to treat molds and rot on crops and seeds. Fungicides may be very specific and control only a few fungi, or general and control a wide range of fungi. They are in the form of wettable powders, dusts, concentrate, and granules. Dangerous fungicides include mancozeb, benomyl, and ziram. Some may contain mercury. Powdered fungicides should not be inhaled. An alternative to fungicide use is to keep excess moisture off of plant leaves. Because some plants do not like to be watered from the top, a drip hose is much better for these types of plants.

HERBICIDES

Herbicides are either selective or nonselective. Selective herbicides kill only broad-leafed dicotyledonous plants. Nonselective herbicides kill any plant with which they come in contact. Herbicides work by preventing photosynthesis, inhibiting enzymes, disrupting cell membranes, or inhibiting root cell division. Some herbicides are applied to the soil before weeds begin to grow (such as atrazine, 2-4,D, and paraquat). Soil-applied herbicides work by inhibiting the growth of roots and new shoots, interfering with photosynthesis, or destroying chlorophyll. Some may be sprayed on the folage (such as sethoxydim, actifluorfen, or paraquat). These work by inhibiting lipid formation, disrupting internal cell membranes, or blocking photosynthesis. Some are applied either to the soil or folage. These work by affecting protein synthesis or plant metabolism and cell division.

Herbicides vary greatly in soil persistence and some may carry over to the next year, especially if there was a drought. One danger of herbicides is that the spray may "drift" to other areas or the person applying the herbicides may become poisoned by direct contact or inhaling it. Dangerous herbicides include 2,4-D; 2,4,5-T; alachlor; amitrole; atrazine; nitrofen; triflualin; hexachlorobenzen; tributyl tin; and zineb. Another danger of herbicides is contamination of surface water and groundwater through stormwater run-off.

Alternatives to Herbicides

The most effective way to remove weeds is to pull them up from the ground or till them away. One way to reduce weeds in the yard without the use of herbicides is to place woven landscape fabric around plants and buildings. The fabric allows air and water to pass through and slows down evaporation.

Mulching will also help keep the weeds down and keep moisture in the soil longer. Mulch is important to control weeds, conserve soil moisture, and improve the nutrient value of soils, but not all mulch is helpful. Toxic or sour mulch can damage or kill plants and lower soil pH. The best way to tell if the mulch is good is to smell it. Good mulch should have an earthy smell like good garden soil or freshly cut wood. Sour mulch smells like vinegar, ammonia, or sulfur. When mulch piles stand too long, summer heat will cause fermentation. Bacteria produce methanol, acetic acid, ammonia, and hydrogen sulfide gas. Acetic acid causes the vinegar smell and hydrogen sulfide causes the sulfur or "rotten egg" smell. When using old vegetation as mulch, do not cover it with plastic or let it stay wet during storage and turn it at least once or twice a month. Only use 1 to 2 inches of mulch around plants, shrubs, or trees. Snakes, lizards, and insects like mulch so it is a good idea not to use it around the foundations of the home.

RODENTICIDES

Rodenticides today consist of anticoagulants and non-anticoagulants. They are in the form of grain-based baits or pellets. The first anticoagulants (warfarin, pindone, diphacinone, and clorophacinone) are known as multiple-feed rodenticides; requiring multiple feedings over several days to a week or more to produce death by internal hemorrhage. When it was found that some rats were resistant to warfarin, second-generation anticoagulants bromadiolone and brodifacoum were developed. Non-anticoagulant rodenticides consist of zinc phosphide, cholecaliferol, and bromethalin. All the non-anticoagulant rodenticides can be used to control anticoagulant resistant rodent populations (Whisson, 1996). The use of rodenticides is a concern because rodents may store them in places other than where the bait was placed. Rodenticides should not be used when there is a concern that pets or young children will find it.

BUILDING BETTER GOLF COURSES
The use of pesticides, the impact on water and soil quality, and irrigation water usage are often cited as public concerns about the golf industry. Although it is true that golf courses use pesticides to maintain their turf and control insects, they are using ounces per square foot as opposed to the pounds per square foot used in the past. The reasons for the decrease include the use of hardier grasses that are easier to sustain with less water and the use of more effective chemicals so they can use less of them. Golf course developers are paying more attention to environmental concerns. For example, some golf courses are built over old landfills to make the land more aesthetically pleasing and useful.

Human Risk of Pesticides

cute problems with pesticides and herbicides concern poisonings. Individuals most likely to experience pesticide poisonings are workers who manufacture pesticides and farmers using large amounts of them. Homeowners may also be exposed to pesticides when using them for lawn and gardens. Children are particularly vulnerable to pesticide poisoning because the same dose in an adult is more harmful in a child. Children also are more likely to play in the dirt, go barefoot, and not wash their hands.

The most toxic pesticides are the organophosphate insecticides, which are toxic to the nervous system. This type of insecticide makes up nearly 40% of all pesticides used and is the most commonly reported worker illness. The particular harm of any pesticide is determined by the toxic qualities of the pesticide, amount of exposure, route of exposure, and the dose of the pesticide taken in. The most dangerous insecticides are carbaryl, chlordane, heptachlor, lindane, mirex, and parathion. The most dangerous herbicides include 2,4-D; 2,4,5-T; alachlor; atrazine; nitrofen; and trifluralin. The EPA has banned the use of chlordane, DDT, aldrin, dieldrin, endrin, heptachlor, and 2,4,5-T (Alexander, 2003). Farmers appear to have a higher risk of lymphoma and prostate cancer than other occupational groups, primarily through pesticide exposure (Tevis, 2002). Lymphoma attacks the immune system. Deaths among farmers with lymphoma are clustered in the Midwest. Farmers should follow instructions, wear protective clothing and gloves while handling pesticides, and change clothes and shower after applying them.

Pesticide poisoning can occur when the pesticide is absorbed on the skin or ingested. Symptoms of pesticide poisoning include headaches, dizziness, severe abdominal pain, muscular twitching, breathing difficulty, convulsions, and coma. Treatment for pesticide poisoning includes the following:

1. Determine the type of pesticide used, how much was taken, and the approximate time of poison contact.

2. Call the poison control center and follow their instructions.

Urushiol
The toxic oil of a poison ivy plant that causes a burning and blistering rash.

Endocrine disrupters
A chemical that mimics the endocrine system producing hormone-like substances; sometimes called "environmental estrogens"; xenestrogens.

Consider the Cost | IS "ORGANICALLY GROWN" BETTER?

Increasing numbers of consumers are purchasing organically grown foods as a way to reduce exposure to potentially harmful chemicals. Many supermarkets now stock organic products in the produce and cereal aisle. Organically grown food is grown and processed without synthetic fertilizers or pesticides. Organic foods cost about 50% more than other foods and consumers should get what they pay for. A 2000 report indicated that organic foods may or may not be free of chemicals. This created concerns that generated new U.S. Department of Agriculture (USDA) rules to "certify" organic products and producers of organic products (Rawson, 1998). The term **organic** means:

- Meat, poultry, and eggs from animals are not given growth hormones or antibiotics. Livestock are given organic feed and live in conditions that allow for exercise, freedom of movement, and the reduction of stress.

- Products are not genetically engineered or irradiated to kill germs.

- Crops are grown on land that has not been fertilized with sewage sludge or chemical fertilizers. Soil is managed through crop rotation, planting cover crops, and the application of plant and animal fertilizer.

- Weeds are controlled by mulching, mowing, hand weeding, or mechanical cultivation, not chemical herbicides.

- Pests and plant diseases are treated primarily with insect predators, traps, natural repellants, and other nonchemical methods.

In addition to producing foods without chemicals or other "unnatural" means, farmers must be able to prove their farmland has been free of pesticides and herbicides for 3 years and utilize practices that conserve soil and water (U.S. Department of Agriculture, 2001). Organic food may not necessarily be more nutritious or safer than conventional products. In fact, without the use of chemicals, the products may spoil faster or bear food-borne illnesses. Consumers should be wary of organic foods and pay attention to the label. The following describes the labeling of organic foods and what it means (Long, 2001):

- Products labeled "100 percent organic" must contain only organically produced ingredients, excluding water and salt.

- Products labeled "organic" must consist of at least 95 percent organically produced ingredients, excluding water and salt.

- "Made with organic ingredients" means that at least 70 percent of the product's ingredients were produced organically.

- Processed products containing less than at least 70 percent organic ingredients cannot use the USDA seal anywhere, but can list organic ingredients individually on the information panel.

Most soils contain pesticides that persist in the environment for many years, therefore it is difficult to find native soil that can provide a truly "organic" environment for plants. Greenhouses probably provide the best control for growing organic plants, but it is not very practical. Certain farming practices that minimize weeds and insects are considered to be organic and this is probably the most-used method of producing organic fruits, vegetables, and grains. How the produce is treated once it leaves the farm may be up to speculation.

Some markets distributing organic foods also market other products such as food supplements, pastries, and other items one would not considered organic. Because organic foods often cost more than "regular" foods, consumers would be wise to determine if the foods they are purchasing really are organically grown and distributed in the same form as when they were harvested. Due to the increased demand for organic foods, it is not likely that organic foods have evaded the usual food preservation and handling procedures as other foods.

Organic produce items can be safer for individuals with food allergies or sensitivity to certain food additives or residues normally found on foods. Organic products are usually more wholesome, meaning they are less likely to be refined and processed.

Sources: Long, 2001; Rawson, 1998; USDA, 2001.

Consider the Cost | ECO-LABELING

Some manufacturers provide information about the effects of their product on the environment through an **eco-label**. Eco-labeling may help a consumer know in advance the harmful effects the chemical may have upon the user and others. Organizations involved with eco-labeling include the EPA, Federal Trade Commission (FTC), the FDA, and the USDA. In the future, consumers may see more efforts to control the use of pesticides and herbicides on food. The United States may also follow guidelines imposed by European countries to ban the use of them altogether. Until then, conservative and appropriate use of chemicals used to control pests should be applied. The best approach, however, is prevention. Control of pests can be managed by effective housekeeping, food storage, and yard maintenance strategies.

Regulation of Pesticides, Fungicides, and Herbicides

The Federal Insecticide, Fungicide and Rodenticide Act (FIFRA, 1996) controls pesticide distribution, sale, and use. Under this law, the EPA was given authority to study the consequences of pesticide use and to require users to register when purchasing pesticides. Users who apply pesticides on a regular basis must also pass certification examinations. All pesticides used in the United States must be registered (licensed) by the EPA. Registration assures that pesticides will be properly labeled and that if in accordance with specifications, will not cause unreasonable harm to the environment.

Concerned about the effects of pesticide residues on food, the Food Quality Protection Act (1996) amended FIFRA providing for the EPA to set allowable pesticide residue levels for food. The EPA is directed to ensure a "reasonable certainty of no harm" from pesticide exposure requiring periodic evaluation until 2006 (Schierow, 1999). The EPA evaluates aggregate and cumulative risks of pesticides through all routes of exposure. An investigation regarding the risks posed by organophosphate insecticides on fruits, vegetables, and grains is ongoing. The primary risk is to children and sanctions have been imposed regarding the use of methyl parathion. When evaluating for potential risk, the EPA uses the following criteria (Schierow, 1999):

- susceptibility of children to exposure and adverse health effects

- potential effects by endocrine disrupters

- potential **teratogenic** effects

- aggregate risk from all sources and routes of exposure

- cumulative risks due to exposure

In 1999, the Consumers Union analyzed data from 27,000 food samples tested by the USDA's Pesticide Data Program from 1994–1997, calculating toxicity indexes (TI) for each food (Groth, Benbrook, & Lutz, 1999). Foods with the highest TI values were fresh peaches, frozen and fresh winter squash, apples, grapes, spinach, pears, and green beans. Up to 37 different pesticide chemicals were detected in apples; more than 20 are found in peaches, pears, and spinach. Only 10 pesticide chemicals were found in broccoli, and fewer than that in apple juice, orange juice, bananas, and corn. Eleven of the highest TI value foods were grown in the United States.

> *Organic*
> A term that implies a food was grown or raised without chemicals such as pesticides, herbicides, steroids, or antibiotics.
>
> *Eco-label*
> A seal or logo indicating that a product has met a set of environmental or social standards.
>
> *Teratogenic*
> Having properties that affect unborn fetuses when the mother is exposed.

Digging Deeper

In the mid-1980s, a species common to Puerto Rico, the coquie frog, came to Hawaii in a shipment of potted plants. The Hawaiian environment had many sources of food (insects, spiders, and mites) with no natural predators for the frogs. By 1998, seven different species of coquies established themselves on Hawaii, with some on Maui, Kauai, and Oahu. Residents and tourists complained about the noise they make, which is from 70 to 90 decibels, equivalent to moderate-to-heavy street traffic. The level is enough to cause hearing problems for those who have to endure it for long periods of time. To make matters worse, the coquie are nocturnal animals, singing their mating songs during the night. Residents would run their air conditioners at night or wear earplugs to soften the noise. Realtors were asked to disclose the presence of coquies on properties for sale, just as they had to list the presence of termites, water damage, or structural flaws.

Trying to catch the frogs by hand was unsuccessful so substances that would poison the frogs and not harm the environment were investigated. When one researcher found that acetaminophen worked as a poison to control the brown tree snake on Guam, he turned his attention to over-the-counter drugs and food additives. It was discovered that the frogs died quickly after being sprayed with a 2% caffeine solution. The EPA agreed to let researchers try the experimental pesticide spray for 1 year. In addition to controlling the frog populations, it also killed garden slugs. After the 1-year period was up, researchers began to explore other alternatives. One that seems to have good potential is citric acid from lemon juice.

Source: Raloff, 2003.

Consider the Cost | THE ENVIRONMENTAL GARDENER

Natural means of controlling indoor pests include:

- Place red chili pepper, dried peppermint, or borax where ants enter the home. Planting mint around the outside of the house will also drive them away.

- Spread a mixture of baking soda, boric acid, and powdered sugar around cockroach areas. Oatmeal mixed with plaster of Paris will also help kill them. Bay leaves in cabinets will keep cockroaches away.

- Brewer's yeast tablets or powder will emit B vitamins with natural odors that keeps fleas away.

- Sticky flypaper can be made by mixing boiled sugar, corn syrup, and water. Cloves can be hung or citrus oil can be placed in the room to keep flies away.

- To keep rabbits and deer away from plants, "paint" them with a mixture of garlic, red pepper, and egg. Sometimes mothballs will help.

- To keep armadillos from tearing up the yard, check to see if the yard has grubs and eliminate the grubs.

Consider the Cost | WHAT I CAN DO ABOUT PEST CONTROL

_____ Use airtight containers for storing food.

_____ Seal cracks around foundations.

_____ Dispose of garbage in a biodegradable plastic bag.

_____ Place garbage in a closed container and haul it away twice a week.

_____ Repair wet areas in the kitchen and bathroom.

_____ Remove any items or drain areas where water may stand for more than 1 day.

_____ Clean up animal food, hair, and feces.

Summary

Pests are a normal part of the ecosystem but they can become a nuisance and transmit diseases. The control of insects is made difficult by changes in the weather. Synthetic chemicals are available to control insect populations, but it is better to find more natural means of control. Most pests look for food and controlling them is a matter of decreasing conditions where they are likely to be drawn to and flourish. The use of pesticides, including insecticides and herbicides, must be carefully monitored because many of them are persistent in the environment and can harm organisms for which they are not intended. Lessons learned from the unrestricted use of DDT provided the need for legislation and regulation by the Environmental Protection Agency. Individuals need to try natural methods of controlling pests. When natural methods are unsuccessful, be careful about the selection, read the directions, and use them according to instructions.

REFERENCES

Alexander, R. (2003). Birth defects caused by herbicides, insecticides, and industrial chemicals that disrupt the endocrine system. *The Consumer Law Page.* Retrieved February 17, 2003, from http://consumerlawpage.com/article/endocrine.shtml

Bell W. J., & Adiyodi, K. G. (1981). *The American cockroach.* London: Chapman and Hall.

Brodgon, W., & McAlister, J. (1998). Insecticide resistance and vector control. *Emerging Infectious Diseases, 4.* Retrieved June 20, 2003 from http://www.cdc.gov/ncidod/eid/vol4no4/brogdon.htm.

Centers for Disease Control (CDC). (2003). Head lice infestation. Retrieved January 29, 2005, from http://www.cdc.gov/ncidod/dpd/parasites/headlice/factsht_head_lice.htm.

Centers for Disease Control (CDC). (2004). Pesticides and public health. Retrieved January 29, 2005, from http://www.epa.gov/history/publications/formative6.htm.

Clements, A. N. 1992. *The biology of mosquitoes, Vol. 1. Development, Nutrition and Reproduction.* New York, NY: Chapman & Hall.

Clemson Extension Home and Garden Information Center. (2004). Mosquitoes. Factsheet HGIC 2504, retrieved from http://hgic.clemson.edu/factsheets/HGIC2504.htm.

CNN.com. (1996). Homeowners worried after pesticide misuse. November 18, 1996. Retrieved from http://www.cnn.com/EARTH/9611/18/pesticide.abuse/.

Conservation Commission of Missouri. (2004). Poison ivy: How to identify and control. Missouri Department of Conservation. Retrieved January 29, 2005, from http://www.conservation.state.mo.us/nathis/plantpage/flora/poivy/.

Core, J. (2003). Hot on the trail of fire ants. *Agricultural Research, 51,* 20.

Crans, W. J. (2004). A classification system for mosquito life cycles: Life cycle types for mosquitoes of the Northeastern United States. *Journal of Vector Ecology, 29,* 1–10. Retrieved January 29, 2005, from http://www-rci.rutgers.edu/~insects/mosclass.htm.

Environmental Protection Agency (EPA). (2004). Pesticides and food: What "integrated pest management" means. Retrieved from http://www.epa.gov/pesticides/food/ipm.htm.

Groth, E., Benbrook, C., & Lutz, K. (1999). Do you know what you're eating? An analysis of U.S. government data on pesticide residues in foods. *Consumers Union Report.*

Jones, S. C. (2004a). Black widow spider. Ohio State University Factsheet HYG-2061A-04. Retrieved January 29, 2005, from http://ohioline.osu.edu/hyg-fact/2000/2061A.html.

Jones, S. C. (2004b). Brown recluse spider. Ohio State University Factsheet HYG-2061-04. Retrieved January 29, 2005, from http://ohioline.osu.edu/hyg-fact/2000/2061.html.

Lewis, V. R. (2001). Pest notes: Termites. UC ANR Publication 7415. University of California: UC Research and Extension Center. Retrieved January 29, 2005, from http://www.ipm.ucdavis.edu/PMG/PESTNOTES/pn7415.html.

Long, C. (2001). Finding truly good food: From organic to authentic. *Mother Earth News,* 189. Retrieved from http://www.motherearthnews.com/arc/5881/.

Manning, A. (2002). USDA gives bite to organic label. *USA Today,* October 16, 2002, D05.

Motavalli, J. (2002). Safer organics. *E: The Environmental Magazine.* July/Aug. Retrieved from http://www.findarticles.com/p/articles/mi_m1594/is_4_13

Public Health Seattle and King County. (2004). How to get rid of rats. Retrieved January 29, 2005, from http://www.metrokc.gov/health/env_hlth/rats.htm.

Raloff, J. (2003). Hawaii's hated frogs: Tiny invaders raise a big ruckus—populations of coquies, frogs native to Puerto Rico, invade Hawaii. *Science News Online,* January 4. Retrieved from http://www.sciencenews.org/articles/20030104/bob9.asp.

Rawson, J. M. (1998). Organic foods and the proposed federal certification and labeling program. 98-264 ENR. CRS Report for congress. Retrieved from http://www.ncseonline.org/NLE/CRSreports/Agriculture/ag-54.cfm.

Rigatuso, R., Bertuluzzo, S., Quattrin, F., & Bertoluzzo, M. (2000). Ant activity associated with a chemical compound. *Journal of Chemical Education, 2,* 183.

Robinson, J., & Meola, R. (1997). Suggestions for indoor and outdoor flea control. UC-034. Texas Agricultural Extension Service: The Texas A & M University System. Retrieved January 29, 2005 from http://entowww.tamu.edu/extension/bulletins/uc/uc-034.html.

Rose, R. I. (2001). Pesticides and public health: Integrated methods of mosquito management. *Emerging Infectious Diseases, 7,* 18–23. Retrieved January 29, 2005, from http://westnilevirusfacts.org/rose.pdf.

Schierow, L. (1999). RS20043: Pesticide residue regulation: Analysis of food quality protection act implementation. CRS Report for Congress. National Council for Science and the Environment. Distributed by the National Library for the Environment. Retrieved January 29, 2005, from http://www.cine.org/nle/pests~10.html.

Schmidt, K. (1995). A new ant on the block. *New Scientists, 148,* 2002–2028.

Solley, G., Vanderwoude, C., & Knight, G. (2002). Anaphylaxis due to red imported fire ant sting. *The Medical Journal of Australia, 175,* 521.

Standing Committee on Environment and Sustainable Development. (2000). History of pesticide use. In *Pesticides: Making the right choice for the protection of health and the environment.* Ottawa, Canada. Retrieved January 29, 2005, from http://www.parl.gc.ca/InfocomDoc/36/2/ENVI/Studies/Reports/envi01-e.html.

Tevis, C. (2002). Rural health: Lymph cancer rates increase significantly in the Midwest. *Successful Farming.*

Texas Parks and Wildlife. (2001). Battling the imported fire ant. Retrieved April 24, 2003, from http://www.dpi.qld.gov.au/fireants/8062.html.

Timm, R. M. (2000). Pest Notes: House mouse. UC ANR Publication 7483. University of California: UC Research and Extension Center. Retrieved from http://www.ipm.ucdavis.edu/PMG/PESTNOTES/pn7483.html.

Tinker, T., Collins, C., King, H. & Hoover M. (2000). Assessing risk communication effectiveness: Perspectives of agency practitioners. *Journal of Hazardous Materials, B73,* 117–127.

Tvedten, S. (2004). Biology and identification of fire ants. In *The best control, 2nd edition.* Retrieved from http://www.thebestcontrol.com/sitemap.htm.

U.S. Department of Agriculture (USDA). (2001). Final organic food standards. *Consumers' Research Magazine, 84,* 6.

Vetter, R. (2001). Kissing bugs and the skin. *Dermatology Online Journal, 7,* 6.

Vredevoe, L. (2004). Background information on the biology of ticks. University of California-Davis, Department of Entomology. Retrieved from http://entomology.ucdavis.edu/faculty/rbkimsey/tickbio.html.

Ware, G. W., & Whitacre, D. M. (2004). *An introduction to insecticides, 4th edition.* Willoughby, OH: Meister Media Worldwide.

Whisson, D. (1996). Rodenticides for control of Norway rats, roof rats, and house mice. Poultry Fact Sheet No. 23. University of California-Davis Cooperative Extension. Retrieved from http://animalscience.ucdavis.edu/Avian/pfS23.htm.

Willoughby, OH. (2005). MeisterPro Information Resources. Retrieved January 29, 2005 from http://www.ipmworld.umn.edu/chapters/ware.htm.

![ASSIGNMENTS]

1. Select a vector-borne illness and learn the effects of the illness and treatment.

2. Select a pesticide and determine what it is used for, its toxicity, and alternatives to its use.

3. Look up a pesticide, fungicide, or herbicide using reputable sources to discover what its hazards are and how to treat a poisoning from the substance.

4. Determine which pesticides described in this chapter are organic and which are inorganic.

5. Identify the types of pests you might encounter inside and outside of your home and develop a plan for controlling them.

6. Determine when the best times would be for a health department to recommend spraying for mosquito control.

7. Find historical information that would explain why servicepeople in World War I were doused with DDT. List possible effects they may have experienced.

8. Explain why children may be more at risk for harm from pesticide residues on produce.

9. Read the label on a pesticide product to see what emergency treatment would be.

10. Locate the poison control center number and call with a nonemergency question regarding a pesticide in your home.

SELECTED ENVIRONMENTAL LAWS

1938 **Federal Food, Drug, and Cosmetic Act (FFDCA)**
Authorized the EPA to set maximum residue levels, or tolerances, especially for infants and young children for pesticides and harmful additives in foods.

1947 **Federal Insecticide, Fungicide, and Rodenticide Act (FIFRA)(PL 80-102)**
Provided for the registration of pesticide materials, and authorized penalties for violation of the Act in order to protect consumers. Amended in 1959 and 1964.

1972 **Federal Environmental Pesticide Control Act (PL 92-516)**
Amends the FIFRA and establishes a program under the direction of the EPA to control the sale, distribution, and application of pesticides. Pesticides are classified for "general" or "restricted" use. The 1972 amendments established, under the Administrator of EPA, a program for controlling the sale, distribution, and application of pesticides through an administrative registration process. The amendments provides for classifying pesticides for "general" or "restricted" use. "Restricted" pesticides may only be applied by or under the direct supervision of a certified applicator.

1990 **The Organic Foods Production Act (Title 21 of PL 101-624)**
Minimum standards for organic farming practices were set so that items labeled "organic" fit the USDA criteria.

1996 **Food Quality Protection Act (FQPA)(PL 104-170)**
Amends the FIFRA and the FFDCA. These amendments fundamentally change the way the EPA regulates pesticides. The requirements included a new safety standard—reasonable certainty of no harm—that must be applied to all pesticides used on foods.

SELECTED PROFESSIONAL JOURNALS

Chemical Week
Chemistry and Ecology
Chemoecology
Ecosystem Health
Ecotoxicology
Ecotoxicology and Environmental Safety
E: Environmental Magazine
Emerging Infectious Diseases
Environmental Pollution
Journal of Environmental Education
Journal of Environmental Health
Journal of Insect Conservation
Mother Earth News
Plant Ecology
Pest Control
Organic Gardening
Science

ADDITIONAL READING

Clemson Extension Service. (2003). *Pest management handbook.* Clemson, SC: Clemson University. Retrieved from http://www.clemson.edu/public.

Toth, S. (1996). Federal pesticide laws and regulations. North Carolina State University and North Carolina Cooperative Extension Service. Retrieved from http://ipm.ncsu.edu/safety/factsheets/laws.pdf.

Pike, D., & Hager, A. (2003). How herbicides work: A short course on how herbicides kill weeds and injure crops. Retrieved February 25, 2003, from http://www.agric.gov.ab/ca/agdex/000/pp6062tc.htm.

Schneider, D., & Freeman, N. (2001). Children's environmental health risks: A state-of-the-art conference. *Archives of Environmental Health, 56,* 103–110.

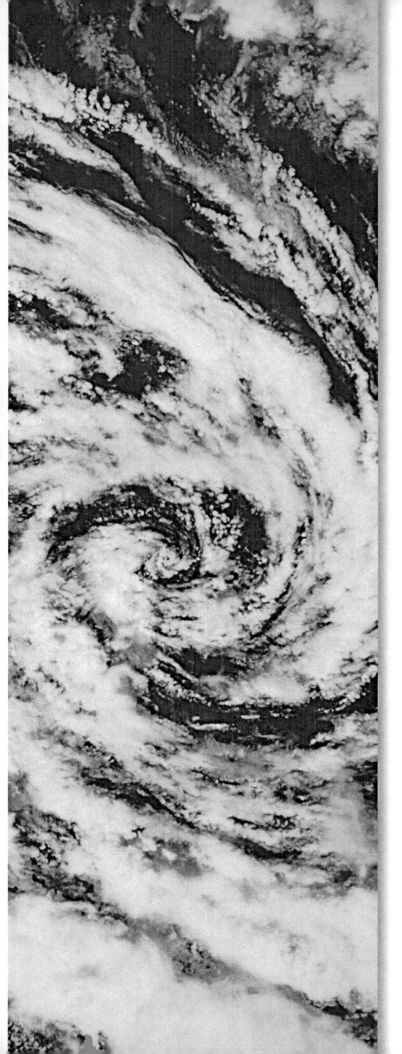

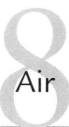

Air

When you can't breathe, nothing else matters.
American Lung Association

When we try to pick out anything by itself, we find it hitched to everything else in the universe.
John Muir (1838–1914)

OBJECTIVES

1. List and describe the four main gases in the air we breathe.

2. Describe how air quality affects human health.

3. Describe the conditions that result in thermal inversion and its effects.

4. List four laws that attempt to control air pollution emissions.

5. Explain the term greenhouse gas and provide an account of the gases that cause it.

6. Provide a brief account of some hazardous air pollutants and their effect on the environment.

7. Describe global attempts to address greenhouse gas emissions.

8. Contrast the difference between good ozone and bad ozone.

9. Debate with a classmate over which causes more air pollution—automobiles or industries.

10. Explain why open burning laws are necessary.

Introduction

The Earth's atmosphere is one of the most important and overlooked resources for life. The atmosphere provides oxygen, insulates the Earth, and controls the **climate**. This chapter provides information about the atmosphere, air quality, and air pollutants.

Atmospheric Air

The atmosphere consists primarily of nitrogen (N), oxygen (O), argon (Ar), and **carbon dioxide (CO_2)**. Other components of the air include neon (Ne), helium (He), krypton (Kr), sulfur dioxide (SO_2), methane (Ch_4), hydrogen (H), **nitrous oxide (NO)**, xenon (X_2), ozone (O_3), nitrous dioxide (NO_2), and iodine (I). In addition to these elements and chemicals, there are trace amounts of **carbon monoxide (CO)** and ammonia. Altitude and temperature changes influence concentrations of each atmospheric gas. Each person breathes in over 3,000 gallons of air per day. The content and quality of air is essential to good health. See Table 8.1 for the percentage of components in clean air.

NITROGEN

Nitrogen is plentiful in the atmosphere primarily because of decomposition of plants and animals. It is also present in the soil and necessary for plants to grow. Nitrogen gas in the atmosphere can only be used by a certain group of bacteria. Atmospheric nitrogen is a volatile compound converted to nitrate (NO_3) by lightning. Coastal fogs are another source of nitrogen. Nitrogen compounds are found in the atmosphere, industrial emissions, and fossil fuel combustion.

2010 HEALTHY PEOPLE OBJECTIVES RELATED TO OUTDOOR AIR QUALITY

8-1 Reduce the proportion of persons exposed to air that does not meet the EPA's health-based standards for harmful air pollutants (particulate matter, nitrogen dioxide, sulfur dioxide, lead).

8-2 Increase use of alternative modes of transportation to reduce motor vehicle emissions and improve the nation's air quality (bicycling, walking, trips by transit).

8-3 Improve the nation's air quality by increasing the use of cleaner alternative fuels (by privately owned cars, buses, trucks, and vans).

8-4 Reduce air toxic emissions to decrease the risk of adverse health effects caused by airborne toxins.

OXYGEN

Oxygen is essential to plants, animals, and humans. The atmosphere contains 21% oxygen. As oxygen is inhaled, oxygen and carbon dioxide are exhaled. Plants create oxygen, carbon dioxide, and hydrogen through a process known as *photosynthesis*. Some gases in the environment can be harmful, depending upon the concentration. These gases are known as **greenhouse gases** because of their ability to trap heat in the troposphere instead of allowing it to radiate into space. This process is quite similiar to the way glass traps heat in a greenhouse. This process has been attributed to global warming and detrimental health effects.

CARBON

As discussed in Chapter 1, carbon is important to life. There is organic carbon and inorganic carbon. Organic carbons are found in all living things. As living things die

---

Climate
Weather conditions such as temperature, precipitation, and wind typical to an area or region.

Carbon dioxide (CO_2)
A colorless, odorless gas formed by respiration, combustion, and decomposition. Composes .03% of air.

Nitrous oxide (NO)
A weak anesthetic gas used since the late 18th century; also known as laughing gas.

Carbon monoxide (CO)
A colorless, odorless gas produced from incomplete combustion. It is toxic and the most commonly inhaled poisonous substance.

Greenhouse gas
Gas that absorbs infrared radiation emitted from the Earth.

TABLE 8-1 Components of Clean Air

Gas	Percent in Atmosphere
Nitrogen (N_2)	78.08
Oxygen (O_2)	20.95
Argon (Ar)	.93
Carbon dioxide (CO_2)	.033
Neon (Ne)	.0018
Helium (He)	.00052
Methane (Ch_4)	.00020
Krypton (Kr)	.00011
Nitrogen dioxide (NO_2)	.00005
Hydrogen (H_2)	.00005

and decompose, organic carbon is returned to the soil. About two-thirds of the carbon in the biosphere is stored in the soil (Alamaras et al, 2000). Carbon is also found in the ocean, primarily from soil runoff.

Inorganic carbon is found in fossil fuels such as coal, oil, and gas. Combustion of these fuels releases carbon back into the atmosphere. Atmospheric carbon is the result when carbon is transferred from soil to water and from incomplete combustion of fossil fuels. The amount of carbon in the atmosphere has been increasing steadily since the Industrial Revolution, and even faster since the 1900s.

Carbon monoxide is a gas that results from incomplete combustion. It binds with the hemoglobin of red blood cells, making it difficult to absorb oxygen. For this reason, it is considered poisonous. Carbon dioxide is a harmless gas resulting from photosynthesis and combustion.

HYDROGEN

Hydrogen is the most abundant of all elements in the universe, making up about 90% of the universe by weight. Hydrogen is an essential component of water (H_2O). Atmospheric hydrogen results from decomposition, evaporation, and burning fuels. Hydrogen is the lightest element and has been used to lift blimps and hot air balloons. Hydrogen has also been used to make the hydrogen bomb. The development of hydrogen cells as an alternative fuel source is promising.

INERT GASES

Argon, neon, krypton, xenon, and helium are inert gases found in the atmosphere. Argon gas is derived from the radioactive decay of potassium. Neon is obtained by the liquefaction of air and is separated from other gases by distillation. Krypton and xenon are obtained as byproducts from the liquefaction and separation of air. Helium is extracted from natural gas.

SULFUR DIOXIDE

Sulfur dioxide is a gas produced when fuels containing sulfur (coal and oil) are burned or from other industrial processes, such as metal smelting (Clean Air Trust, 2005). The effects of sulfur dioxide are problematic for plants, animals, and humans. Sulfur dioxide is a contributor to acid rain and breathing problems.

NITROUS OXIDE AND NITROUS DIOXIDE

Nitrous oxide is a type of gas emitted during natural processes such as volcanic emissions and lightning, agricultural processes such as bacterial growth and anaerobic fermentation of crops, industrial activities such as the burning of solid waste and fossil fuels, and from automobile exhaust. Nitrous oxide and nitrous dioxide are usually found together. Nitrous oxide is oxidized to NO_2, a precursor of ozone. The term NO_x is used to describe both when they are discussed in air pollution literature. NO_xs react in the air to form nitric acid, a corrosive and toxic organic nitrate found in smog and acid rain. Health problems may result to those who work with explosives, as well as welders, fire fighters, military, and aerospace personnel (Peterson & Cairns, 2003).

METHANE

Methane is colorless, odorless, flammable, and lighter than air. Next to nitrous oxide, it is the next most detrimental greenhouse gas, 25 times more effective than carbon dioxide at trapping heat in the atmosphere, creating the **greenhouse effect**. Scientists estimate that atmospheric methane levels have risen to five times the levels it was in 1860. Because methane is produced by aerobic fermentation and decomposition of wastes, scientists attribute the increase in atmospheric methane to activities such as landfills, natural gas systems, rice farming, livestock farming, biomass burning, coal mining, and wastewater. Methane is sometimes referred to as *marsh gas*. Methane production is related to population growth. Some say that the animal waste from livestock farming has increased because increased numbers of consumers demand beef and milk products.

ABOUT NEON SIGNS

Before there were neon signs in America, there were commercial sign tubes that used carbon dioxide. Neon gas, which produces a red color, was discovered by William Ramsey and M.W. Travers in 1898 in London (Jefferson Lab, 2005). Using other gases, different colors can be produced such as blue (mercury), white (CO_2), and gold (helium). The first neon sign was displayed by inventor Georges Claude in Paris in 1910 (Bellis, 2005). In 1912, Georges Claude and his company sold two neon signs to a Packard car dealership in Los Angeles for $24,000.

ARE YOU AT RISK FOR SKIN CANCER?

Check all of the following that apply.

_____ Family history of skin cancer

_____ Fair skin

_____ Early exposure to the sun (in infancy and childhood)

_____ Prolonged exposure to the sun

_____ Two or more painful, blistering sunburns before the age of 18

_____ Moles on the body (created from sun exposure and worsened by sun exposure)

For this cancer, age doesn't matter! Twenty-year-olds and younger have been diagnosed with skin cancers and melanomas (Melanoma Research Foundation, 2005).

Like carbon dioxide, methane is not all bad. It can be used for fuel and burnt to serve as a natural gas to heat homes and commercial buildings. It can also be used in the generation of electric power. Attempts are being made to retrieve methane from coal mines and landfills as an alternate source of energy fuel.

The Ozone Layer

The EPA says when it comes to ozone, it is "good up high—bad nearby" (EPA, 2003). Stratospheric ozone (the up high) is considered good ozone. Ninety percent of the Earth's ozone is in the stratosphere, absorbing ultraviolet radiation from the sun. There is some concern that the ozone layer is thinning or that there are "holes" in the ozone layer. Ozone levels in the atmosphere are affected by the presence of **chlorofluorocarbons (CFCs)** and other toxic gases. For every level of ozone that is destroyed, the increase of ultraviolet (UV) radiation problems doubles. Exposure to UV rays is a concern, particularly in higher altitudes and near the water.

There are three types of UV light: UVA, UVB, and UVC (CDC, 2004). The most harmful of these is UVB because it has harmful effects on crops, marine organisms, human skin, and DNA. The amount of UVB light is highly dependent upon cloud cover, latitude, and elevation. In high-latitude regions of the world, the sun is always low in the sky and UVB light has to pass through more of the atmosphere before reaching the Earth's surface. In high-latitude areas, UVB rays pass through less of the atmosphere's protection. It is estimated that for each mile increase in altitude above sea level, UVB exposure is increased by 17% (Scotto et al., 1988).

Skin cancer is the one of the most common cancers in the United States. There are three types of skin cancer: (1) basal cell, (2) squamous cell cancers (often not malignant), and (3) melanoma (a potentially malignant and fatal type of cancer). The incidence rate of melanoma has increased steadily since the 1930s due to the change in clothing and exposure to sun (Centers for Disease Control, 1995; Geller, 1998). Exposure to UV rays can also be harmful to the eyes, particularly when the sun is reflected by snow or water. Overexposure to sunlight contributes to the incidence of cataracts. Another effect of increased atmospheric ozone is decreased immunity from disease.

Ozone "down low" (in the troposphere) is a potential hazard because it is linked with respiratory problems and is difficult to control. Even the smallest amounts cause breathing difficulties in a person with **chronic obstructive pulmonary disease (COPD)**. Ground-level ozone is the primary component in **smog**. Smog reduces visibility, retards crop and tree growth, and impairs health. Ground-level ozone is formed when other pollutants such as **volatile organic compounds (VOCs)** are emitted into the air. VOCs are released from burning fuels, paint thinners, degreasers, and other solvents as vapors or gases.

Greenhouse effect
When heat energy reflected by the Earth is absorbed by gases (carbon dioxide, CFCs, methane, and water vapor) trapping the warmth in the atmosphere.

Chlorofluorocarbons (CFCs)
Synthetic, nontoxic, easily liquefied chemicals consisting of carbon, hydrogen, chlorine, and fluorine. CFCs not only trap heat in the atmosphere, but also destroy the ozone layer.

Chronic obstructive pulmonary disease (COPD)
Pulmonary disease that has developed over time; reduces the capacity to breathe without restriction; includes asthma, emphysema, and chronic bronchitis.

Smog
A term used when smoke and fog are combined in the air.

Volatile organic compounds (VOCs)
Carbon-containing chemicals found in paint thinners, degreasers, solvents, and emissions from burning fuels; becomes a gas at room temperature.

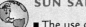

SUN SAFETY

- The use of sunscreens (SPF 15 or higher) can help, but not when exposure to sunlight is longer because of a false sense of protection.

- For those with a family or personal history of skin cancers, protective clothing and seeking shade is advised.

- Wear a cap to protect your head. Skin cancers can develop on the scalp.

- Wear UV protected sunglasses, preferably gray in color.

Source: The Skin Cancer Foundation. http://www.skincancer.org/prevention/index.php.

MIASMA AND YELLOW FEVER
In 1793, the city of Philadelphia experienced a yellow fever epidemic killing 10% of the population. Dr. Benjamin Rush believed the disease was caused by miasma from the malodorous air caused by rotting coffee on the shipyard docks. Citizens fired guns and pistols, hoping to push the disease out of the air. People walked outside with handkerchiefs over their mouths and noses. However, the disease was spread by mosquitoes. Spread of the disease slowed with the first frost, once the mosquitoes started dying off. The disease was eventually controlled by cleaning the streets, establishing standards for the depths of wells and privies, draining stagnant water, and forcing freshwater through the sewer systems (University of Pennsylvania, 2005).

Air Pollution

ir quality is compromised when pollutants are dispersed through the air, particularly in urban areas (Figure 8-1). **Air pollution** is related to climate, humidity, concentration of industrial emissions, population size, **thermal inversion**, stagnant air masses, and seasonal **airborne** pollens, dust, molds, spores, and the ozone (Table 8-2). Poor air quality is related to respiratory diseases (such as bronchitis and lung cancer), eye irritation, and a weakened immune system. The effects of pollutants vary with each individual and are affected by the type of pollutant, prior exposure, sensitivity, and the presence of airway reactive diseases such as asthma and emphysema. Pollutants such as lead may cause neurological damage, kidney disease, and affect fetal development. In addition, toxic materials in polluted air cause death from cancer.

Air pollution has existed due to natural sources such as decaying organic matter, volcanic eruptions, and forest fires. It wasn't until the late nineteenth century that air pollution was recognized as a global problem. The Industrial Revolution created a noticeable change in air quality, particularly in areas inhabited by great numbers of people. Factories and the burning of fossil fuels by many households added particulate matter and gases into the atmosphere, making breathing difficult. The invention of the automobile also has had disastrous effects on air quality. One of the first recorded incidents of citizens becoming sick from air pollution was in London in 1952 when four days of "pea-soup" smog caused an estimated 4,000 deaths (Logan, 1953).

Other incidents include:

- In 1948, a similar "killer smog" emerged in Donora, Pennsylvania, making 7,000 people ill and leaving 20 dead as sulfur dioxide, nitrogen oxides, and metal dust spewed from the local steel plant (EPA, 2000; Reese, 1999).

- In 1953, air pollution killed 200 people in New York City.

- In 1954, Los Angeles shut down industry and schools due to air pollution (Atwood & Kelly, 1997).

- In 1963, New York City experienced air pollution that killed 405 people (American Lung Association, 2002). At least 1 death was attributed to the heavy particulate matter and gases.

Taking Action Against Air Pollution

arly measures to restrict air pollution for health reasons began when cities such as Los Angeles passed their own "smoke emission control" regulations in 1947. There were heated debates about voluntary reduction of air pollution by industries and the need for legislation. When the Air Pollution Control Act of 1947 was established by California lawmakers, local air pollution control districts were developed. **Air quality standards** created by this act continue to be the basis of many air pollution regulatory programs.

FIGURE 8-1 Location of Nonattainment Areas for Criteria Pollutants, September 2001 The EPA has established standards that determine levels of pollution that are harmful to health.
Source: Environmental Protection Agency, http://www.epa.gov/airtrends/data/maps.html.

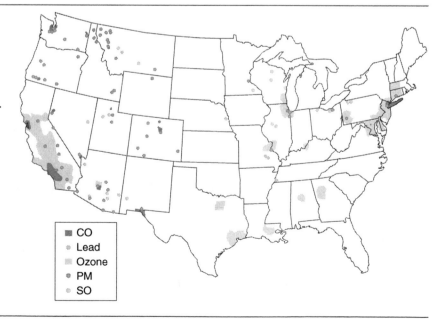

Legend:
- CO
- Lead
- Ozone
- PM
- SO

In 1955 the Air Pollution Control Act (PL 84-159) was passed directing the U.S. Public Health Service to conduct research on the effects of air pollution and provide individual states with assistance and training related to air pollution. As a result of this, automobile emissions were recognized as a major part of the problem. The Air Pollution Control Act was amended in 1960 and the **Clean Air Act** (PL 88-206) was passed in 1963 to control emissions from industries and power plants. Amendments were added in 1965, 1966, 1967, and 1969, calling for control of automobile emissions, expansions of local air pollution control programs, the establishment of air quality control standards and deadlines, and the authorization of research on low emission fuels.

The Motor Vehicle Air Pollution Control Act of 1965 (PL 89-272, an amendment to the Clean Air Act of 1963) called for federal **emission standards** for automobiles rather than allowing states to determine their own levels. By 1965, the automobile industry announced plans to manufacture automobiles with emission controls. The 1970 Clean Air Act (PL 91-604) amendments increased federal enforcement authority and established uniform National **Ambient Air** Quality Standards (NAAQS) for six criteria pollutants. The 1977 amendments authorized the EPA to regulate chemicals suspected of destroying stratospheric ozone. The Clean Air Act of 1990 (PL 101-549) raised automobile emissions standards and set a definite

---

TABLE 8-2   Sources of Air Pollution

Point sources	power plants, steel mills, other industries
Area sources	dust, humidity, solid waste
Biogenic sources	forest fires, volcanoes, tree pollen, vegetation
Mobile sources	cars, trucks, planes, construction equipment

Air pollution
The contamination of the atmosphere by pollutants from industry, fuel exhaust, and other pollution-creating processes. The five primary air pollutants are carbon monoxide, hydrocarbons, nitrogen compounds, particulate matter, and sulfur dioxide.

Thermal inversion
When a stable, slow-moving air mass forms a dense, cool layer of air near the Earth with warmer air above trapping pollutants thus causing illness.

Airborne
Carried by or through the air.

Air quality standards
The maximum allowable concentration of pollutants during a specific time in a specific area.

Clean Air Act
Originally passed in 1963 and amended in 1970, 1977, and 1990 giving the U.S. Environmental Protection Agency (EPA) responsibility for setting air quality standards.

Emission standards
The maximum amount of air pollution legally permitted to be discharged from a single source.

Ambient air
Outside air.

THERMAL INVERSION
In October of 1948, a cloud of gas from Donora Zinc Works, a steel plant, hovered over the town of Donora, Pennsylvania. A layer of cold air trapped the effluent in the air from heavy industry, cars, and furnaces of the citizens, resulting in a thermal inversion. The thermal inversion lasted 4 days. Twenty people died, 14,000 became ill, and 6,000 required medical treatment. Half of them required hospitalization. The local steel plant spewed sulfur dioxide, nitrogen oxides, and metal dust into the air. Ruth Poems, from the EPA, said that the Donora tragedy was the first time that public officials recognized the direct link between air pollution and public health, and mobilized to do anything about it (Shrenk et al., 1949). Public outcry over the incident forced the federal government to begin studying air pollution, its causes, effects, and how to control it. This led to the Air Pollution Control Act of 1955, the ancestor of the Clear Air Act of 1970.

Asthma is an illness that is characterized by coughing and wheezing and affects about 3 million children and 7 million adults in the United States. Asthma has increased the past 15 years in the United States and other developed countries despite significant improvements in outdoor air quality. The significance of this is that the incidence of other pulmonary diseases, such as tuberculosis and pneumonia, is decreasing.

Some speculate that asthma is a result of an underutilized immune system that overreacts to irritants, producing antibodies that release histamine and other inflammatory substances in the airway passages. Others speculate that society is spending a greater number of hours indoors, exposed to indoor allergens such as dust mites, cockroaches, molds, pollens, and harmful chemicals.

It is apparent that changes in outdoor air quality also are important in the development of asthmatic attacks, some of which lead to death. Researchers observed that emergency room visits for asthma occurred 28% more frequently when ozone levels were elevated (Weisel et al., 1995).

timetable to tighten control. This legislation encouraged the use of low-sulfur fuels as well as alternative fuels to reduce sulfur dioxide in the atmosphere. The government also called for a reduction in the amount of chlorofluorocarbons (CFCs) being used to prevent ozone depletion (American Meteorological Society, 2005). State and local air pollution control agencies regulate ambient concentration limits (ACLs) regarding the amount of particulate matter released into the air. The six key pollutants, selected according to their health effects on humans as well as the environment, are: carbon monoxide, lead, nitrogen dioxide, ozone, particulate matter, and sulfur dioxide.

Even with these initiatives, air pollution continues to be a significant problem in urban areas. In some areas, visible pollution called the "pink haze" is noticeable due to the high levels of air pollution. Haze is the result of a **photochemical process** between light, gas, and pollutants in the air. Haze impairs visibility for airplane pilots and disperses across canyons and valleys in mountainous areas (Spurny, 1996). Air travel also contributes to air pollution. Jet fuel consumption has risen 65 percent since 1970 putting tons of nitrous dioxides into the troposphere. Estimates are that air traffic is responsible for about 3% of greenhouse gases.

Digging Deeper — SIX CRITERIA AIR POLLUTANTS AND HEALTH EFFECTS

Carbon monoxide (CO) reduces oxygen delivery of red blood cells to the body's organs and tissues. The threat is most serious for those with cardiovascular disease. Exposures to elevated CO concentrations are associated with impaired visual perception, work capacity, manual dexterity, learning ability, and performance of complex tasks. CO is a by-product of incomplete combustion.

Lead accumulates in blood, bone, and soft tissues. It also affects the kidneys, liver, nervous system, and blood-forming organs. Excess exposure may cause seizures, mental retardation, and/or behavioral disorders. Due to the damage of the brain and nervous system, lead poisoning is the most common and most devastating disease affecting young children. Until unleaded gasoline was available, the primary source of lead pollution was gasoline.

Nitrogen oxides are produced from vehicles and power plants. They are converted to nitrogen dioxide, a precursor to acid precipitation. Nitrogen dioxide can irritate the lungs and lower resistance to respiratory infections.

Ozone damages lung tissue, reduces lung function, and sensitizes lungs to other irritants. Asthmatics, children, and the elderly are particularly affected.

Particulate matter (PM) consists of dust, smoke, ashes, and soot from burning. Some particles can be seen and others are microscopic. PM hangs in the air; it creates a haze, limiting visibility. Airborne particulates can lead to respiratory symptoms, aggravate cardiovascular disease, alter immune defenses, damage lung tissue, and produce cancers. Individuals with COPD or cardiovascular disease are particularly susceptible.

Sulfur dioxide affects breathing and produces respiratory illness. Individuals most affected include asthmatics, individuals with chronic lung disease, cardiovascular disease, children, and the elderly.

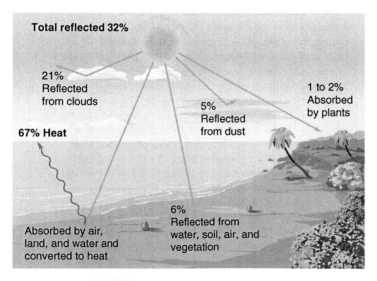

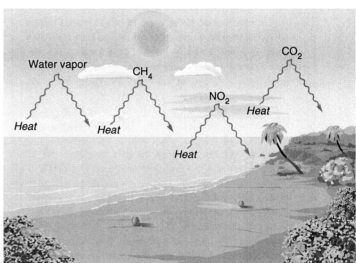

FIGURE 8-2 **Greenhouse Effect** Like a greenhouse, gases are trapped in the atmosphere, causing things to "heat up."

Greenhouse Gases

The greenhouse effect is the natural process of allowing some of the sun's energy to reach the Earth's surface through gases in the atmosphere (Figure 8-2). Without it, the Earth's climate would be 33° C (or 60° F) cold, and life as we know it would not exist. The enhanced greenhouse effect is an increase in this natural heat-trapping phenomena caused by anthropogenic emissions of greenhouse gases such as carbon dioxide, methane, nitrous dioxide, chlorofluorocarbons, and halocarbons. The term greenhouse gases is used to describe these emissions because they produce air-warming effects similar to that seen in greenhouses. The gases that are produced capture wavelengths of infrared radiation, changing rainfall and temperature patterns.

The effects of greenhouse gases can be observed by trends in global warming. As a result of global warming, climate changes are occurring, ice caps are melting, sea levels are rising, and air quality is deteriorating. As a result of these climate changes (creating more storms and rainfall in some areas, drought in others), plant and animal life is affected because they cannot survive in areas where the climate changes. Hot stagnant air and poor air quality aggravates respiratory diseases and increases diseases spread by insects.

No one knows how much the climate will change (Figure 8-3), how much the human contribution to greenhouse gases will affect it, or what the long-term effects of global warming will be on ecosystems, species distribution, and human civilization. Not all regions will experience equal warming. Some areas may become much hotter and drier, while others will actually experience colder weather. Current models predict a rise in global sea levels over the next century, high enough to put the homes of a third-world population underwater (Few, 2003). Other predictions include flooding of coastlines, severe storms, changes in precipitation patterns, and widespread changes in the existing ecological balance. Infectious diseases may increase due to an expansion of habitat for disease vectors such as mosquitoes (Shope, 1991). Many species may be unable to adapt to these changes in the climate and may become extinct.

The Intergovernmental Panel on Climate Change (IPCC) was established in 1988 by the World Meteorological Organization (WMO) and the United Nations Environment Programme (UNEP). The IPPC has published three documents assessing the state of world climate change, based upon peer reviewed and published scientific/technical literature. The first report stated that the twentieth century was the hottest in the past thousand years, with the 9 hottest years on record occurring

Photochemical process
A change in air color and density due to reactions of pollutants in the air.

FIGURE 8-3 **Global Temperature Changes**
The greenhouse effect increases global temperature change, causing ice caps to melt and sea levels to rise.
Source: National Climatic Data Center. Retrieved from http://www.ncdc.noaa.gov/oa/climate/globtemp.html.

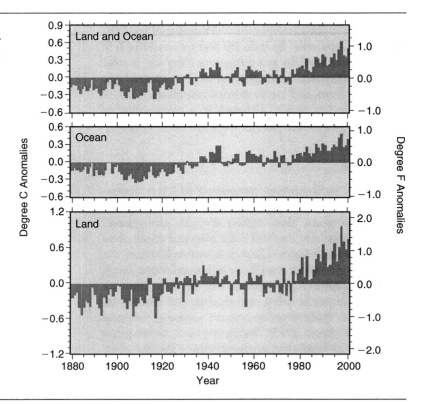

since 1987, and 1998 the hottest year ever (IPCC, 2001). Scientists estimate that surface warming will occur around the globe, ranging from 1.8 to 6.3° F.

The greenhouse effect is enhanced by burning fossil fuels (coal, oil, and natural gas). These fuels consist of stored carbon, formed from organic matter millions of years ago. When they are burned, carbon is returned to the atmosphere in the form of carbon dioxide, a gas that contributes most to the enhanced greenhouse effect. Each year, fossil fuel use adds significant amounts of carbon to the atmosphere (U.S. Climate Change Science Program, 2003). Deforestation also contributes to greenhouse gases in the atmosphere. When forests are cut down and burned, it increases atmospheric carbon and reduces an important carbon storage reservoir so that less carbon is absorbed from the atmosphere.

CARBON DIOXIDE

Natural processes add and remove about the same amount of carbon from the atmosphere. Plant respiration, sea-surface exchange of gases, and the natural decay of residue give off carbon dioxide, while plant photosynthesis and the oceans absorb it from the atmosphere. In nature, surface water often becomes acidic because atmospheric CO_2 dissolves in it.

Carbon dioxide is the most prevalent of the greenhouse gases. The amount of carbon in the atmosphere has changed noticeably in the past 150 years, increasing about 30% since the Industrial Revolution (McElroy, 2002). Nearly all scientists believe that this increase is a result of human contributions. The leading source of carbon dioxide in the atmosphere is the burning of fossil fuels (gas, oil, and coal) by industry and automobiles. It is also used commercially as a refrigerant ("dry ice" is solid CO_2), in carbonated beverages, and in fire extinguishers. It does not burn, and under normal conditions it is stable, inert, and nontoxic. Although it is more common than other greenhouse gases, it has a less harmful effect.

METHANE

Methane is an important component of lower atmospheric ozone. It is 21 times more effective at trapping heat in the atmosphere than carbon dioxide. Atmospheric methane levels have doubled since 1860 and continue to rise (Wuebbels & Hayhoe, 2002). Scientists attribute the increase in atmospheric methane to human sources such as landfills, natural gas systems, rice farming, livestock farming, biomass burning, coal mining, and wastewater. In 1993, rice fields were the primary source of methane production (Neue, 1993). Today, livestock farming has surpassed rice farming in methane production. Some say the blame for emissions from animal waste decomposition is on consumers who demand beef and milk products. About 40% of methane is produced by agriculture with the greatest source from ruminant animals that produce methane gas (Rosenzweig & Hillel, 1998).

Fortunately methane, like carbon dioxide, is not all bad. It can be used for fuel to heat homes and commercial buildings. It can also be used to generate electric power. Attempts are being made to retrieve methane from coal mines and landfills as an alternate source of energy fuel.

NITROUS DIOXIDE

Nitrous dioxide is formed by natural biological sources but is increased by human activities. It is only one-thousandth as common as carbon dioxide, but is 200 to 300 times as effective at trapping heat and remains in the atmosphere far longer than carbon dioxide. The major source of NO_2 emissions are agriculture, industry, and emissions from **catalytic converters** on automobiles. Nitrous dioxide levels can also be increased from the use of nitrogen fertilizers, agricultural waste, sewage, and decomposition of fossil fuels.

HALOCARBONS

Halocarbons include chlorofluorocarbons (CFCs), hydrochlorofluorocarbons (HCFCs), **halons**, and other chemicals that deplete the stratospheric ozone layer. From the 1800s, toxic gases such as ammonia, butane, methyl chloride, and sulfur dioxide were used in refrigerators. In 1930, Thomas Midgley, an American chemist, invented freon, the first CFC. Freon was dubbed a "miracle compound" at the time because it was nontoxic, nonflammable, noncorrosive, stable, and inexpensive to produce. It was used as a refrigerant and spray propellent (Simeonov, 2005). It wasn't discovered until several decades later that it remained high in the stratosphere.

Halon contains bromine, more damaging than chlorine to the ozone layer. Halon is used primarily for fighting fires. CFCs are found in plastics (polystyrene), insulation, and solvents. They are used in refrigerators, air conditioners, fire extinguishers, blowing agents for foams and packing materials, and aerosols. Halons and CFCs enhance the greenhouse effect through ozone loss. CFCs have warming effects ranging from 3,000 to 13,000 times that of carbon dioxide, and persist up to 400 years. CFCs have received great attention because they are extremely stable. It takes CFCs 6 to 8 years to reach the stratosphere. Once there, they break down into chlorine, fluorine, and carbon. In the 1970s, the United States and other countries began to ban the use of CFCs in aerosol sprays. Although CFCs have been banned in many countries, they are still used in others.

HAZARDOUS AIR POLLUTANTS

Hazardous air pollutants (HAPs) cause severe health effects and damage the ecosystem. The 1990 amendments to the Clean Air Act identified 188 HAPs.

These substances are emitted from many different industrial and vehicle sources. Substances such as arsenic, benzene, and beryllium are described here.

Arsenic

Arsenic is one of the world's most potent poisons. Arsenic occurs naturally in soil, rocks, water, air, plants, and animals. For most people living in the United States, arsenic exposure comes primarily from drinking water due to natural erosion processes. Approximately 90% of all arsenic used in the United States is used as a wood preservative. It may be released when wood products containing arsenic are burned. Prior to the introduction of DDT in the 1940s, most pesticides were made from inorganic arsenic compounds. It is linked to skin, bladder, and lung cancer.

Benzene

Benzene is a known carcinogen frequently used in manufacturing rubber, paint, plastics, resins, drugs, pesticides, synthetics, and other products. It is also present in tobacco smoke, gasoline, and automobile exhaust. It is highly combustible, dissolves in water, and evaporates quickly in the air. It can enter the environment through spills, volcanic eruptions, forest fires, and emissions from manufacturing plants. Humans most often come into contact with benzene either by breathing it in, drinking contaminated water, or through skin absorption. Benzene can be found outdoors and indoors. Outdoor air may contain low levels of benzene from automobile service stations, exhaust from motor vehicles, air at waste sites, and industrial emissions. Indoor air may contain benzene from tobacco smoke, glues, paints, furniture wax, and detergents. Benzene can also be found in well water from leaking underground storage tanks or leaching from hazardous waste sites. The highest exposure is for those who work with benzene in industrial sites. Long-term exposure to benzene causes harm to bone marrow and a decrease in red blood cells, leading to anemia. It can also cause cancer and excessive bleeding, and decrease immunity.

Beryllium

Beryllium is a hard, grayish metal found in mineral rocks, coal, soil, and volcanic dust. Beryllium is used in nuclear weapons and reactors, aircraft and space vehicle structures, instruments, X-ray machines, and mirrors. Beryllium alloys are used in automobiles, computers, sports equipment (golf clubs and bicycle frames), and dental bridges. Beryllium dust enters the air from burning coal and oil. This beryllium dust eventually settles over the land and water and is harmful if breathed. Long-term exposure can increase the risk of developing lung cancer in people.

Acid Rain

Gases, such as sulfur dioxide and nitrogen dioxide, contribute to air and water quality. Sulfur dioxide is emitted from the burning of fossil fuels and volcanic activity. Electric utility plants powered by coal or oil account for about 70% of sulfur dioxide emissions and 30% of nitrogen oxide emissions in the United States each year (Reese, 1999). Inhaling sulfur dioxide results in serious respiratory problems. When mixed with water, an exothermic reaction occurs, reacting with skin, paper, animal, and plant matter. Nitrogen dioxide forms in the atmosphere when nitrogen oxide is oxidized. Nitrogen dioxide is a major component of smog, **acid rain**, and haze. The primary source of this compound is fuel combustion. When sulfur dioxide and nitrogen dioxide gases are mixed, they become harmful acids (sulfuric acid and nitric acid). When they are combined with hydrocarbons and ozone in the atmosphere, there is a photochemical conversion caused by the sun, resulting in acid rain.

Catalytic converter
A pollution control device installed on gas-powered vehicles; reduces emissions of carbon monoxide and hydrocarbons; generates up to five times more nitrous dioxide with the device than without the device.

Halons
Substances used in fire fighting that stay in the atmosphere for an extended period of time depleting the ozone layer.

Acid rain
Rain, snow, hail, or fog with a low pH resulting from pollutants in the air, especially sulfur dioxide and nitrogen dioxides. Caused by emissions from the burning of fossil fuels such as coal, oil, and natural gas. When sulfur dioxide and nitrogen dioxide compounds react with sunlight, secondary pollutants such as sulfuric acid and nitric acid are formed.

The pH of acid rain is less than 5.0; the pH of distilled water is 7. Each change of 1 pH is equivalent to a 10-fold increase in acidity. The effects of acid rain include damage to aquatic ecosystems; damage to crops, plant life, and forests; and deterioration of buildings. In the 1980s, the most acidic rain ever noted fell in Wheeling, West Virginia. It had a pH of 1.4, making it almost as acidic as battery acid (Scienceshorts.com, 2005). A National Surface Waters Survey found that hundreds of lakes in New York's Adirondack Mountains were too acidic to support sensitive fish species like the brook trout. Of the 1,000 lakes included in the study, 75% were affected by acid rain (Fuller, 2000).

Acid rain was first observed in the mid-1800s in Manchester, England and is widespread in northern Europe and eastern North America (Schindler, 1988). Acid rain can be in the form of rain, snow, or fog, and converts air pollution into water pollution. When acid rain falls to the ground, lakes and streams become acidic.

Disaster Air Pollution Concerns

National disasters such as forest fires, dust storms, and volcanic eruptions contribute to air pollution. Humans also contribute to air pollution by burning wood in fireplaces, charcoal in outdoor grills, and spraying aerosols. The threat of a fire is always a concern due to the number of gases, particulate matter, and chemicals that rise in the air.

Sometimes catastrophic events take place that contribute significantly to air pollution problems of a city, state, region, or nation. The collapse of the World Trade Center in 2001 in New York City (Figure 8-4) caused tons

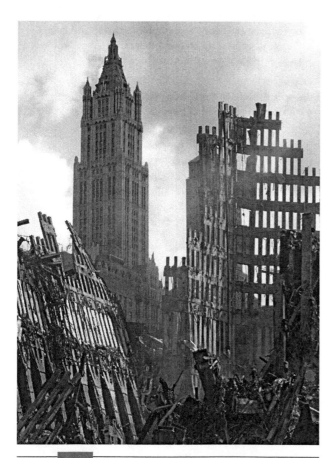

FIGURE 8-4 **Collapsed World Trade Center, September 11, 2001** Man-made disasters contribute to air pollution and change lives forever.

of pulverized and incinerated materials to permeate the air. Particles from building materials, furniture, plastics, jet fuel, and many other items created a dust cloud that enveloped lower Manhattan. Additional pollutants were released by the fire that persisted for 3 months; clean-up processes continued months after that. Rescue workers, tower survivors, area residents, and others were exposed to high concentrations of gaseous and corrosive particulate matter, including soot and dust. The U.S. National Institute of Environmental Health Sciences set up a team to collect dust samples during the clean-up. Asbestos, fiberglass, dioxin, freon, heavy metals, and volatile gases such as benzene were just some of the hazardous substances that caused the "World Trade Center cough" (Chen & Thurston, 2002).

Efforts for Cleaner Air

The United States has taken responsibility for its air pollution problems for the past 50 years. The Air Pollution Control Act of 1955 provided funds for federal research in air pollution. The Clean Air Act of 1963 was the first legislation regarding air pollution control establishing a federal program within the U.S. Public Health Service to research techniques for monitoring and controlling air pollution. In 1967 the Air Quality Act expanded federal government activities to monitor ambient air and stationary sources of air pollution. The Clean Air Act of 1970 authorized the development of federal and state regulations to limit emissions from stationary and mobile sources. The National Ambient Air Quality Standards (NAAQS) and National Emission Standards for Hazardous Air Pollutants

 SELECTED CHRONOLOGY OF AIR POLLUTION CONTROL

1947 California became the first state to address the problem of air pollution prohibiting the release of particles that would constitute a "nuisance to life."

1955 Air Pollution Control Act became law (amended in 1960).

1963 The Clean Air Act enacted.

1965 Motor Vehicle Air Pollution Control Act (PL 89-272) passed.

1970 National Ambient Air Quality Standards for six criteria pollutants were established.

1985 Montreal Protocol eventually banned the use of CFCs.

1990 Tightened Clean Air Act standards mandating reformulated gasoline and set emissions limits for hazardous air pollutants (HAPs).

1997 Kyoto Protocol called for the reduction of six greenhouse gases.

(NESHAP) were initiated. About the same time the National Environmental Policy Act established the Environmental Protection Agency (EPA) to implement requirements included in the Clean Air Act. The 1977 amendments set provisions to prevent significant deterioration of air quality. The 1990 amendments increased the authority and responsibility for the federal government to control acid rain and toxic air pollutants to protect the ozone layer.

Chapter 2 provided information about global efforts to control air pollution and prevent global warming problems. The Montreal Protocol of 1987 called for reduced production of CFCs. The Kyoto Protocol of 1997 called for the reduction of six greenhouse gas emissions. President George W. Bush rejected the Kyoto Protocol, saying the United States would combat global warming in other ways. In spite of that setback, more than 170 other nations proceeded with the treaty (Lindsay, 2001). In response to global concerns, President Bush created the Clear Skies Act of 2003 creating a mandate that power plant emissions comply with the National Ambient Air Quality Standards for sulfur dioxide, nitrogen oxides, and mercury.

Air Pollution Across the Globe

The primary sources of air pollution in the United States are industries, power plants, and automobiles (Figure 8-5). Although all countries are affected, the most problematic air pollution is found in countries in the early stages of industrialization. For example, China is the second largest user of energy in the world after the United States, but it is heavily reliant on coal (EIA, 2005), a very inefficient and wasteful form of energy. Five of China's largest cities are among the 10 most polluted cities in the world. By the year 2015, China's carbon emissions are expected to increase approximately 4% annually due to rapid economic growth and increase in coal use.

India, Brazil, and other developing countries also have problems with air pollution. Citizens have adjusted to living in haze and carry cloths to cover their faces. Unleaded fuel in many areas is expensive and hard to find. Inefficient scooters also spew out pollutants. In addition to the burning of fossil fuels, the burning of forests also creates air pollution that sometimes shuts down airports and factories, and harms crops and tourism. In 1998, millions of people in Mexico and Texas choked from the smoke and cinders that hung over the area for days (NASA, 1998).

Methods for Reduction of Pollution

Some ways to reduce the contribution of greenhouse gases include setting strict emissions standards, reducing fossil fuel use, developing alternative sources of energy, removing carbon dioxide from emissions at the source, eliminating the use of chlorofluorocarbons, slowing or mitigating deforestation, and developing agricultural techniques that release less carbon dioxide to the atmosphere. These changes would have far-reaching impacts on the current use of energy, affecting industries and the economy. Some point out that developing new technology to reduce global dependence on fossil fuels could spur economic growth, but critics contend that the costs of implementing an effective program would be too high (Hopkins, 2003).

CONTROL OF AUTOMOBILE EMISSIONS

In a typical city, automobile exhaust contributes up to 80% of nitrogen oxides, 90% of carbon monoxide emissions in the air, and a significant amount of hydrocarbons and airborne particles (Reese, 1999) (Figure 8-6). The av-

FIGURE 8-5 CO Emissions by Source Category, 2000 Air Trends
Source: Environmental Protection Agency, http://www.epa.gov/airtrends/data/dl_graph.html.

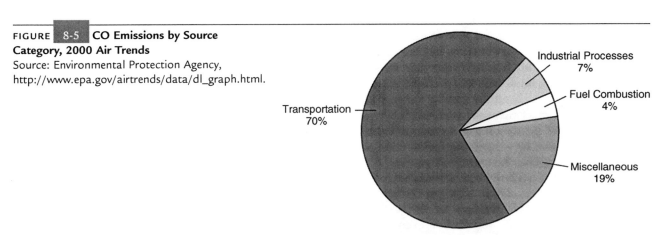

Transportation 70%

Industrial Processes 7%

Fuel Combustion 4%

Miscellaneous 19%

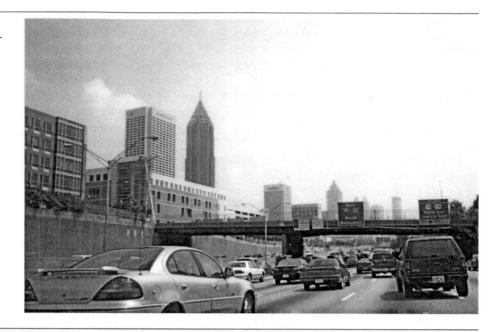

erage automobile operates at 15% efficiency, with sport utility vehicles (SUVs) and light trucks being the least efficient (Motavalli & Reese, 1999).

Since 1969, the U.S. vehicle population has grown six times faster than the human population, 2.5 times faster than the number of households, and double the rate of new drivers. As Matthew L. Wald put it in *The New York Times*, "They bid fair to become the dominant life form." Despite being only 5% of the world's population, Americans own 34% of the planet's cars and drive an estimated 2 trillion miles annually. Over the past 30 years, vehicle miles traveled have gone up 116%. Motor vehicles account for nearly 90% of the energy consumed for travel (Motavalli & Reese, 1999).

Automobile manufacturers have added catalytic converters, fuel injection systems, and even made smaller engines to improve on gas efficiency. Catalytic converters, installed on the tailpipes of automobiles, have been the most successful means of controlling smog. Emissions standards (Figure 8-7) for new vehicles have also been a way of decreasing pollutants, but the standards for trucks and SUVs are less restrictive than standards for cars. Small SUVs, mini-vans, and pickup trucks must meet the same standards set for cars by the year 2007. Large SUVs must meet the same standard by the year 2009. Reformulated gasoline is also a means of reducing automobile emissions by oxygenating fuel to make combustion more complete. Reformulated gasoline (RFG) contains ethanol and has lower octane levels but is sometimes more expensive. Cities with particularly high ozone levels require the purchase of RFGs. Denver, known for its "brown cloud" was the first to enact a program where all fuels sold at gasoline stations were required to have 3% oxygen content (Anderson et al., 1997).

VOLUNTARY ACTIONS BY INDUSTRIES

Some factories that emit particulate matter have installed electrostatic precipitators and filters to smokestacks. In order to reduce sulfur dioxide, scrubbers have been used. Pollution-control equipment, improvements in energy efficiency, and the use of alternative fuels provide ways to control air pollution, but none of them are 100% effective. States with particularly high air pollution have taken the initiative to monitor and reduce air pollution, not without resistance from industries and residents. The health care costs from respiratory illnesses alone ought to be an incentive to reduce emissions, but oftentimes economic development is favored over the health of an "average" individual.

OPEN BURNING LAWS

Most communities have open burning laws specifying when or where open burning is permitted or when a permit can be issued to an individual. Open burning is permitted for burning yard waste such as weed, branches, leaves, and untreated wood products but should not be used to burn household trash. This is important because household trash contains rubber, plastic, and other solid waste that may release toxic chemicals, such as dioxins, cadmium, or hydrocarbons, into the environment. Alternatives to burning include taking waste to the landfill, composting, mulching, or plowing it into the soil.

FIGURE **8-7** **U.S. Mobile Source Carbon Monoxide Emissions Impact of Emission Control Programs**
Source: Environmental Protection Agency, http://www.epa.gov/otaq/inventory/overview/images/charts/emissiontrends_allmobile_co-2.gif.

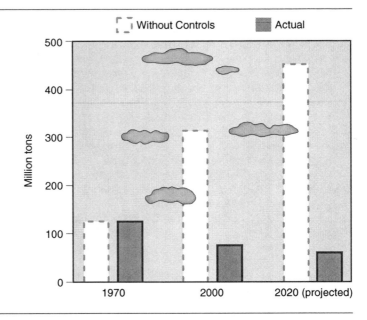

Consider the Cost

WHAT CAN I DO FOR AIR POLLUTION?

_____ Stop using aerosols.

_____ Stop smoking and ask others not to smoke when I'm around.

_____ Keep the muffler and exhaust system on the car in good working condition.

_____ Open windows for fresh air at home, work, and school.

_____ Use cleaning chemicals in ventilated conditions.

_____ Dust, vacuum, and clean living quarters at least once per week.

_____ Remove pets and plants from indoors.

Summary

The composition of the air is extremely important to the prevention of chronic respiratory disease, destruction of vegetation, and maintenance of an environment conducive to health. Air quality must be monitored and maintained by curtailing some of the industries that pollute the heaviest. Each nation has a responsibility to its citizens and other countries to produce without pollution.

Air is composed of natural elements necessary to sustain life in the trophosphere and atmosphere. The influence of human activities has increased the amount of gases known to trap heat, reduce the protective ozone layer, and increase global temperatures. Air pollution is a concern, particularly because of the increased number of automobiles and industries emitting gases and particulate matter that cause respiratory problems. Several air pollutants are being carefully monitored by local, state, and federal governmental officials. The problem is so widespread and leaders from countries around the world have voiced their concerns in an effort to work collaboratively and solve the problem. Without the continuing support and conservative practices of individuals, this goal would not be achievable.

REFERENCES

Allmaras, R., Schomberg, H., Douglas, C. Jr., & Dao, T. (2000). Soil organic carbon sequestration potential of adopting conservation tillage in U.S. croplands. *Journal of Soil and Water Conservation, 55*, 365–73.

American Hydrogen Association. (2005). The Hindenberg fire: Hydrogen too dangerous for the public to use. Retrieved from http://www.clean-air.org/hindenberg.htm.

American Lung Association of California. (2002). Milestones in air pollution history. Retrieved from http://www.californialung.org/spotlight/cleanair02_milestones.html.

American Meteorological Society. (2005). Legislation: A look at U.S. air pollution laws and their amendments. Retrieved from http://www.ametsoc.org/sloan/cleanair/cleanairlegisl.html.

Anderson, L., Lanning, J., Wilkes, E., Wolfe, P., & Jones, R. (1997). Effects of using oxygenated fuels on carbon monoxide, formaldehyde, and acetaldehyde concentrations in Denver. Paper presented at the Air & Waste Management Association, June 8–13. Toronto, Ontario, Canada. 97-RP139.05. Retrieved from http://carbon.cudenver.edu/~landerso/97rp13905.htm.

Atwood, S., & Kelly, B. (1997). The Southland's war on smog: Fifty years of progress toward clean air. Diamond Bar, CA: South Atlantic Air Quality Management District. Retrieved from http://www.aqmd.gov/monthly/marchcov.html.

Bellis, M. (2005). The history of neon signs. Part 1: Georges Claude invents the first neon lamp. Retrieved from http://inventors.about.com/library/weekly/aa980107.htm.

Canadian Center for Occupational Health and Safety. (2004). CHEMINFO: Methane gas. Retrieved from http://www.intox.org/databank/documents/chemical/methane/cie75.htm.

Centers for Disease Control. (1995). Deaths from melanoma—United States, 1973–1992. *Morbidity and Mortality Weekly Report, 44,* 337, 343–347.

Centers for Disease Control. (2004). Cancer prevention and control: Questions and answers. Retrieved from http:www.cdc.gov/ChooseYourCover/qanda.htm#uv.

Clean Air Trust. (2005). Sulfur dioxide. Retrieved from http://www.cleanairtrust.org/sulfurdioxide.html.

Chen, L., & Thurston, G. (2002). World Trade Center cough. *Lancet, 350,* 37–39.

Dao, J. (2000). Acid rain law found to fail in Adirondacks. *New York Times, 149,* A1.

Energy Information Administration. (2005). China's energy demand now exceeds domestic supply. Retrieved from http://www.eia.doe.gov/emeu/cabs/archives/china/part2.html.

Environmental Protection Agency. (2000). Killer smog triggered pollution control. Retrieved from http://www.epa.gov/epahome/other3_0810.htm.

Environmental Protection Agency (2003). Ozone: Good up high, bad nearby. EPA-document 451/K-03-001, June 2003. Retrieved from http://www.epa.gov/oar/oaqps/gooduphigh/.

Estes, J., & Billy Smith, B. (1997). *A Melancholy Scene of Devastation: The Public Response to the 1793 Philadelphia Yellow Fever,* pg. 7. Canton, MA: College of Physicians of Philadelphia.

Few, R. (2003). Flooding, vulnerability and coping strategies: Local responses to a global threat. *Progress in Development Studies, 3,* 43–58.

Foster, K., Jenkins, M., Toogood, A. (1988). The Philadelphia yellow fever epidemic of 1793, *Scientific American, 279,* 88–93.

Fuller, J. (2000). Clean Air Act amendments provide the muscle to fight pollution. *Global Issues: Green Cities: Urban environmental issues, 5.* Retrieved from http://usinfo.state.gov/journals/itgic/0300/ijge/gj-07.htm.

Geller, A. (1998). Skin cancer prevention education interventions. Summary of the National Forum for Skin Cancer Prevention in Health, Physical Education, Recreation, and Youth Sports. Reston, VA: American Association for Health Education.

Gordon, J. (1993). The American environment. *American Heritage, 44,* 30–48.

Gould, P. (2000). Race, commerce, and the literature of yellow fever in early national Philadelphia, *Early American Literature, 35,* 157–186.

Hopkins, B. (2003). Renewable energy and state economics. Lexington, KY: The Council of State Governments. Retrieved from http://www.csg.org/NR/rdonlyres/eojdro6vzmmepzgmgxyzo44okq3qe7jt3.

Intergovernmental Panel on Climate Change. (2001). Observed climate variability and change. In *Climate Change 2001: Working Group I: The Scientific Basis.* Retrieved from http://www.ipcc.ch/.

Jefferson Lab. (2005). It's elemental: Neon. Retrieved from http://education.jlab.org/itselemental/ele010.html.

Lindsay, H. E. (2001). Global warming and the Kyoto Protocol. *Cambridge Scientific Abstracts, Environmental Policy Issues, Hot Topic Series.* Retrieved from http://www.csa.com/hottopics/ern/01jul/overview.html.

Logan, W. (1953). Mortality in the London fog incident, 1952. *Lancet, 1,* 336–338.

McElroy, M. B. (2002). *The atmospheric environment: Effects of human activity.* Princeton: Princeton University Press, 2002.

Melanoma Research Foundation. (2005). The melanoma fact sheet. Retrieved from http://www.melanoma.org/mrf_facts.pdf.

Motavalli, J., & Reese, A. (1999). Moving targets. *Environmental Magazine, 10.* Retrieved from http://www.emagazine.com/oldissues/november-december_1999/1199feat1sb1.html.

Muir, J. (1911). *My first summer in the Sierra.* The quote is found in Chapter 6 Mount Hoffman and Lake Tenaya. Boston, MA: Houghton Mifflin.

National Aeronautical and Space Administration. (1998). Mexico fires—May 1998. Retrieved from http://www.odysseyofthemind.com/mexico.htm.

Neue, H. 1993. Methane emission from rice fields: Wetland rice fields may make a major contribution to global warming. *BioScience, 43,* 466–473.

Peterson, J., & Cairns, C. (2003). Nitrous dioxide toxicity. Retrieved from E-Medicine at http://master.emedicine.com/emerg/topic847.htm.

Reese, A. (1999). Bad air days: Air pollution in the United States. *The Environmental Magazine, 10,* 28–38.

Rosenzweig C., & Hillel, D. (1998). *Climate Change and the Global Harvest: Potential Impacts of the Greenhouse Effect on Agriculture.* New York: Oxford University Press.

Schindler, D. W. (1988). Effects of acid rain on freshwater ecosystems. *Science, 239,* 149–157.

Schrenk, H., Heimann, H., Clayton, G., Gafafer, W., & Wesler, H. (1949). *Air pollution in Donora, Pennsylvania. Epidemiology of the unusual smog episode of October 1948.* Washington, DC: U.S. Government Printing Office.

Scienceshorts.com. (2005). Acid rain. Retrieved from http://www.scienceshorts.com/articles/Acid%20Rain.htm.

Scotto, J., Cotton, G., Urbach, F., Berger, D., & Fears, T. (1988). Biologically effective ultraviolet radiation: Surface measurements in the United States, 1974–1985. *Science, 239,* 762–764.

Shope, R. (1991). Global climate change and infectious diseases. *Environmental Health Perspectives, 96,* 171–174.

Simeonov, V. (2005). Environmental history of the 20th century, pg. 11. Retrieved from http://www.pg.gda.pl/chem/Kierunki/environ_hist_Simeonov.pdf.

The Skin Cancer Foundation. (2005). Sun safety. Retrieved from http://www.skincancer.org/prevention/index.php.

Spurny, K. R. (1996). Atmospheric particulate pollutants and environmental health. *Archives of Environmental Health, 51,* 415–417.

U.S. Climate Change Science Program. (2003). Chapter 7, Carbon cycle. In Strategic plan for the climate change science program: Final report. Washington, DC: U.S. Climate Change Science Program. Retrieved from http://www.climatescience.gov/Library/stratplan2003/final/ccspstratplan2003-chap7.htm.

University of Pennsylvania. (2005). The yellow fever epidemic of 1793. Retrieved from http://www.sas.upenn.edu/~yehchris/yellowfever.html.

Wagner, D. (1997). Clean air at what cost? New anti-pollution standards from the Environmental Protection Agency. *Insight on the News, 13,* 8–9.

Weisel, C.L., Cody, R.P., & Lioy, P.J. (1995). Relationship between summertime ambient ozone levels and emergency department visits for asthma in Central New Jersey. *Environmental Health Perspectives, 103* (Suppl. 2), 97–102.

Wuebbels, D. J., & Hayhoe, K. (2002). Atmospheric methane and global change. *Earth Science Reviews, 57,* 177–210.

ASSIGNMENTS

1. Call the local health department and find out how air pollution is monitored in the city in which you live.

2. Use several resources such as SCORECARD, GEOCITIES, and AIRNOW to determine the air quality in your location compared to other states and cities.

3. Visit a Web site such as http://www.skincancer.org or http://www.cancer.org to learn more about skin cancer risks, what it looks like, and how to prevent it.

4. Discuss automobile emissions laws in the state in which you live.

5. Utilize a Web site like GreenVehicles http://www.epa.gov/greenvehicles/ to find out how energy efficient your automobile is. Compare your results with others in the class.

6. Compare the contents, price, and performance of various types of fuels sold at gasoline stations.

7. Utilize the environmental science search engine www.envirolink.org to learn more about the harmful effects of air pollution from the 9/11 incident in New York City.

8. Write an essay about the causes and effects of asthma.

9. Investigate hybrid cars or alternative fuels and determine criteria you would use before deciding to buy or use one.

10. Select one of the HAPS from the list found at http://www.epa.gov/ttn/atw/188polls.html and find out what products contain them.

SELECTED ENVIRONMENTAL LAWS

1955 *Air Pollution Control Act (PL 84-159)*
The federal government's first attempt to consider the problem of air pollution. This law authorized the Public Health Service to begin air pollution research and provided some technical assistance to state and local governments.

1963 *The Clean Air Act (PL 88-206)*
The purpose of this act was to prevent the deterioration of air quality by setting emissions standards for power plants and steel mills. In 1965 the Motor Vehicle Air Pollution Control Act (PL 89-272) set standards for auto emissions. In 1967 the Air Quality Act (PL 90-148) set quality standards with deadlines. PL 91-604 was enacted in 1970 to prevent the deterioration of air quality by setting national ambient air quality standards. PL 101-549 was enacted in 1990 to raise automobile emissions standards, encourage the use of low-sulfur fuels as well as alternative fuels, and called for a reduction in chlorofluorocarbons to prevent ozone depletion.

SELECTED PROFESSIONAL JOURNALS

Atmospheric Environment
Aviation, Space, and Environmental Medicine
Ecology
Environmental Pollution
Environmental Science and Technology
Journal of the Air and Waste Management Association
Journal of Environmental Quality
Particulate Science and Technology
Respiratory Cell and Molecular Biology
Respiratory Physiology
Water, Air, and Soil Pollution

ADDITIONAL READING

Davis, Devra. (2002). *When smoke ran like water: Tales of environmental deception and the battle against pollution.* New York, NY: Basic Books.

Rock, M. *The Automobile and the Environment.* New York: Chelsea House, 1992.

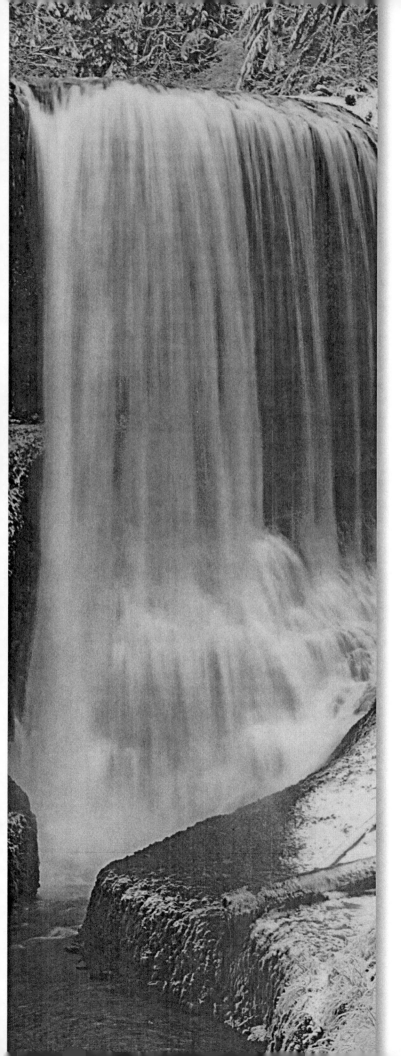

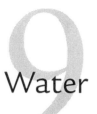

Water

Water, water, everywhere, and all the boards did shrink;
water, water, everywhere nor any drop to drink.
Samuel Taylor Coleridge (1772–1834)

OBJECTIVES

1. Contrast problems for wildlife in freshwater and saltwater environments.

2. Differentiate sources of surface water from groundwater.

3. Explain what estuaries are and why they are important.

4. Explain why wetland areas are important and give examples of different types.

5. Describe what an aquifer is and how the water rises to the surface.

6. Explain what a watershed is and its importance.

7. Provide an explanation of aquaculture and reasons for its development.

8. Compare ocean water pollution issues, freshwater pollution issues, and groundwater pollution issues.

9. Differentiate point source and nonpoint source pollution.

10. Discuss drinking water quality issue and threats to drinking water safety.

Introduction

quatic ecosystems need water to support the plants, animals, and fish living in them. There are four types of *aquatic* ecosystems: rivers and streams, lakes, freshwater **wetlands**, and coastal or marine. Each ecosystem has its own unique characteristics that sustain the biodiversity of species different from the other ecosystems. Freshwater species cannot live in saltwater environments, and saltwater species cannot live in freshwater environments. Aquatic ecosystems are vulnerable to climate changes, perhaps more than any other ecosystem. Without water, there are no aquatic ecosystems. The ecosystems of **aquatic life** are extremely important because they provide food for millions of people on this planet.

Water: A Natural Habitat

here are basically two types of water: saltwater and freshwater. Over 97% of the Earth's water is saltwater, providing a habitat for **marine life** (Earth Ministry, 2005). Saltwater is found in oceans and seas. Whales, walruses, seals, manatees, dolphins, sharks, tuna, shrimp, clams, lobsters, and many other species inhabit the oceans. So vast is the ocean that there are probably species that have not been discovered. Many species have been used for food. Some species have been over-farmed or over-fished so that they are becoming harder for those in the fishing industry to find; some are endangered.

Saltwater sources provide a means of transporting goods and citizens from one country to another. Unfortunately, it also has been used as a dumping ground. Containers full of hazardous waste have been dumped offshore (Moreno, 2000). Urban garbage and sewage are routinely dumped. Some cities have disposed of old subway cars, buses, and other means of public transportation in ocean depths. Cruise ships, a fast-growing industry, also dump sewage and garbage (IMO, 2000). Ship accidents and off-shore drilling have contaminated ocean water with oil, radioactivity, and chemicals. Warmer coastal waters have changed reproductive patterns of shellfish, making it more difficult for those fishermen to make a living. Coral reefs are inhabited with new bacteria that destroy it and the species it shelters.

Only 3% of the Earth's water is freshwater (Earth Forum, 2005). Freshwater provides a habitat for fish, birds, frogs, plants, and other species and is found in rivers, streams, lakes, ponds, and underground **aquifers**. Almost 2% of freshwater supply is unavailable because it is frozen in polar ice caps and glaciers. The amount of water on Earth does not increase. There are 6 billion people in the world today. If growth continues the way it has, by the year 2050 there will be 9 billion people. If water consumption continues at the current rate, 2.7 billion people will face severe water shortages by the year 2025 (Postel, 2001). Someday water will become as valued as iron or oil. All over the globe, usable water is being pumped out of the Earth faster than it can be replenished. Severe water scarcity presents the single biggest threat to future food production (Postel, 2001). Many freshwater sources are stressed beyond their limits.

"Water wars" over ocean transportation have been present for centuries. On land, water rights have been legally disputed between landowners, industries, and communities. In the United States, some states have

2010 HEALTHY PEOPLE OBJECTIVES

WATER QUALITY

8-5 Safe drinking water
   Increase the proportion of persons served by community water systems who receive a supply of drinking water that meets the regulations of the Safe Drinking Water Act.

8-6 Waterborne disease outbreaks
   Reduce waterborne disease outbreaks arising from water intended for drinking among persons served by community water systems.

8-7 Water conservation
   Reduce per capital domestic water withdrawals.

8-8 Surface water health risks
   Increase the proportion of assessed rivers, lakes, and estuaries that are safe for fishing and recreational purposes.

8-9 Beach closings
   Reduce the number of beach closings that result from the presence of harmful bacteria.

8-10 Toxic chemicals
   Reduce the potential human exposure to persistent chemicals by decreasing fish contaminant levels.

Wetlands
Areas covered with water for periods long enough to support plants that thrive in wet soils; bogs, swamps, marshes, and wet meadows; many wetlands may be seasonally dry or lack noticeable vegetation during certain seasons.

Aquatic life
Plants, animals, and fish living in or on the water.

Marine life
Plants, animals, and fish inhabiting the oceans and seas.

Aquifers
Underground geologic formations in which the cracks in rock, sand, soil, or gravel are filled with water.

fought over the use of rivers and aquifers. The state of Colorado is most famous for water rights issues. As settlers were acutely aware of how important the water supply was for survival, they homesteaded river banks. Some dredged areas diverting water away from the primary source in order to irrigate crops. As industries became established and required large supplies of water, water rights were threatened, particularly during a **drought**. Many lawsuits claimed that industries violated water rights laws when they diverted water away from its primary source (Walley, 1999). Water rights are especially important in 19 Western states, including California, Idaho, and Utah. Increasingly more states and communities are experiencing or facing similar issues. As populations increase in urban settings, cities and industries compete with farmers for water resources.

Water: A Natural Resource

long with land, minerals, and energy, water is one of for Earth's most valuable resources. Without water, humans would only survive 3 to 4 days (Irvin, 1999). Nearly every living thing depends on moisture to survive. Most people consider water to be a renewable resource; indeed, water can be used and reused, disposed of and deposited back to Earth again. After reading about the hydrologic cycle in Chapter 1, it would seem that the supply is endless. In fact, only 1% of Earth's water can be consumed by humans, and it is in short supply as populations grow rapidly, municipal water consumption increases, global warming and drought continue, irrigation increases, and pollution continues (Hinrichsen, et al., 1998). Pollution and global warming have changed weather patterns and ecological processes that sustain life. After describing different types of water and their uses, the issues of pollution and waterborne illnesses will be discussed.

Types of Water

pproximately 71% of the Earth's surface is covered with water. There are two types of water on Earth: surface water and groundwater. **Surface water** is found in oceans, rivers, streams, lakes, ponds, and wetlands and can be saltwater or freshwater. Surface waters provide transportation, food, and can be used as a source for municipal water supplies.

 HOW DOES WATER FLOW?
Water flows to the Pacific on the west side of the continental divide and toward the Atlantic on the east of the continental divide.

SURFACE WATER

Ocean Waters

Ocean water comprises 97.4% of the Earth's water. Ocean water is very salty and as is cannot be used for human consumption. There is no cheap and effective method of **desalinization**, although in coastal areas where water is becoming scarce, cities are considering it.

Estuaries

Estuaries are areas where saltwater and freshwater meet, providing a valuable habitat important to sustaining fish and other aquatic populations. Rivers and streams provide the freshwater and the ocean brings the tide in and out to provide the saltwater. The Chesapeake Bay is one of the largest and most productive estuaries in the world, supporting over 2,700 species of plants and animals (Chesapeake Bay Program, 2002).

Rivers, Streams, Lakes, and Ponds

Rainfall or snowmelt either seeps into the ground and is stored in an aquifer or it becomes runoff flowing into rivers and lakes. The water is usually flowing from one source into another. Creeks merge into rivers and streams, and rivers eventually flow into the ocean. Large

Desalinization is a process used to extract salt from saltwater so it can be used for drinking, irrigation, and industrial uses. Only 1% of the water people use is desalinated, and most of that is produced in desert and island areas. The primary reason why desalinization is not widely used is because of the time and expense it takes to remove the salt from saltwater. The principal methods used for desalinization include distillation, electrodialysis, freezing, ion exchange, and reverse osmosis. During the distillation process, saltwater is heated to make the water evaporate, leaving the salt behind. The desalinated vapor is then condensed to form water. Unfortunately, fossil fuels are used to produce the heat for the process. India and Africa have used distillation processes. Another method is electrodialysis. Ions in the saltwater are attracted to semipermeable membranes, leaving desalinated water outside the membrane. Again, this process requires fuel. The most promising approach is reverse osmosis. Pressure is applied to saltwater to force it through a special membrane. Only water flows through, leaving the salt behind. Reverse osmosis costs less than half of the cost of distillation and is being used to remove salts from the Colorado River. In Hawaii, an ocean thermal energy conversion plant has been built using steam for energy, then condensing the steam into freshwater. California and Florida are also experimenting with desalinization processes that might make it more affordable and efficient (Montaigne, 2002).

rivers may branch out into tributaries that divert water out toward other areas of land (Figure 9-1). If natural tributaries do not provide water in certain areas or if the rivers frequently rise about the riverbank and flood land used for homes or farmland, channels can be dredged, diverting the overflow into areas where it will do more good than harm. A major river, including its main channels, backwaters, all tributaries, wetlands, and terrestrial habitats contribute to its drainage and flow.

If water flows to a place surrounded by higher land and no outlet, a lake is formed. Flat land with a depression can become a pond. Whether flowing water becomes a creek, stream, lake, or pond depends on the **water table** lying beneath the land. When the water table is high, the ground is saturated from the aquifer underneath, making ground unstable. Over time and in areas with heavy rainfall, creeks and streams can cut into the land even farther into aquifers making a strong current that widens and deepens the river even farther.

Wetlands

There are four types of wetlands: **marshes, swamps, bogs**, and **fens**. Not all wetlands are wet all the time. Marshes are wet most of the time and have various types of grasses and trees in them (Figure 9-2). Some are along the coast and others are in floodplains or along rivers and lakes. The Florida everglades is a marsh. Prairies and plains have areas that are wet during certain seasons. They are sometimes referred to as *prairie potholes* or *wet plains*. Swamps are known for their standing water, trees, and shrubs. Georgia has the Okofenokee Swamp

Drought
A period of several months when precipitation is significantly less than normal.

Surface water
Freshwater not absorbed into the Earth or returned to the atmosphere as part of the water cycle; streams, rivers, ponds, lakes, and reservoirs; only about .02% of all water on Earth is surface water.

Desalinization
The removal of salt from saltwater sources for drinking.

Water table
The depth or level below which the ground is saturated with water.

Marshes
Saltwater or freshwater wetlands characterized by grasses and sedges.

Swamps
Areas fed by streams or springs that are flooded most of the year; swamp vegetation prevents downstream floods and is a natural purifier of organic waste.

Bogs
Raised areas of wet earth, roots, grass, decaying moss, and other vegetable matter with a spongy consistency, found in a marsh or swamp; a type of wetland where soil is soggy, strongly acidic, and low in nutrients.

Fens
Low lands covered wholly or partly with water (German and Old English term).

FIGURE 9-1 **River** Once clear and free-flowing, rivers are struggling to keep up with the demands of irrigation, urban sprawl, and tourism.

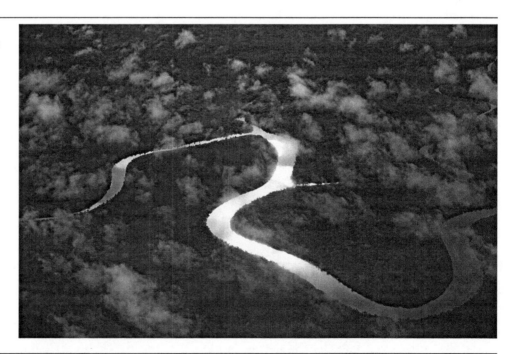

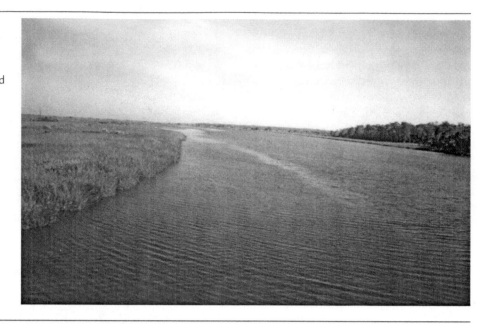

and Virginia the Great Dismal Swamp. In Louisiana, they are referred to as *bayous*. Bogs are known for their evergreen trees, shrubs, and spongy peat and sphagnum. Bogs are known for their favorable habitat for growing blueberries, cranberries, and pitcher plants. They are found from Maine to the Carolinas. Peat bogs are found in cooler latitudes such as the northern U.S. and Siberia. Fens are noted for their grasses, reeds, and wildflowers. They are usually found in states with cool climates and higher altitudes such as New York, Michigan, Minnesota and Oregon.

Wetlands are considered a transition zone between water and land. Wetlands assist with the hydrological and nutrient cycles mentioned in Chapter 1. Because of the varieties of species that live in wetlands, they are sometimes referred to as the "nurseries of life." As urban developments consume more land, many native species seek refuge in wetlands areas. Unfortunately, about 60,000 acres of wetlands are lost each year in the United States. Wetland loss along the coast can be attributed to human population growth, urban development, changes in sea level, and erosion from coastal storms (NOAA, 2004). Wetlands are important because they improve drinking water, reduce flood damage, and enhance recreational opportunities. They absorb large quantities of water because of their sponge-like capabilities. The loss of any wetlands to urban development is a great tragedy.

GROUNDWATER

Groundwater is freshwater found underground in large reservoirs surrounded by rock called aquifers. An *aquifer* is like a sponge filled with wet gravel with areas in between filled with water. Precipitation and streams and lakes **recharge** the water supplies in aquifers, but at a much slower rate than is being removed. The largest aquifer is in known as the Ogallala aquifer and extends under several Midwestern states (Figure 9-3).

- The Ogallala aquifer is the largest single water-bearing unit in North America. It stretches from Texas to South Dakota with the largest portion lying under Nebraska. Most of the water from this aquifer is used for irrigation. There is a major concern as water levels continue to drop due to irrigation of semi-arid regions and drought (U.S. Water News Online, 2003).

- The Sparta aquifer provides water to Arkansas, Louisiana, Mississippi, and Tennessee. Geologists have recorded large withdrawals from the Memphis area, causing water levels to decrease by 7 feet (USGS, 2004).

Depletion of water from aquifers is becoming a major concern because it cannot be replenished or recharged by rainfall as quickly as it is being pumped out.

Groundwater becomes surface water when it is brought to the surface by springs through rock faults or fractures, forming a brook, pond, wetland, bog, or marsh. The type of soil and rock where the water is found is important to water quality.

Water Tables

ater tables lay beneath the topsoil and between the saturated and unsaturated zone under the topsoil

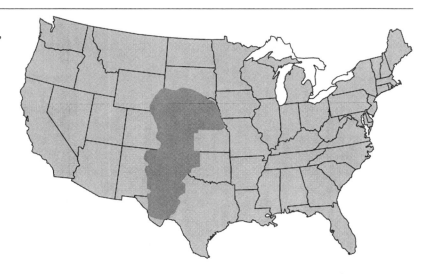

FIGURE 9-4 **Water Table** Underground water
supplies should be determined before building to
prevent damage due to potential flooding or shifting
foundations.
Source: U.S. Geological Survey, Water Science for
Schools, http://ga.water.usgs.gov/edu/earthrivers.html.

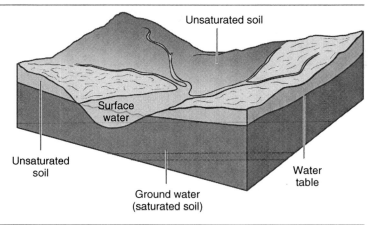

(Figure 9-4). Water tables are not at the same levels because they are dependent upon their water sources. Areas that flood may have fluctuating water tables, depending upon the wet and the dry season. Before building a home or digging a **well**, it is important to know where the water table is.

Watersheds

In order to protect surface water, watersheds have been developed. A **watershed** is an area of land that drains to a body of water such as a stream, lake, pond, wetland, or **estuary**. Watersheds benefit from the ability of wetlands to filter nutrients and mediate water and soil chemistry. Watershed ponds are often created in areas where there is a depression or near

Groundwater
Water beneath the Earth's surface between soil and rock; supplies wells and springs for drinking water.

Recharge
To fill, as water seeps into the ground to fill aquifers and groundwater supplies.

Well
A deep hole dug in the ground to obtain water and other substances.

Watershed
The geographic region within which water drains into a particular body of water.

Estuary
Inland marine waterways dominated by grass or grass-like plants and lay between barrier islands and beaches; an inlet where the salty tide of the ocean meets the freshwater current of a river, lake, or stream.

a stream. In rural areas, watershed ponds are used for fish farming or conservation projects. Dams or levees are built to capture the water. Watershed ponds are built with overflow pipes and can be drained when needed. The water quality in ponds depends upon rainfall and land uses. Watershed ponds in urban areas are created to catch **storm water runoff**.

There are often boundary issues concerning the use of water for drinking, recreation, flood control, agriculture, ecosystem maintenance, hydropower, and other things managed by federal, state, and local officials, and governing bodies. **Watershed districts** serve as a voice for anyone affected by the jurisdiction or use of water and adjacent land for any purpose.

Freshwater Uses

ater is needed for many things. In addition to providing habitat for biodiversity, transportation, flood control, and recreation, water is needed for human activities such as household consumption, irrigation, aquaculture, power generation, and industrial uses.

The average American citizen probably does not appreciate the abundance of freshwater the country has. Globally 1.2 billion people drink unclean water (Czarra, 2002-03). About 2.5 billion lack proper toilets or sewage systems. More than 5 million people die each year from waterborne illnesses. Areas like Africa, the Middle East, and South Asia are especially short of drinkable water. In these areas, freshwater is hard to maintain because the land is so dry.

BIOINVASION OF WATERS
Zebra mussels, native to eastern Europe, were first discovered in the Great Lakes in 1988. Since then, they have spread rapidly and become a pest with great potential for changing aquatic ecosystems. First, the mussels easily attach to vessels that transports them many miles from where they first appeared in the country. Second, mussels have larvae that spread quickly and settle in large colonies. Third, they can attach to any hard surface. They have plagued aquatic systems and water intake systems, impeding water source supplies. They foul the water, remove edible algae, and reduce native clam populations by attaching to them and competing with them for food. Their large numbers push native fish out of their ecosystems. The fouled water can plug engine cooling systems for some boats. Once they have colonized a lake or river system, there is no means to control or eliminate them. The solution to the zebra mussels dilemma will not be over any time soon (Chou, 1999).

Water usage is monitored by the U.S. Geological Survey (USGS) and information is published every 5 years. In the United States, the use of *surface water* is classified as instream or off-stream. **In-stream** means the water is used at its source; for example, a power plant utilizes water from a river or stream to cool its nuclear reactors or generators. **Off-stream** use means the water is channeled away from its source; for example, for agricultural irrigation.

In order, the largest uses of water are (1) agriculture, (2) industry, and (3) household use. Freshwater usage in the United States has increased dramatically from 1950 to 1980, particularly for livestock and household use (Brown, 1999).

AGRICULTURAL USE

The primary uses for water in agriculture are to irrigate crops, provide water for livestock, and parks and golf course maintenance. Irrigation is the biggest single use of water consumption in the United States. Today, irrigation accounts for two thirds of water use worldwide (Postel, 2005). With about 40% of the world's food grown in irrigated soils. Farmers can reap two to three harvests each year and get higher crop yields with irrigation. Because of irrigation, the global grain production has tripled since 1950. The U.S. Department of Agriculture monitors irrigation and produces a report every 5 years. Food crops need large quantities of water, particularly in dry climates or areas with clay soil. In dry climates, water evaporates, limiting the number of species that can provide food. Clay soils fail to hold moisture and crops require more water than areas with **loamy** soil.

Irrigation is the biggest single use of water consumption in the United States. The availability of water resources is becoming crucial in western and southern states where the population growth is booming. Some areas in the western states are experiencing droughts and irrigation levels are low. When water levels in irrigation ditches are low, **stagnant** water creates breeding areas for mosquitoes that carry infectious diseases. In addition to monitoring low irrigation water, farmers need to inspect their irrigation systems to eliminate seepage, run-off, and soil erosion from too much water use. The Soil Conservation Service has been working with those in the Colorado River Basin and Uinta Basin in Utah to assist in practices such as land leveling, structures for water control and measurement, and reduced salt loading, which help to better utilize the natural resouces.

INDUSTRIAL USE

Industrial use includes the cooling down of generators for power plants and processes in manufacturing. Solvents used to degrease machinery and wastes from older manufacturing operations are still emitted in some areas. Sometimes mercury and dioxins are emitted as by-products of industrial processes. Mining activities use water to cool drills, machines, and transport raw materials out of the mine. Mining operations have been known to dump iron hydroxide and sulfuric acid into streams lowering the pH and eliminating aquatic life.

HOUSEHOLD USE

Household use includes water for drinking, washing, and other uses. The typical person uses about 100 to 150 gallons of water daily or about 23,000 gallons per year (Rogers & Sothers, 1995). Most of water use is for:

- flushing the toilet
- personal bathing and hand washing
- laundry
- kitchen tasks
- other uses, such as watering the lawn and washing the car

AQUACULTURE

Aquaculture in the United States began in the 1850s as a commercial enterprise when the spawning and growing of brook trout was desirable as a food source. After finding that aquaculture could be profitable, the species have expanded to include finfish, shellfish, crustaceans, reptiles, and various aquatic plants. Some are produced for a food source, pets, bait, and for sport fishing. Others are used for research purposes. Aquaculture is regulated by the nation's first federal conservation agency, the U.S. Fish and Fisheries Commission, established in 1871. Today it is known as the National Marine Fisheries Service and it regulates marine commercial fishers. The U.S. Fish and Wildlife Service (USFWS) is responsible for regulating freshwater fish and recreational fishing. For some species of fish, such as the Chinook and coho salmon, the two agencies share responsibilities.

Private hatcheries produce fish for food, bait, as aquarium pets, and for stocking private waters. Public fish hatcheries produce "wild" fish for stocking public waters to enhance or restore recreational or commercial fisheries. In 1973, the Endangered Species Act became a catalyst for shifting the goals of public hatcheries from stocking sport fish to propagating endangered and threatened species. Any species of fish living in a natural pond can be grown in a levee pond, including channel catfish, hybrid striped bass, shrimp, crawfish, perch, and several types of bait fish. Water quality is especially important to aquacultures providing fish for food. Fish can be grown in watershed levee ponds, flowing water systems, or recirculating water systems, depending on the type of fish. Some species of salmon and redfish are grown in net pens or cages suspended in ocean water because the species require normal tidewater processes to flourish. Floating and bottom water systems are used to produce shellfish such as mussels, clams, and oysters.

HYDROELECTRIC GENERATION

Hydroelectric plants require the construction of a dam and **reservoir**. The Hoover Dam was constructed on the Colorado River in the 1930s to generate power, to control floods, for irrigation, and for recreation. The United States is considered a world leader in building dams, but Russia, China, and other countries have a greater number of them. Although dams are useful, increasing the water supply to one user means decreasing it for other users. Dams reduce land and natural habitats. In particular, ecosystems are damaged or destroyed. Because their habitats are destroyed, hundreds of species of freshwater fish are threatened or endangered. An example of this is the squaw fish, native to Colorado. This particular fish extends from 4 to 6 feet in length and often becomes trapped in channels for dams so they cannot reproduce.

Global Warming Issues

Scientists have been monitoring the effects of global warming on surface and ground water supplies. Increased climate temperature increases evaporation of water stores and changes the habitat for microscopic organisms that aquatic life need. Changes have already been observed in fish and plant

Storm water runoff
Water that flows downhill to a stream, lake, or ocean; usually carries soil, plant nutrients, pesticides, urban litter, and other residues.

Watershed district
A political subdivision of the state where the conservation, development, and proper management of natural resources is a priority.

In-stream
The use of surface water at its source; e.g., stream water used to cool nuclear reactors at a power plant.

Off-stream
The use of surface water channeled away from its source; e.g., irrigation.

Loam
A type of soil with clay, sand, and organic matter; a very fertile type of soil.

Stagnant
Not moving or glowing, motionless.

Reservoir
A body of water stored for future use.

Many take the Earth's water supply for granted. Society expects water to come forth each time the tap is turned on. It is a good idea to read the water meter or water bill each month to check how much water the household is using. The amount of water used often can be reduced by fixing leaky toilets, faucets, or pipes, installing water-efficient shower heads and faucets, and other water-saving habits. Leaky faucets can usually be fixed by tightening the connections or replacing a worn washer. A toilet that leaks can waste as much as 200 gallons of water per day. To determine if there is a silent leak in the toilet, put a few drops of food coloring in the tank before going to bed. If there is color in the bowl the next morning, the toilet has a leak. Inventors have been designing new toilet systems that decrease the amount of water used to flush toilets. Biological toilets, composting toilets, incinerating toilets, oil-flushed toilets, and vacuum-disposal systems also are being tested.

Flow restrictors are inexpensive and easy to install for faucets, but should not be used in water lines leading to washing machines, dishwasher, lawn-watering systems, or garbage disposers. Shower heads can be purchased with a shut-off valve that temporarily stops water while shampooing. Aerators can be installed to fit into the end of a faucet so the water stream seems the same as a faucet without flow restriction.

When building or remodeling, toilets, showers, water heaters, washing machines, and dishwashers that have water-saving mechanisms should be considered. Low-flow toilets use only 1.6 gallons of water per flush (gpf) compared to an older toilet that uses 5 to 7 gpf. Showers that use 2.5 gallons of water per minute (gpm) can be used instead of regular showers that use 5 to 10 gpm. If a person does not have the luxury of replacing or buying new plumbing devices, the water bill can still be reduced by the following strategies:

- Set a timer for 4 minutes to take a shower.

- Do not let the water run while shaving, brushing teeth, or washing the face or hands.

- Turn the water off when shampooing or shaving.

- Keep the water level less than 5 inches for a bath.

- Reduce the number of showers or baths taken. A sponge bath uses less water.

- Flush the toilet after every 2 to 3 uses or when solid waste is present. Do not put facial tissue in the toilet and flush each time the nose is blown.

- Use the dishwasher for full loads. Scrape dishes before putting them in the dishwasher instead of rinsing.

- Select the shortest dishwashing cycle. If pots and pans have excess residue, wash them by hand.

- Large serving and cooking dishes that take up space in the dishwasher can be washed by hand.

- When hand-washing dishes, rinse them in a basin of water rather than running water.

- Store bottles of water in the refrigerator instead of running water until it is cold enough for drinking.

- When doing laundry, select the water level for the amount of laundry or only wash full loads.

- Wash clothes only when truly soiled. Garments can often be worn a few times before laundering.

- Hand wash several items at the same time (e.g., pantyhose or stockings).

- Use a spray nozzle that shuts off when washing the car. Wet the car, soap the car while the water is turned off, and then rinse the car.

- Water plants and grass only when it is necessary. Make sure the driveway and sidewalks are not "watered."

- Water the lawn or plants early in the morning using a drip-hose instead of a sprinkler.

- Mulch plants, trees, and shrubs to hold in the moisture.

- Remove weeds that use water and nutrients.

- Reduce the size of the lawn or consider Xeriscaping with plants, trees, and shrubs that require little water.

HOW SAFE ARE OUR BEACHES?
The EPA has a Beach Watch Program that provides information about beaches along coasts, inland waterways, and the Great Lakes. Records are kept regarding beach advisories and closings from the previous season. Data from 2002 indicate that over 80% of beach advisories were for elevated bacteria levels. The primary identifiable sources were from storm water runoff, wildlife excretions, boat discharges, and sewage. More than half of the pollutants could not be identified. Source: EPA, 2005.

species. In ocean waters, sea levels are rising as polar ice caps melt. Increased water temperatures have changed aquatic environments, particularly when algae flourish in the warmer waters. With more algae, the rate of photosynthesis increases, causing plants to grow and die faster. When the plants die, the increased water temperatures speed up bacterial decomposition and create a higher demand for oxygen. Warm water also increases metabolic rates of aquatic animals and the demand for oxygen. Species numbers may decrease if they are not able to reproduce in warm water and many are susceptible to disease. Sudden changes may cause thermal shock and death (Stevens Institute of Technology, 2004). Of course, warmer waters mean that other fish can migrate into the area, but experts are reluctant to make predictions whether it would be for the better or worse.

Water Pollution Issues

 SURFACE WATER POLLUTION

Sometimes chemicals are discharged into surface waters by industries.

Ocean Pollution

The ocean has been a depository of waste for a long time. Sewage, toxic waste, and other harmful materials were dumped into ocean waters until 1988. Today, most of what is dumped into the ocean is **sediment** from dredging other bodies of water to provide better channels for boats to pass through. The U.S. Army Corps of Engineers is responsible for the dredging and dumping activities. Most of the sediment goes to the ocean floor far from the shoreline. Substances such as gasoline, oil, other types of fuel, human waste, and other materials are left behind by naval carriers, submarines, cruise ships, barges, and other oceangoing vessels. Some coastal cities discharge storm water **runoff** onto beaches. *Marine pollution* is an invasion of the marine environment by something that doesn't belong there. Many species of marine life do not tolerate polluted coastal waters because of warmer than usual waters, lower concentrations of **dissolved oxygen** (**DO**), or lack of species they normally feed on. Destruction of natural habitat destroys species.

In 1989, the *Exxon Valdez* spilled 11 million gallons of crude oil near Prince William Sound, Alaska. Few can forget the images of dead and dying wildlife covered with oil. Ten years later oil continued to leach from area beaches and aftereffects indicated recovery was still several years in the making. As tragic as this was at the time, oil spills continue to happen nearly every day. Tankers, barges, pipelines, refineries, and offshore oil drilling are sources of oil leaks. Oil floats on water and spreads rapidly in a thin layer called an *oil slick*. The layer becomes thinner and thinner, eventually looking like a rainbow on top of the water creating a sheen. Oil spills are especially harmful to birds and animals that frequent ocean surfaces. Skimmers, sponges, chemicals, and vacuums are just some of the ways that oil spills are managed.

Newspaper headlines reveal dead seals, dolphins, and whales that wash up on the shoreline due to disease or the effects of pollution. Scientists speculate water pollution as the cause of these sea creatures' demise, a problem that allows viruses to destroy the creatures immune systems, thus succumbing to diseases. Over 700 dead bottlenose dolphins

NEWS RELEASE
EPA SEWAGE PROPOSAL SEEN NEAR COMPLETE: A long-stalled regulation aimed at limiting the amount of raw sewage discharged into America's waterways is in the final stages of analysis and will be released to the White House Office of Management and Budget for approval in the next two weeks, a U.S. EPA official said last week. The new sanitary sewage overflow (SSO) rule, developed during the Clinton administration, seeks to address a problem that has been hampering progress on water quality since the enactment of the Clean Water Act 30 years ago. EPA has been slow to act on the problem because of the cost to local communities of bringing the discharges under control.
Source: Greenwire, 2002.

that washed up on the coast of New Jersey in 1987 were found to harbor up to 50 times the danger levels of toxic PCBs (International Dolphin Watch, 2005). These are symptomatic of the human problem on a larger scale. Oils and chemicals can kill birds, plants, and fish. Untreated **sewage** can spread disease and contaminate shellfish beds. Sea turtles can mistake plastic bags for jellyfish and eat them. Birds, seals, dolphins, turtles, and other animals can get caught in fishing lines, nets, and suffocate or become crippled.

Because of different incidents polluting ocean waters, there are laws to guard against ocean pollution. In 1972, the Marine Protection, Research, and Sanctuaries Act was enacted to regulate intentional disposal of materials in the ocean and to authorize research. The EPA, the U.S. Army Corps of Engineers, the National Oceanic and Atmospheric Administration, and the U.S. Coast Guard regulates permits and enforces the ban on dumping radiological and chemical waste, biological warfare agents, high-level radioactive waste, and medical wastes. In 1997 the act was amended to ban the dumping of municipal sewage sludge

---

Sediment
Soil, sand, and minerals washed from land into water, usually after rain; destroys aquatic life.

Runoff
The portion of rainfall, melted snow, or irrigation water that flows across land, picking up pollutants from air or land, and eventually runs into streams.

Dissolved oxygen (DO)
The amount of free oxygen dissolved in water that sustains aquatic life; low DO is generally due to excessive organic matter present in water as a result of inadequate waste treatment and runoff.

Sewage
Mostly liquid waste, including human waste, transported by sewers and treated in a sewage treatment plant.

and industrial waste. In response to the *Valdez* spill, Congress passed the Oil Pollution Act of 1990 (PL 101-380), requiring companies involved in storing and transporting oil to have plans to clean up oil spills on land or in water. The Coast Guard must approve the cleanup plans while the EPA oversees the cleanups on land and in waterways.

Freshwater Pollution

Pollution of freshwater is a serious issue. A leading cause of water pollution is sediment carried by wind or runoff from urban development. When silt is deposited into water, fish and vegetation are affected. Fish suffocate or die from disease, and vegetation either becomes overgrown or gets killed out. Environmental science specialists often refer to the biochemical oxygen demand (BOD) needed by aquatic species. A high BOD is an indicator that microorganisms are in the water, trying to manage decaying material and pollutants. When runoff includes fertilizers or sewage, vegetation can mature rapidly, die, decay, and contribute to stagnant, smelly, and aesthetically unappealing waters.

Sewage is also discharged into **waterways**. Pathogens from sewage are carried into bodies of water, making it poor for many uses. In certain areas, consumption of shellfish carries a warning. Heavy metals can also pollute the water from industrial discharges and atmospheric deposits from power plants and incinerators. Even under normal circumstances, surface water can become contaminated by floods, fertilizers, pesticides, urban runoff, sewage, and deposits from the atmosphere.

Flooding

The overflow of water from flooding can affect human health in many ways. It is the most common of all environmental hazards, adversely affecting millions of people worldwide. Floods occur due to heavy rains but certain areas are more prone to flooding when areas with a high *water table* are developed for urban housing. When an area floods, many drinking water supplies become contaminated. As stagnant water pools are left standing for several days, mosquitoes and other disease-carrying insects multiply, and individuals may acquire infections from unsanitary living conditions (Roberts, Confalonieri, & Aron, 2001). Floodwaters also carry sewage, oil, fertilizers, pesticides, and other pollutants to wells and municipal drinking water supplies.

Irrigation, Pesticides, Fertilizers, and Animal Waste

Irrigation of crops and grasses contribute to major water losses from run-off, seepage, and evaporation. In addition, irrigation creates other problems such as soil erosion and water pollution. Water pollutants from agricultural uses include sediment, pesticides, fertilizers, organic wastes, and salts from soils. Organic waste from animals is a big problem because it can contaminate water supplies when run-off seeps through the soil and invades groundwater supplies.

Urban Run-Off and Deposits from the Atmosphere

Urban sprawl has created many opportunities for pollution. Residues, such as gasoline, oil, rubber, and other materials, are left on streets and highways from automobiles. When it rains, storm water washes these materials, sewage, and other debris into water sources, creating water pollution problems (Figure 9-5). In coastal areas, the runoff is shunted to areas where bacteria deposits make

FIGURE **9-5** **Stormwater Drain** In urban areas these are needed to control stormwater runoff to prevent flooding in residential and business areas.

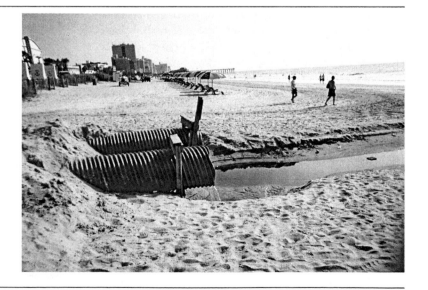

the water unsafe for swimming. Beach advisories often inform swimmers not to get into ocean waters within 24 hours after a storm for that reason (US EPA, 2002). Air pollutants from automobiles and factories also contribute to acid rain, which can make surface waters acidic and create unsafe water supplies for wildlife.

GROUND WATER POLLUTION

Aquifers are essential to life above the ground by providing water to drink, replenishing rivers and wetlands, and their effects on rainfall and climate. Groundwater in aquifers or wells can become contaminated by anything that enters the groundwater source or anything that percolates or **leaches** down through the soil. A primary cause of groundwater contamination are underground storage tanks containing toxic chemicals, septic systems, landfills, large industrial facilities, fertilizers, and oil spills. Underground storage tanks contain petroleum products and hazardous chemicals. Leaking pits, ponds, and lagoons in urban areas where wastewater is "treated" are also a major source of ground water pollution. When rainfall is heavy or if flooding occurs, overflow from septic and **sewer systems** can get into groundwater supplies. Toxic substances can also reach aquifers from the surface when substances are poured on the ground and it percolates through the soil.

Point Source Versus Nonpoint Source

Origins that are well-defined by a pipe, ditch, or tank are known as *point source pollution*. Origins that are not identifiable because of runoff or seepage are known as *nonpoint source pollution*.

🌎 THE CUYAHOGA RIVER
In Ohio's early history, the Cuyahoga River provided transportation into the wilderness from Lake Erie. The city of Cleveland, located on this great river, grew into a mighty industrial city. By the mid-twentieth century, the river was not only a major artery for transportation, but it also carried the effluent of area industries. The river became turbid and rank with chemicals and sewage. On June 22, 1969, the Cuyahoga River burst into flames because of the ignitable oil and debris from smelting that was associated with a local mining operation. Today, the water sparkles, boaters enjoy the water, and 27 species of fish have returned to inhabit the waters.
Source: Gordon, 1993.

POINT SOURCE POLLUTION

Factories account for nearly all of the **point source pollution** origins; the majority is wastewater discharging from manufacturing and power plants. Some of the wastewater is contaminated with mercury, dioxins, and other harmful pollutants. Some refinery businesses discharge crude oil by-products into surface waters. The logging industry leaves behind many wood materials that cannot be used to make furniture, paper, or other wood products. The problem is that there are limitations to what the government can do about these problems. The EPA has set standards for pollutants using total maximum daily loads (TMDLs). A *TMDL* is the amount of a single pollutant that is allowed from point and nonpoint pollution sources.

NONPOINT SOURCE POLLUTION

Agriculture accounts for 50 to 70% of the nation's usage of surface water and is a **nonpoint source polluter**. Agricultural sources of ground water pollution include farm chemicals (fertilizers and pesticides), soil erosion, and manure. Runoff from agricultural land and other properties carries nitrogen and phosphorus into surface water and groundwater supplies that cause vegetation to grow out of control due to increases in nitrogen.

Urban activities also contribute a substantial amount of pollution from all different kinds of sources. Storm water runoff consists of sediment, sand, dirt, road salt, oil, grease, pesticides, fertilizers, leaves, seeds, bark, grass clippings, animal and bird wastes, and raw sewage. Con-

---

Waterways
Navigable bodies of water, such as a river.

Leach
Occurs when water moves through landfills or soils and the chemicals in the soil dissolve in the water and contaminate groundwater; the substance moving through the soil is known as *lechate*.

Sewer system
Piping arrangements that carry sewage away from homes to sewage treatment plants.

Point source pollution
Pollution that comes from a specific, identifiable source, such as a pipe, tank, pit, ditch, or channel to a body of water.

Nonpoint source pollution
Pollution from diffuse sources (rather than specific). Stormwater run-off from large land areas may contain pollutants that contaminate surface and ground water over a large area. Common nonpoint sources of pollution include agriculture, forestry, urban sprawl, mining, construction, dams, and saltwater intrusion.

struction sites contaminate waterways with cement wash, asphalt, paint, cleaning solvents, oil, tar, and pesticides. Other sources of groundwater pollution include waste treatment facilities, landfills, septic systems, sewer systems, and in some areas, graveyards. Leakage of underground storage tanks and pipelines, oil spills on the ground, mining, and de-icing of highways also pollute groundwater.

Water Pollution Measures

The first law regulating water supplies was known as the Federal Water Pollution Control Act (PL 845, 1948), which was later renamed the Clean Water Act (PL 95-217, 1977). This act still regulates the restoration and maintenance of water integrity used for recreational purposes. The Clean Water Act maintained that "no one has the right to pollute" and created goals to eliminate all pollutants discharged into waterways by 1985. The main objective was to restore and maintain the integrity of navigable waters in the United States in order to protect fish, shellfish, wildlife, and recreation on the water (Figure 9-6). Waters were also to be restored so they were safe for fishing and swimming activities. The act required states to monitor their own waters and set their own standards regarding chemical discharges and deteriorating conditions. The goals are still being monitored by the EPA, U.S. Geological Society, and state agencies with the responsibility for enforcing the Clean Water Act.

The Clean Water Act also provides guidelines for groundwater protection programs. Other acts have also included groundwater protection measures. The 1974 Safe Drinking Water Act (42 USC 3000) focused on all waters potentially designed for drinking water use whether aboveground or underground. The 1976 Resource Conservation and Recovery Act (RCRA) provides for the cleanup of leading underground storage tanks. The Comprehensive Environmental Response, Compensation, and Liability Act (CERCLA, PL 96-510, also known as Superfund) requires the clean-up of hazardous wastes that can seep into groundwater. The 1996 Federal Insecticide, Fungicide, and Rodenticide Act (FIFRA, 61 Stat 163; amended to PL 100-532) regulates chemicals used on farms.

Recreational Waters

The demand for outdoor recreation areas for swimming, boating, fishing, picnicking, and camping have increased. The Natural Resources Commission works with local health departments to promote watershed protection and control storm water runoff so that waters are swimmable and fishable. Recreational water quality is an increasingly important issue, particularly in states where tourism is a strong base for the economy. Contamination by chemicals, over-vegetation, and pathogens must be kept to a minimum. Most surface waters (lakes, streams, ponds, rivers, and the ocean) are monitored for po-

FIGURE 9-6 **Tennessee River** The Tennessee River flows southwest from the Appalachian Mountains. The Cherokee Dam controls flooding for the Tennessee Valley Authority.

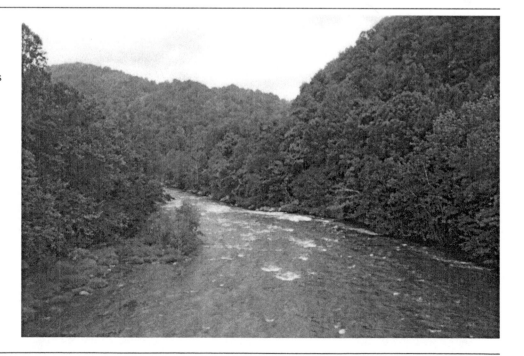

tential problems particularly from point source and nonpoint source pollution origins.

The Coast Guard regulates boating activity in U.S. waters as well as shore side and offshore facilities to prevent pollution incidents. The Coast Guard has emergency plans for oil spills and hazardous substances found near the waterways. The Sea Partners Campaign is the U.S. Coast Guard's marine environmental protection outreach and education program. The purpose of this campaign is to raise public awareness concerning marine pollution issues, to educate waterway users about environmental laws, and to encourage citizens to take personal responsibility for protecting the country's waterways.

Municipal, resort, and hotel facilities for swimming are also inspected regularly to assure water safety. Acidity and alkalinity (pH) levels should range between 6.5 and 8.5. **Turbidity** is important because cloudy waters contain more sediment and pathogens than clear water. When turbidity is a problem, a "clarifier" is added to make the water appear cleaner. Chlorine is added to most swimming pools to control bacterial contamination and growth harmful to humans. Chlorine levels must be carefully controlled as under-chlorination causes red eyes from irritation when bacteria are still present in the water. Chlorine can be added in gas or powder form, and the handling of either is dangerous because of its corrosive nature. All swimming pools are required to have filters that circulate the water, cleaning out debris and other materials that might encourage bacterial growth. The filters usually use sand or diatomaceous earth (a clay powder-like substance) that must be cleaned or replaced on a regular basis. The cleaning of filters requires "backwashing," which rinses water through the filter in order to clean it. The backwash goes into the sewer system or street rather than back into the pool. After backwashing, more sand or diatomaceous earth is added.

Drinking Water

aw or treated water considered safe for drinking and cooking is known as **potable** water to environmental science and sanitation profes-

sionals. Potable water supplies can be contaminated with bacteria, chemicals, metals, and radioactive particles.

BACTERIA

Microbial agents such as bacteria, viruses, or parasites can be found in drinking water even if the water is checked regularly. Most water treatment facilities test for coliform (*E. coli*) bacteria contaminating water supplies by sewage leaks. *Cryptosporidium* is another parasite that is found in surface water. Water treatment programs usually do not test for it because it takes several days to detect. *Cryptosporidium* is resistant to chlorination. Organisms such as this can be killed by boiling water for 1 minute.

A common parasite is *Giardia lamblia,* believed to be the most frequent cause of waterborne illness in the United States. The usual cause is contamination with human or animal waste. Symptoms include abdominal pain, vomiting, and diarrhea. Health effects from drinking contaminated water can occur over a short period of time or a long period of time depending on the type of pollutant. Bacterial infections are often obvious soon after the water is consumed, but the effects of chemicals in drinking water may not be apparent until years after exposure.

CHEMICALS

Pesticides and fertilizers are the most common types of chemicals found in drinking water. In an effort to control heavy mosquito populations, oil and larvicides may be used in standing waters. (See Chapter 5.)

Nitrates

Nitrogen is essential to sustain life. In order to boost plant production, farmers increase the amount of nitrogen in the soil by applying anhydrous ammonia (NH_3) to the ground. When applied to the soil, plants utilize nitrogen and break it into nitrates. However, the primary sources of nitrates in water include fertilizer or feedlot runoff, septic system sewage, and airborne fallout from factories or motor vehicles. The accumulation of nitrates in drinking water is not desirable. Nitrates convert to nitrites in the stomach, attaching to the hemoglobin, thus reducing the oxygen-carrying ability of blood. Nitrates in drinking water can cause "blue baby disease" if it gets into the intestinal tract of infants 6 months and younger.

Turbidity
A measure of the amount of material suspended in water.

Potable
Water quality having good taste, odor, and microbiological quality; drinkable water.

METALS

Heavy metals such as lead and mercury are found in water supplies. Lead may be found in drinking water due to its passage through antiquated plumbing systems. Copper pipes were often soldered together with lead. Brass fixtures also may have been molded with lead. Usually this is not a problem unless these pipes and fixtures become corroded. Because lead is highly toxic, particularly for children, the Lead Contamination Control Act of 1988 (PL 100-572) requires the testing and remedying of lead contamination in drinking water in schools and day care centers. Water coolers with lead-lined storage tanks or parts are also to be tested, recalled, repaired, or replaced or noncompliers will receive heavy penalties. Plumbing in new homes today cannot have lead in them; today PVC pipes are used. Other sources of lead in drinking water include smelting, refineries, steelworks, batteries, iron foundries, and copper mines.

Mercury can evaporate in water or in soil and is usually found in water supplies from smelting operations, cement manufacturing, landfills, sewage, and motor vehicle emissions. The danger with mercury is that it accumulates in the tissues of fish in contaminated waters. When the fish are consumed by humans, mercury poisoning can be very harmful.

RADIOACTIVE PARTICLES

Radioactive particles found in drinking water come from two sources: natural and man-made. Naturally occurring radioactivity is found in bedrock. Uranium, radon, and radium are found in rock and soils surrounding aquifers and in creek beds and river basins. Man-made radioactivity is usually found in surface waters. While it is startling to think we may actually be drinking a carcinogenic substance, it is impossible to eliminate all contaminants from drinking water (Howd, 2002). Various levels of radioactivity in water are considered "acceptable."

PHARMACEUTICALS

Since 1990, the presence of pharmaceuticals in waste and drinking water has become a concern (Jorgensen & Halling-Sorensen, 2000). The first United States study was

in 1999 when water was tested by the USGS. In 81% of the surface water samples, nonprescription drugs were present. Apparently 48% of the samples had antibiotics and 32% had other prescription drugs (Ash, Mauck, & Morgan, 2002; Kolpin, et al., 2002). The highest total concentration noted was steroids (Erickson, 2002). The presence of these medicines was due to veterinary, aquaculture, and human use. The drugs enter the water either through the toilet or drain, spraying or dipping, hospital waste (Kummerer, 2001), or landfill leachate. This reveals that staggering amounts of medications are being discarded inappropriately. The use of the drug prior to disposal is important. Drugs may be unused, excreted, or become biologically active. Never flush medicines down the toilet. Some medicines are transformed in the sewer system or water so they are harmless, and others become more potent. Major concerns about the presence of medications in water supplies are **bioaccumulation** and **bioconcentration**. The lack of data leaves researchers with an "educated guess" at this point. There have been no toxic effects reported from medicines in drinking water, but toxicity levels and degradation of medicines needs to be assessed further. Researchers have been concerned about the "feminization of fish" noted in European rivers since the 1980s (Christensen, 1998). The problem is that this phenomenon may also be attributed to endocrine disruptors found in the water. It is known that antibiotics may lead to antibiotic resistant strains of bacteria and anaphylactic reactions (Kolpin, 2002).

Drinking Water Systems

RURAL DRINKING WATER SYSTEMS

Primary sources of drinking water for rural areas are private wells and rural water systems (Figure 9-7). Over 42 million people in the United States, or 15% of the total population, get their water from private wells, cisterns, or streams. A *cistern* is a large tank open at the top used to gather rainwater for watering crops or lawn. Private

---

DANGERS OF LEAD POISONING:
Lowered intelligence, impaired learning and language skills
Loss of hearing, reduced attention span, poor school performance
Damage to the brain and central nervous system
Possible miscarriage, premature birth, and impaired fetal development
High blood pressure, fatigue, and hearing loss

IS THERE ANYTHING WRONG WITH YOUR WATER?
Fill a clear glass with water and check for the following:
_____ chlorine smell
_____ salty taste
_____ noticeable odor
_____ cloudiness (turbidity)
Check the toilet tank, sinks, shower, bath tub, and other porcelain appliances for:
_____ reddish-brown stains (iron)
_____ blue/green stains (copper)
_____ white stains (calcium and magnesium)

---

wells can be dug by hand or with powered tools. Wells bring water to the surface using pumps.

Private wells are not regulated and property owners must monitor their own water. If individuals experience gastrointestinal symptoms, a health department official can be called upon to test for contamination. In most cases, well water does not need chlorination unless **fecal coliform bacteria** are found. The shallower the well, the greater the potential for contamination. The best site for digging a well is as far away from a septic system as possible. Well locations should be at least 50 feet away from bodies of water, barns, septic tanks, and at least 100 feet from gardens and other areas that may pollute *groundwater* supplies. In areas at risk for potential flooding, the well should be on higher ground. Wells must have a cap over it to keep insects and other surface contaminants out of the water supply. The well should extend at least 12 inches above the ground to prevent rainwater runoff from flowing into the well.

Every state has developed rural water systems that monitor water supplies and water quality. Many rural residents need access to larger quantities of water than average wells for putting out fires, irrigation, and other uses. Water lines and pipes with hydrants are constructed in areas where many rural residents live outside of municipal water supply areas. In less populated areas, rural water association members strive to test water regularly to assure water quality.

MUNICIPAL WATER SUPPLY SYSTEMS

The primary sources of drinking water in urban areas are municipal water supplies (Figure 9-8). Municipal water systems transport water through aqueducts or pipes to a **water treatment plant** that screens the water for large objects, eliminates gases, and adds oxygen. Lime or soda is added to **hard water** to remove the calcium and magnesium. The water is sent to basins where heavy particles (floc) settle to the bottom and are removed. The water is then sent through filters to remove small particles and

Bioaccumulation
Increase in concentration of a pollutant from the environment to the first organism in the food chain.

Bioconcentration
The increase in concentration of a chemical in an organism resulting from tissue absorption levels exceeding the rate of metabolism and excretion; the biocentration factor (BCF) is used to describe the accumulation of chemicals in organisms, primarily aquatic life living in contaminated environments.

Fecal coliform bacteria
A variety of organisms common to the intestinal tracts of people and animals; an indicator of pollution and potentially dangerous bacterial contamination.

Water treatment plant
A facility where source water is cleaned and disinfected to meet drinking water standards.

Hard water
A term used to describe water with high dissolved mineral content such as magnesium and calcium; whereas "soft" water has a low dissolved mineral content.

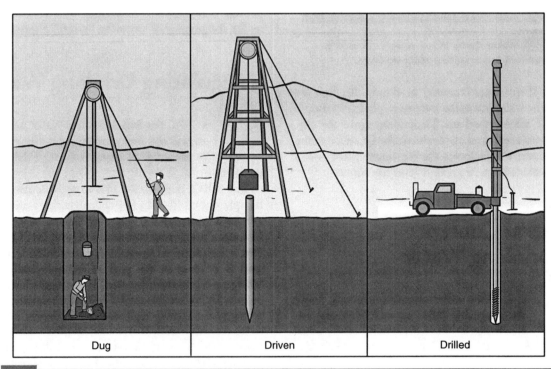

| Dug | Driven | Drilled |

FIGURE **9-7** **Types of Wells** Dug, driven, and drilled.
Source: U.S. Geological Survey, http://ga.water.usgs.gov/edu/earthgwwells.html.

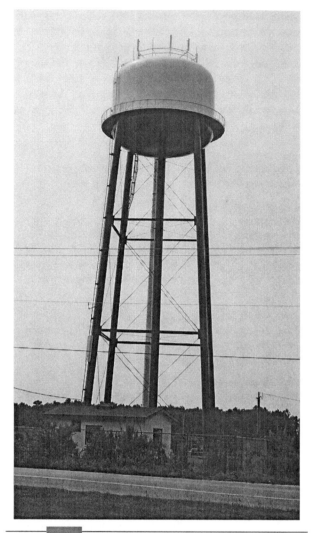

FIGURE 9-8 **Water Tower** Water towers are used in small communities and influence water pressure.

pathogens. If the water is murky or cloudy, clarifiers are added. As the water leaves the treatment plant, chlorine is used to kill microorganisms. Depending upon the city, fluoride to reduce dental cavities may also be added to the water. The water then leaves the treatment plant and is stored in water towers or ground-level containers.

Mineral Content of Drinking Water

all drinking water contains minerals. Some are acceptable (like zinc and selenium) because they enhance the quality of the water or contribute to good health. Other minerals are not desirable because they give the water a bad taste or odor (such as iron, manganese, or sulfur) or because they are harmful to health. It is possible to tell that the water con-

tains minerals by observing stains on porcelain fixtures in plumbing. A reddish-brown stain indicates iron content. This is not a bad thing because the human body requires iron and iron can be absorbed in any form. The only problem is the stain on plumbing appliances. A blue-green stain, however, is an indication that cooper is present in the water. This is not a good thing. Copper is a toxic material but was commonly used in plumbing systems. Older homes may have copper pipes that have corroded and have released copper into the drinking water.

A "rotten egg" odor is an indication that hydrogen sulfide is in the water. From time to time, especially when water resources are low, drinking water may have a peculiar taste and may be cloudy. This is an indication that bacteria or organic matter is in the water. Various types of water filters can be used to remove the bad taste and some of the particles that make the water look cleaner, but water filters cannot remove bacteria, viruses, or chemicals from contaminated drinking water.

In some areas, the water is considered "hard." Hard water may contain magnesium or calcium. It is often considered undesirable because it can stain porcelain and corrode pipes. In other areas of the country, water is considered hard if phosphorus and iron deposits are noted on porcelain plumbing fixtures. Hard water makes it difficult to remove soap scum from clothing, hair, and skin, but this is not necessarily harmful. It does, however, erode plumbing and the appliances that use water such as hot water heaters, dishwashers, and washing machines. In an effort to reduce wear and tear on household appliances and plumbing, and to feel cleaner, some individuals install soft water dispensers. Soft water dispensers distribute salts into the water for the purpose of removing harmful minerals.

Regulating Drinking Water

in 1974, the Safe Drinking Water Act (SDWA) created the first mandatory national program to protect public health through drinking water safety.

The SDWA requires the EPA to regulate contaminants that present health risks in public drinking water supplies. For each contaminant requiring federal regulation, the EPA sets a **maximum contaminant level (MCL)** goal. The EPA is then required to establish an enforceable limit. This level is as close to the goal as technologically feasible, taking costs into consideration. These regulations not only include MCLs but also established requirements for monitoring and analyzing regulated contaminants in drinking water, reporting analytical results, keeping records, and notifying the public when a water system fails to meet federal standards. The SDWA gave the EPA the authority to delegate the primary responsibility for enforcing drinking water regulations to states, territories, or tribes.

The Safe Drinking Water Act of 1974 (PL 93-523) and the Safe Drinking Water Act Amendments of 1996 (PL 104-182) require communities to test drinking water to make sure it is safe. Since passage of the SDWA, there has been a three-time increase in the number of contaminants regulated. Many of these new regulations occurred in 1986 when the act was reauthorized. Amendments to SDWA in 1996 enhanced the existing law by recognizing source water protection, operator training, funding for water system improvements, and public information as important components of safe drinking water.

Threats to Drinking Water Safety

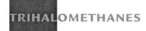

TRIHALOMETHANES

Trihalomethanes (THMs) are a by-product of chlorine and organic matter. There are some concerns that THMs may cause cancer and miscarriages in humans (Capece, 2003). In situations where they are detected, another type of **disinfection** method, such as ozone, is used.

ANTIQUATED MUNICIPAL WATER SYSTEMS

Municipal water systems were not intended to last forever, but many communities do not budget for the replacement of worn-out water systems. The cost of repairing and replacing long-neglected water mains and treatment plants in thousands of cities and towns nationwide is estimated to be as much as $1 trillion (Ausubel & Herman, 1988). In most cases, consumers experience rising water bills due to the cost of repairing and replacing these long-neglected water mains and treatment plants.

BIOTERRORISM THREATS TO WATER SUPPLIES

Water provides an easy way to distribute biological or chemical agents for terrorism; sabotage of the food supply has already occurred (Khan, Swerdlow, & Juranek, 2001; Stern, 1999). In June of 2002, the Public Health, Security and Bioterrorism Preparedness and Response Act (PL 107-188), amended the Safe Drinking Water Act requiring all public water suppliers serving populations greater than 3,300 to complete vulnerability assessments and to develop or modify emergency response plans (Greenblatt, Donohue, & Wagner, 2003). Emergency response plans must provide details about response, recovery, and remediation if a contamination or disruption should occur. More information is needed by local officials regarding the inadequacy of current disinfection and inspection methods against contamination of biological

and chemical disease agents. Enhanced surveillance and response activities provide ways in which illnesses can be detected and treated, but by no means is it preventive.

Acceptable Levels of Water Contaminants?

Contaminants can still be found in municipal water supplies, even after processing. Pollutants are monitored but may be allowed because the substances have permissible MCLs that allow a certain amount in drinking water. There are regulated MCLs and unregulated drinking water contaminants. The list of contaminants and their MCLs is long, but they can be grouped into six categories:

1. microorganisms
2. disinfectants
3. disinfection by-products
4. inorganic chemicals
5. organic chemicals
6. radionuclides

Every 5 years, the EPA is required to list unregulated drinking water contaminants that pose potential health risks.

Future Water Supply Strategies

With all the technology available to us, it would seem that we could generate our own pure water supply without harming the environment or ourselves. Although it is true that certain processes, such as incineration, photosynthesis, and chemical reactions produce water as a

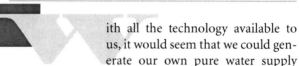

Maximum contaminant level (MCL)
The highest (maximum) level of a contaminant allowed in a public water system under federal or state regulations.

Trihalomethanes (THMs)
A group of volatile organic chemicals (VOCs) formed when chlorine, added to drinking water during disinfection, reacts with naturally occurring organic matter.

Disinfection
The process of killing microorganisms to make water safe to drink.

by-product, it would be impossible to generate new sources of water without harming the water supplies already in place. Air pollution often results in water pollution. Chemical processes also pollute water sources. Water generated from photosynthesis usually evaporates and is lost. To date, no one has found a way to generate water without harming something else.

The hydrologic cycle helps restore water supplies in order to sustain life. It does not, however, produce new water sources. The best strategy to have would be to get more use out of each drop of water. Although rainfall generates water and replenishes aquifers and other bodies of water, it cannot keep up with the rate at which water is drawn from the Earth. Natural water resources that once seem abundant are short in supply as some areas become heavily populated. In urban areas, water conservation is becoming the norm during warmer months in an effort to assure that water is available for everyone, not just those who can afford to waste it. Water can be recycled by cleansing **wastewater** and making it drinkable.

Summary

ater is necessary for life and is a renewable resource. Unfortunately most of the water seen is not drinkable. Some of the water is harmful due to urban runoff, bacteria, sewage, flooding, toxic discharges from industries, and oil spills from transportation vehicles. The water ecosystem is important but is jeopardized by pollutants and invasive species such as the water hyacinth and nutria described in Chapter 1. Rural and municipal water systems have been developed to provide drinkable water

---

Wastewater
Water that has been used either in the home or to manufacture a product and requires treatment and purification before it can be used again.

to citizens and livestock. The water treatment process is complicated and requires continued monitoring. Even with as many controls as available, water is not pure and may have "acceptable" levels of contaminants. Water is a precious commodity that requires conservation. Until more water-efficient appliances are developed, the best way to reduce the use of freshwater is to use it prudently. Conservative use of water can reduce water bills and help preserve the environment for other species.

REFERENCES

Arnaiz, E. (1998). Home water treatment systems: Water filters and purification. Michigan's Drinking Water. Retrieved from http://www.gem.msu.edu/gw/wtr_trt.html.

Ash, R., Mauck, B., & Morgan, M. (2002). Antibiotic resistance of gram-negative bacteria in rivers, United States. *Emerging Infectious Diseases, 8,* 713–716.

Ausubel, J., & Herman, R. (1988). *Cities and their vital systems: Infrastructure past, present, and future.* National Academy of Engineering. Washington, DC: National Academy Press.

Brown, T. (1999). Past and future freshwater use in the United States: A technical document supporting the 2000 USDA Forest Service RPA Assessment. Technical report RMRS-GTR-39. Fort Collins, CO: U.S. Department of Agriculture, Forest Service, Rocky Mountain Research Station.

Capece, J. (2003). Trihalomethanes and our water supply. Retrieved from http://www.southerndatastream.com/thm/.

Centers for Disease Control. (2002). Waterborne diseases. Retrieved April 14, 2003 from http://www.cdc.gov/ncidod/dbmd/diseaseinfor.htm.

Chesapeake Bay Program. (2002). About the Chesapeake Bay. Retrieved from http://www.chesapeakebay.net/about.htm.

Chou, P. (1999). What is the current status of the "invasion" of non-native zebra mussels in the Great Lakes? Has the invasion been stopped or controlled? And what ecological damage has this creature caused other than the clogging of drainage pipes? *ScientificAmerican.com.* Retrieved from http://www.sciam.com/print_version.cfm?articleID= 000279F1-D7F7-1C71-9EB7809EC588F2D7.

Christensen, F. (1998). Pharmaceuticals in the environment—A human risk? *Regulatory Toxicology and Pharmacology, 28,* 212–221.

Colorado Department of Public Health. (2005). Household medical waste management. Compliance Bulletin: Solid Waste SW 005. Retrieved from http://www.cdphe.state.co.us/hm/infecthm.pdf.

Czarra, F. (2002-2003). Fresh water—Enough for you and me? Occasional papers of the American Forum for Global Education, 174. Retrieved from http://www.globaled.org/final174.pdf.

Earth Forum. (2005). Distribution of the world's water. Houston Museum of Science. Retrieved from http://earth.rice.edu/mtpe/hydro/hydrosphere/hot/freshwater/0water_chart.html.

Earth Ministry. (2005). Conservation and care. Retrieved from http://www.earthministry.org/Congregations/water.htm.

Environmental Protection Agency (EPA). (2005). Beach standards, monitoring, and notification. Retrieved from http://www.epa.gov/ost/beaches/.

Environmental Protection Agency (2003). List of drinking water contaminants. Retrieved April 29, 2003 from http://www.epa.gov/safewater/mcl.html.

Erickson, B. (2002). Analyzing the ignored environmental contaminants. *Environmental Science and Technology, 36,* Supplement A, 140–145.

Gordon, J. (1993). The American environment. *American Heritage, 44,* 30–48.

Greenblatt, M., Donohue, J., & Wagner, K. (2003). Homeland security for drinking water supplies. Westford, MA: ENSR International. Retrieved from http://www.environmental-expert.com/articles/article1264/article1264.htm.

Greenwire. (2002). The Environmental News Daily. Retrieved October 29, 2002 from http://www.eenews.net/subscriber/search/swishe-search.cgi?maxhits=&hitsperpage=&q= epa+sewage+proposal&frommonth=01&fromdate= 01&fromyear=2002&tomonth=12&todate=21&toyear=2002.

Hinrichsen, D., Robey, B., & Upadhyay, U. (1997). Solutions for a water-short world. Population Reports, Series M, No. 14. Baltimore: Johns Hopkins School of Public Health, Population Information Program. Retrieved from http://www.infoforhealth.org/pr/m14edsum.shtml.

Howd, R. (2002). Can we protect everybody from drinking water contaminants? *Journal of Toxicology, 21,* 389–395.

International Dolphin Watch. (2005). Dolphins in danger. Retrieved from http://www.idw.org/html/dolphins_in_danger.html.

International Maritime Organization. (2000). Prevention of pollution by sewage from ships. Retrieved from http://www.imo.org/home.asp.

Irvin, J. (1999). How long can a human live without water and food? Retrieved from www.madsci.org/posts/archives/sep99/93754022.Gb.r.html.

Jorgensen, S. & Halling-Sorensen, B. (2000). Drugs in the environment. *Chemosphere, 40,* 691–699.

Khan, A., Swerdlow, D., & Juranek, D. (2001). Precautions against biological and chemical terrorism directed at food and water supplies. *Public Health Reports, 116,* 3–14.

Kolpin, D., Furlong, E., Meyer, M., Thurman, E., Zaugg, S., Barber, L., et al. (2002). Pharmaceuticals, hormones, and other organic wastewater contaminants in U.S. streams, 1999–2000: A national reconnaissance. *Environmental Science and Technology, 36,* 1202–1211.

Kummerer, K. (2001). Drugs in the environment: Emission of drugs, diagnostic aids, and disinfectants into wastewater by hospitals in relation to other sources: A review. *Chemosphere, 45,* 957–969.

Lavelle, M. (2002). Watering hole. *U.S. News & World Report, 133,* Issue 19.

Montaigne, F. (2002). Water pressure. *National Geographic, 202,* 2–34.

Moreno, M. (2000). Hazardous waste cleanup continues: Containers, some full of unsafe material, wash up on Matagorda Island. *Corpus Christi Caller-Times,* Wednesday, October 4. Retrieved from http://www.cbautos.com/2000/october/04/today/local_ne/5743.html.

NOAA. (2004). Use of water level and datum information in NOAA. *NOAA Magazine,* January 14. Retrieved from http://www.magazine.noaa.gov/stories/mag126.htm.

Parrott, K., Roberts, T., & Ross, B. (1999). Household water quality: Emergency supplies of water drinking and food preparation. Virginia Cooperative Extension Publication 346–579. Retrieved from http://www.ext.vt.edu/pubs/housing/356-479/356-479.pdf.

Poff, N., Brinson, M., & Day, J. (2002). Aquatic ecosystems and global climate change. Report prepared for the Pew Center on Global Climate Change. Retrieved June 25, 3003 from http://www.pewclimate.org/projects/aquatic.cfm.

Postel, S. (2001). Growing more food with less water. *Scientific American,* February 18. Retrieved June 23, 2003 from http://www.scientificamerican.com.

Postel, S. (2001). Special report: Safeguarding our water, growing more food with less water. *Scientific American,* February. Retrieved from http://www.sciam.com/2001/0201issue/0201postel.html.

Postel, S. (2005). Quote as Director of Global Water Policy Project. Retrieved from http://www.thinkpopulation.org/pages/water.htm.

Roberts, L., Confalonieri, U., & Aron, J. (2001). Too little, too much: How the quantity of water affects human health. In Aron, J., & Patz, J. *Ecosystem change and public health: A global perspective,* pgs. 409–429. Baltimore, MD: Johns Hopkins University Press.

Rogers, D., & Sothers, W. (1995). Irrigation management series, L-910. Manhattan, KS: Kansas State University Cooperative Extension Service. Retrieved from http://www.oznet.ksu.edu/library/AGENG2/L910.PDF.

Stern, J. (1999) The prospect of domestic bioterrorism. *Emerging Infectious Diseases, Special Issue, 5,* 517–522.

Stevens Institute of Technology. (2004). The global water sampling project: An investigation of water quality. CIESE Collaborative Project. Retrieved from http://njnie.dl.stevenstech.edu/curriculum/waterproj/temperature.shtml.

U.S. Environmental Protection Agency. (2002). Before you go to the beach. Brochure from the Office of Water, USEPA Publication 4101M.

U.S. Geological Survey. (2003). Ground-water depletion across the nation. USGS Fact Sheet 103-03, November 2003. Retrieved from http://water.usgs.gov/pubs/fs/fs-103-03/.

U.S. Water News Online. (2003). Scientists say drought accelerating depletion of Ogallala Aquifer. *U.S. Water News Online, February.* Retrieved from http://www.uswaternews.com/archives/arcsupply/3scisay2.html.

Walley, (1999). The water rights rebellion. Press release, The Paragon Foundation. Retrieved from http://www.furcommission.com/resource/perspect999ay.htm.

ASSIGNMENTS

1. Compare four different types of bottled water for cost, type of water bottled, and particulate matter in the bottom of the bottle; or compare three different types of water-filtering devices for cost, convenience, water clarity, and taste.

2. Call the local fish and wildlife commission to find out what type of wildlife inhabit local bodies of water.

3. Search the Internet to learn what types of aquatic life are considered endangered or threatened.

4. Ask your local county extension agent to sample your water supply or tell you about the characteristics in local drinking water.

5. Visit the Safe Drinking Water Web site sponsored by the EPA to view the list of MCLs.

6. Determine whether you should purchase bottled water or drink water from the municipal water system.

7. Investigate the symptoms of contaminated drinking water and the appropriate action to take to prepare a class presentation.

8. Consider a trip to a lake, river, or beach and use information from this chapter and Chapter 4 to determine whether or not the water is safe for recreational sports such as swimming, boating, or camping.

9. Call the local wildlife and fisheries office in your state to learn where fishing is prohibited in your area due to polluted waters.

10. Discuss one of the following laws regarding water quality in class.

11. Select a governmental Web site and develop a short report on the agency and activities associated with water resources.

SELECTED ENVIRONMENTAL LAWS

1948 ***Water Pollution Control Act (PL 80-845)***
Law concerned with pollution in streams, lakes, and estuaries. Revised in 1972 (Federal Water Pollution Control Act (*PL 92-500*) to include programs for water quality improvements. Amended again in 1977 Clean Water Act (*PL 95-217*) to impose a greater number of stringent requirements on industries and cities to meet the statutory goal of zero pollutant discharge. Provisions were also made for federal financial assistance to municipal wastewater treatment construction. In 1987, it was amended again (*Water Quality Act PL 100-4*) to establish a program for controlling toxic pollutant discharges, to implement programs to control nonpoint source pollution and runoff. In 2000 Congress passed The Beaches Environmental Assessment and Coastal Health Act (*PL 106-284*) to upgrade water quality standards and coastal waters monitoring programs.

1954 ***The Watershed Protection and Flood Prevention Act (PL 83-566)***
Passed to protect streams and flood plains from erosion and sedimentation caused by severe flooding.

1965 ***Water Quality Act (PL 89-234)***
Revised in 1970 by the Water Quality Improvement Act (*PL 91-224*) requiring owners of vessels to clean up or cover the cost of cleaning up water polluted by discharges from their vessels.

1972 ***The Marine Protection, Research, and Sanctuaries Act***
Authorized the EPA to regulate ocean dumping of in-

dustrial wastes, sewage sludge, and other wastes through a permit program. In 1983 a 2-year restriction prohibited dumping any low-level radioactive waste in the ocean (*PL 97-424*). *PL 100-688* prohibited dumping of dumping sewage sludge and industrial wastes. *PL 102-580* amended the law to allow the EPA to designate dumping sites and identify "critical sites where dumping was not appropriate."

1974 *Safe Drinking Water Act (PL 93-523; 42 U.S.C. 300f-j-26)*
Law passed to protect the quality of drinking water; made provision of maximum limits for contaminants (MLC) in public drinking water and techniques for their removal; amended in 1986.

1990 *Oil Pollution Act (PL 101-380)*
Determination of oil pollution sources, liability, and means of compensation for damage incurred.

1996 *Federal Insecticide, Fungicide, and Rodenticide Act (PL 95-516; 7 U.S.C. 136-136y); also known as FIFRA*
FIFRA supplies legal requirements to have pesticides registered, classified, labeled, distributed, and properly used to protect humans and the environment from adverse effects of insecticides, fungicides, and rodenticides.

SELECTED PROFESSIONAL JOURNALS

Biocycle
Coastal Management
Ecology
Estuaries
Environmental Management
Environmental Science and Technology
Functional Ecology
Hydrological Processes
IMO News Magazine
Journal of Aquatic Ecosystem Stress & Recovery
Journal of Coastal Research
Journal of the American Water Resource Association
Journal of the American Water Works Association
Journal of the Water Environment Federation
Journal of Water Resources Planning and Management
Marine Pollution Bulletin
Science
Water Environment and Technology
Water Environmental Research
Water Management
Water Research
Water Resources Bulletin
Water Resources Research
Water Science and Technology
Wetlands

ADDITIONAL READINGS

Chapelle, F., & Landmeyer, J. (1997). *The hidden sea: Ground water, springs, and Wells.* Tucson, AR: Geoscience Press.
Mitsch, W., & Gosselink, J. (2000) *Westlands,* 3rd edition. New York: John Wiley & Sons, Inc.
National Research Council. (2001). *Compensating for wetland losses under the Clean Water Act.* Washington, DC: National Academy Press.

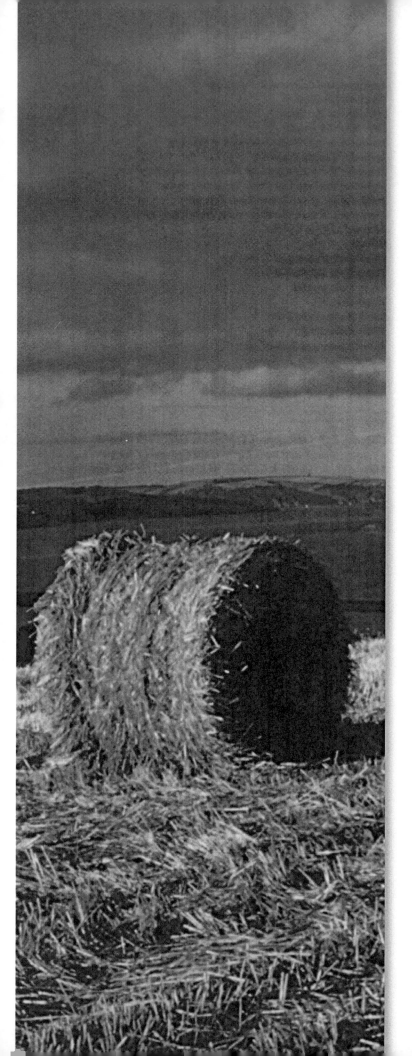

10

Land

We abuse land because we regard it as a commodity that belongs to us. When we see land as a community to which we belong, we may begin to use it with love and respect.

Aldo Leopold (1887–1948)

OBJECTIVES

1. List agencies assigned the responsibility for preserving and managing public lands.

2. Explain how deforestation and forest fires cause problems with land quality.

3. Provide reasons for coastal erosion and methods used to defer it.

4. Explain the concern over riparian rights.

5. Describe land concerns regarding mining practices.

6. Describe factors that lead to desertification.

7. Explain why the composition of soil is important.

8. Provide evidence that the use of fertilizers and pesticides are harmful.

9. Explain hazards associated with brownfields.

10. Describe hazards associated with the management of biosolids.

Introduction

and is just as important as air and water in sustaining life. The quality of land is important to the types of food available, the nutrient content of foods, susceptibility to water pollution, shelter requirements, and safety from external elements. Land quality differs from place to place and is one of society's greatest natural resources. It is renewable, as long as it is not degraded to the point of no return. People have profoundly affected the **topography** and quality of land since the beginning of time.

It is estimated that people migrate from one area to another, one country to another, and one continent to another because of scarce resources. Lack of water, **desertification**, natural disasters, deforestation, depleted soils, pollution, and contamination are just some of the reasons why people migrate in the hopes of finding better opportunities and quality of life. Population growth and land degradation are interrelated. Estimates are that 10% of the Earth's surface is at least moderately degraded, some areas so severely degraded that biotic functions have been completely destroyed, losing its natural productivity (World Resources Institute, 2005). Figure 10-1 shows areas of the world where soil degradation is severe.

Certain ecosystems or biomes are more vulnerable than others. Tropical rain forests, wetlands, grasslands, and tundra are more easily disturbed and take longer to recover. Deforestation, draining of wetlands, overgrazing of livestock herds, and poor agricultural practices are the primary reasons for land degradation. In addition to concern for the impact degradation has on biomes, the economy of these areas depends on productivity of the land.

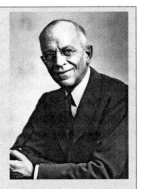

Aldo Leopold (1887–1948) was a forester who advocated total protection of certain wilderness areas, including predators. He is best known for writing *A Sand County Almanac* (1949), a volume of nature sketches and philosophical essays expressing an ecological attitude toward people and the land. He advocated what he called "the land ethic," which said that anything harming an ecosystem is ethically and aesthetically wrong.
Source: The Aldo Leopold Foundation. Retrieved from http://www.aldoleopold.org/Biography/Biography.htm.

Land Definitions

he land has varying altitudes, soil composition, and capabilities of restoring our natural resources. Each region in the United States has unique characteristics and biotic qualities according to the type of land.

MOUNTAINS

Mountain areas span over one fifth of the Earth's landscape and are home to nearly one tenth of the Earth's population (Kone, 2002). Society depends on mountainous areas for water, timber, minerals, and grasslands. By definition mountains must be at least 300 meters high and are susceptible to earthquakes, volcanic eruptions, landslides, **avalanches**, and floods. Mountains attract precipitation and account for variations in temperature,

Topography
Detailed description or representation of the physical features of a region.

Desertification
The process of becoming a desert either from mismanagement of land, drought, or climate change.

Avalanche
Large masses of ice, snow, and mud sliding down a mountain.

 "Other holidays repose upon the past. Arbor Day proposes for the future."
J. Sterling Morton (1832–1903)

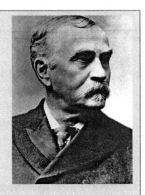

J. Sterling Morton moved his family from Detroit, Michigan, to the Nebraska Territory, once a treeless plain. A newspaper editor, he rose to the position of secretary of the Nebraska Territory. He encouraged residents to plant trees to prevent the loss of *topsoil,* for fuel, and for building materials. He proposed a "tree planting holiday" that was signed by the governor and celebrated on April 8, 1872. The holiday is still promoted by The National Arbor Foundation of Nebraska City, Nebraska. Today Arbor Day is celebrated each year on the last Friday in April, except in areas where planting is best another time of the year.
Source: The history of Arbor Day by the National Arbor Day Foundation. Retrieved from http://www.gardengrove.com/treehist.htm.

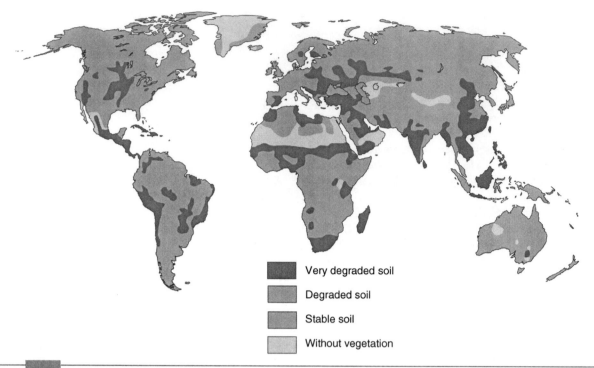

	Very degraded soil
	Degraded soil
	Stable soil
	Without vegetation

FIGURE 10-1 **World Soil Degradation Map**
Source: UNEP Global Resource Information Database (GRID), Arendal, http://www.gm-unccd.org/English/Field/soil.htm.
Reprinted with permission.

wind, and moisture. Wild plants found in mountainous areas also provide important sources of food and medicine. Mountainous areas attract mining operations, hydroelectric and other types of power plants, and tourists.

FORESTS

Twenty-five years ago forests covered slightly over one quarter of the world's land area; now they cover one fifth (Peterson, 2000). The number of forest acres, however, is decreasing as much as 28 million acres per year. Over half of U.S. forests have been destroyed by logging, road construction, mining, forest fires, ski resorts, off-road vehicles, and other human activities (Wear & Greis, 2001). The removal of trees is a major cause of soil **erosion** and landslides. Trees are important for many other reasons, including serving as the habitat for certain species and providing oxygen generated from their photosynthesis processes.

Between 1960 and 1990, tropical forests were destroyed in Asia, Latin America, Africa, the Amazon Basin of South America, and Mexico to clear land for agriculture or for use as firewood and charcoal for fuels. This is unfortunate because of the plant and animal species as well as the atmospheric carbon dioxide absorption benefits that are lost. In addition, soils from forests often are not as fertile as other soils for growing crops and are susceptible to flooding and erosion.

Deforestation is the permanent decline of trees to less than 10% of the forest's original extent (FAO, 2001, 2003). The process usually means burning trees for their removal. Only the United States and Europe have programs to sustain forests to provide timber for building materials, furniture, paper, fuel, and other uses. Nearly 60% of the United States commercial forestland is privately owned. The Soil Conservation Service (SCS) works with owners to maintain woodland resources. They analyze soil productivity to determine the relationship between tree growth and soil types. When trees are removed by logging companies, they are replanted. However, successful reforestation requires years to accomplish and trees are being removed faster than they can be regrown.

WETLANDS

Wetlands were mentioned in Chapter 8 and are explained further here. Wetlands comprise 5 to 9% of the lower 48 states and 40% of Alaska (USGS, 2005). Wetlands may be along coastlines or inland; they may contain saltwater or freshwater. Wetlands are distinguished according to their plant, bird, fish, and animal life and may be referred to as

FIGURE 10-2 **Wetlands**
Wetlands provide nature's
way of shielding land from
erosion and flooding due to
heavy rains.

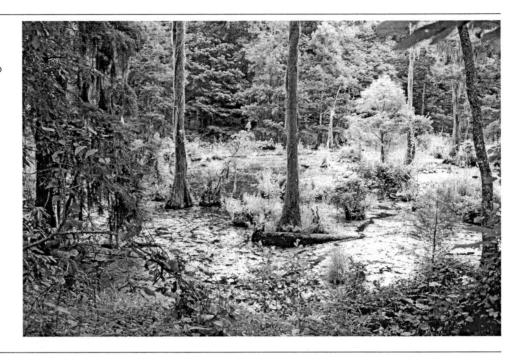

marshes, swamps (or bayous), bogs, and fens. Once regarded as useless swamps and breeding grounds for mosquitoes, alligators, crocodiles, and snakes, wetlands have
had a bad reputation. In fact, wetlands are saturated by
moisture for plants such as rice, blackberries, cranberries,
sphagnum moss, peat moss, and cypress tress. Wetlands are
nutrient-rich, providing habitats for numerous species of
plant, fish, and animal life. One in five species considered to
be endangered depends on the wetlands to survive (EPA,
1995). Nearly two thirds of fish and shellfish require wetlands to reproduce and grow large enough to survive deeper
waters. Over 60 to 90% of commercial fisheries depend on
coastal wetlands. Coastal wetlands have some of the highest
rates of plant productivity. Inland wetlands provide valuable habitat for migratory birds. The difference between
where wetlands begin and where dry land begins is often
debated, resulting in disputes by property owners, builders,
and government officials.

Wetlands also provide a natural method of filtering
pollutants out of the water, converting them to less harmful forms. Wetlands also provide a buffer for flooding,
protect coastlines, and provide recreational opportunities
such as hunting, fishing, canoeing, boating, kayaking, and
skiing. In the past, wetlands were drained for agriculture,
mining, forestry, oil and gas extraction, or urban developments. Some of the wetlands were dredged to make
way for marinas, canals, and ports for boaters. One of the
largest wetlands is in the Florida Everglades. Almost every
state, including dryer states, has wetlands.

In 1977, President Carter issued Executive Order
11990 requiring that federal agencies identify and reduce
potential impacts on wetlands from proposed activities.

Wetlands provide a natural reservoir for flood waters, diverting it from populated areas. Before construction of a
project can be approved in a wetland, it must be demonstrated that no reasonable alternative is available. When
wetland use cannot be avoided, action must be taken to
minimize the damage by repairing the harm or replacing

 REGENERATED LAND
Even the effects of natural disasters can be overcome through conservation efforts and time.
When Mount St. Helens erupted in 1980 in southwestern
Washington, mud, rocks, and lava destroyed plant and
animal life for 15 miles. By the early 1990s, 83 of the
256 plant species present prior to the eruption have
emerged through the layers of volcanic debris. It is apparent that plant life can regenerate itself given time. There
are also examples of plant life transforming barren areas
such as those destroyed by forest fires. After the 1988
fires in Yellowstone National Park, plant life was restored.
In Vermont, trees were planted on abandoned farmland
to begin "new" forests. Older lakes filling with sediment
can convert to marshlands, providing new habitats.

Erosion
The wearing away of rock or soil by the gradual detach-
ment of soil or rock fragments by water, wind, ice, and
other forces.

Deforestation
The removal of trees from a forest area by cutting or
burning to less than 10% of the virgin forest.

the wetlands with an equal or greater acreage. Federal agencies are required to identify and reduce potential impacts on wetlands from proposed activities.

Land Preservation

In order to help protect U.S. natural resources, land was set aside for protection. The land was designated for national forests, national parks, wildlife refuges, wilderness areas, and historic sites. Over 726 million acres have been set aside and are managed by federal government agencies (National Resources Defense Council, 1996).

Today, beautiful areas of the United States are reserved for use as national parks for the public to enjoy. It was not always that way. In 1916, three agencies were in conflict about how forest land should be set aside and used. At that time, the U.S. Department of the Interior was responsible for 12 national parks, 19 national monuments, and 2 reservations. The U.S. Forest Service managed the Grand Canyon and Olympic National Park near Olympus for timber harvest. Then Congress passed the National Park Service Act, establishing the National Park Service for the management and protection of national parks, monuments, and reservations. The authors of the act were well aware of the conflicts between the concepts of use and preservation, but they also knew that Congress would never agree to exclude these areas from public use. The law mandated the National Park Service to conserve the scenery and the natural and historic objects and the wildlife therein and to

In the United States, George Perkins Marsh (1812–1929) was the first to raise concerns about the destructive impact of human activities on the environment. In 1847, Marsh gave a speech to the Agricultural Society of Rutland County, Vermont, calling attention to deforestation. He advocated a conservationist approach to the management of forested lands in his book, *Man and Nature or The Earth as Modified by Human Action*. Source: Clark University (2005).

Gifford Pinchot (1865–1946) is known as America's first professionally trained forester. He is remembered as a conservationist because he led an era where the cutting of trees became controversial. He fought for wiser use of natural resources. In 1898 he was appointed chief of the Division of Forestry for the Department of Agriculture by President Theodore Roosevelt. During his term as chief forester, the number of state parks swelled from 32 to 149 and covered 193 million acres. Source: Department of Environmental Protection, Pennsylvania (2005).

FIGURE **10-3** **National Forest and Grasslands**
Source: U.S. National Forest Service.

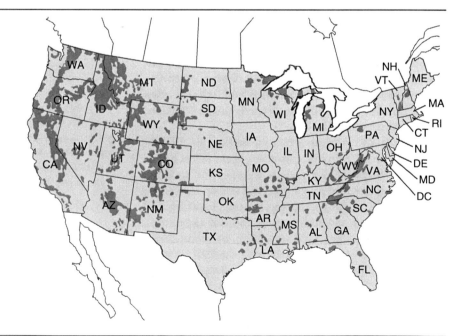

provide for the enjoyment of the same in such manner and by such means as will leave them unimpaired for the enjoyment of future generations.

This carefully chosen language has weathered numerous lawsuits that have, in general, served to strengthen the National Park Service's resource protection powers. Public lands are provided to protect natural resources and ecosystem species as well as provide recreational and other outdoor opportunities.

Effects of Land Usage

 n addition to concerns about the destruction of wetlands, forests, and national parks, the use and abuse of land contributes to environmental health concerns. Overgrazing, mining, erosion, and land pollution cause populations to be exposed to food shortages, impure water, and contaminants.

SOIL EROSION

A major concern regarding land use is the potential for erosion. Erosion normally occurs due to wind, water, and other natural forces. When forests and native grasses are destroyed, rainfall is heavy and erosion is a possibility. Erosion results in sediment formation in waterways and water supplies.

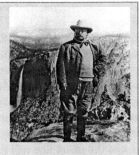

President Theodore Roosevelt visited the "Badlands" of North Dakota in 1883 for hunting and became enamored of the area. Roosevelt is considered a leader in wilderness recreation for the enhancement of personal growth. During his presidency (1901–1909), he helped establish the U.S. Forest Service and the National Wildlife Refuge System. By establishing five national parks, the national forest system was increased by 400%. One of the places saved under the Antiquities Act of 1906, established to create national monuments, was the Grand Canyon. As a result of his efforts, there are now 51 wildlife refuges and 150 national forests in the United States. As a tribute, Theodore Roosevelt National Park is located in Medora, North Dakota.
Source: National Park Service (2005).

COASTAL EROSION

According to the U.S. Army Corps of Engineers, 43% of the lower 48 United States experience significant erosion problems. Over 2,600 miles of beachfront are identified as having critical erosion problems (Public Works, 1997). A beach is like a "river of sand" flowing in a zigzag path

FIGURE 10-4 **Threat to Coastal Ecosystems**
Condominiums and hotels provide economic growth on the coast, and harm to the beaches.

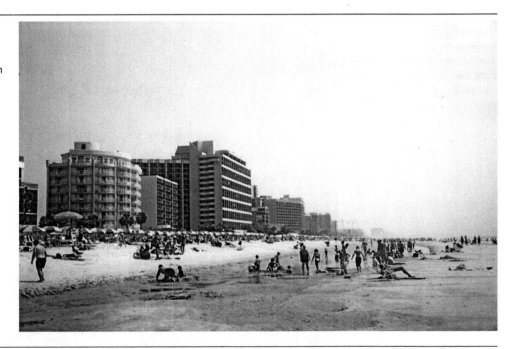

along a shoreline. The **swash zone** is denoted as where water rushes in and out from action of the waves. Disruption of this natural flow causes sand buildup along some beaches and to be lost on others. Breakwaters, **groins**, and **jetties** are artificial structures perpendicular to the shore line and designed to prevent beach erosion. Sometimes beachfront landowners want to build **seawalls** to ward off waves and to prevent their beach from being washed away. The problem is that beaches down the shore line will then be deprived of their natural sand flow and erode.

Coastal erosion has been a problem for some time. Ocean waves and storms attack beaches and bluffs along ocean shorelines. Shorelines are dynamic and diverse, shaped by natural processes as well as human development. Some of the variations include:

- **Barrier islands** are located along the Atlantic and Gulf of Mexico coasts.

- Along the Carolinas, there are strand beaches attached to the mainland.

- Outer Cape Cod, Long Island, the Great Lakes, and the Pacific coast have bluffs and cliffs.

> Wilderness, in the elegant words of the 1964 U.S. Wilderness Act, is land "where man himself is a visitor and does not remain" (McCarthy, 2002). Wilderness areas are critical for protecting biodiversity. Tropical rain forests, covering only 6% of the planet, are home to more than half of all known species. Source: McCarthy (2002).

- There are pocket beaches between headlands in southern New England, California, and Oregon. Central and Eastern Maine have crystalline bedrock bordering the ocean.

- Southern Florida has coral reefs and **mangroves**. Southern Louisiana and areas on the land side of barrier beaches have coastal wetlands.

Barrier islands have been retreating inland as much as 2 to 3 feet per year in response to slowly rising sea levels (Dunn et al., 2000). In some locations, cliffs along the Pacific coastline have retreated tens of feet. Bluffs and dune erosion rates vary. A continued threat to coastal beaches is the rising sea level due to global warming. Coastal areas are—or should be—very protective of the natural habitat that helps prevent beach erosion.

The dunes ecosystem is especially important. Coastal dunes range from a small hill to 50 feet in height. Coastal dunes erode from the effects of waves and wind. The dunes are built naturally when sand is blown into a vegetated area on the beach and act as dikes against flooding. Heavy vehicle or foot traffic can destroy the natural vegetation holding a dune in place. New construction may also flatten dunes. When dunes are flattened, beaches are lost.

Littoral drift is another reason sand is lost along beaches. Waves approaching the beach at an angle stir up sand and carry it away from its normal location. The harshness of the salt spray from oceans makes it difficult to grow many species along beaches. Native plants are the best means of protecting beaches. The Soil Conservation Service (SCS) uses plants to help control dune erosion. Native and naturalized dune plants are protected and cultivated. Sea oats, salt grass, and trees and shrubs of varying species

FIGURE 10-5 **Coastal Conservation**
Sand dunes protect beaches from erosion by sea oats and seabeach amaranth.

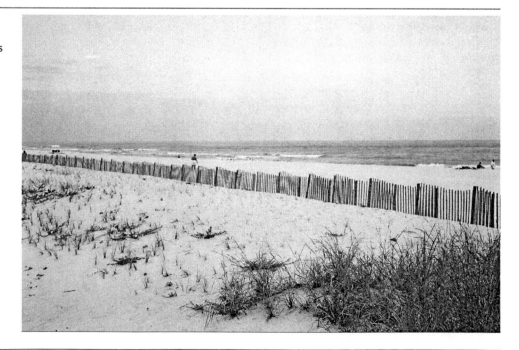

must be protected. Where beach vegetation is still developing, access walkways and sand-trapping fences are used to hold dune sand in its place.

New developments along the coast are dredging artificial channels to give boat owners direct access to the coast. The dredging and removal of material destroys the natural barrier protecting beachfronts from storms. Ocean currents deposit moving sands into the newly dredged channel rather than moving it along the coast. Beaches along the channels have more sand and areas down current are deprived of sand. Dredging the channel regularly is not economically feasible and is only a temporary solution to a long-term problem. Lawsuits often result. The Army Corps of Engineers has been rebuilding and renourishing eroded beaches since the 1950s. Under the Coastal Barrier Resources Act of 1983, the Coastal Barrier Resources System protects barrier island habitats and discourages development. The costs are offset by federal funds, but state governments must also contribute. Along coastal areas, particularly tourist areas, **beach renourishment** is a major concern. Without beach renourishment, or replacing sand that is misplaced or washed away, there would be no tourists for beaches, and homeowners would lose their beachfront property. Finding sand resources offshore is a continuing problem. A major concern is the cost of transporting replacement sand by truck or barges.

OVERGRAZING

The activity most devastating to soil degradation is overgrazing. Too many cattle, goats, or sheep depletes the land surfaces of plants holding its soil in place. Under natural conditions, moderate grazing of grasslands is not harmful, but when livestock managers increase the number of ani-

Swash zone
The narrow zone on the shore where water rushes up and back on the beach.

Groin
On a beach it is a small jetty extending from a shore to protect the beach against erosion or to trap shifting sands.

Jetties
Structures extending into a sea, lake, or river to influence the tide or current, or protect a harbor.

Seawall
A special type of retaining wall along the beachfront that is designed to withstand wave force; usually prohibited.

Barrier island
An offshore island composed primarily of sand; provides protection from the sea for marsh and mainland areas. A *transgressive barrier island* lacks dune or stable vegetation; storm waters wash over it, causing it to change shape dramatically; an unstable island.

Mangroves
A tropical forest found on the coast; the mangrove tree is a species found in Florida and other coastal states.

Littoral drift
A phenomenon where sand drifts at an angle, carrying it away from its normal location.

Beach renourishment
The artificial establishment and periodic addition of sand to a beach done in such as a way as to create a dry sand beach at all stages of the tide.

TRASHING OUR BEACHES
An increasing problem associated with tourism on the nation's beaches is the disposal of *solid waste*. *Littering* is illegal and individuals can face a fine of up to $1,000. Improper disposal of waste on the beach contributes to water pollution, wildlife endangerment, and ruins the beauty of areas we should be able to enjoy. Some parks require visitors to pick up all trash before leaving an area. It should not be the responsibility of park or city personnel to clean up human body and animal wastes, cigarette butts, beer bottles, cans, and other materials that could be disposed of safely. In most tourist communities, the amount of trash exceeds the number of people employed to clean it up. Residents wanting to keep the area clean for all to enjoy sometimes have to organize volunteers to help pick trash out of lakes, rivers, marshes, and roadsides. There are many organizations such as Surfriders, Inc., with concerned individuals who try and help keep the beaches clean.

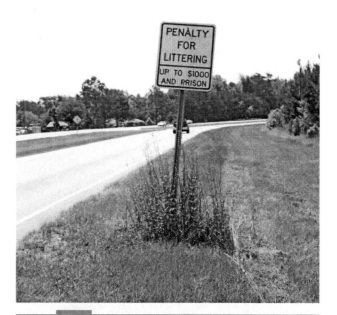

FIGURE 10-6 Signs warning of fines are one way of creating awareness and decreasing littering on highways.

mals feeding on an area, grass is depleted. Native plants give way to weeds. As soil is exposed to wind and water, it becomes barren or rocky, unable to support vegetation that supports animal life. Overgrazing is the most potent force in desertification, or changing a biosystem into a desert, in the United States. Half of U.S. rangeland is severely degraded (Durning & Brough, 1991). Livestock grazing is a major cause of species endangerment (Tazik & Martin, 2002).

In addition to land issues, overgrazing causes water problems. Vegetation bordering streams and lakes has been destroyed by residents with **riparian rights.** Oversized herds of livestock congregate in or along waterways, eating and trampling vegetation, damaging river banks and polluting the water. As a result, soil from riverbanks erode and become shallower and warmer from sedimentation. Water becomes more turbid harming aquatic life and creating conditions for harmful microorganisms that make the water from lakes, rivers, and streams harmful to humans. Overgrazing is now regarded as the main reason for the decline of native trout populations in the western states. Many areas of the western states contain *Giardia,* a protozoan causing diarrhea among local residents and tourists.

MINING

The United States is the world's largest producer of clay, copper, gypsum, lithium, magnesium, phosphate, salt, silica, and sulfur, and the world's second largest producer of coal and gold (Colorado Mining Association, 2003). Mining is a major industry, generating $323 billion in business income, $112 in personal income, and $25 billion in state and local government revenues (Colorado Mining Association, 2005). Materials are extracted from underground by various mining techniques. These include **placer, hydraulic,** hard rock, and open pit. *Placer mining* includes panning, dredging, sluicing, rocker, and picking. *Hydraulic mining* is the most destructive way to mine leaving the land unuseable. **Hard rock mining** digs into

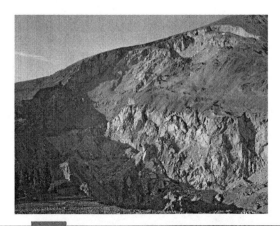

FIGURE 10-7 **Climax Mine in Colorado** One of the largest mines in the Midwest, the climax mine is an example of how mining influences ecosystems and contributes to landslides.

solid rock to find minerals in ore form. Miners use picks, shovels, rock drills, dynamite, and other tools to find the ore. Tunnels or shafts are dug. *Open pit mines* are used most often but are very destructive to the land.

Mining is destructive to the land, forests, rivers, plants, and animals. Hundreds of acres of open mining pits have been left behind. Heavy metals, acids, and other materials also are left behind. Vegetation, essential to prevent soil erosion, has been destroyed. Restoring vegetation from mined surfaces is difficult because organic matter, nutrients, and water needed for plant growth is either acidic or **alkaline** (Walker & Powell, 2001).

Summitville, Colorado, is one of the most expensive mining disaster sites in U.S. history (Hunter, 2000). Once a gold mining site, heavy metals and the acid used to extract gold from the rock seeped into the land and rivers. The site has been cleaned up using **Superfund** monies. There are 209 other Superfund sites in Colorado, many of them mine areas, including the California Gulch project and Eagle Mine site. California Gulch is in Leadville, Colorado, where soil and water were contaminated with lead and acid. The Eagle Mine site is near Vail, Colorado. Metals such as arsenic, cadmium, copper, lead, and zinc were found in the soil and water. Fish were killed and drinking water in nearby communities was threatened.

More than 70 million Americans live within 4 miles of a Superfund site (National Environmental Trust, 2005). Superfund cleanup is intended to reduce or eliminate risk to human or environmental health, not restore an area to its former condition. The cleanup process begins with citizen groups, state agencies, and the EPA reporting the site. Each site is evaluated to determine whether it should be placed on the National Priorities List according to the cause of contamination, seriousness (extent and possible threats), and cleanup alternatives. After a Superfund site is cleaned, activities continue to maintain the cleanup.

Tailings consist of rock and other materials left over from mining after the ore has been extracted. Tailings can amount to hundreds of thousands of tons per year at one site (The National Online, 2003). Tailings from uranium mines include radioactive materials such as thorium-230, radium-226, radon-222, and polonium-210, which are harmful to living things (Edwards, 1998). Other materials found in tailings that are harmful to human health include aluminum, arsenic, beryllium, cadmium, chromium, copper, iron, lead, manganese, mercury, selenium, tetrachloroethene, thorium, and zinc. A major concern with the finely ground tailings is environmental contamination from wind or water erosion (Schippers et al., 2000).

Heap leaching is a process used with very low-grade ore. Ground-up rock is piled into heaps and sprayed with cyanide and water that **leaches** the gold or other mineral from the rock onto leach pads. **Slurry** is created when the finely ground-up tailings are mixed with water, creating a thin, watery mixture contaminated with other materials such as cyanide or uranium. Concerns about mining include the possibility that hazardous elements from mines leach into ground and surface waters as well as the soil. Slurry from uranium tailings (uranium-234, radium-226, and radon-222) are a special problem. Radium causes lymphoma, bone cancer, and leukemia. Radon causes lung cancer.

Mining of lead is another concern. Positive relationships between mining activities, lead concentrations in soil, and elevated blood levels in children have been recorded (Lynch et al., 2000). Children living close to the Big River Mine Tailings in Missouri site had higher levels of lead in the blood, presumably from indoor dust and playing in their yards (Mugueytio et al., 1998).

DESERTIFICATION

Global warming may cause heavy rainfall in some areas and drought in others. Resulting floods may pollute waters, erode land, and bring diseases. The cutting of forests further increases the risk of flooding. Abusive land practices such as overgrazing livestock, barren **brownfields**, and mining discharges create unfavorable conditions that may drastically change the productivity and livability of the land. As populations continue to grow in grassland and tundra areas, water supplies become reduced. In areas where rainfall is significantly below normal, grasslands and semiarid regions may turn into deserts. Wind erosion, salinization, and the accumulation of toxic substances in the soil will always pose a threat to soil and land quality.

Preservation of Wildlife

very year, acres of vital wildlife areas, including land and water, are converted for human use. The draining of wetlands, use of herbicides and pesticides, and emission from fossil fuel combustion has destroyed the habitats of many species. Water shortages and global warming also threaten many species in some areas or cause them to migrate into other more fertile areas. The migration of elk herds in the Rocky Mountain National Forest are now considered a threat to other plants and animals (Wade, 2003). In 2002, approximately 3,000 elk living near Estes Park, Colorado, contributed to a 20% reduction in willow trees and 40% in aspen trees. Elk are considered migratory animals who move about to mate and to look food. The Division of Wildlife considered control measures such as injectable birth control, limited elk hunting in the park area, and the reintroduction of gray wolves.

Soil Composition

oil consists of inorganic and organic matter. Inorganic materials are released when rock surfaces are broken down by heat, water, explosions, or weathering. Organic matter is contributed by decaying microorganisms, insects, birds, reptiles, plants,

Riparian rights
The right to utilize land and water adjacent to owned property such as rivers, lakes, streams, and oceans; owners are allowed to build docks, boat, swim, and utilize the area for recreation and business purposes. *Riparian rights* also entitle landowners to have an unpolluted stream come into their property.

Placer mining
A process of mining valuable minerals from soil, marine, or glacial deposits containing particles of valuable minerals by washing or dredging; as in gold mining.

Hydraulic mining
A system of mining using the force of a jet of water to wash down a bank of gold-bearing gravel or dirt.

Hard rock mining
A technique used to remove large ore bodies by creating underground "rooms" or stopes supported by pillars of standing rock. Because it is costly, this type of mining is used primarily for mining valuable minerals such as gold and diamonds.

Alkaline
The opposite of acidic. Having a pH greater than 7.

Superfund
Also known as the Comprehensive Environmental Response, Compensation and Liability Act (CERCLA); was passed by Congress in 1980 to help pay for the management and cleanup of hazardous waste sites.

Tailings
Waste material that is left after the majority of the ore has been extracted.

Heap leaching
A process of leaching valuable metals from a heap of crushed ore, as leaching solutions percolate downward through the heap, and collected from a sloping, impermeable liner.

Leach
When a liquid filters down through a material; to lose soluble matter as a result of the filtering through of water.

Slurry
A watery mixture of insoluble matter such as mud or lime.

Brownfields
A large parcel of industrial land that was polluted and then abandoned.

FIGURE 10-8 **Farming** Tractors provide the means of tilling land so topsoil is not lost and crops are profitable.

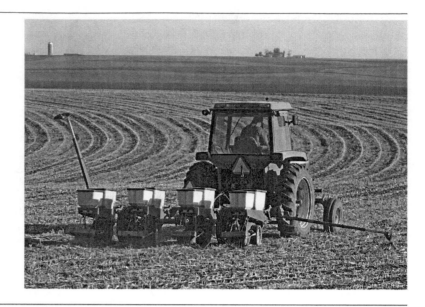

and animals and their waste products. Soil contains valuable nutrients needed by plants to produce food for plants and animals. Soil conditions determine the viability of organisms within an ecosystem. Minor disruptions can threaten, disturb, or destroy plant, animal, and human inhabitants. Humans exert enormous pressure upon soil and its ecosystems. Mismanagement of soils can deplete or contaminate soil constitution. Mining, ranching, farming, and industrial uses of land must protect the land on which they depend. Flooding, overgrazing, and chemical pollution destroys valuable soil, making it difficult for soils to continue to produce valuable products. Forest fires threaten entire ecosystems, contribute to erosion, and pollute the air and land. Soil degradation, desertification, and contamination are not in the best interests of human survival or quality of life.

Soil surveys conducted by the SCS describe the physical and chemical characteristics of soils. When a survey is done, engineers determine the soil's texture, structure, chemical composition, depth, slope, degree of erosion, and other features. It is important to identify farmland, pastureland, flood-prone areas, wetlands, saline and alkaline areas, and forest land. This information is imperative to determine proper land use and management by farmers, ranchers, city planners, land developers, building contractors, and others. Soil surveys assist in planning roads and airports, reducing flooding, controlling sediment, protecting wildlife, establishing parks, and the planning for businesses and industries.

Topsoil is especially important to agriculture and management of large areas for building developments. In order for food-producing plants to grow, sufficient rainfall, sunlight, and nutrients are needed. Soil macronutrients include carbon, hydrogen, oxygen, nitrogen, phosphorus, potassium, calcium, magnesium, and sulfur.

Trace elements include iron, copper, manganese, zinc, chlorine, and iodine. Topsoil also provides moisture needed by plants. It is easily eroded without proper management. As topsoil becomes thinner and thinner until it disappears completely, it leaves only unproductive subsoil or bare rock. When it rains, water will drain through topsoil into the subsoil. Some soil loss is natural, but human activities have destroyed soil in amounts that exceed the development of new soil. Under natural conditions, through the gradual decomposition of organic matter, it takes 200 to 1,000 years to form an inch of topsoil. Topsoil loss has a direct negative impact on soil productivity. Topsoil around the world, particularly in agricultural areas, is thinning at an alarming rate, destroying billions of acres of cultivated land. The Food and Agriculture Organization of the United Nations has warned Third World countries that soil erosion will result in less food to feed expanding populations (FAO, 2001).

Farmland and Topsoil Issues

Agriculture depends on the quality of the top 6 to 8 inches of soil, known as topsoil. Approximately 25% of U.S. cropland is highly erodible (Claussen et al., 2004). Midwestern states with farmland are susceptible to erosion and runoff because crops are planted in rows. During the 1930s farmland and grasslands in the Great Plains of the central United States was plowed. A lack of rainfall and high winds blew topsoil away, creating the "Dust Bowl." Crops withered and livestock died. It is estimated that 200,000 people abandoned their farms and moved westward to California (PBS, 2005). Beginning in 1935, the Soil Conservation Service (SCS)

182   ENVIRONMENTAL HEALTH

Many people would like to have a soil test done to determine the type of soil and nutrient content in order to grow plants. It is important to know how to fertilize the soil so that problems associated with underfertilizing or overfertilizing do not occur. Soil samples can be taken at any time of the year. It is best to sample the soil before planting a garden or lawn so that the fertilizer will have time to establish in the soil. A soil test requires 12 or more samples combined as one composite sample. Dry soil should be taken from the *root zone*, a depth of 2 to 3 inches, with a clean garden trowel. Keep track of where the soil came from. When the samples are combined, they should be mixed thoroughly. Soil samples can be sent to the local county extension service for analysis. The report will tell the pH value; levels of phosphorus, potassium, calcium, magnesium, zinc, and manganese in the soil; and make a recommendation for the amount and type of fertilizer and/or lime needed to add to the soil for optimum plant growth.

The pH scale ranges from 0 to 14 with 7 as neutral. Less than 7 indicates acidity and greater than 7 indicates alkaline soil. Some plants thrive in acid soils with a pH of 5.0 to 5.5 pH. Plant nutrients include primary, secondary, and micronutrients. Nitrogen (N), phosphorus (P), and potassium (K) are primary nutrients needed in fairly large quantities. Calcium (Ca), magnesium (Mg), and sulfur (S) are secondary nutrients. Zinc (Zn) and manganese (Mn) are micronutrients. Nitrogen (N) testing is not recommended because nitrogen is water soluble and rapidly moves through the soil with rainfall and irritation, causing the amount in the root zone to fluctuate over time.

Source: Clemson Extension (2003).

---

was created to monitor soil erosion. Cooperative Extension agents and SCS officials encouraged farmers to plant trees for windbreaks, create terraces, contour strip-crop, and develop waterways to prevent soil erosion. Windbreaks are still encouraged to control wind erosion, provide wildlife habitat, and make the land more attractive. Windbreaks also trap snow, providing moisture for plants and groundwater supplies in the spring and summer when it melts. Crops are rotated so that nutrients removed by some crops are replaced by others. Alfalfa, brome grass, and other types of hay can provide a protective cover for topsoil.

In order to encourage the growth and development of more nutrient-dense soil, farmers were encouraged to leave vegetation from last year's crop to decompose in the field. Old crop residues help retain soil composition by decreasing wind access to topsoil, and restricting runoff. Conservation tillage practices for corn and soybean crops were encouraged that included "no till" (meaning seeds are planted in undisturbed residue of an old crop); "ridge till" (where seeds were planted in ridges left from the previous year's crop after plowing), and "mulch till" (seeds are planted in a field with a minimum amount of residue) (Midwest Plan Service, 1992). The Food Security Act of 1985 (PL 99-198, also known as The Farm Act) created the Conservation Reserve Program (CRP, Title XII, 16 USC 3831) in order to provide financial incentives to farmers in order to decrease soil loss and erosion. Landowners were paid to leave erodible or environmentally sensitive land, converting them to pastures or woodlands. The Federal Agriculture Improvement and Reform Act of 1996 (PL 104-127, also known as the Farm Bill) provided for the modification of agricultural programs by defining farmlands and delineating wetlands.

Fertilizers are used to enhance the soil to increase crop production. The United States is the largest producer of fertilizers in the world. Use of fertilizers skyrocketed after World War II to boost food production. The most common nutrients in fertilizers include nitrogen, phosphorus, and potassium. Nitrogen is a concern because it can accumulate in water. Nitrogen and phosphorous pollution can trigger **eutrophication** (the growth of algae that depletes oxygen in the water), thus killing aquatic species. The addition of chemical nitrogen and potash for topsoil to maintain good harvests cannot replace nutrients lost through erosion or the organic matter necessary to maintain healthy soil structure. Some researchers say that heavy fertilizer use can actually damage the soil by disrupting natural nutrient cycles (Hayes, 1981).

CHANGES IN FARMING PRACTICES

In the 1970s, high commodity prices and the demand to feed growing populations overseas called for a "green revolution" aimed at boosting farm production (Rosset et al. 2000). Soil erosion was increased again as plants and trees were removed in favor of continuous production of corn and soybeans. Pastures were converted to farmland, fields were plowed and left dormant until spring, crop rotation was abandoned, and even though

Topsoil
The top layer of soil containing valuable nutrients.

Fertilizer
A material added to soil to increase its fertility.

Eutrophication
The aging process by which lakes are fertilized with nutrients so they evolve into marshes or bogs.

the push was on to produce, farmland production decreased due to erosion and poor soil quality. Soils became compacted and soil nutrients were depleted as crops were repeatedly grown on the same land. Farmers used manure and chemical fertilizers to improve crop production from poor soils.

Crop yields have increased dramatically due to better farming practices, hybrid seeds, the use of pesticides, and the use of nitrogen fertilizers. It is unlikely that such a dramatic increase will be seen again. The amount of land once used for farming, is developing into subdivisions, malls, and industrial uses. Water tables are falling as aquifers are being depleted. Soil fertility has been maximized with nitrogen, potash, and other chemical and potash applications. Adverse climate changes due to global warming result in drought in some areas and heavy rainfall in others. Because crop yields per acre are not likely to increase, the best solution to assure an adequate food supply would be to stabilize population growth and reverse land degradation. People move from one area to another because water is scarce, soils are depleted, forests are removed, and once fertile land becomes a desert. So long as population growth is allowed to continue as it has in the past, the amount of food available to each person is a concern.

Land Pollution

The mismanagement of land by mining, agriculture, and urban sprawl are major concerns regarding soil quantity and quality. Soil pollution has been and continues to be another problem. The disposal of toxic waste underground and above ground has been resisted and continues to be hotly debated. Municipal sewage disposed of above ground contributes to a type of "toxic sludge" when it rains. When toxic materials are discharged into the ground, they do not break down. They accumulate with time. Prevention is far better than remediation.

BROWNFIELDS

In various parts of the United States, former industrial or commercial sites, known as *brownfields*, are abandoned properties polluted with **hazardous substances** or contaminants, covered with trash, polluted, or left idle (EPA, 2005). Those who manage the property can be held liable for the cost of cleanup. Reclamation programs have tried to use the abandoned sites in order to give the area a new look, create jobs, and increase tax revenues. The Taxpayer Relief Acts (PL 105-34 and PL 105-32) provided tax incentives to encourage the cleanup and redevelopment of brownfields. Expenses associated with the cleanup of brownfield areas are tax deductible. The Small Business

Liability Relief and Brownfields Revitalization Act (PL 107-118) was signed in 2001 to exempt homeowners, small businesses, and nonprofit generators of municipal **solid waste** from liability for Superfund response costs due to cleanup of hazardous waste (EPA, 2002).

HUMAN WASTE DISCHARGES

When sewage is treated by wastewater treatment plants, water is returned to the waterways, but the solid material, known as sludge, is discharged to land called drying beds. Another word for this sludge is **biosolids**. The discharge of biosolids is a controversial subject. In the United States, 60% of wastewater treatment biosolids are discharged onto land (Apedaile, 2001). One reason for this is because they contain high concentrations of nutrients essential to crop growth, such as nitrogen and phosphorus. The practice of recycling biosolids seems to make sense because they can replace the use of inorganic fertilizers. The EPA established rules regarding the tillage of sludge into the soil for fertilizers. It limits public access to drying fields, the grazing of cattle, and the planting of crops. In addition, **buffer strip zones** must separate sludge-treated land from slopes, creeks, and homes. Wastewater treatment plants and sludge-hauling companies are required to keep records for the EPA's review.

Biosolids present a major public health issue as residents complain about the smell and potential health hazards. In addition to local residents, agencies such as the National Research Council, the Sierra Club, Centers for Disease Control and Prevention, and the National Academy of Sciences have raised concerns. Two concerns related to land use of biosolids include the source of the sewage used and the potential for harmful pathogens which could present airborne and waterborne illnesses. Most scientists are unconcerned because most of the pathogens in biosolids are unable to survive the soil environment. Soil is said to filter bacteria and absorb viruses (Gerba et al., 1975). But the risk of some bacteria and viruses being released into the environment before it is filtered through soil is always possible.

The Clean Water Act of 1972 classified sludge into two classes: (1) Class A biosolids with undetectable pathogens, and (2) Class B biosolids with detectable levels of pathogens. The risk of biosolid pathogens has been tested in a few studies. Dowd et al. (2003) conducted a risk assessment and determined the potential risk of airborne pathogens to site workers handling Class B biosolids. The National Institute of Safety and Health recommends that workers use protective equipment and use good hygienic practices (NIOSH, 2000). In 2003 the EPA made a statement that "no toxic substances have been detected that warrant regulation of sewage sludge, and land application of sewage sludge is still an appropriate choice for communities" (McGiley, 2003). The use of biosolids as fertilizer continues in the United States, Canada, and other countries requiring surveillance and careful studies to determine the risk to public health.

Natural Disasters

The discussion of land as it pertains to the people who live there is not complete without attention to geographic and climactic hazards specific to various regions of the United States. Many move from one area to another without regard for potential hazards. The type of land and weather of any given area is important when selecting an appropriate type of home.

FOREST AND WILD FIRES

Areas experiencing drought are especially likely to be at risk for forest fires. Dry wood, lack of water, and a spark is all that it takes.

Some fires are necessary in order to burn leftover logging materials, clear brush, control undergrowth, encourage new growth, get rid of diseased trees, and reduce insect populations. Some tree species, such as the lodgepole pine, need heat to reproduce. When the pinecone gets hot enough, the cone opens and seed spread across the forest floor allowing more growth. Fires that are deliberately set by forest authorities and monitored by firefighters are called "controlled' or "prescribed" fires (Thorsen and Kirkbride, 1998). Weather conditions are taken into consideration before the fire is set.

Once the fire is over, heavy rains can produce mudslides when vegetation that normally holds the soil in place are lost. The resulting soil is less fertile because nutrients are destroyed from the heat and topsoil is washed away by subsequent rainfall.

EARTHQUAKES

Earthquakes can occur almost anywhere at any time. It is estimated that there are 500,000 detectable earthquakes in the world each year. One-fifth of those can be felt, and 100 of them cause damage (PBS, 2005). Earthquakes can be anticipated, but not predicted. In the United States, eastern and western states are most at risk. The repercussions of earthquakes include landslides and **liquefaction**.

Hazardous substance
Substances, that if used improperly, may be dangerous to human health and/or the environment.

Solid waste
Trash and garbage—solid, liquid, and semisolid—or contained gaseous material from industrial, commercial, mining, agricultural, and community activities.

Biosolids
Solid waste matter from sewage systems discharged onto land; biosolids contain pathogens.

Buffer strip zone
Strips of grass or other erosion resistant vegetation between a waterway and an area of greater intensive land use.

Liquefaction
When particles of soil separate, creating a loose slurry of moving soil, destroying everything nearby; caused by an earthquake.

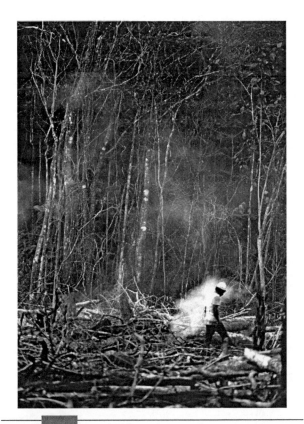

FIGURE 10-9 Recovery from a forest fire can take years.

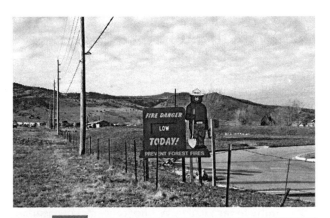

FIGURE 10-10 Smokey the Bear reminds us that humans are the cause of most forest fires.

When liquefaction occurs, loose, moist soil or sand is shaken so hard that the grains separate, turning the earth into a soft, fluid mass that can swallow an entire building. When there is an earthquake under the ocean, a large wave of sea water, known as a tsunami, occurs (USGS, 2005).

TORNADOES

A tornado is a violently rotating column of air capable of destruction in paths up to 1 mile wide and 50 miles long (Storm Prediction Center, 2005). With wind speeds of 250 mph or more, the tornado extends from a thunderstorm. Sometimes there may be two or more tornadoes sighted at the same time. Tornadoes forming over warm water are called *waterspouts,* which can move from the ocean inland, causing damage and injuries. In an average year, 800-1,000 tornadoes are reported nationwide (National Severe Storms Laboratory, 2005).

FLOODS

Flooding is one of the most destructive of all geologic hazards in the United States, causing over $1 billion in property damage each year (FEMA, 2005). Areas more susceptible to flooding than others are called **floodplains.** Floodplains are low-lying lands near rivers, lakes, or oceans that periodically flood and are classified according to the probability they will be flooded. A 100-year floodplain has a 1% chance of flooding any given year (Houston Stormwater Management Program, 2005). The U.S. Army Corps of Engineers has attempted to reduce the likelihood of flooding, but cannot prevent it.

Floodplains are assessed and documented by governmental officials in order to avoid adverse impacts associated with occupancy and modification of flood plains. When selecting a home site or considering purchasing a home near areas close to water the potential buyer should determine whether or not the home is likely to be flooded. This is a major determinant in securing home owner's insurance. The city or county planning office has flood zone maps and can provide information to the public. Most home insurance policies do not cover flood damage.

HURRICANES

Hurricanes are also known as cyclones because the winds rotate around an eye (NOAA, 2005). Hurricanes occur in coastal areas on the Atlantic and consist of a storm surge and heavy winds. The storm surge can increase the average sea level by 15 feet or more, pushing water toward the shore. Strong winds cause great damage, even in inland locations, destroying trees and homes. Great damage can occur from flying debris. A hurricane making landfall may have at least one tornado. Hurricanes produce so much rain that communities hundreds of miles from the coast can experience major flooding problems. In addition, tropical storms or tropical depressions with heavy and persistent rains are less destructive than hurricanes. The main concern about hurricanes is the inland flooding. Floods result in contaminated water, structural damage, and pests such as rodents and snakes.

SUBSIDENCE

Subsidence is the tendency of soil to sink or collapse. The sinking can be naturally produced from caves caused by groundwater dissolving bedrock. The most common reason for subsidence is a manmade void from abandoned mines and draining groundwater levels during droughts. Most abandoned or inactive mines have deep, vertical shafts that can suddenly reopen.

Sinkholes develop when water moves through soluble rock underground, forming caves. Most sinkholes are less than 10 feet in diameter. A visual inspection of the area does not always reveal whether there was mining in the past or whether or not tunnels exist under a property. Geological surveys can predict areas most likely to develop sinkholes.

LANDSLIDES AND AVALANCHES

Landslides and avalanches contribute to deaths and home destruction. A *landslide* is the rapid downward and outward movement of rock, soil, and vegetation. An *avalanche* is the rapid downward and outward movement of snow and ice. Not all landslides are sudden. **Soil creep,** a movement of wet soil on slopes from freezing and thawing, can have the same destructive effect on structures. Most losses occur in cities with homes built on gently sloping hillsides. All landslides are triggered by weaknesses in the rock and soil, earthquake activity, heavy rainfall or snowmelt, or construction that changes critical aspects of the environment. If trees on a slope show signs of a struggle to grow vertically, this is an indicator of soil movement. Another clue on a slope is a swath of young

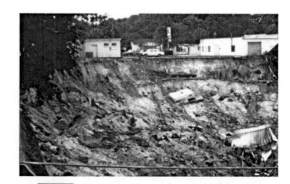

FIGURE 10-11 **Sinkhole in Florida** When the ground underneath softens due to geological movements, surface soil can fall suddenly.

trees showing where trees may have been previously destroyed by a landslide or avalanche. A bulge in a hillside may indicate a potential landslide.

Buying and Selling Land

Most individuals in the United States purchase land or property, yet many do not know about potential geologic hazards or the potential for purchasing land that is contaminated or soil problems that can make building or living in their "dream home" a major problem.

Geologic hazards are natural processes that threaten man and property. A building's true foundation is the soil or the rock beneath the concrete. Damage from swelling soils is caused by the soil composition and moisture change in the ground. When wet, soil can swell 20% to 50%, exerting enough pressure to lift and buckle floors and foundations. Damage also occurs to sidewalks and driveways.

To learn about soil, the first step is to visit the Natural Resources Conservation Service (NRCS) or the Soil Survey Section (formerly the Soil Conservation Services) in the county where the building will be constructed. A state geological survey provides information about problem areas. Check to see whether the builder tested the soil prior to building. If not, insist on having appropriate soil tests made. Tests should be made of the soil or rock underlying the foundation. Buyers of existing homes should also use this information to provide knowledge about potential problems and detect existing problems in a building.

A major concern is purchasing contaminated land. Some subdivisions are built on old **landfill** sites, old arse-

Floodplains
Land that is likely to be submerged by floodwaters in times of heavy rainfall or storms.

Hurricanes
A severe tropical cyclone with heavy rains, thunder, lightning, and winds moving at 74 miles (118 kilometers) per hour or greater; generally occur in the western Atlantic.

Subsidence
To sink or fall.

Landslide
A downward movement of large masses of rock and dirt on a slope.

Soil creep
A creep of soil on even slopes; often accelerated in the spring by freezing and thawing.

Geologic hazards
Hazardous situations as a result of natural land and water forms; such as, landslides, earthquakes, tsunamis, volcanic eruptions, and mudslides; sometimes referred to as natural disasters.

Landfill
A large waste site with the Earth scooped out. The sides and bottom are lined with clay and a vinyl liner. Waste is dumped and sand is used to help divert water and other materials that leach through the soil.

FIGURE 10-12 **Love Canal Cleanup** Residents in the Love Canal area had to evacuate so Superfund efforts could clean up toxic materials.

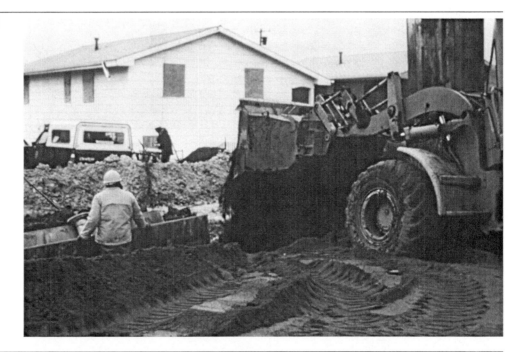

In 1892, the construction of Love Canal began when a developer by the name of William T. Love began building a canal to connect the upper and lower parts of the Niagara River in New York. It was never finished. From 1920 to 1953, the Love Canal was used by Hooker Chemical Company to dump over 20,000 tons of hazardous wastes. The area was then covered with dirt presumed safe, and sold to the city for $1. Homes were built on the land and residents moved in. Then leaking drums of hazardous materials began to surface. When residents complained about health problems in 1978, health department officials recognized the hazards and evacuated residents. Residents received over $20 million in settlement money from the company and the city of Niagara Falls (Columbia Encyclopedia, 2001). In addition, the company agreed to pay the state of New York $98 million and the federal government $129 million toward the costs incurred during the cleanup of the area. This incident lead to the creation of EPA's Superfund, which makes responsible parties liable for the cleanup of environmental hazards. Money was used to buy homes, demolish them, and clean up chemicals in the area. In 1990, residents began moving back into their homes. In 1997, the New York Department of Health received $3 million to study the health effects of residents who lived in the area from 1940 to 1978, their children, and their grandchildren.

Sources: Beck (1979) and Columbia Encyclopedia (2001).

nal or bombing sites, former feed lots or animal containment sites, or land contaminated by chemicals or radioactive materials. A home built on an old landfill may shift as the ground settles, causing cracks in foundation or basement walls. Old pieces of scrap materials can be dug up when landscaping or gardening. Sellers are required to report known defects in the home, but are not required to volunteer information about environmental hazards to potential buyers. It is a good idea to inquire among realtors, local businesspeople, and neighbors about the history of the land. When asked, the seller must provide a truthful answer or they can be charged with fraud. However, it is possible that even the seller is unaware of a potential or existing problem.

The most common land contaminants include pesticides, gasoline, or manure. Another major concern is the mixing of chemicals or the rinsing of chemical tanks near a groundwater source. This is much more harmful than application of chemicals on crops. Another major source of land contamination is leakage from underground storage tanks or pipes. If a seller reports an underground tank, it should be removed or filled with inert material and sealed.

Potential buyers should look for odors, holes, pits, and unusual colors of soil and then request additional information. Dead or decaying trees, shrubs, or other vegetation also may provide clues that something about the property is unusual. Inspect adjoining properties to see if there are other potential sources of contamination to the land under consideration. Any bid on property should include a contingency that states the property must be free of potential problems and must pass an inspection by a disinterested party, designated by the buyer. If the land is potential farmland, the county extension agent could provide useful information. If the buyer discovers something during purchase negotiations, they can request that the owners clean up the land before the sale is completed.

If this is not done prior to acceptance of the bid, the buyer may be liable for any cleanup expenses. Sometimes an "innocent purchaser defense" can be used if the buyer is required to cleanup newly purchased property. This might work if the appropriate inquiries into the previous ownership and uses of the property were made and the buyer did not know or have reason to know of contamination at the time of purchase (Creath, 1996).

There are other land issues that potential owners should investigate such as riparian rights, **setbacks**, and **easements**. A survey of the land is always a good idea before making an offer or buying a property.

More to Consider

Land is a natural resource and a valuable commodity. Ideally, the best location for a city or town is one where the environment is least likely to be disturbed—but most cities are already established and expanding. When it comes to determining where someone wants to live, location is everything. Some areas are more susceptible to natural disasters than others. If a homeowner chooses to live there, it is a good idea to buy a home that can withstand a major storm and be prepared for evacuation or emergency situations.

Summary

Land is an important natural resource that erodes and becomes less productive through natural disasters and processes. It can even be made into desert land if it is overutilized. The use of water; discharge of waste, fertilizers, and pesticides; and mil-

1864 Congress gave Yosemite Valley to the state of California to use as a park.

1872 Yellowstone became the world's first official national park.

1872 A mining law was passed under which companies and individuals could buy the mining rights for public land thought to contain minerals for $5 per acre or less.

1890 The Forest Reserve Act created forest reserves and the National Forest System. This was considered the end of the American frontier.

1892 The Sierra Club was founded by John Muir, Robert Underwood Johnson, and William Colby.

1897 Forest Management Act authorizes commercial use of public forests.

1901 Anthracite coal strike leaves millions without heat increasing interest in alternative energy such as wind, tidal, and solar power.

1935 Wilderness Society co-founded by Aldo Leopold and Arthur Carhardt.

1946 U.S. Bureau of Land Management established.

1947 Everglades National Park established.

1951 The Nature Conservancy founded.

1964 Congress creates the National Wilderness Preservation System.

1968 Redwood National Park was established in California.

1970 The first Earth Day was organized.

1973 Congress approves the Alaska Oil pipeline.

1980 President Carter announced the relocation of 700 families in the Love Canal area of Niagara Falls, New York, exposed to toxic wastes.

1988 Beaches were closed along the East Coast due to contaminated medical waste.

1989 Congress voted to halt timber production in Alaska's Tsongass National Forest, the last undisturbed temperate rain forest in the U. S.

2001 Over 210 million gallons of toxic coal sludge, contaminated with poisonous heavy metals, breaks through the dam wall in Inez, Kentucky.

Source: Environmental History Timeline, http://www.radford.edu/~wkovarik/envhist/.

Consider the Cost

WHAT I CAN DO ABOUT LAND USAGE

_____ Buy recycled paper products.
_____ Read the newspaper online rather than buying the paper.
_____ Plant a tree each year.
_____ Do not buy drinks in cans or plastic bottles.

_____ Do not deposit cigarettes or other trash on the beaches.
_____ Donate used magazines to medical facilities or clinics.
_____ Donate items to charities such as Habitat for Humanity.

_____ Clean up litter and campfire waste while camping.
_____ Don't litter.

itary, farming, and mining practices are very important to maintaining soil quality and keeping hazardous situations from harming humans and animals. Attempts from conservationists have resulted in preservation of public lands and national parks. Potential homeowners should be aware of potential hazards they might not be able to manage by hiring a home inspector and by purchasing insurance.

pliance in U.S. agricultural policy: Past performance and future potential. AER-832. USDA/ERS. June 2004. Available from www.ers.usda.gov/publications/aer832.

Clark University. (2005). George Perkins Marsh: Renaissance Vermonter. The George Perkins Marsh Institute, Clark University, VT. Retrieved from http://www.clarku.edu/departments/marsh/georgemarsh.shtml.

Clemson Extension. (2003). Soil testing. Home and Garden Information Center. HGIC

REFERENCES

Apedaile, E. (2001). A perspective on biosolids management. The Canadian Journal of Infectious Diseases, 12. Retrieved from http://www.wessuc.com/Downloads/BiosolidsPerspective.pdf.

Beck, E. (1979). The Love Canal tragedy. EPA Journal. Retrieved from http://www.epa.gov/history/topics/lovecanal/01.htm.

Claassen, R., Breneman, V., Bucholtz, S., Cattaneo, A., Johansson, R., & Morehart, M. (2004). Environmental com-

Setback
A legally defined distance from a specific point, such as a street, golf course, beach, or other public area, where buildings are not allowed to encroach.

Easement
The legal right to cross-over or go into another person's property; usually associated with the development of roads, utilities, and other services.

Colorado Mining Association. (2005). Colorado mining facts. Retrieved from http://www.coloradomining.org/COMiningFacts.html.

Colorado Mining Association (2003). Colorado Mining Facts, TRI data for Colorado. Retrieved March 8, 2003 from http://www.coloradomining.org/COMiningFacts.html.

Columbia Encyclopedia. (2001). Love Canal. Retrieved from http://www.bartleby.com/65/lo/Lovecana.html.

Creath, W. (1996). Home buyers' guide to geologic hazards. An AIPG Issues and Answers Publication. Arvada, CO: American Institute of Professional Geologists.

Department of Environmental Protection, Pennsylvania. (2005). Gifford Pinchot. Pennsylvania's Environmental Heritage. Retrieved from http://www.dep.state.pa.us/dep/PA_Env-Her/pinchot_bio.htm.

Dowd, S., Gerba, I., & Pillai, S. (2000). Biological transport modeling and risk assessment in relation to biosolids placement. *Journal of Environmental Quality, 29,* 343–348.

Dunn, S., Friedman, R., & Baish, S. (2000). Coastal erosion. *Environment, September.* Retrieved from http://www.findarticles.com/p/articles/mi_m1076/is_7_42/ai_64718895.

Durning, A., & Brough, H. (1991). Taking stock: Animal farming and the environment. Washington, D.C., USA : Worldwatch Institute.

Edwards, G. (1998). Uranium: A discussion guide. Canadian Coalition for Nuclear Responsibility. Retrieved from http://www.ccnr.org/nfb_uranium_3.html#F.1.

Environmental Protection Agency. (1995). *America's wetlands: Our vital link between land and water.* Office of Water, Office of Wetlands, Oceans and Watersheds. EPA843-K-95-001. Retrieved from http://www.epa.gov/owow/wetlands/fish.html.

Environmental Protection Agency. (2005). Brownfields definition. Retrieved from http://www.epa.gov/swerosps/bf/glossary.htm.

Environmental Protection Agency. (2002). Brownfields Federal Partnership Action Agenda. Retrieved from http://www.epa.gov/brownfields/pdf/fedparaa.pdf.

Environmental Protection Agency. (2003). Brownfields Regional Assessment Pilot Fact Sheet. Retrieved 8/18/2003 from http://www.epa.gov/brownfields/.

Federal Emergency Management Agency. (2005). Backgrounder: Floods and flash floods. Retrieved from http://www.fema.gov/hazards/floods/flood.shtm.

Food and Agriculture Organization. (2001). Ethical issues in food and agriculture. Rome, Italy: United Nations. Retrieved from http://www.fao.org/documents/show_cdr.asp?url_file=/docrep/003/x9601e/x9601e00.htm.

Food and Agriculture Organization. (2001) State of the world's forests. Rome, Italy: United Nations. Retrieved from http://www.fao.org/documents/show_cdr.asp?url_file=/docrep/003/y0900e/y0900e05.htm.

Gerba, C., Wallis, C., & Melnick, J. (1975). Fate of wastewater bacteria and viruses in soil. *Journal of Irrigation and Drainage Division, 101,* 157–174.

Hayes, J. (Ed.).(1981). *Will there be enough food?* Washington, DC: U.S. Department of Agriculture.

Houston Stormwater Management Program. (2005). About floodplains. Retrieved from http://www.swmp.org/floodplains/about.htm.

Hunter, M. (2000). Colorado considers a mining ban. *High Country News, June 19.* Retrieved from http://www.hcn.org/servlets/hcn.Article?article_id=5876.

Kone, I. (2001). Environment and sustainable development. Paper presented at the Sustainable Development, Governance and Globalization conference, Nairobi, Kenya. Retrieved from http://www.worldsummit2002.org/texts/IbaKone.pdf.

Lynch, R., Malcoe, L., Skaggs, & Kegler, M. (200). The relationship between residential lead exposures and elevated blood lead levels in a rural mining community. *Environmental Health, 63,* 9–15.

McCarthy, T. (2002). Special report: Let them run wild. *Time Magazine.* Retrieved from http://www.time.com/time/2002/greencentury/encontents.html.

McGinley, S. (2003). Biosolids safe for land application, UA researchers find. Retrieved from http://www.biosolids.com/Features/archives/000543.shtml.

Midwest Plan Service. (1992). Conservation tillage systems and management: Crop residue management with no-till, ridge-till, mulch-till. Ames, IA: Agricultural and Biosystems Engineering Department, Iowa State University.

Murgueytio, A., Evans, R., Sterling, D., Clardy S., Shadel B., & Clements B. (1998). Relationship between lead mining and blood lead levels in children. *Archives of Environmental Health, 53,* 414–423.

National Environmental Trust. (2005). Superfund in crisis. Retrieved from http://www.net.org/superfund/.

National Park Service. (2005). Theodore Roosevelt. National Park Service, Department of the Interior. Retrieved from http://www.nps.gov/thro/.

National Resources Defense Council. (1996). Federal land management. Based on *Selling Our Heritage: Congressional Plans for America's Public Lands,* a July 1995 report by the Natural Resources Defense Council.Retrieved from http://www.nrdc.org/land/use/fagency.asp.

National Severe Storms Laboratory. (2005). Tornadoes. Retrieved from the National Weather Service at http://www.nssl.noaa.gov/researchitems/tornadoes.shtml.

NIOSH. (2000). Workers exposed to class B biosolids during application. Pub. No. 2000-158. Washington, DC: United Department of Health and Human Services.

NOAA. (2005). Hurricanes. Retrieved from http://hurricanes.noaa.gov/.

Peterson, T. (2000). *Forests, biodiversity, and resource change.* Taken from Viewing global change, universal timelines, and the promise. Retrieved from http://www.windowview.org/WV.files/global.change/biodiversity.html.

Public Broadcasting Service. (2005). The American Experience: Mass exodus from the plains. Retrieved from http://www.pbs.org/wgbh/amex/dustbowl/peopleevents/pandeAMEX08.html.

Public Broadcasting Service. (2005). The restless planet: Earthquakes. Retrieved from Savage Earth, WNET: New York, http://www.thirteen.org/savageearth/earthquakes/index.html.

Public Works (1997). New beach erosion control system. *Public Works,* March 01. Retrieved from http://static.elibrary.com/p/publicworks/march011997/newbeacherosioncontrolsystemstablerdiscerosioncont/index.html.

Rosset, P., Collins, J., & Lappe, F. (2000). Lessons from the green revolution. Tikkun Magazine. Publication of Food

First, Institute for Food and Food Policy. Retrieved from http://www.foodfirst.org/media/display.php?id=148.

Schippers, A., Jozsa, P., & Sand, W. (2000). Microbiological pyrite oxidation in a mine tailings heap and its relevance to the death of vegetation. *Geomicrobiology Journal, 7,* 151–162.

Smil, V. (1991). *General energetics: Energy in the biosphere and civilization.* New York: Wiley.

Storm Prediction Center. (2005). The online tornado FAQ. Retrieved fromhttp://www.spc.noaa.gov/faq/tornado/#The%20Basics.

Tazik, D., & Martin, C. (2002). Threatened and endangered species on U.S. Department of Defense lands in the arid west, USA. Arid Land Research and Management, 16, 259–276.

Texas Environmental Profiles. (2005). Retrieved from http://www.texasep.org/html/lnd/lnd_3for_legis.html.

The National Online. (2003). Mining, tailings and cyanide. Retrieved March 8, 2003 from http://tv.chbc.ca/national/pgminfo/ugly/mining.html.

Thorsen, J., & Kirkbride, E. (1998). Prescribed fire and public education. *Fire Management Notes, 58,* 27–29.

U.S. Geological Survey. (2005). Cool earthquake facts. Retrieved from http://earthquake.usgs.gov/4kids/facts.html.

USGS. (2005).Wetlands: Losses in the United States. Summary of findings 17802 to 1980s. Northern Prairie Wildlife Research Center. Retrieved from http://www.npwrc.usgs.gov/resource/othrdata/wetloss/findings.htm.

Wade, K. (2003).Elk and vegetation management plan: Environmental impact statement, Rocky Mountain National Park, Colorado. *Federal Register, 68,* 32084-32086. Retrieved from http://www.epa.gov/fedrgstr/EPA-IMPACT/2003/May/Day-29/i13338.htm.

Walker, L., & Powell, E. (2001). Soil water retention on gold mind surfaces in the Mojave Desert. Restoration Ecology, 9. Retrieved from http://www.blackwell-synergy.com/links/doi/10,1046/j,1526-100x.2001.009001095.x/abs/.

Wear, D., & Greis, J. (2001). The southern forest resource assessment summary report. USDA Forest Service. Draft retrieved from http://www.srs.fs.usda.gov/sustain/draft/summry/summary.htm.

World Resources Institute. (2005). Minimizing soil degradation. Retrieved from http://newsroom.wri.org/media_kits_text.cfm?contentID=849.

1. Use the Internet to research information about the potential for earthquakes, tornadoes, hurricanes, floods, wildfires, volcanic eruptions, and/or other hazards specific to your geographical area.

2. Visit the EPA's Envirofacts Web site to learn if there are any environmental hazards near your home or city.

3. Find professional journal articles and do research on areas you might want to visit, including beaches, mountains, national parks, or national forests.

4. Visit your local county extension agent and have your soil tested.

5. Interview a real estate agent and find out what they must, by law, disclose about a property and what does not need to be revealed.

6. Find locations of brownfields, old arsenals, old toxic waste dump sites, or other "contaminated" land sites near your home.

7. As a class, organize and determine a theme for the next Earth Day and create ways to get others to respect the country's natural resources and practice conservation behaviors.

8. On the Internet locate the national parks.

9. Do additional research about warnings, damage, and preparation for one of the natural disasters discussed in the chapter.

1916 *The National Park Service Organic Act (16 U.S.C. 1)*
Created the establishment of the U.S. National Park Service and other purposes.

1964 *Wilderness Act (PL 88-577)*
Defines wilderness as "land where man himself is a visitor and does not remain. Established the National Wilderness Preservation System (NWPS) to oversee all national forest land designated as "wilderness" or "wild," protecting them from commercial use or the construction of buildings and permanent roads and recreational facilities. It also placed strong restrictions on mineral extraction rights. In 1970, *PL 91-504* called for the review of every roadless area and island to recommend the area for inclusion in the National Wilderness Preservation System. The *Wilderness Act of 1978 (PL 98-625)* authorized $1.2 billion for national parks projects in 44 states.

1966 *National Wildlife Refuge System Administration Act (amended PL 89-669)*
Provides guidelines for the management of wildlife refuge areas for the protection and conservation of fish and wildlife threatened with extinction.

1968 *Wild and Scenic Rivers Preservation Act (PL 90-542)*
Provides for a national wild and scenic rivers system and other purposes.

1969 *The National Environmental Policy Act (PL 91-190)*
Created the Environmental Protection Agency.

1972 *Coastal Zone Management Act (PL 92-583)*
Provides federal assistance to states for managing coastal areas.

1973 *Open Mining Land Reclamation Act (PL 95-87)*
Established requirements that mining operations for coal, sand, gravel, gold, silver, and so forth must have a permit and land reclamation timelines. By 1975, all western states except Arizona had adopted some form of mining and reclamation standards and regulations.

1976 *Federal Land Policy and Management Act (PL 94-579)*
Established the Bureau of Land Management to oversee use of public land.

1977 *Surface Mining Control and Reclamation Act (PL 95-87, amended 1982, 1984, 1986, 1987, 1990, and 1992)*
Established a nationwide program to protect society and the environment from the adverse effects of surface coal mining operations protect the rights of surface landowners, assured that adequate procedures are taken to reclaim surface areas, assured the nation's coal supply and encouraged full utilization of coal resources through the development and application of underground extraction technologies.

1978 *Uranium Mill Tailings Radiation Control Act (PL 95-604)*
Requires the remediation of former uranium mill processing and disposal sites.

1980 *The Alaska Land Protection Act (PL 96-487)*
Designated over 100 million acres of parks, wildlife refuges, and wilderness areas.

1980 *Comprehensive Environmental Response, Compensation and Liability Act (CERCLA or Superfund; PL 96-510)*
Requires cleanup of existing disposal sites; establishes financial responsibility for the sites. Amended by Superfund Amendment and Reauthorization Act (SARA) in 1986.

1980 *Farmland Protection Policy Act (PL 97-98)*
Minimized the extent to which federal programs contribute to the unnecessary and irreversible conversion of farmland to nonagricultural uses.

1985 *Food Security Act (PL 99-198)*
Created the Conservation Reserve Program and financial incentives for farmers to take their land out of production and use it for pastures or woodlands.

1986 *Coastal Barrier Resources Act (PL 97-348)*
Protects undeveloped coastal barriers and related areas by prohibiting funding of various projects areas that might support development. **The Great Lakes Coastal Barrier Act of 1988 (PL 100-707)** required that a map be prepared with inclusion of undeveloped barriers along the Great Lakes. **The Coastal Barrier Improvement Act of 1990 (PL 101-591)** included additional areas along the Great Lakes, Puerto Rico, the Florida Keys, the Virgin Islands, and secondary barriers within large embayments.

1994 *California Desert Protection Act (PL 103-433)*
Established the Death Valley and Joshua Tree National Parks and the Mojave National Preserve in the California desert and ensured that Indian people had access to the lands designated for traditional cultural and religious purposes.

SELECTED PROFESSIONAL JOURNALS

Bulletin of Environmental Contamination and Toxicology
Civil Engineering
Journal of Environmental Engineering
Water, Air, and Soil Pollution

ADDITIONAL READING

Albright, H. (1985). *The birth of the National Park Service: The founding years, 1912-33*. Howe Brothers, Salt Lake City, Chicago.

Creath, W. (1996). Home buyers' guide to geologic hazards. An AIPG Issues and Answers Publication. Arvada, CO: American Institute of Professional Geologists.

Marsh, G. P., and D. Lowenthal. *Man and Nature: Or Physical Geography As Modified By Human Action*. Seatle, WA: University of Washington Press, 2003.

Muir, J. (2001). *Our National Parks*. Washington, D.C.: Ross & Perry.

O'Leary, R., R. Durant, D. Fiorino, and P. Weiland. *Managing for the Environment: Understanding the Legal, Organizational, And Policy Challenges*. San Francisco: Jossey-Bass Publishers, 1998.

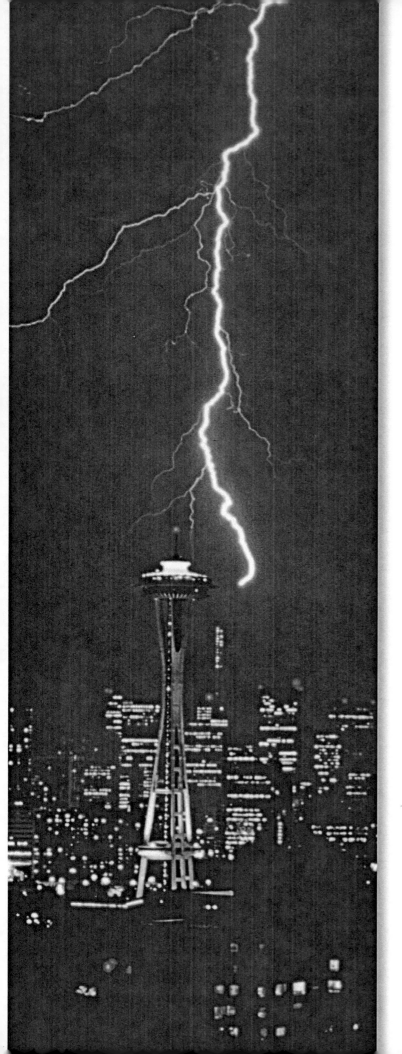

11

Energy

To play safe, I prefer to accept only one type of power: the power of art over trash, the triumph of magic over the brute.

Vladimir Nabokov (1899–1977)

OBJECTIVES

1. Give a historical account regarding the use of fuel sources by humans.

2. Describe the use of fossil fuels and why there is a concern regarding their use.

3. Explain how fuel usage endangers whale populations.

4. Explain why gasoline had to be rationed in the United States during the 1970s.

5. Describe the source of oil spills and environmental problems resulting from them.

6. Explain concerns regarding nonfossil fuel sources such as nuclear energy.

7. List sources of alternative energy fuels with the advantages and disadvantages of each.

8. Provide a list of ingredients for gasoline.

9. Provide alternative sources of fuel for automobiles and their prospective uses.

10. Give an account of other strategies to reduce the demand for gasoline.

Introduction

The earliest source for fuel was probably wood, used for heat. When **steam** engines were invented, coal provided the most efficient fuel and by the beginning of the twentieth century, coal was preferred over wood. Because coal produces harmful gas emissions and particulate matter, **petroleum** products became more popular for fuel in the 1950s through the 1970s. Until then supplies of coal and **oil** seemed abundant and the cost was relatively inexpensive. In the 1960s the average price of crude oil was $3 per barrel. Because the price of oil continued to rise due to increased demands and costs of drilling oil, the U.S. became active in protecting oil reserves in the Middle East, where two thirds of the world's oil reserves exist. In 1960, as Middle East oil-exporting countries experienced increasing demand for their crude oil, Iran, Iraq, Kuwait, Saudi Arabia, and Venezuela formed the Organization of Petroleum Exporting Countries (OPEC). In 1973 Syria and Egypt attacked Israel. When the U.S. and several other countries in the Western world supported Israel, OPEC imposed an embargo on the countries supporting Israel. This was known as the Arab Oil Embargo. By 1974, the price of crude oil quadrupled to $12 per barrel (William, 2002).

The Iran/Iraq War (1979–1980) resulted in a drop in crude oil production. By 1981 the war pushed the price of crude oil in the United States to $35 per barrel, creating an "energy crisis." The defeat of Iran increased the United States' support for Iraq, which possessed the second largest oil preserve in the world. Oil producers ExxonMobil, BP Amoco, Shell, and Chevron Texaco have found the quality of oil to be very good and profitable because it could be produced for less than $1.50 per barrel. Political unrest and corruption in the Middle East have made access to the oil fields a continuing battle. When Saddam Hussein attacked Kuwait, initiating the Gulf War of 1991, another oil crisis ensued (D'Amato, 2001). United States troops were deployed and continue to occupy the Middle East today. The price of crude oil in 2005 is $46 per barrel in the United States (EIA, 2005).

Activity in the Middle East has created awareness regarding the importance to developing alternative sources of energy to supplement and perhaps one day replace the use of **fossil fuels**. In the 1970s, there were long lines for **gasoline** and **thermostats** were set lower in an effort to conserve fuel and keep costs down. When oil prices dropped in the late 1970s, the Carter administration provided funding for alternative energy sources. In 1978 Congress passed the Public Utilities Regulatory Policies Act (PL 95-617) exempting small producers from utility regulations and requiring local utilities to purchase energy from **renewable** sources. Today legislation has mandated that automobile manufacturers produce passenger cars that are increasingly energy efficient and financial incentives have been in place for industries to use alternative energy sources.

Even though automobiles generate less pollution than they did 10 years ago, there are many more cars on the road today. The need to find more environmentally friendly sources of fuel is becoming more necessary as population demands increase and air pollution continues to affect climactic changes. Fuel is needed to produce electricity, provide an energy source to fuel automobiles and other machines, and to create products for industrial, business, and home use. According to the U.S. Energy Information Administration, the demand for electricity worldwide will increase by about 54% over the next 20 years due to projected population increases (IAGS, 2004). Electricity for

2010 HEALTHY PEOPLE OBJECTIVES

8-1 Reduce harmful air pollutants.
8-2 Alternative modes of transportation such as bicycling, walking, public transit systems, and telecommuting.
8-3 Improve the Nation's air quality by increasing the use of alternative fuel vehicles (AFVs) and cleaner alternative fuels.
8-4 Reduce airborne toxins.

Steam
Vapor that forms when water is heated to boiling; able to drive pistons or turn the blade of a turbine.

Petroleum
Also known as crude oil; a natural, flammable, liquid hydrocarbon mixture found principally beneath the Earth's surface; processed to make gasoline, natural gas, naphtha, fuel, and lubricating oils.

Oil
Greasy, combustible substances obtained from animal, vegetable, and mineral sources; liquid at ordinary temperatures; can be dissolved in solvents.

Fossil fuels
Coal, oil, natural gas, and other combustible materials originating from ancient plant and animal life; a nonrenewable energy source.

Gasoline
A volatile flammable liquid mixture of hydrocarbons (hexane, heptane, octane, etc.) produced from refined crude oil; used as a fuel in internal combustion engines.

Thermostat
An automatic device for regulating the temperature of a heating and cooling system.

Renewable
Resources that can be replenished with proper management and wise use, such as sunlight, water, geothermal heat, and biomass.

homes and industry can be generated, but it requires a primary fuel source in order to do so. Primary sources of fuel to generate energy include the fossil fuels. These sources are considered natural resources that have evolved over many centuries and supplies cannot be diminished. In addition, fossil fuels must be burned using **combustion**. Unfortunately, the combustion process is not clean because particulate matter and gases are produced as a result of the burning process. Fossil fuel sources for energy include coal, oil, **natural gas**, and uranium (Figure 11-1).

Fossil Fuels

COAL

Coal was formed 400 million years ago from the remains of decayed plants that converted to carbon with help from the sun. It is sometimes referred to as "buried sunshine." As the surface of the Earth changed over time, sand, clay, and other mineral matter buried soggy **peat**. Over time, the weight of sedimentary rocks and sandstone formed squeezed water from the peat. Coal is still

being formed in areas such as the Great Dismal Swamp of North Carolina and Virginia, Okefenokee Swamp of Georgia, and the Everglades in Florida. Scientists estimate that 3 to 7 feet of compacted plant matter is required to form 1 foot of bituminous coal.

Coal must be mined from underground sources. French explorers discovered coal sources in the United States on the Illinois River in 1679. The earliest recorded commercial mining operation began near Richmond, Virginia, in 1748 (Gerard, 1997). From 1850 to 1950 coal was the country's primary energy source for fuel. Today the United States is the second largest coal exporter in the world, after Australia (National Mining Association, 1995). The largest reserves are in Montana, Illinois, and Wyoming (American Coal Foundation, 2005) (Figure 11-2). The American Coal Foundation estimates there is still enough coal for another 250 to 300 years at the current rate of use (American Coal Foundation, 2002). There is 12 times as much energy in the United States coal reserves as all the oil in Saudi Arabia; however, much of it cannot be mined because it is too costly or current technology does not allow it.

Today coal supplies more than half of the country's electric power generation. The rest is used for the steel industry and exported to other countries. Coal is ranked

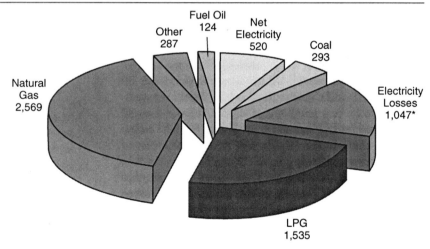

FIGURE 11-1 **Energy Use by Fuel (in Trillion Btu), 1994**
Note: * denotes losses incurred during transmission, distribution, and generation of electricity.
Source: Energy Information Administration. Retrieved from http://www.eia.doe.gov/emeu/mecs/iab/chemicals/page2a.html.

Total Energy Consumed
6,375 trillion Btu (with electrical losses)*

Consider the Cost HOW MUCH ENERGY DO YOU USE?

Many of us take our use of energy for granted until we see our electric bills. Electricity to our homes is monitored by a meter outside of the house. In urban communities, meter readers visit and report numbers to the electric company for billing. In other communities, the resident may be required to read the meter. It is a good idea to check your own meter to see if the meter was read correctly and to monitor electrical usage. Your electrical bill should state the number of kilowatt hours used per day. It would be a good idea to check this each month and attempt to keep it as low as possible.

according to the amount of energy it contains per unit of weight, expressed in **British thermal units (BTU)** per pound. The higher the carbon content, the more heat it generates. Ninety percent of the coal used is bituminous and subbituminous coal. Bituminous coal (45 to 86% carbon; 15,000 BTU per pound) is the most plentiful form of coal in the United States and predominates in the eastern and Mid-Atlantic coal fields. Subbituminous coal (35 to 45% carbon; 8,300–10,000 BTU per pound) is generally found in the western states and Alaska. Lignite coal (25 to 35% carbon; 4,000–8,300 BTU per pound) is the "youngest" of the coals and found in Texas, Montana, North Dakota, and some Gulf Coast states. Anthracite coal has the highest carbon content (86 to 89%; 15,000 BTU per pound) and produces the most heat. It is found in Pennsylvania. Coal is transported from one state to another by railroad cars or barges on waterways.

Coal under the surface must be uncovered and removed by large machines. This process, the leading method for coal mining today, is called **surface mining** (also known as *strip mining*). Surface mining accounts for 61% of coal produced in the United States, producing

Combustion
Burning of coal, wood, or other material, resulting in the release of energy in the form of heat and light. A major contributor to air pollution.

Natural gas
An odorless, colorless, tasteless, nontoxic, clean-burning fossil fuel consisting mainly of methane, a hydrocarbon produced by coal gasification; may contain ethane, propane, butane, pentane, helium, and hexane.

Peat
A wet vegetable substance made of roots, fibers, and moss in various stages of decomposition; usually found in bogs or swamps. It was often dried and used for fuel.

British thermal unit (BTU)
The amount of heat needed to increase the temperature of 1 pound of water 1 degree.

Surface mining
Also known as strip mining, a mining technique that removes large amounts of soil and sub-soil in order to extract coal close to the Earth's surface.

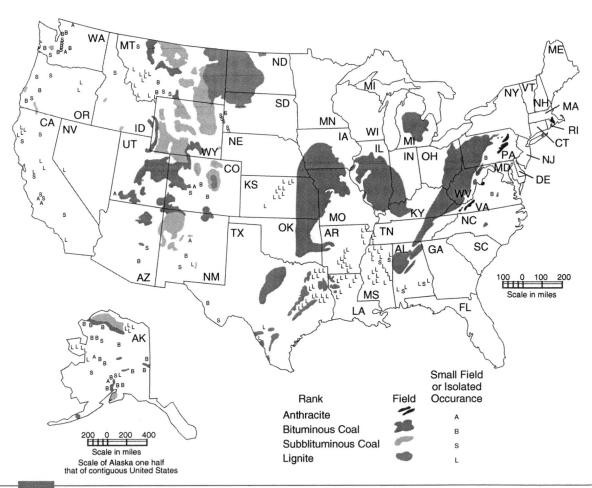

Rank	Field	Small Field or Isolated Occurance
Anthracite		A
Bituminous Coal		B
Subblituminous Coal		S
Lignite		L

200 0 200 400
Scale in miles
Scale of Alaska one half that of contiguous United States

100 0 100 200
Scale in miles

FIGURE 11-2 **Coal-bearing Areas of the United States**
Source: Energy Information Administration. (1999). U.S. coal reserves, 1997 update. http://www.eia.doe.gov/cneaf/coal/reserves/front-1.html.

more than 1 billion tons each year. Topsoil and subsoil are removed and set aside to be used for land reclamation later. Large shovels remove rock and other materials to expose the coal bed. Smaller shovels load the coal onto large trucks that remove coal from the pit.

Where the coal is too deep or the land is too hilly for surface mining, underground mining is used (Figure 11-3). Most underground mines are east of the Mississippi, especially in the Appalachian mountain states. Approximately one third of the nation's coal comes from underground mines (Asbury et al., 2002). The most common type of underground mine is the shaft mine. To reach the coal, mine shafts are cut by machines. In conventional mining, a machine cuts into the coal and holes are drilled for explosives to blast loose chunks of coal. Machines scoop the coal onto conveyors which dump it into shuttle cars that haul the coal out through the shaft. Another technique for underground mining, is known as **longwall mining**. A machine shears back and forth along the wall of coal, cutting chunks and removing them on a conveyor.

Coal is known as a "dirty fuel" because of fly ash, the dark material (known as **soot**) given off when coal is burned, and sulfur emissions. Because coal contains sulfur, when it is burned, it produces sulfur oxides. Emissions of these substances is much less than it was before the 1970s because of emissions control techniques such as precipitators and scrubbers. Precipitators produce a negative charge that causes ash particles to stick to collecting plates so they can be disposed of later. **Flue gas scrubbers** cause flue gases to react with lime, forming calcium sulfite or calcium sulfate (gypsum), which can be sold for other uses. Another way to reduce sulfur emissions is to wash the coal after it is mined and before it is burned. Other techniques can also be used to control the production of greenhouse gases (such as sulfur dioxide and carbon dioxide). The cleanest and most efficient method is coal **gasification**. Coal gasification uses steam from burning coal to turn power **generators**.

PETROLEUM

Petroleum is a dark oil, also referred to as crude oil. It is refined by distillation to make kerosene, gasoline, and other oil products. Approximately 700 million gallons of oil are used in the United States each day. Globally, nearly 3 billion gallons are used every day (National Ocean Service, 2004). Oil products are used to fuel automobiles, heat homes, lubricate machinery, produce electricity, and make asphalt, plastics, medicines, ink, fertilizers, pesticides, paints, varnishes, and other materials. Oil is found beneath the Earth's surface.

Prior to the 1800s, indoor light was provided by candles, torches, and oil-burning lamps. When it was discovered that whale oil had less odor and smoke than other oils, it became very popular. Right whales provided oil as a machine lubricant. Sperm whale oil was the best for lamps. Of the two, sperm whale oil was the most expensive, costing $3 per gallon. It was recorded that about 15,000 right whales were killed per year (San Joaquin Geological Society, 2002). Some species became endangered, close to extinction. When the public became aware of the whale's plight, concern for other endangered species followed.

Around 1854 a Yale chemist, Benjamin Silliman, found that crude oil ($100 per barrel at the time) could be refined and made into kerosene, and the demand for whale oil significantly decreased (Armentano, 1981). Kerosene, known as coal oil, was less expensive, had a longer shelf life, and smelled better when it burned. In 1878 the electric light bulb was invented by Thomas Edison, significantly reducing the need for kerosene for lighting.

FIGURE 11-3 **Climax Mine** Mining provides access to fossil fuels.

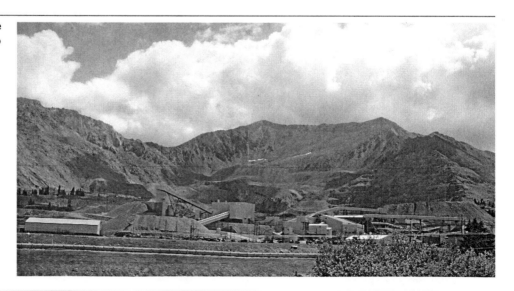

In western Pennsylvania pits were built next to Oil Creek to make oil float to the surface. To extract the petroleum, blankets were thrown on the water soaking up the oil. The oil was then wrung out of the blankets and sold for $2 per gallon. The oil was promoted as a miracle drug, curing wounds, rashes, pimples, scratches, and other skin afflictions. In 1859, the first oil well in the United States, near Titusville, Pennsylvania, hit oil 70 feet below the ground. When the internal combustion engine was invented in the early 1900s, petroleum production was in high demand.

By the early 1950s, the demand for coal lessened for transportation, home heating, and industrial needs as petroleum, natural gas, and **propane** became more popular. Because of the increased need for oil, the United States began to import it from other countries. Since the 1970s, domestic production of oil in the United States has declined. Oil and natural gas supplies tightened while prices surged and the nation learned a painful lesson about dependence on foreign energy. By the 1990s, the United States has imported more oil than it produces (Bush, 2002). In 2002, the world consumed 74 million barrels of oil daily. The United States is the world's largest consumer, burning 19 million barrels of oil (Flavin, 2002). The increased dependence on foreign oil raises concerns about national military and economic security.

The largest producers of oil in the world are Saudi Arabia and the former Soviet Union (Flavin, 2002). Nearly one third of the world's oil comes from offshore wells in the North Sea, the Persian Gulf, and the Gulf of Mexico. If consumers choose to reduce the nation's dependence on imports, each must reduce petroleum consumption. Possible solutions include taxing oil products, rationing them, and improving the way that they are used.

Much of the underground oil is trapped in pores of rocks and wells that must be drilled to draw it to the surface. At first, oil wells were drilled where oil seeped from the ground. Today, gravity meters, magnetometers, seismographs, CAT and MRI imaging, and other technologies are used by geologists to determine where the oil may lay. A well is drilled using a rotary tool with diamond bit drills. **Drilling mud** composed of clay, water, and chemicals, are used to keep the drill bit cool. In the United States, the average well is more than 1 mile deep. Drilling rigs measure underground pressure and use special valves to prevent **gushers** from wasting oil. Carbon dioxide, other gases, water, or chemicals are injected to maintain well pressure. Crude oil must be refined before it can be used for fuel.

Longwall mining
A type of mining where a machine shears back and forth along the wall of coal, cutting chunks and moving them to a conveyor belt.

Soot
A fine, black powder formed by or separated from fuel during combustion.

Flue gas scrubbers
A device installed in a smokestack or chimney that removes impurities from the smoke.

Gasification
The conversion of a solid fuel to a gas that in turn is used to produce electric power.

Generator
A device that converts mechanical energy into electrical energy such as steam turning turbines to produce electrical current. A small quantity generator is used by schools, hospitals, or businesses and generates less than 1,000 kilograms of hazardous waste per month.

Propane
A colorless gas found in natural gas and petroleum, used as fuel.

Drilling mud
A mixture of clays, chemicals, and water used for mining.

Gushers
An abundantly flowing gas or oil well.

 A barrel of oil is equal to 42 gallons. Although barrels are no longer used to ship oil, the term is still used as a volume of measurement for oil.

AMERICA'S MOST FAMOUS "GUSHER"
The amazing Lakeview Gusher started spewing crude oil in March of 1910. The San Joaquin Valley in California has had many gushers. The Shamrock gusher began in 1986 and the Midway gusher came in 1909. Oil shot into the air at an estimated 125,000 barrels a day from a column of oil and sand 20 feet in diameter and 200 feet high. The gushing continued at a reduced rate for 18 months and released approximately 9.4 million barrels. Half the oil was captured but the rest flowed into rivers, land, and the air.
Source: Weiss, 2003.

 Fuel oils include:
Kerosene
Coal oil
Jet fuel
Diesel fuel
Home heating oil
Gas oil
Heavy residual fuel oil
Marine diesel fuel
Propane
Butane

Petroleum products used for fuel are known as **fuel oils**. Fuel oils can be used in furnaces, stoves, heaters, engines, lamps, and solvents (ATSDR, 1996). Fuel oils contain a mixtures of **aliphatic** (open chain and cyclic compounds that are similar to open chain compounds) and **aromatic** (benzene and compounds similar to benzene) petroleum hydrocarbons. In addition, they may contain small amounts of nitrogen, sulfur, and other elements as additives. The exact chemical composition of each of the fuel oils may vary somewhat, depending on the source and other factors.

All fuel oils are liquids at room temperature, although they can evaporate, depending on the temperature (ATSDR, 1996). When they evaporate, some of the chemicals react with sunlight (photo oxidation). Most fuel oils are yellowish to light brown in color. They generally have an odor, are flammable, and burn at temperatures between 177° and 329° C (Tripathi, 2001). Breathing fuel oil may cause nausea, increase blood pressure, and cause eye irritation (bloodshot). Breathing kerosene can affect the nervous system with effects such as headache, light-headedness, anorexia, poor coordination, and difficulty in concentration. When kerosene gets on your skin for short periods, it can make the skin itchy, red, and sore, sometimes forming blisters. Numerous cases of children drinking kerosene have been reported. Drinking kerosene may cause vomiting, diarrhea, swelling of the stomach, stomach cramps, coughing, drowsiness, restlessness, irritability, and unconsciousness (ASTDR, 1996). It may be difficult to breathe and breathing may be painful. Coughing, pneumonia, and difficult or painful breathing indicate kerosene has entered the lungs.

Thomas Midgeley, one of the developers of tetraethyl leaded gasoline suffered ill effects in 1923. In 1924, five workers at several Standard Oil refineries in New Jersey and Ohio died while making tetraethyl lead gasoline additive in unsafe conditions. Seven other workers had died previously at General Motors and DuPont plants. In 1925, five more tetraethyl lead workers died in a New Jersey DuPont plant. The U.S. Surgeon General investigated the problem but leaded gasoline stayed on the market until 1986. November of 1973, the EPA released a health document titled *EPA's Position on the Health Implications of Airborne Lead* confirming that lead from automobile exhaust was a direct public health threat. Thanks to the Clean Air Act of 1970, the EPA could call for a gradual reduction in lead content of gasoline, starting January of 1975. Beginning in 1975 cars were equipped with pollution-reducing catalytic converters designed to run only on unleaded fuel.
Source: Lewis, 1985.

Nonfossil Fuels

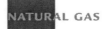

NATURAL GAS

Natural gas provides about one fourth of all the energy used in the United States (Udall & Andrews, 2001). The United States produces 19.9% of the world's natural gas although it holds 3.1% of the world's natural gas reserves (EIA, 2004). The only country that exceeds the United States in natural gas production is the former Soviet Union. Natural gas is located underground where oil supplies are found. Methane gas is separated from oil and compressed for later use. Natural gas is usually more expensive than fuel oils or electricity. Most of the natural gas supplies in the United States are from Alaska, Louisiana, New Mexico, Oklahoma, and Texas. It is transported in underground pipes. Natural gas is colorless and odorless, but it is harmful. To protect citizens and natural gas workers, sulfur has been added so when a "rotten egg" smell is evident, it is known that there is a natural gas leak and action can be taken to correct it.

Natural gas is not available in all areas of the country, particularly in areas where water tables are high. The first recorded use of natural gas in the United States was for streetlights in Baltimore, Maryland in 1816. Natural gas produces almost no pollutants or ash when burned. Natural gas is expected to be the fastest growing component of world primary energy consumption (EIA, 2004).

URANIUM

Uranium-235 is a primary source for nuclear power. Uranium is found in the ground and is mined, transported, and stored. It requires very careful handling because it is **radioactive**. The fuel cycle associated with nuclear power includes refinement or enrichment, the generation of power, the processing of spent fuel rods, and the management of *radioactive waste*. The refinement process limits uranium fuel to 4% and is in a form that is resistant to water and sealed inside corrosion-resistant metal tubes. The process of using radioactive materials for power is known as **nuclear fission**. As uranium-235 disintegrates or "decays," radioactive waves generate heat, until atoms becomes stable. The **nuclear reactor** controls the disintegration of the uranium and produces steam that turns a **turbine** and generator to provide electricity. The **half life** of a radioactive substance is a way of calculating the amount of time for half of the atoms of a radionuclide to decay or become stable. Although the substance is less harmful than it was in its previous state, it is still a hazardous material and must be carefully stored and disposed.

Environmental Health Concerns

PROBLEMS WITH COAL AND URANIUM MINING OPERATIONS

Before Superfund, mining operations accounted for some of the worst land, water, and air pollution in the United States (Murphy, 2000). Because of this, the coal mining industry is regulated by several agencies. Mining companies may be required to pay $10,000 per acre to cover the cost of land reclamation so the land can be contoured to its original state, be productive, and provide wildlife habitats. There are abandoned mines in some areas of the country because requirements were not as strict for land reclamation as they are today. To restore these orphan lands, coal producers pay a special tax for every ton of coal they produce which is set aside into the Abandoned Mine Lands Fund, administered by the federal government, and distributed to states initiating land reclamation projects. This fund was set up in the 1970s when Congress enacted the Surface Mining Control and Reclamation Act (SMCRA) mandating strict regulation of surface mining. Each state is responsible for enforcing SMCRA standards, but where there are no programs for enforcement, the Office of Surface Mining Reclamation and Enforcement in the Department of Interior enforces the law.

 In 1939, an air pollution disaster in St. Louis occurred when the city switched from soft coal to hard coal and fuel oil to reduce the amount of industrial smoke. In 1941, St. Louis adopted the first strict smoke control ordinance for a large city in the United States.

 Selected legislative acts affecting mining include:
Wilderness Act of 1964
National Trails System Act of 1968
Wild and Scenic Rivers Act of 1968
Bald Eagle Protection Act of 1969
National Environmental Policy Act of 1969
Clean Air Act of 1970
Resource Conservation and Recovery Act of 1970
Clean Water Act of 1972
Safe Drinking Water Act of 1974
Archeological and Historical Preservation Act of 1974
National Forests Management Act of 1976
Noise Control Act of 1976
Soil and Water Resources Conservation Act of 1977

PROBLEMS WITH PETROLEUM PRODUCTION

Another environmental concern with respect to petroleum production, aside from the depletion of a nonrenewable resource, is the impact on the environment. Over two million petroleum wells have been drilled in the United States and about 800,000 of them are still active (EIA, 2005) (Figure 11-4). In the past 150 years, petroleum production has polluted land, waterways, oceans, and the atmosphere. The primary issues concern abandoned oil fields, old petroleum storage facilities, and transportation accidents (Table 11-1). Abandoned facilities leave potential hazards to the environment and local

Fuel oil
A liquid petroleum product used to generate heat or power.

Aliphatic
Material that has carbon atoms linked in open chains.

Aromatic
Having a strong fragrance; relating to or containing one or more benzene rings.

Radioactive
Materials exhibiting spontaneous emissions of alpha, beta, or gamma rays from unstable nuclei; hazardous to humans and other living organisms.

Nuclear fission
The splitting of an atomic nucleus causing the release of large amounts of energy.

Nuclear reactor
A facility where energy is derived from fission.

Turbine
A rotary engine powered by steam or fluid; used to power a generator to produce electricity.

Half-life
The average lifetime of a radioactive substance or an unstable subatomic particle.

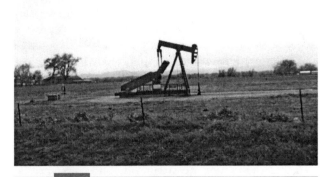

FIGURE 11-4 **Oil Well in Colorado** Small oil wells can be found in rural areas of the United States.

TABLE 11-1 Major Oil Spills

March 1967	*Torrey Canyon* ran aground off the Sicily Islands spilling 38 million gallons of crude oil
December 1976	*Argo Merchant* ran aground near Nantucket Island spilling 7.7 million gallons of fuel oil
April 1977	Blowout of a well in Ekofish leaking 81 million gallons
March 1978	*Amoco Candiz* wrecked off the Brittany coast spilling 68 million gallons
June 1979	An exploratory oil well in the Gulf of Mexico blew out spilling 140 million gallons of crude oil
July 1979	*Atlantic Empress* and *Aegean Captain* collided off Barbados spilling 46 million gallons of crude oil with an additional 41 million gallons spilled while being towed
February 1983	A field platform spilled 80 million gallons of oil in the Persian Gulf
August 1983	*Castillo de Bellver* caught fire spilling 78 million gallons of oil off the coast of Cape Town, South Africa
November 1988	*Odyssey* spilled 43 million gallons of oil off Newfoundland
March 1989	*Exxon Valdez* spilled more than 10 million gallons of oil near Prince William Sound, Alaska causing the worst oil spill in U.S. history
December 1989	*Kharg-5* exploded causing 19 million gallons of crude oil to spill New Las Palmas, Canary Islands
June 1990	*Mega Bor* experienced an explosion and fire releasing 5.1 million gallons of oil near Galvaston, Texas
January 1991	Iraqui tankers deliberately released 240 to 260 millions of crude oil into the Persian Gulf during the Gulf War
April 1991	*Haven* spilled 42 million gallons near Genoa, Italy
May 1991	*ABT Summer* exploded and leaked 15 to 78 million gallons of oil near Angola
March 1992	An oil well spilled 88 million gallons in Uzbekistan
August 1993	*Bouchard B155, Balsa 37,* and *Ocean 255* tankers collided spilling 336,000 gallons of fuel oil near Tampa, Florida
September 1994	A Russian dam burst spilling approximately 2 million barrels
February 1996	*Sea Empress* ran aground spilling 70,000 tons of crude oil near Milford Haven, Wales
December 1999	*Erika* broke apart spilling 3 million gallons of heavy oil near the French Atlantic coast
January 2000	A ruptured pipeline owned by Petrobras spewed 343,200 gallons of heavy oil near Rio de Janeiro
November 2000	*Westchester* ran aground near Port Sulphur, Louisiana dumping 567,000 gallons of crude oil, the largest spill in U.S. waters since *Exxon Valdez*
November 2002	*Prestige* was damaged and sank; 20 million gallons of oil remains underwater

Source: Info Please Almanac. Retrieved from http://www.infoplease.com/ipa/A0001451.html. Reprinted with permission.

citizens. Leakage of underground tanks can pollute water supplies. Transportation of petroleum products poses a major hazard when an accident causes a spill.

The primary reason for oil spills today is an accident that occurs during oil transportation. The possibility of an oil tanker accident is likely as nearly half of the world's seaborne trade concerns crude oil or petroleum products. Oil tankers are also the largest ships built, carrying more than one million barrels of oil at a time (Figure 11-5). Large oil spills at sea and in harbors cause severe pollution and destruction of marine life and lower coastal property values. These incidents prompted Congress to enact the Oil Pollution Act of 1990 to reduce and plan for

oil spills. Guidelines were established by the U.S. Coast Guard, the EPA, and the Mineral Management Service. To prevent or limit the size of oil spills, single-hulled tankers are being replaced with double-hulled tankers.

Oil spills present a major environmental hazard. When spilled on the ground, some of the chemicals slowly leach through the soil to pollute groundwater. Chemicals that attach to the soil may remain for more than a decade. When spilled into streams, rivers, lakes, or oceans, some of the chemicals evaporate while other chemicals dissolve in the water. Bacteria and fungi can break down some of the chemicals; however, this may take up to a year to occur. Oil floats on the water and is flammable. In the event

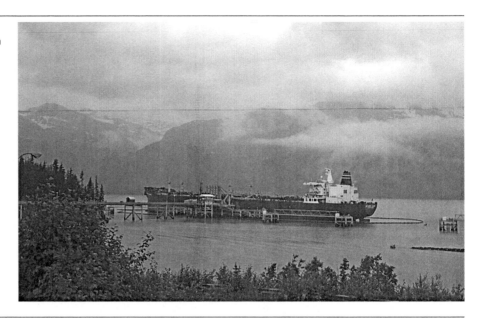

WHAT TO DO DURING A POWER OUTAGE

A storm, accident, or excessive power demands may result in a power **outage**. A power outage is a major inconvenience putting a stop to most businesses, homeowner activities, and recreational activities. A grocery store, restaurant, or home may be especially concerned about food storage. Do not open the refrigerator or freezer door frequently. If the power outage is less than 2 hours, the food will not spoil. If the outage will be for more than 2 to 4 hours, pack refrigerated items such as dairy products, meat products, eggs, and leftovers into a cooler of ice. A freezer that is half full will hold the cold for up to 24 hours and a full freezer for 48 hours. It is a good idea to keep canned or boxed food products that can be eaten cold or heated on an outdoor grill. Propane and charcoal grills should never be used indoors because the incomplete combustion will give off carbon monoxide. Source: USDA, 2004.

of an oil spill, local, state, and federal officials must be called to respond. Skimmers, absorbents, dispersants, burning, pressure washing, vacuuming, and shovels are just some of the ways that oil spills are managed.

PROBLEMS WITH POWER PLANTS

Electrical power plants use coal, steam, oil, and radioactive materials to move generators to create and transmit electrical power to businesses and residents. Most power plants are built along rivers, streams, or lakes where water can be used to cool the generators so they can run longer. The heated water expelled by power plants has been a concern for environmentalists and wildlife conservationists for several years.

In 1957, the first commercial nuclear reactor in the United States went on line in Shippingport, Pennsylvania.

Nuclear Power

About 20% of United States electricity is generated by nuclear power reactors (NEI, 2005). The ability to use nuclear power reduces reliance on fossil fuels. Many fear the possibility of radiation exposure from nuclear power plants. In actuality, nuclear power plant operations account for less than .01% of the total radiation exposure. Workers of nuclear power plants receive higher doses, but the overall dose is still low. In 1979, the EPA issued environmental standards protecting the public and workers from radiation from **nuclear energy** facilities. In 1987, the EPA issued standards for nuclear, medical, industrial, mining, and waste management worker exposure to radiation. In 1989, standards for radionuclide emissions from federal and industrial facilities were issued.

Safety in nuclear power plants is absolutely essential. The nuclear plant must be designed for safety and employees must be highly trained. In the United States, nuclear reactors are enclosed in massive concrete (Figure 11-6) and steel containment structures designed to prevent nuclear accidents that can release radioactive

Outage
The discontinuance or temporary loss of electrical power.

Nuclear energy
Energy produced by changes in the nucleus of an atom by fission of a heavy nucleus or by fusion of light nuclei into heavy ones; accompanied by loss of mass.

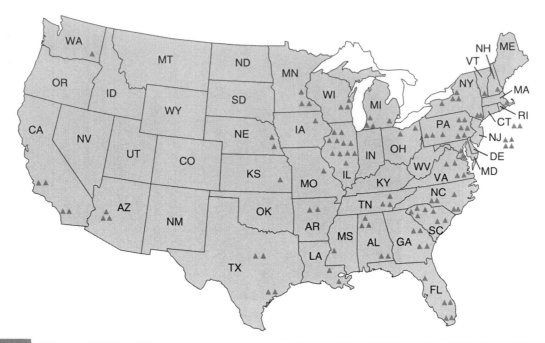

FIGURE 11-6 Locations of Operating Nuclear Power Reactors
Source: U.S. Nuclear Regulatory Commission. Retrieved from http://www.nrc.gov/info-finder/reactor/.

FIGURE 11-7 Three-Mile Island Reactors in Pennsylvania Nuclear reactors must meet NRC standards in order to operate without danger to the public.

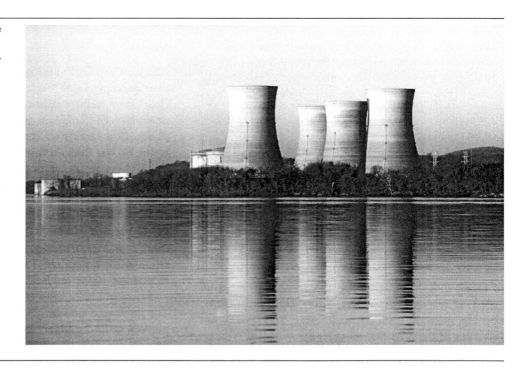

materials in the environment (Figure 11-7). Most nuclear power plants were opened with a 40-year license, meaning that they were meant to operate for only 40 years before they were to be decommissioned (shut down and sealed). Nuclear power plants are heavily scrutinized for potential problems and periodically closed for repairs, assuring that no problems will affect surrounding communities or citizens. Some nuclear power plants have been maintained so well that their 40-year license has been extended.

The Nuclear Regulatory Commission (NRC) is the federal agency responsible for implementing the EPA's radiation exposure standards through regulation of nuclear power reactors and many other uses of radiation. The NRC was created as an independent agency by the Energy Reorganization Act of 1974, which abolished the Atomic

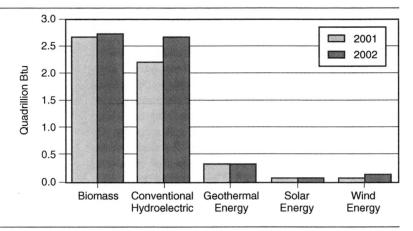

FIGURE 11-8 Renewable Energy Consumption by Source, 2001 and 2002
Source: Energy Information Administration. Retrieved from http://www.eia.doe.gov/cneaf/solar.renewables/page/rea_data/chapter1.html.

Energy Commission (AEC) initiated in 1947 (Dept. of Energy, 2005). This act, along with the Atomic Energy Act of 1954 provides for the regulations of commercial nuclear power plants (NRC, 2000). The NRC inspects nuclear facilities, training, procedures, and other aspects of nuclear power plants with strict regulations and penalties to prevent incidents in the United States similar to the 1986 incident in Chernobyl. The Department of Energy (DOE) implements the standards at facilities under their direction.

Renewable Energy Sources

Innovations in energy production have created renewable energy sources (Figure 11-8). The sun, wind, water, vegetation, and heat from the Earth provide virtually unlimited sources for power. Each of these energy sources has advantages and disadvantages, but they provide hope that there are fuel sources more environmentally friendly and cheaper than fossil fuels. In 2001, renewable energy accounted for 6% of U.S. energy consumption (EIA, 2004). Renewable energy sources include biomass (wood, wood waste, municipal solid waste, landfill gas, ethanol, and other biomass), hydropower, geothermal, wind, and solar (solar thermal and photovoltaic) and wind (Table 11-2).

WOOD

Wood for fuel comes from forest land, private land clearing, and from urban tree and landscaping. Waste wood from manufacturing, construction, and demolition is also used for fuel. Wood is considered a "renewable" resource because trees are planted to replace those cut down for manufacturing and fuel uses. The type of wood used for fuel is important. Hard woods (such as walnut, oak, and elm) burn longer than soft woods (such as pine and cedar). In addition, wood should be "cured" by dry-

TABLE 11-2 World's Largest Hydroelectric Plants (Over 4,000 MW Capacity)

Name of dam	Location	Rated capacity (MW) Present	Rated capacity (MW) Ultimate	Year of initial operation
Itaipu	Brazil/Paraguay	12,600	14,000	1983
Guri	Venezuela	10,000	10,000	1986
Grand Coulee	Washington	6,494	6,494	1942
Sayano-Shushensk	Russia	6,400	6,400	1989
Krasnoyarsk	Russia	6,000	6,000	1968
Churchill Falls	Canada	5,428	5,428	1971
La Grande 2	Canada	5,328	5,328	1979
Bratsk	Russia	4,500	4,500	1961
Moxoto	Brazil	4,328	4,328	n.a.
Ust-Ilim	Russia	4,320	4,320	1977
Tucurui	Brazil	4,245	8,370	1984

Note: MW = megawatts; n.a. = not available.
Source: International Hydropower Association. World's Largest Hydroelectric Plants. Retrieved from http://www.infoplease.com/ipa/A0001336.html. Reprinted with permission.

ing it outdoors for several months before burning. The problem with burning wood is that the incomplete combustion process leaves behind ashes, soot, and carbon monoxide, resulting in indoor and outdoor air pollution. Sparks may also leap from a fire, causing burns or accidental fires. The burning of wood is considered an inefficient fuel source because it may take as many as 10 to 30 years to replace the wood burned in one tree.

WASTE INCINERATION

The burning of solid waste reduces the volume of solid waste by 90% and can provide steam or electrical power. There are two designs: mass burn and refuse-derived fuel. Most waste-to-energy plants use the mass burn system. The waste does not have to be sorted or prepared except for removing noncombustible or oversized objects. Waste is transported to the plant and dropped into a storage pit where it is then moved by crane into the combustion zone. Refuse-derived fuel systems require that the waste be sorted, shredded, and "fluffed" by breaking up clumps and adding water before it is burned. It can also be compressed into pellets for later use. Neither of these methods is without disadvantages. Because garbage is burned, ashes still need to be disposed of, noise is generated from the machines required to process it, and there are still emission of particulate matter and dioxin.

HYDROPOWER

Hydroelectric energy is generated by using the large quantities of water from a reservoir behind a dam to turn turbines and generate electricity. Hydroelectric power is the world's largest renewable source of energy and considered a clean source of energy. Hydropower does not generate waste or produce air pollution. Unlike fossil fuel plants that are only 50% efficient, hydro turbines convert as much as 90% of available energy into electricity. The United States is second in the world, behind Canada, in the amount of hydropower it produces. Hydropower contributes between 8–12% of U.S. electrical generation (National Hydropower Association, 2005). It accounts for 15% of the world's electrical supply.

The first use of moving water for production of electricity was a waterwheel on the Fox River in Wisconsin in 1882 (Lamark et al., 1998). After that, hydroelectric plants were established along Niagara Falls in New York. At that time, the hydroelectric plants proved to be more efficient than fossil fuel plants. The most well-known and frequently visited dams in the United States are the Hoover and Grand Coolie dams. The Hoover Dam (formerly known as the Boulder Canyon Dam) was designed to capture water power from Lake Mead and the Colorado River near the Arizona–Nevada border (Figure 11-9). The dam was finished in 1936 and was intended to provide power to cities in California, Arizona, and Nevada. The Grand Coolie Dam was designed to provide power and irrigation for farmland and wildlife. It is located on the Columbia River between Seattle and Spokane, Washington. It was completed in 1975 and is said to be the largest concrete structure in the United States.

Hydroelectric plants have a poor reputation among environmentalists and land owners. Primary concerns include the effect on watersheds, flooding of usable land, decayed vegetation submerged by the flooding, and the effect on global warming. Water needed to generate the electricity is diverted away from the farms, ranches, streams, waterfalls, and wildlife that depend on it. New projects require an **environmental impact study** weighing the impact on the environment with the gains in providing power from an alternative source.

GEOTHERMAL ENERGY

Geothermal energy utilizes heat trapped in rock formations such as hot springs, geysers, and **fumaroles** (holes in or near volcanoes where vapor escapes) to provide hot water or steam for heat. The steam is then directed to turbines that generate electricity. Different types of geothermal energy include hydrothermal, dry rock, geopressurized, and magma reservoirs. Most of the nation's geothermal sites are west of the Mississippi River. Geothermal plants are expensive because they need to be built near the source and sometimes arsenic or boron are found in geothermal water.

SOLAR POWER

Solar power initiatives have been in place for years. Energy from the sun can be collected from passive or active systems. **Passive solar systems** absorb heat through windows. When a building is designed with solar power in mind, large windows on the south side of the building and materials that absorb and slowly release the sun's heat are used. An **active solar system** uses solar collectors, pumps, and valves to transfer energy from the sun to a storage place (U.S. Department of Energy, 2004). There are several different types of solar collectors. A flat plate collector (Figure 11-10) is the most common.

The solar collector has a clear or translucent cover that lets in solar energy. There is a dark surface (absorber plate) that soaks up heat with insulation on the back, preventing the heat from escaping. Heat is transferred to a "working fluid" (heated air or liquid) and transferred by vents and pipes to a storage facility to be used for power

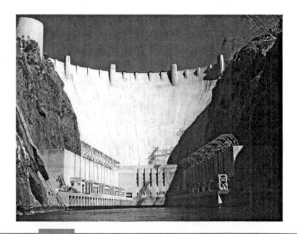

FIGURE 11-9 **Hoover Dam** One of the largest dams in the United States, Hoover Dam provides hydroelectricity to several areas.

on cloudy days. This system is usually installed at the site where it is used. The most common use for **solar panels** is to heat water. Solar panels do not have moving parts so that they last for a long time. More expensive panels generate more power from each square foot of area. In order to use solar panels, you must have a clear area with no trees or shadows, facing south to mount the panels.

A **solar thermal energy system** collects solar energy at a central location and is used by several customers. A solar thermal energy system uses mirrors or lenses to track the sun's position so that rays are focused on the **solar collectors** that contain fluid. The sunlight is intensified in order to heat water or other fluids to more than 750° F. The resulting steam powers an electric generator. In this type of system, the collected energy powers irrigation pumps, provides electricity for small communities, or captures normally wasted heat from the sun in industrial areas. Other solar thermal energy systems include solar ponds and trough systems.

Photovoltaic (PV) cell solar energy systems convert sunlight directly into electricity without the use of mechanical generators. PV cells have no moving parts, are easy to install, require little maintenance, last up to 20 years, and do not pollute the air. Small PV cells are used for calculators or watches. Larger PV cells are used to provide electricity for rural households, recreational vehicles, and businesses. The maximum amount of power is produced around noon when sunlight is the most intense. PV systems produce electricity only when the sun is shining, therefore a backup energy supply during darkness or cloudy days is needed.

At this time, solar power costs more than three times as much as fossil fuel energy. Most users of solar power have their own solar collection systems. All or some of

Hydroelectric energy
Electric energy produced by a turbine generator powered by water.

Environmental impact study
A survey conducted to determine the conditions of a proposed construction site, analyzing the impact the site will have on the environment, and proposing measures the company will take to compensate for any ecological loss.

Fumaroles
Holes in or near volcanoes where vapor escapes.

Passive solar system
Solar heat absorbed through glass panels to heat water and store hot water.

Active solar system
The use of solar collectors, pumps, and valves to transfer solar energy to a storage place.

Solar panel
A battery of solar cells. A solar cell converts radiant energy from the sun into electrical energy using the photovoltaic process.

Solar thermal energy system
A system of mirrors or lenses used to draw the sun's rays to panels that collect solar energy.

Solar collector
A box, frame, or room that collects rays from the sun to produce heat. Clear covers let in solar energy, dark surfaces (absorber plates) soak up heat. Vents and pipes carry heated air or liquid from inside the collector to where it will be used.

FIGURE 11-10 **Solar Panels in Kansas**

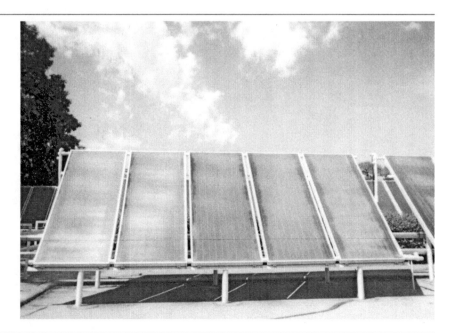

the electricity is stored in a bank of large batteries. The generated and stored electricity is in the form of **direct current (DC)** like a car **battery** and must be converted to the **alternating current (AC)** for home use. If the system is connected to the power grid, the inverter converts the current. When grid power blacks out, the inverter draws power from the batteries. In remote or rural areas, homeowners have a gasoline or propane generator to fill the batteries in the event there is no sun or wind to generate new power. Batteries are heavy, expensive, wear out, and are filled with acid and lead.

WIND POWER

Wind energy is really a form of solar energy because wind is created when the atmosphere is unevenly heated by the sun. Winds are also influenced by terrain, water, weather patterns, vegetation, and other factors. Early wind machines known as **windmills** dating back to medieval ages were used to pump water and grind grain (Berry, 2004). State-of-the-art windmills today resemble airplane propellers because they are aerodynamic and made from fiberglass (Figure 11-11). Wind turbines take up space. They must be at least 30 feet higher than any building, hill, or tree within 500 feet (Sullivan, 2005). They have moving parts that require maintenance and wear out or break.

Unlike solar power, wind systems can produce energy at night as well as during the day. It is considered an efficient source of power and less costly to install and generate power than coal or nuclear facilities. Areas most suited for wind machines are areas free of obstructions to the wind with open plains, tablelands, hilltops, ridge crests, and mountain summit terrain. Land with class 4 power is found in the Great Plains, Great Lakes, and coastal areas of Texas and the Northeast (Elliott et al., 1986). More than half of the land in Wyoming and Montana has a class 4 or greater annual average for wind power. The only problem with wind energy is that the wind does not always blow. Some residents do not like wind machines because they create a "whirring" noise and birds or bats can fly into the blades. Wind will probably become a more popular energy source because wind is free, and it does not emit pollutants.

New Fuel Sources

BIOENERGY

Bioenergy refers to energy generated using biomass materials such as wood, agricultural plant and animal waste, seaweed, algae, solid waste, and garbage. Raw materials

---

 LIGHTNING

Can we use the energy in lightning as an alternate power source? Probably not, for three reasons. First, no one knows exactly where lightning will strike because it is unpredictable. Second, conventional storage devices, such as batteries, do not accommodate the magnitude of a powerful flash that only lasts a fraction of a second. Finally, about half of the energy from a lightning strike dissipates into light, noise, and electromagnetic waves.

FIGURE **11-11** **Wind Machines** Wind machines in the plains areas provide an alternative power source.

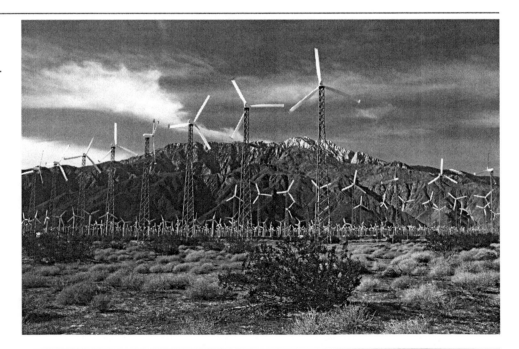

are converted into liquid or gaseous biofuels or burned in their present state to provide heat, electricity, or power. By-products of biomass conversation can be used for fertilizers and chemicals. There are two types of biomass **conversion**: thermochemical and biochemical. Thermochemical conversion burns chopped up wood and agricultural waste to produce chemical reactions in order to produce steam, electricity, or heat. Gasification or carbonization uses heat to break biomass down into a different types of fuel, such as converting wood to charcoal. Biochemical conversion uses enzymes, fungi, or microorganisms to convert biomass (manure, paper, algae) into either liquid or gaseous fuels. An example would be the containment of methane gas from sewage treatment facilities. Another biochemical conversion process uses fermentation to decompose sugar cane, grains, potatoes, and other starchy crops to make ethyl alcohol (**ethanol**) and carbon dioxide.

LANDFILL GAS RECOVERY

As garbage decomposes, methane is produced and because it is flammable, it can be used for fuel in the same way as natural gas. The process of methane production is slow, however, and methane can leak into the environment. See Chapter 14 for more details.

Fuels for Automobiles

lthough the generation of electrical power for heat, industrial uses, and home uses is important to fuel consumption in the United States, the provision of fuel for transportation and other machine uses is also important. The primary fuel source for machines is oil, providing 97% of transportation fuels (Gonzales, 2002). Crude oil is converted to gasoline when it is distilled. In the early 1800s, gasoline was a by-product of kerosene distillation that was thrown away because there were few gas-burning engines. When gas-burning engines for automobiles and farm equipment became common after World War I and World War II, the demand for gasoline increased. The consumption of gasoline presents many concerns in this country (Figure 11-12). The primary concerns include poor fuel efficiency of the gasoline engines in most transportation vehicles and pollution due to incomplete combustion and vehicle emissions. It has been estimated that the gasoline engine utilizes only 35–55% of the fuel passing through its cylinders (Fusaro, 1997). Current strategies include improving gasoline composition to boost fuel efficiency, developing alternative fuels, and developing hybrid or **alternative fuel vehicles (AFVs)** to replace current automotive engines.

The formulation of gasoline is important to fuel efficiency and environmental impact. Gasoline engine efficiency has been a concern for a long time. Gasoline engines compress fuel before it is ignited, causing engine "knocking," which damages the engine. Raising the **octane** levels of gasoline improves the problem and increases gasoline efficiency. The octane level tells how much the fuel can be compressed before it ignites. In general, the higher the octane level in fuel, the slower the fuel is burned during the compression cycle, meaning better fuel economy and cleaner emissions (Bellis, 2005). In addition to the type of fuel used, engine design is important. In the 1980s engines were designed to use fuel injectors to control the air/fuel mix, important to fuel efficiency.

Chemical emissions are also very important to environmental health. During World War II, it was discovered that adding tetraethyl lead to gasoline (known at the time as *ethyl* or *leaded* gasoline) significantly improved the octane rating of gasoline. Unfortunately lead emissions were found to be toxic to many living things, including

---

Direct current (DC)
An electric current that flows in only one direction through a circuit as from a battery.

Battery
Stores and discharges energy with the capacity of six volts or more through the use of lead, sulfuric acid, or cadmium.

Alternating current (AC)
An electric current with its direction reversed at regular intervals. Electric current in the United States alternates with a frequency of 60 hertz or cycles per second. Some European countries use 50 hertz.

Windmill
A machine for doing work using wind as an energy source. Newer windmills are referred to as wind machines.

Bioenergy
Energy generated using biomass materials such as wood, plant waste, animal waste, solid waste, and garbage.

Conversion
The use of one energy source to produce another.

Ethanol
A colorless, volatile, flammable liquid in liquors and solvents; also known as ethyl alcohol or grain alcohol.

Alternative fuel vehicle (AFV)
A vehicle that uses nonpetroleum-based fuel such as ethanol, compressed natural gas, hydrogen cells, compressed air, or water.

Octane
A term used to indicate the resistance of a fuel to burn or detonation. The higher the octane rating, the slower the fuel is burned.

FIGURE 11-12 **Gasoline
Pumps** Gasoline is provided
in different formulas.

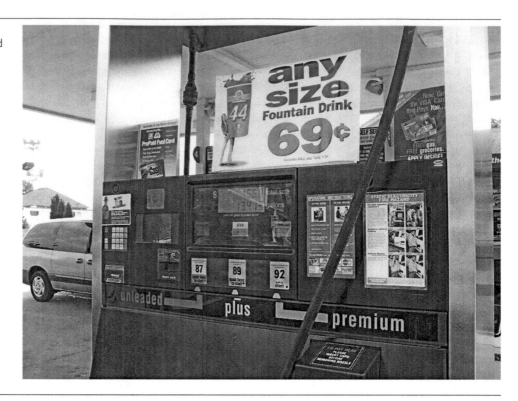

humans. Lead in gasoline has been phased out of production since the 1970s for automobile use and gasoline has become more expensive to produce. Another gasoline additive found to boost octane levels was methyl tertiary butyl ether (MTBE), used since 1979. It is suspected to be carcinogenic but is still used, particularly in areas where there are high levels of unhealthy air pollution (EPA, 2003). Ethanol is now a popular fuel additive, but it is somewhat more expensive than MTBE, increasing the cost of gasoline (Lave et al., 2001).

Reformulated gasoline (RFG) is gasoline blended with oxygen compounds added to burn cleaner and reduce smog-forming and toxic pollutants in the air. Some communities with the worst smog pollution are required by The Clean Air Act Amendments of 1990 to use RFG in order to reduce harmful emissions of ozone.

The Importance of Fuel Efficient Machines

Fuel efficiency in automobiles is a major concern to most consumers so that more mileage can be produced from less fuel. Fuel resources were a concern during war times and the Great Depression, but the shortage did not receive national attention until the Oil Embargo of 1973. When Arab leaders limited the supply of oil and increased prices, consumers were upset. As a result, several efforts have been in place to reduce the demand for domestic and foreign oil.

The U.S. Congress passed the 1975 Automobile Fuel Efficiency Act (PL 96-426). This act set fuel economy standards requiring automakers to increase the average mileage per gallon (mpg) of new cars. As a result, lighter vehicles were produced. This does not solve the problem, however, because many people prefer larger vehicles such as trucks, minivans, and sport utility vehicles (SUVs). Many car manufacturers believe that features of a vehicle, such as **horsepower** and acceleration, are more important to consumers than fuel efficiency.

President George W. Bush established the National Energy Policy Development Group in an effort to increase funding for energy efficiency programs, encourage the development of fuel-efficient vehicles, create tax credits to encourage consumer conservation, and expand the Department of Energy conservation programs (National Energy Policy Development Group, 2001). As part of the Energy Policy and Conservation Act of 1975 (PL 94-163) corporate average fuel economy (CAFE) standards were established to reduce greenhouse gas emissions (Agras, 1999). Automobile efficiency standards increased the minimum of 18 miles per gallon (mpg) for passenger cars in 1978 to 27.5 mph by 1985. Standards for light trucks and sport utility vehicles (SUVs) began at 17.2 mpg in 1979 to 20.7 mpg in 2002 (Bamberger, 2002). By 2007, the standard will be increased to 22.2 mpg or automakers out of compliance will be issued a fine (Dinan & Austin, 2004).

Strategies to Reduce the Demand for Gasoline by Consumers

In addition to setting standards for vehicles with better fuel efficiency, additional strategies were aimed at consumer use such as reducing the speed limit, taxing gasoline, advocating the use of carpools, using alternative fuels, and developing alternative fuel vehicles (AFVs). In 1974 the national maximum speed limit (NMSL) of 55 mph was initiated to reduce the consumption of fuel and reduce the frequency and severity of crashes. Although the number of fatal crashes decreased dramatically, the speed limit was allowed to increase on rural interstates in 1987. In 1995 Congress suspended the NMSL, giving states the responsibility for setting their own speed limits. Many states are at their pre-1974 settings.

Gasoline taxes were another form of encouraging drivers to be more prudent. Federal gasoline taxes date back to 1932 and are used to support highways and mass transit systems. The Congressional Budget Office (CBO) estimated the gasoline tax would reduce gasoline consumption by 10%, more than an increase in CAFE standards (Dinan & Austin, 2004). The average gasoline tax today is 41 cents per gallon, with 18.4 cents per gallon going to the federal government. The rest goes to local and state agencies. Authorities suggest the gasoline tax is a very effective way of decreasing demand by consumers who now drive vehicles with better fuel efficiency. It has been suggested that gasoline taxes continue to rise while building vehicles with even better fuel efficiency (31.3 mph for cars and 24.5 for light trucks and SUVs). The increased cost is estimated to be $900 per vehicle with $230 of the cost charged to consumers (Dinan & Austin, 2004). They rationalize that consumers would be willing to pay for more expensive vehicles if it required less gasoline to drive it.

Some communities advocate the use of carpools. A **carpool** is a group of individuals with the same or similar destination who take turns using their vehicles to drive the others to work. Carpools reduce money spent on gas, toll fees, and parking spaces in urban areas. Alternatives to carpooling include the use of public transportation (subway, train, or bus), bicycling, or walking to work (Haberkorn, 2004).

Alternatives to gasoline such as gasohol, propane, natural gas, batteries, **hydrogen cells**, water, compressed air, and renewable energy sources are being used, but to a much lesser degree due to cost, practicality, and lack of consumer confidence.

ALTERNATIVE FUEL VEHICLES

The search for a vehicle that provides cheaper transportation has been in the development stages since the first automobile was built. Electric and hybrid cars are still in the development stages.

Electric Cars

The first attempt to provide an automobile using an alternative fuel source was the electric automobile. The development of the electric car began in the 1830s when Robert Anderson of Scotland invented a simple horseless carriage. Electric cars became popular in France and Great Britain. Americans became interested in electric cars in the 1890s when an electric tricycle was built by A.L. Ryker. In the 1900s electrified carriages and surreys could move at 14 mph and could go 18 miles. By 1900, electric cars outsold all other types of cars as they had less vibration, smell, and noise. They did not need manual starting with a hand crank or to change gears. President Dwight Eisenhower enjoyed driving an electric car made in 1914 by Rauch and Lang. The car was not very practical, however, because it could not exceed the speed of 20 miles per hour (Postcard from Eisenhower Museum, no date). In 1916 a hybrid car with an internal combustion engine and an electric motor was developed (History of the Electric Car 1890–1930, 2005).

Electric cars improved on speed and appearances in the 1970s, but they were never popular because they needed to be recharged every 70 to 100 miles and did not have air conditioning. Compared to gasoline-powered cars, electric cars are less noisy, cost less to refuel, and have fewer parts that break or wear. Today electric cars look and perform similar to other vehicles on highways but are limited to 50 to 150 miles between recharges (Anonymous, 2005).

Hybrid Cars

The Partnership for a New Generation of Vehicles (PNGV) initiative was established by the Clinton administration to encourage the development of automobiles that travel three times farther on a gallon of gas and spew fewer pollutants (Malakoff, 1999). The result was the development of hybrid vehicles that use more than one energy source to operate. Available since 1999, hybrid cars combine a gasoline engine with a battery-powered elec-

---

Horsepower
The power needed to lift 500 pounds 1 foot high in 1 second (746 watts).

Carpool
A group of people who travel together in one car to save money and gasoline.

Hydrogen cell
A battery-like container filled with hydrogen; used as an alternative fuel source.

tric motor. The first hybrid to be unveiled was the Toyota Prius, introduced in 1997 that got 67 mpg with 90% less pollutants than non-hybrid vehicles (Normile, 1999). The Honda Insight was introduced a short time later. The Honda Insight uses gasoline and electricity generated from a battery that is recharged by the forward motion of the three-cylinder car. Gas mileage is 60 to 66 mpg compared to 32 to 37 mpg for a gasoline version of the same model. Toyota and Honda vehicles burn gasoline for highway cruising with an electric motor that gives it an extra nudge up hills or when accelerating. Electric power from a battery also fuels the car while idling. The compression ignition direct injection (CIDI) still emits pollutants such as nitrogen oxide and soot beyond acceptable standards. The battery packs are heavy, contain lead, have up to 500 volts, and cost $1,000 to $2,000.

Advantages to having a hybrid car include:

- Better gas mileage and less pollution per mile than conventional gasoline engines.

- Consumers who buy hybrid cars get a federal tax deduction through the year 2006. The savings depends upon the tax bracket you are in. Some states offer an additional tax deduction.

- More automobile makers are producing hybrid cars. Ford has recently developed an SUV hybrid version of the Escape. GMC and Chevy offer hybrid pickup trucks, C15 Silverado and C15 Sierra. Lexus and Saturn have announced plans to develop hybrid SUVs.

Disadvantages to having a hybrid car include:

- Hybrid cars currently cost $3,500 to $6,000 more per car. It could take the average driver (15,000 miles per year) between 10 to 14 years to break even, unless gas prices increase.

- The circuitry required in battery-supported hybrid cars poses some electrical hazards to rescue personnel in the event of a crash (Associated Press, 2004).

ALTERNATIVE FUELS

Alternative fuels are being developed today to reduce emissions causing air pollution. Alternative fuels include **clean fuels**, such as alcohol fuels, natural gas, and hydrogen. Although they may have some advantages, they are not without problems.

Alcohol Fuels

There are three types of alcohol fuels: ethanol, gasohol, and **methanol**. *Ethanol* is made from fermented corn (biomass). The production of ethanol is popular among farmers because it creates another market for their agricultural products. **Gasohol** has been promoted as another alternative fuel source. Gasohol is a blend of 10%

ethanol and 90% unleaded gasoline. In an effort to reduce the nation's dependence on imported oil, President Jimmy Carter issued an Executive Order (#12261, 1981) so that federal agencies purchased gasohol when the price was equal to or lower than gasoline (Federal Register, 1981). In spite of governmental encouragement to use gasohol, its use is limited because of cost and unavailability. Agricultural states are still promoting its development and use.

Methanol reduces ozone formation, but increases formaldehyde emissions, is more harmful to the skin than gasoline, and more of it is needed than gasoline to propel an engine.

Natural Gas

Natural gas is considered an alternative fuel because it is cleaner than coal or oil to burn. It is clean, but not completely pollution free because natural gas reduces hydrocarbons and carbon monoxide by-products, but increases nitrous dioxide.

Natural gas primarily consists of methane but can include thane, propane, butane, and pentane. As mentioned earlier, natural gas was used in this country in the seventeenth century for streetlights. Then in 1885, Robert Bunsen found a way to mix natural gas with air to create a flame used for heating and cooking, giving birth to the Bunsen burner. After that, researchers discovered natural gas had many capabilities as a gas, a compressed gas, as a liquid, and as a fuel cell.

Hydrogen

Hydrogen has been promoted as the "fuel of the future" because it is abundant, clean, and inexpensive. Hydrogen is abundant in the atmosphere and hydrogen fuel can be obtained from ordinary water, methanol, natural gas, and biomass (Thomas et al., 1998). The problem is that it is easier to make hydrogen from natural gas and other fossil fuels than from water or biomass. Because it is a gas, it is also very light. It is carbon-free so that when it is used, there is no pollution. In addition, a hydrogen **fuel cell** uses 45 to 58% of the fuel used to make the vehicle move, making it twice as efficient as gasoline as a fuel source. Some consider it to be the ideal fuel.

Hydrogen can be stored in *fuel cells* of almost any size, making them more adaptable than combustible engines. Hydrogen fuel cells work by mixing hydrogen and air in a mixing chamber to produce water and electricity. The chemical reaction produces low heat and there is no combustion, making it a clean process. Electricity is only generated when the fuel is flowing. Hydrogen fuel cells have been used by NASA since the early Apollo missions and are still used today to create electricity on space shuttles and international space stations. Hydrogen fuel cells are used to power homes, buildings, and automobiles. The main disadvantages of hydrogen fuel cells to power automobiles include the high cost and lack of refueling stations.

Other alternative fuels are being considered using compressed air, wind, sunlight, and water.

Summary

nergy resources have switched over the past 200 years from wood, to coal, and then to oil. Although efforts are in place to reduce air pollution from the burning of fossil fuels, decrease the likelihood of oil spills and nuclear accidents, and prevent underground pipeline leaks, the amount of fossil fuels are diminishing. The need to find alternative fuels is increasing as fossil fuel sources become scarcer and prices rise higher. There are those who predict that the "age of petroleum" may be over and plastic materials may become more expensive than recycled materials. There are others who insist there is an abundant supply but for now it is inaccessible.

Energy use is expected to increase in the next two decades, at a rate much faster than it can be replaced (Maugeri, 2004). The development and production of renewable energy requires significant financial, governmental, and public support. Some states allow a tax write-off for those who use alternative fuels in accordance with the Energy Policy Act of 1992 (PL 102-486). Research and development regarding renewable energy should also be endorsed and supported by energy companies. Until there is another energy shortage, predictions are that consumer and provider use of alternative fuel or renewable energy will be slow in advancing.

REFERENCES

Agency for Toxic Substances and Disease Registry. (1996). ToxFacts for fuel oils. CAS# 8008-20-6, 70892-10-3, 68476-30-2, 68476-34-6, 68476-31-3. Retrieved from http://www.atsdr.cdc.gov/tfacts75.html.

Agras, J. (1999). The Kyoto Protocol, CAFE standards, and gasoline taxes. _Contemporary Economic Policy, 17,_ 296.

American Coal Foundation. (2005). Coal: Ancient gift serving modern man. Retrieved from Kentucky Educational Television website at http://www.ket.org/Trips/Coal/AGSMM/agsmmwhere.html.

Anonymous. (1998). Oil harvest: Pennsylvania oil pits. _Discover,_ July. Retrieved from http://www.findarticles.com/p/articles/mi_m1511/is_n7_v19/ai_20870319.

Anonymous. (2005). Surface mining, _Coal Leader._ Retrieved from http://www.coalleader.com/surface_mining.htm.

Anonymous. (2005). The history of electric vehicles: The early years—Electric cars (1890–1930). Retrieved from http://inventors.about.com/library/weekly/aacarselectrica.htm.

Anonymous. (2005). The history of electric vehicles: Recent years—1990 to 1998. Retrieved from http://inventors.about.com/library/weekly/aacarselectrica.htm.

Armentano, D. T. (1981). The petroleum industry: A historical study in power. _The Cato Journal, 1,_ 53–85. Retrieved from http://www.catojournal.com/pubs/journal/cj1n1/cj1n1-4.pdf.

Asbury, B., Cigla, M., & Balci, C. (2002). Design methodology, testing and evaluation of a continuous miner cutterhead for dust reduction in underground coal mining. Preprint 02-136. Paper presented for the Society of Mechanical Engineers, February 26-27, 2002. Phoenix, AR. Retrieved from http://www.mines.edu/research/wmrc/Webpage/RP-3_dust_files/Publications/RP3%20TP1%202002.pdf.

Clean fuels
Low pollution fuels like ethanol or compressed natural gas that replace traditional fuels.

Methanol
A colorless, flammable liquid, used as an antifreeze, solvent, or fuel; a type of alcohol; the liquid form of methane.

Gasohol
A mixture of 90% gasoline and 10% ethanol, used to replace pure gasoline.

Fuel cell
A device combining fuel and oxygen to produce chemical energy converted to electrical energy.

Associated Press. (2004). Rescue workers preparing for more accidents involving hybrid cars. May 4, 2004 report. *ABC Action News,* Tampa, St. Petersburg. Retrieved from http://www.wfts.com/stories/2004/05/040504hybrids.shtml.

Bamberger, R. (2002). Automobile and light truck fuel economy. Is CAFÉ up to standards? Issue Brief for Congress, Received through the Congressional Research Service (CRS), Library of Congress. Web. Order Code IB90122. Retrieved from http://www.cnie.org/nle/crsreports/air/air-10.pdf.

Bellis, M. (2005). History of gasoline. Retrieved from http://inventors.about.com/library/inventors/blgasoline.htm.

Berry, M. (2004). History of windmills. Retrieved from http://www.windmillworld.com/windmills/history.htm.

Bush, G. W. (2002). State of the union address given January 29, 2002. Retrieved from http://www.newsaic.com/ressou2002.html.

D'Amato, P. (2001). U.S. intervention in the Middle East: Blood for oil. International Socialist Review, 15. Retrieved from http://isreview.org/issues/15/blood_for_oil.shtml.

Department of Energy. (2005). Historical records of the atomic energy commission. Website of the Office of Scientific and Technical Information, OpenNet. Retrieved from http://www.osti.gov/opennet/nsi_desc.html.

Dinan, T., & Austin, D. (2004). Fuel economy standards vs. a gasoline tax. Almanac of Policy Issues, March 9, 2004. U.S. Congressional Budget Office. Retrieved from http://www.policyalmanac.org/environment/archive/fuel_economy.shtml.

Eisenhower Museum. (No date). Postcard. Salina: KS.

Elliott, D., Holladay, C., Barchet, W., Foote, H., & Sandusky, W. (1986). Wind energy resource atlas. Prepared by Pacific Northwest Laboratory, Richland, WA for the Department of Energy. Retrieved from http://rredc.nrel.gov/wind/pubs/atlas/appendix_E.html.

Energy Information Administration. (2005). Short-term energy outlook: Crude oil and petroleum products. Retrieved from http://www.eia.doe.gov/emeu/steo/pub/contents.html.

Energy Information Administration. (2005). Country analysis brief: United States of America. Retrieved from http://www.eia.doe.gov/emeu/cabs/usa.html.

Energy Information Administration. (2004). International Energy Outlook 2004: Natural gas. Retrieved from http://www.eia.doe.gov/oiaf/ieo/nat_gas.html.

Energy Information Administration. (2004). U. S. renewable energy consumption. http://www.eia.doe.gov/cneaf/solar.renewables/page/rea_data/chapter1.html.

Environmental Protection Agency. (2003). Gasoline. Retrieved from http://www.epa.gov/mtbe/gas.htm.

Executive Order 12261. (1981). Gasohol in Federal motor vehicles. *Federal Register, January 8,* 46 FR 2023. Retrieved from http://www.archives.gov/federal_register/codification/executive_order/12261.html.

Flavin, C. (2002). 21st century energy security: The challenge and the opportunity. Speech presented by the President of the Worldwatch Institute, April 30, 2002. Retrieved from http://www.sustainable.ch/pdf/info/flavin_script.pdf.

Florida Energy Extension Service & Cook, G. (1990). The Middle East oil crisis. *Energy Efficiency and Environmental News.* Newsletter of the Florida Energy Extension Service,

Florida Cooperative Extension Service, Institute of Food and Agricultural Sciences, University of Florida.

Fusaro, B. (1997). Chapter 7: Energy principles. In *Environmental Math.* Retrieved from http://web.math.fsu.edu/~fusaro/DL/chapter7.html.

Gerard, A. (1997). A chronology and overview of the U. S. coal market. Retrieved from http://www.eia.doe.gov/cneaf/coal/chron/chronc.html.

Gonzales, M. (2002). Black gold: The economics of oil in North Dakota. *North Dakota Geological Survey Newsletter, 29,* 1-5. Retrieved from http://www.state.nd.us/ndgs/Newsletter/nl02s/PDF/blkgold.pdf.

Haberkorn, J. (2004). D. C. drivers find new ways to work. *Washington Times, June 17,* 2004. Retrieved from http://www.washtimes.com/business/20040616-092638-9964r.htm.

Institute for the Analysis of Global Security. (2004). Highlights from the Department of Energy's international energy outlook 2004-2025. Energy Security, May 24. Retrieved from http://www.iags.org/n0524044.htm.

International Dolphin Watch. (2005). The dophin die-off. Retrieved from http://www.idw.org/html/dolphins_in_danger.html.

Lamark, B., Lindberg, A., Wegelin, R., & Engstedt, L. (1998). Hydro-electric power, technical and insurance development. Presentation IMIA 16-71 (98)E at the IMIA meeting in Interlaken, Switzerland. Retrieved from http://www.imia.com/documents/hydro.htm#2.

Lave, L., Griffin, W., & Maclean, H. (2001). The ethanol answer to carbon emissions. *Issues in Science and Technology Online, Winter* issue. Retrieved from http://www.issues.org/18.2/lave.html.

Lewis, J. (1985). Lead poisoning: A historical perspective. EPA Journal, May. Retrieved from http://www.epa.gov/history/topics/perspect/lead.htm.

Malakoff, D. (1999). U. S. supercars: Around the corner or running on empty? *Science, 285,* 680.

Maugeri, L. (2004). Science and Industry: Oil: Never cry wolf—Why the Petroleum Age is far from over. *Science, 304,* 1114–1115. Retrieved from http://www.sciencemag.org/cgi/content/summary/304/5674/1114.

Murphy, K. (2000). A deep and wide mining scar in Idaho. Reprinted from the Los Angeles Times. Retrieved from an edition of *Transitions, 14.* http://www.landscouncil.org/transitions/tr0003/.

National Energy Policy Development Group. (2001). Reliable, affordable, and environmentally sound energy for America's future. Washington, DC: Superintendent of Documents, U.S. Government Printing Service. Retrieved from http://www.whitehouse.gov/energy/National-Energy-Policy.pdf.

National Gas Supply Association. (2005). Overview of natural gas. Retrieved from http://www.naturalgas.org/overview/background.asp.

National Hydropower Association. (2005). Hydro facts. Retrieved from http://www.hydro.org/.

National Mining Association. (1995). U.S. is world's second largest coal producer. PolicyFAX Factsheet #2322107. Washington DC: National Mining Association. Retrieved from http://www.heartland.org/pdf/23221g.pdf.

National Ocean Service. (2004). What's the story on oil spills. Retrieved from http://response.restoration.noaa.gov/kids/spills.html.

Normile, D. (1999). Toyota's hybrid hits the streets first. *Science, 285,* 681.

Nuclear Energy Institute. (2005). Nuclear energy and the enivronment: Key facts. Retrieved from http://www.nei.org.

Nuclear Regulatory Commission. (2000). Mission and organization. Retrieved 3/27/2000 from http://www.nrc.gov/NRC/WHATIS/mission.html.

Postcard. (no date). Dwight Eisenhower Museum, Abilene, KS.

San Joaquin Geological Society. (2002). The history of the oil industry. Retrieved from http://www.sjgs.com/history.html.

Slusher, J. (1995). Wood fuel for heating. University of Missouri Extension Service. Retrieved from http://muextension.missouri.edu/xplor/agguides/forestry/g05450.htm.

Srinivasan, R. (2002). Characteristics of traffic flow and safety in 55 and 65 mph speed limits: Literature review and suggestions for future research. FHWA-NJ 2002-18. Retrieved from http://tid1s0.engr.ccny.cuny.edu/research/assets/1/trafficflow1.html.

Sullivan, D. (2005). Farming the wind: The nuts and bolts of blade design, site selection and tower technology. On-farm wind power: part 2 of a 3 part series. Retrieved from http://www.newfarm.org/features/0504/wind2.shtml.

Thomas, C., Kuhn, I., James, B., Lomax Jr., F., & Baum, G. (1998). Affordable hydrogen supply: Pathways for fuel cell vehicles. *International Journal of Hydrogen Energy, 23,* 507–516. Retrieved from http://www.directedtechnologies.com.

Tripathi, R. (2002). Fuel oils. Prepared for the Virginia Department of Health, Richmond, VA. Retrieved from http://www.vdh.virginia.gov/hhcontrol/fueloill.pdf.

Udall, R., & Andrews, S. (2001). Methane madness: A natural gas primer. Produced by the Community Office for Resource Efficiency (CORE): Aspen, CO. Retrieved from http://dieoff.com/page230.pdf.

United States Department of Energy. (2004). Solar heating basics. Retrieved from the Energy Technology Program website at www.eren.doe.gov/RE/solar.html.

U.S. Department of Agriculture. (2004). Emergency preparedness: Keeping food safe during an emergency. Retrieved from http://www.fsis.usda.gov/Fact_Sheets/keeping_food_Safe_during_an_emergency/index.asp.

Weiss, D. (2003). Ecology Hall of Fame. Environmental Movement Timeline: A history of the American environmental movement. Retrieved from http://www.ectopia.org/ehof/timelintext.html.

Williams, J. (2002). Oil price history and analysis. *Energy Economics Newsletter.* Retrieved from http://www.wtrg.com/prices.htm.

SELECTED ENVIRONMENTAL LAWS

1954 ***Atomic Energy Act of 1954***
Regulates civilian and military uses of nuclear materials. Anyone using nuclear fuel is required to have the facility licensed and it is to be governed by established rules and regulations. An amendment was added later to establish compensation for and limits on liability for injury to persons or property caused by nuclear accidents.

1969 ***National Environmental Policy Act (NEPA)***
Mandates preliminary evaluation of projects and processes for potential environmental impact.

1973 ***Open Mining Land Reclamation Act***
Established requirements that mining operations for coal, sand, gravel, gold, silver, and so forth must have a permit and land reclamation timelines. By 1975, all western states except Arizona had adopted some form of mining and reclamation standards and regulations.

1974 ***Energy Reorganization Act***
Created the Nuclear Regulatory Commission (NRC) and moved the Atomic Energy Commissions' (AEC) regulatory function to the NRC.

1974 ***Energy Supply and Coordination Act (PL 93-319)***
Directed NIEHS to study the effects of chronic exposure to sulfur oxides.

1975 ***Energy Policy and Conservation Act of 1975 (PL 94-163)***
Established corporate average fuel economy (CAFE) standards for new passenger cars after 1978. The current standard is 27.5 mpg for passenger automobiles and 20.7 mpg for light trucks and sports utility vehicles (SUVs).

1977 ***Surface Mining Control and Reclamation Act (PL 95-164)***
Appointed an advisory committee on coal and other mine health research.

1990 ***Oil Pollution Act***
Provides for prevention and planning for incidents, such as the *Exxon Valdez* oil spill.

1992 ***Energy Policy Act (PL 102-486)***
Provides for the restructure of energy markets in the United States, calling for energy efficiency programs, the use of alternative fuels and renewable energy, research and development, tax credits, and exemptions.

SELECTED PROFESSIONAL JOURNALS

Energy Research News
E Source
The Energy Journal

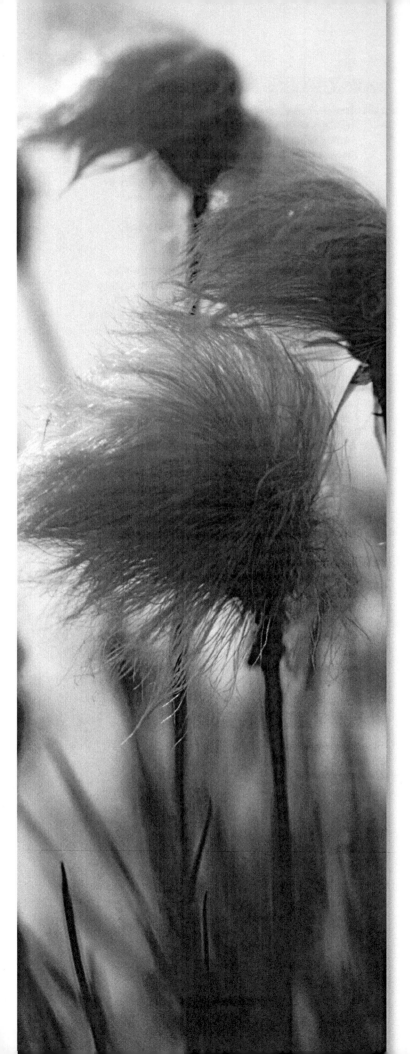

Radiation

There is no safe level of exposure and there is no dose of (ionizing) radiation so low that the risk of a malignancy is zero.

Dr. Karl Morgan, father of health physics

OBJECTIVES

1. Define the terms radiation, ultraviolet light, infrared, rems, radioisotopes, photons, ion, anode, cathode, volts, microwave, and electromagnetic.

2. Describe natural sources of radioactivity.

3. List devices used to measure radioactivity and exposure.

4. Differentiate ionizing radiation and nonionizing radiation exposure according to health effects.

5. Explain the terms deterministic effects, threshold effects, nonthreshold effects, and cumulative effects.

6. Describe different types of light and any potentially harmful effects of exposure.

7. Explain health-harming effects of acoustic noise.

8. Debate the use of ultrasonic devices for medical diagnostic procedures.

9. Discuss your conclusions about potential damage from increased exposure to electromagnetic waves.

10. List sources of daily radioactivity exposure and ways to decrease health risks associated with it.

Introduction

ll plants, animals, and humans are constantly exposed to radiation from natural or artificial sources (Figure 12-1). Scientists estimate the average U.S. citizen receives a dose of about 360 **millirems** of radiation per year (EPA, 2004). There are multiple ways in which an individual can be exposed to radiation.

Eighty percent of our exposure comes from natural sources. Natural sources include ultraviolet light from the sun, radon gas from the soil, or uranium in rocks and soil. Of these, approximately 55% of exposure is from radon gas. Artificial sources include manmade sources such as communications devices (televisions, radios, computers, cellular phones), microwaves, **X-rays**, and medical devices (EPA, 2000). About 18% to 20% of radiation exposure comes from manmade sources. Manmade sources have increased after William Roentgen discovered X-rays and their capabilities in 1895. Irene and Frederick Joliot-Curie discovered radioactive elements could be produced from stable elements in 1896 and since then, radiation has become a part of our daily lives (EPA, 2002).

Understanding Radiation

ll matter is composed of atoms (Figure 12-2). Atoms consist of a nucleus that contains protons, neutrons, and electrons. Unstable atoms with too many or too few neutrons, also known as **radioisotopes**, emit particles or energy waves, known as **electromagnetic waves**, in order to become more stable. The type of radiation emitted depends on the type of instability. There is **nonionizing radiation** and **ionizing radiation**. Nonionizing radia-

---

Millirems
One thousandth of a rem.

X-rays
Extremely high frequencies and short wavelengths capable of forming ions by breaking molecules or removing electrons.

Radioisotopes
Isotopes that are radioactive.

Electromagnetic waves (EMWs)
Waves sent through space or matter by oscillating electric and magnetic fields.

Nonionizing radiation
Electromagnetic and light waves that do not emit photons.

Ionizing radiation
Radiation that becomes electrically charged either under the influence of radiation or electronic discharge; the ions interact with matter to produce charged particles.

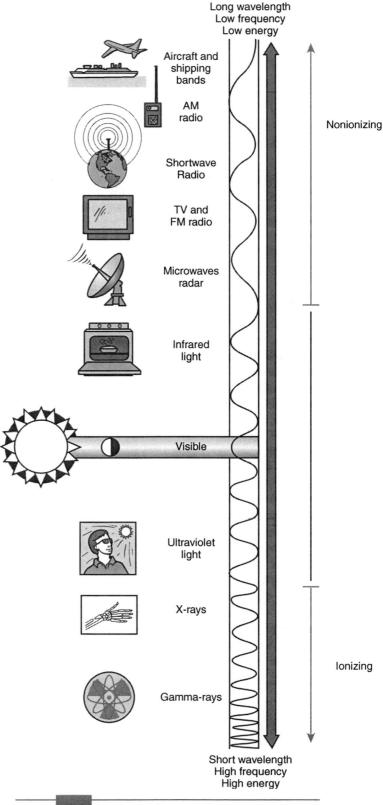

FIGURE 12-1 **Spectrum of Frequencies**
Source: National Aeronautics and Space Administration. (2005). Retrieved from http://imagine.gsfc.nasa.gov/docs/science/know_11/emspectrum.html.

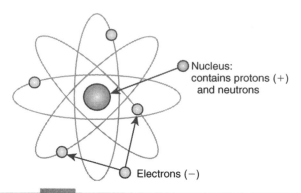

Nucleus: contains protons (+) and neutrons

Electrons (−)

FIGURE **12-2** **Structure of an Atom** The structure of an atom is important because it determines the presence of radioactivity.
Source: Environmental Protection Agency. (2004). Retrieved from http://www.epa.gov/radiation/students/what.html.

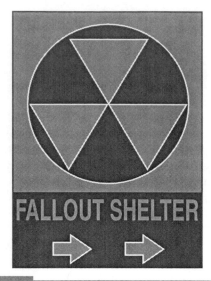

FALLOUT SHELTER

FIGURE **12-3** **Radiation Sign**
Source: Environmental Protection Agency. (2005). Retrieved from http://www.epa.gov/radiation/students/symbols.html.

tion does not have charged photons and includes ultraviolet (UV) light, visible light, infrared light, microwave, and radio frequencies. Ionizing radiation is electronically charged with photons and interacts with matter in such a way that particles are changed. Ionizing radiation is used for the production of nuclear power, diagnostics such as X-rays, and medical treatment (such as radiation therapy for cancer). Ionizing radiation requires special handling because the effects of exposure are cumulative with time.

Signs for fallout shelters (Figure 12-3) were popular in the 1960s when the Cuban Missile Crisis posed an international threat of nuclear war. Schools hosted drills much like the fire drills and tornado drills we have today.

Electromagnetic waves are emitted through space at the speed of light in the form of **photons**. Each photon has a particular **frequency** and wavelength expressed in electron volts (eV). Waves emitted by electromagnetic photons vary in length as exhibited by the electromagnetic spectrum. Electromagnetic waves with longer frequency, lower-energy range do not possess sufficient energy to be ionizing. The longest waves are associated

NUCLEAR REACTOR ACCIDENTS
At least four major accidents have occurred since the use of nuclear power began:

- 1957 Windscale, England

- 1979 Three Mile Island power plant in Pennsylvania

- 1986 Chernobyl in the former Soviet Union

- 1986 Hanford nuclear facility in Richland, Washington, reported to have been releasing radioactive material into the environment for a period of years

with communication devices such as radio, television, computers, and telephones. Microwaves are shorter and associated with wireless transmissions for radar detection equipment, microwave ovens, wireless telephones, and wireless computers. Light rays include infrared light (which is invisible but produces heat), visible light (such as sunlight and incandescent or fluorescent light), and lasers. Shorter lights, such as X-rays and gamma rays, cannot be seen, but can penetrate human tissues and be used for nuclear energy. The short wave, high frequency, high energy electromagnetic waves have sufficient energy to ionize.

Measurement of Radioactivity and Radiation Exposure

The measurement of ionizing radiation is especially important because of the potential harm. Ionizing radiation emits charged particles known as photons. When photons are emitted, the radiation disintegrates, reducing the charge or radioactive mass (Curtis, 1999). The rate at which radioisotopes decay is known as a Becquerel (Bq) or a curie (Ci).

$$1 \text{ Becquerel (Bq)} = 1 \text{ dps}$$
$$1 \text{ Curie (Ci)} = 3.7 \times 10^{10} \text{ dps}$$

The rate of decay is especially important for nuclear sources.

Ionizing radiation can be measured using the following techniques:

■ *Gas detector.* A gas detector is comprised of an **anode, cathode,** voltage supply, and ammeter. Gas detectors measure the voltage initiated when a photon ionizes a gas molecule. A gas detector has an ionization chamber that collects voltage on the anode and replaces electrons from the cathode. Ionization chamber survey meters measure external radiation dose rates emitted.

■ *Scintillation counters.* The device converts energy particles to visible light. A "cocktail" comprised of a solvent and **scintillate** is placed into a vial. The vial is lowered into the light-tight chamber with two photomultiplier tubes (PMTs). The photons of the radioactive sample interact with electrons of the scintillator, creating flashes of light and their intensities.

■ *Proportional counters.* Rather than collecting the electrical current (voltage), each ionizing particle causes a cascade of secondary ionizing events that detected as an electrical pulse. Proportional counters are used to measure contamination in laboratory and environmental settings.

■ *Geiger-Mueller detector.* When the voltage produced by radioactivity is high enough, particles can become completely ionized in the tube, generating a large electrical pulse. The pulse is measured by a Geiger-Mueller or GM detector. GM detectors are commonly used as survey instrument detectors because the instrument is relatively inexpensive, lightweight, and rugged. GM survey meters are often used to determine whether or not an area has been contaminated with radioactive particles.

■ *Film badge.* Photographic film is used to determine the dosage of radiation to which an individual may be exposed. An ionizing particle disrupts silver bromide crystals in the film, allowing silver to be precipitated onto the film during processing. The greater the dose of radiation, the darker the image. This type of film is used to obtain an X-ray image when directed by radiology personnel. The same type of film is sandwiched between metal and plastic filters in a plastic holder to measure penetrating and nonpenetrating doses of radiation exposure.

■ *Dosimeter.* Crystals used to store ionizing radiation trap electrons and are measured as visible light. The process is called *thermoluminescent dosimetry (TLD).* **Dosimeters** are used to measure exposure to small, high-activity exposure to radiation for those who work with nuclear energy.

Proportional counters and ionizing (gas) chamber instruments are used to measure higher levels of radiation (Table 12-1). Scintillation detectors and proportional

TABLE 12-1 Devices Used to Measure Radioactivity

Type of Radiation Measured	Measurement Device
Alpha	Proportional or scintillation counters
Beta, Gamma	Geiger-Mueller or proportional counters
X-ray, Gamma	Ionization chambers
Neutrons	Proportional counters

counters are used to measure beta radiation in laboratory conditions. Proportional counters and Geiger counters are used in environmental settings. The Geiger-Mueller counter only approximates radiation exposure levels and is used as a means of locating radioactive contamination. Dosimeters and film badges are worn by nuclear and radiological workers to measure daily radioactive exposure. Exposure to radiation is important, particularly for those who work near it daily.

In a nuclear power plant or similar business, a health physicist would monitor radiological exposure to employees and maintain records, as well as establish emergency procedures in the event of radiation contamination. In a medical facility, radiation employees would wear a badge, similar to a dosimeter worn by nuclear power plant workers, that indicates exposure on a daily basis. In public health departments, environmental health divisions have a radiological health division. The purpose of this division of environmental health services is to assist in the detection of radioactive contamination; scrutinize the installation, maintenance, and operation of X-ray equipment; determine health hazards associated with exposure to radiation; and develop and implement programs to reduce exposure or help protect against radiation expo-

Photons
Electromagnetic waves of ionizing materials.

Frequency
A term used to describe the number of alternating cycles that occur in a given time; expressed in Hertz or Hz.

Anode
A positively charged terminal of a battery.

Cathode
A negatively charged terminal of a battery.

Scintillate
A substance causing fluorescence when struck by a charged particle or high-energy photon.

Dosimeter
A device for measuring the total absorbed dose from exposure to ionizing radiation.

sure. Radiological health professionals also need to protect themselves against and monitor their own exposure to ionizing radiation.

Sources of Ionizing Exposure

The primary source of ionizing exposure is determined by one's occupation. Nuclear power plants, nuclear testing, and nuclear accidents are sources of ionizing radiation. Nuclear medicine using X-rays, CT scans, magnetic resonance imaging (MRIs) for diagnostic purposes and cancer treatments are an occupational source of ionizing radiation. Radon is also another ionizing type of radiation. It is found in the ground.

ABOUT CT SCANS

Known as computed tomography (CT) imaging, CT devices use X-rays to produce three-dimensional images of the human body. CT scans are similar to X-ray scans but take longer because the body is "sliced" into parts in order to see things in more detail and more clearly than X-rays. CT was invented in 1972 by British engineer Godfrey Hounsfield. The first CT scanner was installed at the Mayo Clinic in 1973 and was first used on the head, then the entire body (Mayo Clinic, 2005). Unlike other medical imaging exams, such as conventional X-ray imaging, CT has the ability to image a combination of soft tissue, bone, and blood vessels. CT scans account for approximately 4% of medical imaging exams, however, research shows that CT scans contribute to 40% of the total amount of radiation received from diagnostic tests. The number of CT scans

MAGNETIC RESONANCE IMAGING (MRI)

In 1977, Dr. Raymond Damadian, Dr. Larry Minkoff, and Dr. Michael Goldsmith performed the first MRI exam after 7 years of development. The MRI machine uses a giant magnet to produce radio waves, causing protons to absorb energy. MRI scans require the body be injected with dye to determine the type of tissue it is examining and build a three-map of tissue types. The dye or contrast materials alter the magnetic field, responding differently to various signals that allow visualization of tissue abnormalities and disease processes. The MRI system can detect organs and the flow of blood. The fact that MRI systems do not use ionizing radiation is a comfort to many patients, as is the fact that MRI contrast materials have a very low incidence of side effects.
Source: University of Louisville (2005).

performed in recent years has also risen dramatically, further creating the need for minimizing radiation exposure during the test.

GEOGRAPHICAL SOURCES

There are many factors that contribute to radiation exposure including the geographical areas where people live. Natural background radiation levels are much higher in certain geographic areas. A person may receive 1 rem in about 9 days on the beach at Guarapari, Brazil, but only 4 rems for the entire year in Kerala, India. In the United States, the dose from natural radiation is higher in states such as Colorado, Wyoming, and South Dakota, because of increased cosmic radiation at higher elevations and naturally high concentrations of uranium and thorium in the soil.

RADON

Radon is a radioactive gas that forms during the decay of uranium-238, naturally found in rocks and soil. Radon has a half-life of only 3.825 days, eventually becoming lead atoms. Radon exposure is the second leading cause of lung cancer, particularly in smokers when it is inhaled and DNA is changed (EPA, 2005). It has been estimated that 500 to 600 miners who worked in uranium mines from 1950 to 1990 died of lung cancer, most associated with radon exposure (Brugge & Goble, 2002).

The radon gas seeps from underground rock into cracks in the basements and foundations of buildings. Testing for radon gas in homes is recommended for those homes with basements, crawl spaces, or cracked slab foundations. County extension agents, public health department workers, and home owners can test for radon by purchasing one of the following from a hardware store and sending it to a laboratory for analysis:

- Charcoal canister or charcoal liquid scintillation devices absorb radon or its products on to the charcoal. In the laboratory, the radioactive particles emitted from the charcoal are counted by a sodium iodide counter or converted to light in a liquid scintillation medium and counted in a scintillation detector.

- Alpha track detectors have a plastic film that gets etched by the alpha particles that strike it. In the laboratory, the plastic is chemically treated to make the tracks visible, and then the tracks are counted.

The guideline for safe exposure to radon in the home is 4 **picocuries** per liter. Radon gas leaking into a home can be inexpensively repaired by sealing cracks with caulk and foam materials.

Health Effects of Ionizing Radiation Exposure

Cell mutations associated with ionizing radiation were first discovered in 1927, creating public health concerns (Muller, 1927). Early experiments with radioactive substances resulted in harmful effects to those exposed to large and repeated doses. A large dose delivered at one time has a greater effect than the same dose administered over time in increments. The basic law of radiobiology states that biological effects from radiation exposure are directly proportional to individual cell mitosis (cell division) and the cell's specific function in an organism. The most sensitive cells are those that rapidly divide such as epidermal skin cells, bone marrow, red blood cells, and sperm cells. The DNA in these cells is damaged as molecular strands break. Although they are nondividing cells, lymphocytes and ova are also very radiosensitive. Rather than affect DNA, the damage is to lipoprotein structures in the nuclear cell membrane. Muscle and nerve cells are the most resistant to damage.

The greatest harm of radiation is during fetal development. The extent of damage reduces as an individual develops and ages. Exposure of children to radiation in utero may result in genetic defects or mental retardation. It has been estimated that the chance of a severe hereditary effect is between 0 and 0.00006 per rem. The normal chance of a birth defect is 0.03, about one fourth of which is considered of genetic origin. Lead aprons are routinely used in X-ray procedures to protect against damage.

The biggest concern from radiation is the risk of developing cancer, a risk much higher than the other negative health effects. The effects of ionizing radiation, used in medical diagnosis (X-rays) and cancer treatment, include increased risk of lung, skin, breast, and thyroid cancer, as well as leukemia.

The Measurement of Radiation Exposure

Radiation exposure is measured according to the dose absorbed (rad) and the dose of equivalency (rem) are used.

- The biological **dose equivalent** of a **Roentgen** is known as a **rem**.

    100 rems = 1 **Sievert** (Sv)

- The absorption of 100 ergs of energy from any radiation in 1 gram of material is a **rad**.

    1 **Joule** (J/kg) = 100 rads = 1 **Gray** (Gy)

The general population is exposed to approximately 200 to 300 medical rem (mrem) per year: 100 rem from radon, 55 rem from terrestrial sources, 30 rem from cosmic sources, 4 rem from fallout, and less than 1 rem from industrial exposure. Industrial exposure includes nuclear reactors, radon in mines, industrial and medical radioisotopes, and high-voltage devices such as X-ray machines, radar generators, video display terminals, and televisions.

Predicting the Effects of Ionizing Radiation

Severity depends on the dose of radiation (Table 12-2). The effects of ionizing radiation are divided into deterministic effects, threshold effects, nonthreshold effects, and cumulative effects.

Picocurie
A unit of measure used to express the results of radioactivity tests in air and water; expressed as picocuries per liter (PCi/l).

Dose equivalent
A measure of biological damage to a human for a particular type of radiation; the product of the absorbed dose and the quality factor; also known as the human-equivalent dose.

Roentgen
A unit of radiation exposure equivalent to 1 electrostatic unit of electricity in 1 cc of dry air; named for German physicist Wilhelm Konrad Roentgen who discovered X-rays.

Rem
The dosage of ionizing radiation that will cause injury to human tissue; roentgen equivalent man.

Sievert (Sv)
A dose equivalent to 100 rems.

Rad
A unit of ionizing radiation absorbed equal to 100 ergs per gram of irradiated material.

Joule
A unit of work equal to one watt-second, named after physicist James Prescott Joule.

Gray (Gy)
A unit of absorbed dosage of ionizing radiation, 100 times the commonly used rad unit; named for radiobiologist Louis Harold Gray.

TABLE 12-2 Measures of Radiation

Dose	Effect
0–25 rads	No observable effect
25–50 rads	Minor temporary blood changes
50–150 rads	Possible nausea and vomiting with reduced WBCs
150–300 rads	Increased severity of the above and diarrhea, malaise, loss of appetite; some death
300–500 rads	Increased severity of above and hemorrhaging, depilation; LD50 at 450–500 rads.
More than 500 rads	Symptoms appear sooner; LD100 approximately 600 rads

Source: OSHA. (1999). Introduction to ionizing radiation. Retrieved from http://www.osha.gov/SLTC/radiationionizing/introtoionizing/ionizinghandout.html.

DETERMINISTIC EFFECTS

Deterministic effects are observable within days to months after an acute radiation dose. Examples include skin reddening or swelling, depilation, or hematological depression. Deterministic effects require a dose that is greater than a threshold, typically greater than tens or hundreds of rad. Much knowledge about the risks from high doses of radiation exposure is based on studies of over 100,000 survivors of atomic bombings at Hiroshima and Nagasaki, Japan, and those exposed to nuclear accidents. A large dose to the whole body (such as 600 rems in 1 day) would probably cause death in about 30 days.

THRESHOLD EFFECTS

Also known as **nonstochastic effects**, threshold effects establish a dose-effect relationship for one individual. The Nuclear Regulatory Commission has set a 5-rem worker dose limit that is considered an acceptable risk. The dose limits for individual organs are below the levels at which biological effects are observed. Thus the risk to individuals at the occupational exposure levels is considered to be very low. However, it is impossible to say that the risk is zero.

NONTHRESHOLD EFFECTS

Also known as **stochastic effects**, these are "all-or-non" outcomes with a predictable outcome based on exposure. This principle is used to determine the risk of developing cancer. The risk of cancer is assumed to be proportional to the dose, assuming there is no minimum threshold. Certain body cells are more susceptible to damage than

Documented cases of long-term exposure to radiation including such people as scientists, miners, and factory workers have provided valuable information. The most important findings were that (EPA, 2000):
1. Any exposure to radiation poses some risk.
2. The risk of cancer from natural sources alone is estimated to be about one in 100 people.
3. The more radiation dose a persons receives, the greater the chance of developing cancer.
4. It is the chance of cancer occurring, not the kind or severity of cancer, that increases as the dose increases.
5. Most cancers do not appear until many years after the radiation dose is received; typically 10–40 years.

others, for that reason, threshold effects are different from one organ to another. Dose limits have been set for the lens of the eye (15 rem each year) and organs (50 rem each year). The estimated average surface skin dose from one radiographic chest X-ray is 0.03 rem. The estimated average surface dose per abdominal X-ray is 0.3 rem. These levels are considered safe because they are beneath the threshold levels.

CUMULATIVE EFFECTS

Exposure to radiation has a **cumulative effect**. The body absorbs radiation, increasing the risk over time as more exposure is added. The effects of ionizing radiation exposure are dependent upon toxic exposure and continued exposure. The more radiation one is exposed to either with short-term exposure or long-term exposure, the greater the chance for damage. Only the chance of cancer increases with repeated exposure over time. The type and severity of cancer cannot be predicted. The normal incidence of fatal cancer in an average North American population sample of 10,000 individuals is about 2000.

Public Health Interventions

Exposure to radiation is monitored by the Occupational Health and Safety Administration (OSHA) for personnel in occupational settings, the Nuclear Regulatory Commission (NRC) for personnel and the public regarding nuclear settings, and the transportation of radioactive waste by the Department of Transportation. These agencies recommended exposure "as low as reasonably achievable" (ALARA).

Health hazards associated with **radioactivity** have been a concern of the U.S. Public Health Service since the establishment of the Bureau of Radiological Health in the Food and Drug Administration. The first large-scale inspection of irradiated food began in 1954 to determine whether fish caught in the Pacific Ocean in areas where they would be subjected to atomic bombing fallout were safe.

The U.S. Public Health Service and other agencies regulate medical procedures that use radiation to reduce unnecessary use and exposure. Researchers began to scrutinize medical devices using radiation for safety and began to measure exposure to X-rays and other sources of radiation. In 1979, the U.S. Public Health Service assisted with the Three Mile Island nuclear reactor incident. The Center for Environmental Health also investigated the chemical dump near Niagara Falls, New York, in 1980 where Love Canal residents experienced negative health effects.

Preventive Measures to Control Radiation Exposure

ontrol of exposure to radiation is based on the assumption that any exposure, no matter how small, involves some risk. Individuals can minimize exposure to radiation by controlling food, air, and water concerns. Preventive strategies include:

■ Limiting the time exposed to radiation. Before receiving X-rays or radiation treatments, it is sensible to discuss the need for and benefits of the procedure and if there are other alternatives.

■ Increase the distance from the radiation source to lessen the effects.

■ Protect against radiation by wearing shields or clothing that can be removed and discarded, or use protective shields on equipment using radioactive materials.

■ Use a HEPA filter in furnace, air conditioners, and air-cleaning systems to catch particulate matter that might be contaminated with radioactive particles.

■ After removing contaminated gloves or clothing, shower carefully and dress in uncontaminated clothing, then check for radioactive levels with a health physicist or radiological health professional.

Solar Radiation

s noted earlier, the scope and types of radiation span the electromagnetic spectrum from the shortest and strongest ionizing rays (gamma rays, X-rays) to visible light rays (ultravio-

TABLE 12-3 Classification of Nonionizing Radiation

Type	Wavelength	Photon energy (in eV)
Ionizing radiation	less than 1 nm	more than 1 keV
Ultraviolet radiation (UV)	1 to 400 nm	0.3 to 1 keV
Visible radiation (VIS)	400 to 780 nm	0.15 to 0.3 eV
Infrared radiation (IR)	780 to 3 nm	0.15 to 40 meV
Microwaves and radio waves	larger than 3 nm	less than 40 meV

let, visible, infrared rays) to microwave and radio waves (Table 12-3). Wavelength increases and frequency (as well as energy and temperature) decrease from gamma rays to radio waves. All of these forms of radiation travel at the speed of light. Ionizing radiation comes from the decay of radioactive particles found in rock, soil, gas, and man-made sources. Another source of radiation is ultraviolet (UV) light from the sun. Most of the solar radiation reaching the surface of the Earth is infrared radiation (55%) and visible light (40%). Approximately 5% of the ground-level solar radiation is ultraviolet radiation, mostly in the UV-A range.

ULTRAVIOLET RADIATION

Ultraviolet light (UV) is between ionizing radiation and nonionizing radiation. UV light travels from the sun to the Earth, passing through the ozone layer filter. Ozone, as you recall, absorbs most of the UV-A light. Sunlight consists of UV-A, UV-B, and UV-C radiation. UV light has wavelengths between 180 to 400 nanometer (nm).

Nonstochastic effect
Also known as the threshold effect, the dose-effect relationship for an individual.

Stochastic effect
A calculated effect dependent upon the preceding effect; a predictable outcome based on exposure calculations.

Cumulative effect
Having an increasing effect with successive doses.

Radioactivity
The decay and emission of ionizing alpha and beta particles and gamma rays from unstable radioactive materials to become more stable.

UV-A light is between 315 to 400 nm, UV-B light is between 280 to 315 nm, and UV-C light is between 180 to 280 nm. UV-A light is sometimes referred to as *black UV light,* UV-B radiation is sometimes referred to as *erythemal UV light,* and UV-C is sometimes referred to as *germicidal UV light.*

Health Risks of UV Light

Each type of UV light has a different effect on living tissue. UV-A light is the least energetic, but can penetrate the skin and cause photoaging damage.

UV-B light causes tanning and sunburn (erythema) and can damage the immune system. Immunosuppression from UV radiation can make the person more susceptible to viruses, bacteria, and parasitic and fungal infections. **Immunosuppression** is also a risk factor for skin cancer and non-Hodgkin's lymphoma. UV-B radiation contributes to photochemical smog.

The highest energy band, UV-C, can damage DNA and other molecules. For that reason, it is used as a germicidal agent.

Direct UV exposure to the eyes can result in blindness. A temporary blindness from damage to the cornea is known as **photokeratitis**, also known as *welder's flash* or *snow blindness* and can occur for at least 24 hours. Damage to the cornea results in extreme pain, excessive tearing, and eyelid spasm. Prolonged exposure can result in lens thickening (cataracts) and damage to the retina. Those who are exposed to UV light must wear protective eye shields. Regardless of the season, sunglasses should be worn outside, particularly in areas where reflection of the sun is likely, such as water or snow. The UV protection factor on sunglasses is very important. Be certain that the sunglasses purchased have a label saying they have UV protection and block 99 to 100% of the sun's rays. If there is no label, do not buy the sunglasses.

Monitoring UV Radiation

Because of the potential harm from UV light, UV radiation is measured all over the world. NOAA has set up monitoring stations all over the United States (Figure 12-4). Measurements from these UV monitoring sites are taken so the National Weather Service can broadcast UV warnings. The amount of UV radiation reaching the Earth depends on the season, time of day, latitude, clouds, and altitude.

ABOUT SUNBURNS AND "TANS"

The skin is made up of two layers, the epidermis and the dermis (Figure 12-5). The **epidermis** is the outer layer and the **dermis** contains nerve endings, sweat glands, and hair follicles. Beneath both layers is subcutaneous fat and blood vessels supplying blood to capillaries in the dermis. The epidermis consists of dead

FIGURE **12-4** **UV Monitoring Sites Operated by U.S. Agencies**
Source: National Oceanic and Atmospheric Association. (2005). Retrieved from http://www.arl.noaa.gov/research/programs/uv.html.

- ■ Environmental Protection Agency Network = Spectral
- ◆ National Science Foundation = Spectral
- ● Smithsonian Institution = Multifilter
- ✪ National Oceanic and Atmospheric Administration–SURFRAD = Broadband
- ● National Oceanic and Atmospheric Administration–ISIS = Broadband
- ● USDA Network = Broadband

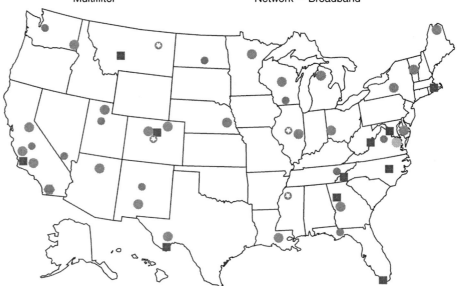

skin and a "living layer" called the **malpighian layer**. The malpighian layer consists of very thin layers.

- The uppermost layer is the **stratum corneum**, an outer layer of dead cells that is seen as the skin. The cells in this layer are filled with **keratin**, a tough protein.

- Underneath the stratum corneum are the granular layer and the spinous layer.

- The basal layer is in direct contact with the dermis. This is where basal cell carcinoma (cancer) begins.

The basal cell layer contains **melanocytes** that produce **melanin**, a pigment necessary for tanning. The number of melanocytes is the same no matter what the skin color. The difference in skin color is due to the amount of melanin produced and the nature of the pigment granules. Melanocytes produce two different

UV-A light
The least energetic light outside the visible spectrum causing damage to the skin; sometimes referred to as black UV light.

UV-B light
Light outside the visible spectrum causing damage to the immune system; sometimes referred to as erythemal UV light

UV-C light
The highest energy band of light outside the visible spectrum causing damage to the DNA; sometimes referred to as germicidal UV light because it can kill molecules.

Immunosuppression
A lowered immune response to a foreign agent in the body.

Photokeratitis
A temporary blindness from prolonged exposure to UV light; also known as welder's flash, snow blindness.

Epidermis
Outermost non-sensitive layer of skin.

Dermis
The deeper layer of skin under the epidermis.

Malpighian layer
Innermost layer of the epidermis.

Stratum corneum
The outermost layer of the epidermis consisting of dead cells that slough off.

Keratin
A fibrous protein insoluble substance found in skin, fingernails, and hair.

Melanocytes
Cells containing melanin in the basal cell layer.

Melanin
A black pigment found in the skin.

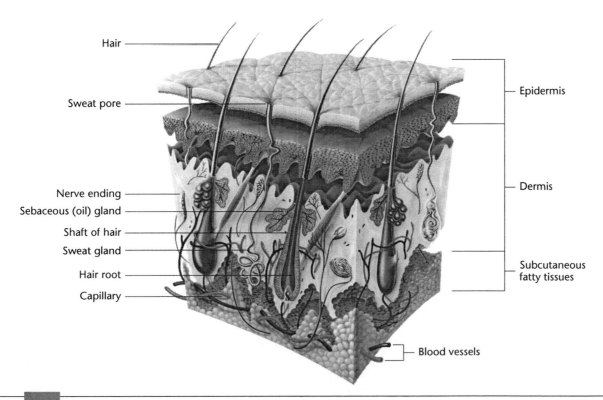

FIGURE 12-5 **Cross Section of Human Skin** UV light can penetrate several layers of skin.

Digging Deeper   ABOUT SUNBLOCKS AND SUNSCREENS

Sunblock and sunscreen products have an "SPF" number on the label, which stands for sun protection factor. A higher number means the product protects longer. For the best sun protection, the FDA recommends:

■ A sunblock or sunscreen product with an SPF of 15 or more.

■ A label that says "broad spectrum," meaning it protects against both UV-A and UV-B rays.

■ A label that says "water resistant" because it stays on the skin longer even if you perspire or swim.

The FDA also recommends putting on the sunscreen at least 15 to 30 minutes before going outside. Apply evenly on all uncovered skin, including eyelids, lips, nose, ears, neck, hands, feet, and the top of your head if you lack hair. However, do not apply sunscreen to babies under 6 months of age.

When wearing sunscreen:

■ Do not rub sunscreen in your eyes.

■ After being in the sun for 1 hour, reapply additional sunscreen.

Sources: American Dermatological Association, American Cancer Society, and Centers for Disease Control.

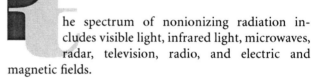

TANNING BEDS

The International Commission on Non-Ionizing Radiation Protection has thoroughly studied the effects of tanning beds on skin cancer risk. Findings are that ten 30-minute sessions in tanning beds per year increase the risk of melanoma by 5%. In addition, there is a "functional decline" in skin texture, known as *premature aging*, that is inescapable from the use of tanning beds. Skin loses elasticity and becomes dry, coarse, and wrinkled. The same effect is achieved as if the person was continually exposed to UV-A radiation for 2 months. There is also evidence that tanning beds accelerate the growth of human viruses, including herpes simplex and HIV.

pigments: **eumelanin** (brown) and **phaeomelanin** (yellow and red). Redheads produce more phaeomelanin and less eumelanin, which is why they do not tan very well. Albinos have no melanin in their skin.

When the skin is subjected to light, the melanocytes do not increase in number, only in activity. Sunburns damage melanocytes. Damage to melanocytes from UV radiation causes cancerous mutations, known as *melanoma*. UV radiation is unable to penetrate most materials and this shielding can prevent damage from the sun's rays. For shielding the skin, clothing and sunblocks are used.

Artificial sources of UV light include welding torches, tanning beds (UV-A and UV-B), black lights (UV-A), curing lamps used by dentists to harden resins, germicidal lamps (UV-B and UV-C), mercury vapor lamps, halogen and xenon lamps, high-intensity discharge lamps (UV-A) used for dermatology, and some types of lasers.

Lasers

asers are beams of light created when light rays are combined into a single light wave. Lasers are in a class all by themselves because they emit ultraviolet (UV), visible light (VIS), or infrared (IR) light as well as generate high temperatures. Laser beams can be used for welding, cutting, drilling, heat treatments, eye surgery, home security systems, and light shows. They can also be used in CD and DVD players, supermarket scanners, facsimile (fax) machines, and printing equipment.

Nonionizing Radiation

The spectrum of nonionizing radiation includes visible light, infrared light, microwaves, radar, television, radio, and electric and magnetic fields.

VISIBLE LIGHT

Visible light (VIS) has longer wavelengths than UV light. Whereas UV light waves are between 180 to 400 nm, visible light (VIS) has wavelengths between 400 to 780 nm. Visible light can be natural or manmade. The type of light generated from its source is dependent upon the level of photon energy produced. The speed of the particles when they collide or vibrate sets a limit on the energy of the photon. The speed is also a measure of temperature. For instance, on a hot day, the particles in the air are moving faster than on a cold day. Visible light includes ultraviolet light, **incandescent light**, **fluorescent light**, and neon light.

Artificial Light

Incandescent light, fluorescent light, and neon light are all produced by humans. Incandescent light is produced by a light bulb with a filament inside that is heated with electricity, producing visible light. A fluorescent light has a tube with a positively charged anode on one end and a negatively charged cathode on the other end with mercury and argon gas suspended between. The tube is coated inside with phosphor that lights up as mercury gas is activated from photons produced from an electrical charge, giving it a slightly purple color. A neon light works in the same manner as a fluorescent light, but with krypton, neon, argon, or mercury gas to give it a different color. The tube in a "black light" is lined with a different substance that blocks most visible light, so only long-wave UV-A light and some blue and violet visible light pass through. Infrared and ultraviolet light are both given off in these types of lighting.

INFRARED LIGHT

This type of light is directed into beams that can detect heat and motion. In fact, heat is a form of infrared light. Infrared technology has many applications. Infrared satellites have been used to monitor the Earth's weather, vegetation, geology, and ocean temperatures. Medical infrared imaging is a useful diagnostic tool. The military, police, and security personnel use infrared cameras. Infrared imaging is also used to detect heat loss in buildings and test electronic systems. Home owners may have infrared light in their home security systems.

Measurement of Light

amma rays and X-rays are measured according to their ionizing factors. Visible light is measured differently; the fundamental unit of optical power for light is the **watt** (W), which has the rate of energy of one joule (J) per second. *Optical power* is a function of both the number of photons and the wavelength. The photometric properties of light are in accordance with what can be seen with the human eye. For visible light, the photometric equivalent of the watt is the **lumen** (lm) (Ryder, 1997).

Electromagnetic Fields

lectromagnetic fields (EMFs) are fields charged with electromagnetic radiation (WHO, 1995). The measurement of electromagnetic fields is considered less important by researchers and health physicists because it is nonionizing radiation. However, in combination with exposure to radiation from natural sources, medical sources, and common household appliances, the relative risk may be higher than we expect. Nonionizing radiation exposure is becoming more important as advancements in technology have made de-

vices that emit radioactive frequencies commonplace. The magnetic component is measured using **amps** per meter (A/m). The strength of an electric field is measured using **volts** per meter (V/m). The frequency is measured using **Hertz (Hz)** and the Tesla (T).

> Health benefits from electric and magnetic fields have been claimed since the 18th century (WHO, 2005). Some medical practitioners use pulsed EMFs in the intermediate range to heal bone healing and stimulate nerve regeneration.

Eumelanin
Brown pigmentation of the skin due to melanin.

Phaeomelanin
Yellow and red pigments of the skin.

Laser
An abbreviation for Light Amplification by Stimulated Emission of Radiation; a laser is a device that uses natural oscillations between atoms and molecules to generate electromagnetic radiation in same spectrum as ultraviolet light, visible light, and infrared light.

Incandescent light
Light created with a light bulb as electricity heats up a metal filament.

Fluorescent light
Light created inside a tube with an anode on one end and a cathode on the other end that distribute electricity through argon and mercury gas; as mercury atoms become excited, photons are produced, the photons strike the phosphor lining inside the tube and emit light. A neon light works in the same way but with argon or krypton gas.

Watt
A metric unit of electrical power; the production of voltage and current (amps); a kilowatt (kW) is 1,000 watts.

Lumen
A unit of illumination.

Amp
A unit of electrical current intensity equal to the rate of flow for an electrical charge per second; a measure of strength of an electric current.

Volt (eV)
Unit of force moving electrical energy through power lines.

Hertz (Hz)
The basic unit of frequency in the International System of Units, equal to one cycle per second.

STATIC ELECTROMAGNETIC FIELDS

Static electromagnetic fields include Earth's magnetic field or magnetic waves from a magnet or battery-operated device. A static field does not vary over time. An example is direct current (DC) electricity current flowing in one direction from the battery to the device, then back to the battery. Household devices with permanent magnets such as audio speaker components and battery-operated motors emit static fields between 1 to 10 **milliT**. Magnetic fields are also used for public transportation. The highest static magnetic field is produced from magnetic resonance imaging (MRI) devices used for medical diagnostics, ranging from 150 to 2000 milliT. Studies have found that magnets slow heart rate (Sait et al., 1999; Zubkova, 1996). It is believed that static electromagnetic fields are not associated with tumors, immune system suppression, change in hormones, or any other ill effects (Moulder, 2000). Experts caution the effect magnetic resonance imaging devices have on cardiac pacemakers (Pavlicek et al., 1983).

PULSED ELECTROMAGNETIC FIELDS

Electrical power and electric appliances provide the main source of pulsed electromagnetic fields (WHO, 2005). An example of a pulsating electromagnetic field is alternating currents (AC) found in electricity, reversing direction at regular intervals. In Europe, electricity changes direction with a frequency of 50 cycles per second or 50 Hz and the field changes direction 50 times every second. AC electricity reverses its direction at regular intervals. In North American electricity has a frequency of 60 Hz. **Pulsed electromagnetic fields** include radiofrequency fields (RFs), intermediate frequency fields (IF), and extremely low frequency fields (ELFs).

Radiofrequency Fields (RF)

Radiofrequency fields (RFs) range from 10 MHz to 300 GHZ. Radio and other forms of wireless technology are the main source of RF fields. The first wireless technology began in 1895 when a German scientist, Heinrich Hertz, developed equipment that could send and detect electromagnetic waves (Briggs, 2001). Beginning in 1894, Guglielmo Marconi (1874–1937) studied his work and became the first person to send a message in Morse code between a transmitter and a receiver (Briggs, 2001). The first telegraph message sent overseas was in 1902. In 1900 Canadian-American physicist Reginald Fessenden (1866–1931) transmitted the first voice message using a spark-gap transmitter. By 1906, both voice and music were transmitted by AM radio waves. The use of radio frequencies continued to include the transmission of pictures when a photograph was sent by wire in 1923 (Bellis, 2005). The first FM station was built in 1939, but the frequency did not become popular until 1960.

A radio wave is propagated by an antenna and there are different frequencies. By tuning a radio to a particular frequency, a person can pick up a signal. The Federal Communications Commission (FCC) regulates the authorization and use of devices that use radio frequencies. The FCC also determines who uses what frequency and for what purpose. Radio frequencies are transmitted in a **band**. Each type of wireless technology has its own band (Table 12-4).

Television towers today emit **very high frequency (VHF)** as well as **ultra-high frequency (UHF)** microwave frequencies. Each television station has its own frequency. A UHF antenna will help pick up more channels on the UHF frequency. Areas with very good television reception have an electric field of 80 decibel (dB) microvolts per meter (m/V), 200 times greater than normal brain magnetic field levels.

Microwaves (MW) are the shortest radio waves, with radiation in the range of 300 MHz to 300 GHz. They are found between radio waves and visible light. Microwaves come from broadcast stations, long-distance telephone equipment, ultra-high frequency (UHF) waves, air traffic control systems, cellular phones, and radar. Microwave radiation occurs naturally in the Earth's atmosphere, but some areas of North America where human-made communication microwaves and high frequency radio waves in the environment are estimated to have 100 to 200,000,000 the natural radio frequency background from the sun (Brodeur, 1977).

The higher the power of communication microwaves, the better the transmission for analog and digital signals. Microwave towers today emit electromagnetic waves to carry over long distances. The primary effect of MW energy is heating. MW radiation is absorbed by the skin. Evidence is accumulating that suggest telecommunication electromagnetic fields increase cancer rates in humans due to the high levels of RFs in the environment and increased exposure in

TABLE 12-4 Common Frequency Bands

Type	Measure
AM radio	535 **kilohertz (KHz)** to 1.7 **megahertz (MHz)**
Short wave radio	5.9 megahertz to 26.1 megahertz
Citizens band (CB) radio	26.96 megahertz to 27.41 megahertz
Television stations (channels 2 through 6)	54 to 88 megahertz
FM radio	88 megahertz to 108 megahertz
Television stations (channels 7 through 13)	174 to 220 megahertz

some populations (Microwave News, 1997). The use of mobile or cellular phones is a concern. Cellular phone radiation (82.5 to 84.5 MHz) has wavelength fields ranging from 355 to 364 millimeters. Electric fields from the antennae of a handheld cellular phone can be as high as 60 volts per meter, more than 1,000,000 times the magnetic field levels found in the brain (Nordenberg, 2000). The brain is particularly susceptible to electromagnetic radiation. The location of the antennae on the phone and the length of time the phone is used are important considerations (Figure 12-6).

Intermediate Frequency Fields (IF)

Intermediate frequency fields (IF) range from 300 Hz to 10 MHz. Those likely to have the highest exposure include hospital and military personnel. Hospital personal working with MRI systems and electromagnetic nerve stimulators should exercise caution. Military personnel working with power units and those who work from high-range broadcasting communication transmitters also have higher exposure than the limits established for reduced risk to health (WHO, 2005). For the rest of us, video display units (computer screens and television sets), anti-theft devices in libraries and stores, and security systems are the main sources of IF fields.

The **cathode ray tube (CRT)** was developed by producing extremely high voltages across two electrodes in a

 During World War II, two scientists invented the magnetron, a tube that produces microwaves to create the use of radar (Ament, 2005). The primary purpose of radar is to detect the presence, direction, or range of moving objects. Radar exposure comes from air traffic control towers, weather radar systems (usually found near air traffic control towers), military bases, boats, and traffic speed control systems.

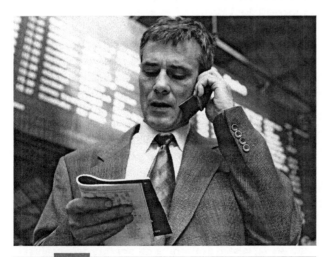

FIGURE 12-6 **Cellular Phone** Electromagnetic waves are transmitted through the antenna.

HOW DO MICROWAVES WORK?
Microwaves vibrate water cells, generating heat. It is important to know this because water must be present when items are heated in a microwave. Without water, things will explode or crack. Water cells are heated from the inside to the outside of items cooked in a microwave. For this reason, it is important to partially cook the food, stir it, and then cook it until it is done.

Food heated by a microwave oven should be allowed to sit 1 minute before eating because water cells can become extremely hot.

Static electromagnetic field
An electrical charge generated from friction.

milliT
Static magnetic fields are measured in Tesla (T). A tesla is equal to 1000 milliT.

Pulsed electromagnetic field
An electrical field that alternates current to run electrical devices.

Band
Radio frequency space on the radio frequency spectrum.

Very high frequency (VHF)
Any radio frequency between 30 and 300 megahertz.

Ultra-high frequency (UHF)
Any radio frequency between 300 and 3,000 megahertz.

Microwave (MW)
The electromagnetic spectrum associated with infrared and radio waves; used for radar, communications, and heating food.

AM radio
A radio signal received within the radio band spectrum of 535 to 1,700 kilohertz, used for AM radio only.

Kilohertz (kHz)
One thousand cycles per second; as in the AM radio band frequency.

Megahertz (MHz)
One million hertz, one million cycles per second, as in the FM radio band frequency.

FM radio
A signal with a frequency between 88 and 108 megahertz; this band of the radio spectrum is used for no other purpose than FM radio broadcasts.

Cathode ray tube (CRT)
A tube that illuminates from a reaction of particle charges and a gas. In a CRT, the anode filament is inside a tube attracting electrons from the cathode, the electrons are focused and accelerated into a beam, the beam flies through the vacuum inside the tube and hits a flat screen coated with phosphor that lights up the screen. The tubes are wrapped in steering coils that create electromagnetic waves horizontally and vertically to produce an image.

glass tube containing gas. Reddish to yellowish-green light (cathode rays) was produced on the glass opposite the cathode or negative electrode. These rays were later found to be beams of high-energy electrons. While experimenting with one of these tubes in 1895, William Konrad Roentgen observed the fluorescence on a nearby zinc sulfide screen. The radiation produced from the cathode rays and exposure to a metal anode created another type of radiation, known as X-rays, which was extremely penetrating. These same rays are used to produce visual images in television sets and computer screens, but they are kept inside the tube, rather than dispersed in the environment. Prior to the 1970s, television screens produced detectable levels of X-rays. Since then manufacturers have improved the X-ray absorbing properties of the front screen so no detectable levels of X-rays have been found (International Non-Ionizing Radiation Committee, 1994; Weiss, 1983). However, computer microprocessors work at speeds of 100 megahertz (100 million cycles per second), generating electromagnetic fields at higher frequencies such as 200 to 300 MHz. Faster microprocessor chips will generate even higher frequencies absorbed by the human body.

Extremely Low Fields (ELFs)

The main sources of ELFs are trains used for public transportation and any device used to generate, distribute, or use electrical power. ELFs can come from household appliances, waterbeds, electric blankets, and electric toothbrushes. Most household appliances use an electric current at a frequency of 50 to 60 Hz. Extremely low frequency fields (ELFs) range from 0-300 Hz. The impact of ELFs has come under scrutiny but is a low priority for research because of the demand for technology today.

HEALTH EFFECTS OF ELECTROMAGNETIC FIELDS

Scientists have known for years that exposure to high levels of electromagnetic fields can interact with biological systems. Researchers found evidence that communication microwaves used in radar and telecommunication systems could damage vegetation (Volkrodt, 1989). In humans, absorption of electromagnetic fields occurs around 70 to 80 megahertz (MHz) in adults and 80 to 150 MHz in children, depending upon their height.

Links to Cancer

The correlation between childhood leukemia and electromagnetic fields from power lines in proximity to their residences was introduced by Wertheimer and Leeper in 1979. In 1986, Savitz found that cancer cases among children who lived close to high-current wires had higher than usual cancer rates. Findings of another study suggested a significant mortality rate from acute myeloidleukemia and other cancers among amateur radio operators (Milham, 1988). A study of 4,000 New York police officers was conducted to determine the extent that radar use may have had harmful effects such as an increased incidence of leukemia or testicular cancer (Lotz et al., 1995). Findings were that radar exposure to officers was very low and no unusual effects were noted among groups. Military personnel exposed to radio frequency and microwave radiation in Poland were found to have higher rates of leukemia and lymphoma, more than eight times higher than expected (Szmiglielski, 1996). Researchers from Australia supported the idea that broadcast towers were possibly related to childhood and adult leukemia rates were greater in communities with broadcast towers than communities that were not exposed (Hocking et al., 1996). In England, a cluster of leukemia and lymphoma cases was reported around an FM radio transmitter with nine times the expected number of leukemia cases (Dolk, 1997a). When the study was repeated examining other types of cancers relevant to tower locations, the results were inconclusive (Dolk, 1997b).

The first microwave oven was invented by Percy Spencer in 1945. The first commercial microwave oven was marked in 1954 but was too large to be practical for consumers. The primary use of microwave ovens is to heat food. A typical home microwave generates 2.45 **gigahertz (gHz)** with energy output between 400 to 1,000 watts. A magnetron tube inside the microwave oven causes a beam to oscillate water molecules in the food at extremely high frequencies. Microwave heating of foods is a form of irradiation. Irradiation by microwaves changes the color, taste, nutritional qualities, and other properties of food. It is known that antibodies in human milk are decreased when heating human breast milk in the microwave, even at low temperatures (Stevenson & Kerner, 1992).

Microwave ovens need to be inspected periodically for leaks in seals around the door or poorly closing doors. Foods heated in the microwave should have some water content and dishes should be microwave safe. Never put metal in a microwave or leave it unattended while food is cooking. Allow food to cool until it is safe to remove. Medical hazards associated with microwave ovens include burns, cataract formation, neurologic injury, and pacemaker dysfunction (Murray, 1984; Pavlicek et al., 1983). Consumers are cautioned to stand 3 feet away from the microwave oven while it is operating, particularly those who are pregnant or have a pacemaker.

Links to Disturbances in the Brain and Soft Tissues of the Body

Researchers found resonant peaks in the brain and eyes at 800 MHz (Anderson & Joyner, 1995). Areas of the brain, particularly the pineal gland, are affected. The pineal gland produces melatonin, a hormone affecting sleep cycles and inhibition of cancer cells. Researchers found that nocturnal melatonin production was suppressed by low frequency magnetic fields (De Guire, 1988; Reiter, 1994). Some speculate that microwaves interfere with the brain's reception of solar rays believed to contribute to the entrainment of human circadian rhythms (Cremer-Bartels et al., 1984). Others have found that pulsating light decreases melatonin levels (Bortkiewicz, et al., 2002).

Others determined that thermal heat generated from these devices, particularly the cellular phone, could cause headaches and acoustic neuroma (Chia, Chia, & Tan, 1999; Lonn et al., 2004; Repacholi & Greenebaum, 1999). There is some evidence that the heat from laptops reduces fertility in male users (Sheynkin et al., 2005).

The Need for More Research

While there has been some research regarding radiofrequency fields, very little research has been done regarding the intermediate frequency fields. The rate of spontaneous abortion and birth defects was reportedly higher for women using video display units (VDUs) for 20 hours per week or longer during the first trimester of pregnancy (Goldhaber et al., 1988). There was also evidence that dermatitis occurred after exposure to VDU (Johansson et al., 1994). There was some evidence among radio and telegraph operators showing increased risk of breast cancer, but causation related to intermediate frequency exposure was not confirmed and there could have been other factors involved (Hardell et al., 1995; Liburdy et al., 1993; Garland et al., 1990). The need for more research is obvious.

POTENTIAL RISK AND STANDARDS FOR ELECTROMAGNETIC RADIOFREQUENCIES

When agencies such as the National Council on Radiation Protection and Measurements (NCRP) the International Commission on Non-Ionizing Radiation Protection (ICNIRP), and the World Health Organization reviewed the literature concerning harmful effects of **radiofrequency radiation (RFR)**, they determined it was not harmful below levels that produced thermal effects. In 1997 the United States Federal Communications Commission (FCC) set the RFR standard at a specific energy absorption rate (SAR) of 4 W/kg, based upon thermal effects of sensitive tissues of the body (brain, testicles, breasts, and lymph glands). Occupational standards set by OSHA are 10 times higher (Mann et al., 2001). Scientists still believe there are nonthermal effects but findings have been inconsistent and difficult to confirm, even in occupational studies where workers were exposed to much higher levels than the average person.

There are no standards in the United States for exposure to intermediate magnetic fields from VDUs. The Swedish government, however, has set standards used by the VDU industry worldwide. Guidelines recommend magnetic fields no stronger than 2.5 milligauss. As more people are exposed to them, particularly at a younger age for extended periods of time, more research needs to be done and emissions may need to be controlled. There is still some concern because microwave emissions are not

Gigahertz (gHz)
One billion hertz.

Radiofrequency (RF) radiation
An electromagnetic wave frequency between audio and infrared.

monitored in our environment. Perhaps one day there will be standards regarding the location of microwave towers near local schools and residences, as well as guidelines for cellular phone use. Until then, precautionary measures such as limiting cellular phone use to just a few minutes, sitting at least five feet from a color television screen or video game, and taking frequent breaks from computer screens are suggested.

Acoustic Sound

coustic sound consists of vibrations or waves heard by the human ear. Sound is measured in terms of frequency and pitch. Frequency is measured in hertz (Hz) and intensity is measured in watts per centimeter squared (W/cm2) or decibels (dB). One hertz is the equivalent of one vibration per second. Pitch and resonance are other qualities of sound. Sound vibrations are detected by inner ear structures that transmit messages to the brain to interpret sound vibrations (Figure 12-7). Unwanted sound is noise. The effects of noise include deafness and psychological stress.

NOISE AND HEARING LOSS

One does not often think of noise as pollution, but is harmful. What may be music to one person may be noise to someone else. Indoor noise can include rock concerts, alarm clocks, telephones, office machines, air conditioners, fans, drills, kitchen noise such as microwave ovens and dishwashers, vacuum cleaners, washing machines and dryers, hair dryers, exhaust fans, people talking loudly, televisions, and stereos. In addition, outdoor noise can permeate indoors from construction, garbage trucks, farm equipment, traffic, aircraft, thunder, fireworks, lawn mowers, yard trimmers, and chain saws.

Health physicists measure noise according to intensity (amplitude or loudness) and frequency (vibration, or compression and expansion of wave pressure). The measure most responsible for hearing loss is amplitude. The louder the noise, less exposure it takes to experience hearing loss. Both measures are considered when determining harmful levels. One may be exposed to extreme levels on a short-term basis and suffer ringing of the ears (tinnitus) and temporary deafness. This phenomenon is known as temporary threshold shift (TTS). Continued exposure to loud noises can result in permanent hearing loss as hair cells in the organ of Corti of the cochleae of the inner ear are destroyed. This type of hearing loss is irreversible.

The Noise Control Act of 1972 made an attempt at regulating noise in the United States. The regulation of noise in the United States declined significantly in 1981 when the Reagan administration viewed noise pollution as a local problem that does not travel far and quickly dissipates. Some states and local municipalities do regulate noise. Citizen action has resulted in "no-noise zones" during certain times of the evening. Noise barriers of concrete or brick are sometimes constructed along new highways to protect neighborhoods from traffic noise. Some neighborhood associations prohibit residents and their guests from driving motorcycles and other loud vehicles in the area. For residents who do not have the advantage of these laws, planting trees or putting up wooden fences to absorb some of the noise is helpful.

Ultrasound

onography has been used by submarines and those studying marine life for some time. Ultrasound or ultrasonography is a medical imaging technique that uses high frequency sound waves and

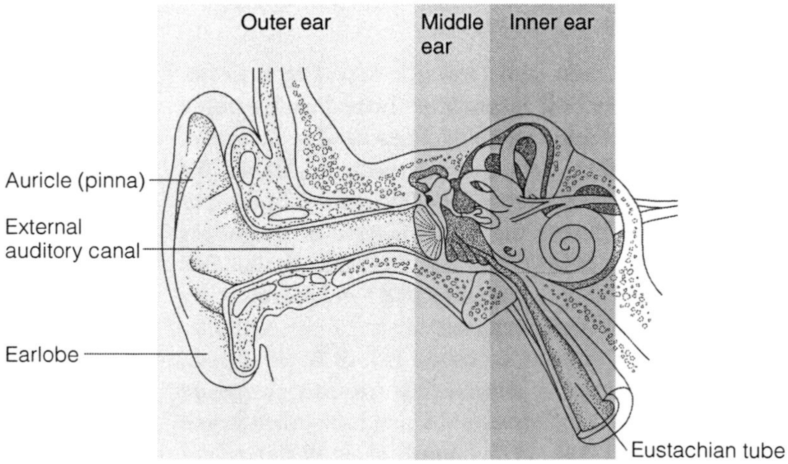

FIGURE 12-7 **Cross Section of Ear Structure** Excessive noise can damage hearing.

- Auricle (pinna)
- External auditory canal
- Earlobe
- Outer ear
- Middle ear
- Inner ear
- Eustachian tube

their echoes. The machine transmits high-frequency (1 to 5 megahertz) sound pulses into the body using a probe. The sound waves strike areas of the body and reflect back to the probe. The machine calculates the distance from the probe to the tissue or organ, displaying the distances and intensities of the "echoes" on the screen, and forming a two-dimensional image on a computer monitor. There have been some safety concerns about the use of ultrasound and the effects it might have on a developing fetus from the heat and bubbles generated internally during the test. Some report effects such as low-birth weight babies but no other ill-effects have been documented in animals or humans.

Public Health Agencies Regulating Radiation

agencies with the authority to regulate medical and radiation-emitting products include the Food and Drug Administration and the Federal Communications Commission. FDA derives its authority to regulate wireless telephones from the Radiation Control provisions of the Federal Food, Drug, and Cosmetic Act (originally enacted as the Radiation Control for Health and Safety Act of 1968). The Center for Devices and Radiological Health is responsible for these duties. FCC derives its authority to regulate wireless telephones from the National Environmental Policy Act (NEPA) of 1969 and the Telecommunications Act of 1996.

The Food and Drug Administration has determined that there is a need for more research regarding the health effects of cellular phones (Nordenberg, 2000). The FDA recommends that concerned cell phone users take the following precautions:

- Reserve cell phones for shorter conversations when a conventional telephone is not available.

- Switch to a type of cell phone with a headset to place more distance between the cell phone antenna than the body or a hands-free headset.

- If the cell phone is for car use only, have the antenna mounted outside the vehicle.

> Wireless phones in the United States are regulated by the Federal Communications Commission (FCC) and the Food and Drug Administration (FDA). The FCC ensures that phones adhere to safety guidelines limiting radiofrequency (RF) energy to safe levels. The FDA monitors the health effects of wireless telephones.

Summary

There are two types of radiation: ionizing and nonionizing. All contain a certain amount of radioactivity. The measurement of the exposure to radioactivity is important, particularly to those who work closely with ionizing radiation. Even among those who do not, radon exposure is a possibility. Exposure to ionizing radiation, even overexposure to sunlight, has negative health consequences to individuals and a developing fetus. For all of us, exposure to radiation has cumulative effects.

The effect of various types of light and electromagnetic waves is also seen in humans. As more technology is available to us, exposure to harmful elements in the environment increase. Research linking the incidence to cancer has been inconclusive, but further studies continue to investigate the effects.

Each individual spends more time indoors than outdoors, exposed to more artificial light, noise, electromagnetic waves, and radiation than ever before. Individuals spend hours each day in front of a television set. Children spend even more hours with videogames and personal computers. In the workplace, computer monitors are on nearly all day long. Outdoors people are exposed to ultraviolet radiation, radio and television frequencies, and satellite and cellular telephone and computer frequencies. It is important to understand how technology may affect human health in the short term and the long term, as well as the health of children and unborn children.

REFERENCES

Ament, P. (2005). Inventor Heinrich Hertz. Retrieved from http://www.ideafinder.com/history/inventors/hertz.htm.

Ament, P. (2005). Microwave oven history. Retrieved from http://www.ideafinder.com/history/inventions/story068.htm.

Anderson, V., & Joyner, K. (1995). Specific absorption rate levels measured in a phantom head exposed to radio frequency transmissions from analog handheld mobile phones. *Bioelectromagnetics, 16,* 60–69.

Bellis, M. (2005). The invention of radio. Retrieved from http://inventors.about.com/library/inventors/blradio.htm.

Bortkiewicz, A., Pilacik, B., Gadzick, E., & Symczak, W. (2002). The excretion of 6-hydroxymelatonin sulfate in healthy young men exposed to electromagnetic fields emitted by cellular phone—an experimental study. *Neuroendocrinology Letters.* Nofer Institute of Occupational Medicine, Lodz, Poland. Retrieved from http://www.ibl-hamburg.com/lit/melatonin/Bortkiewicz-2002.pdf.

Briggs, H. (2001). Profile: Marcoi, the wireless pioneer. BBC News, December. Retrieved from http://news.bbc.co.uk/1/hi/sci/tech/1702037.stm.

Brodeur, P. (1977). *The zapping of America,* pg. 13. New York: W. W. Norton and Company.

Brugge, D., & Goble, R. (2002). The history of uranium mining and the Navajo people. *American Journal of Public Health, 92,* 1410–1419.

Chia, S., Chia, H., & Tan, J. (1999). Prevalence of headache among handheld cellular telephone users in Singapore: A Community Study. *Environmental Health Perspectives, 108,* 1059–1062.

Cremer-Bartels, G., Krause, K., Mitoskas, G., & Brodersen, D. (1984). Magnetic field of earth as additional zeitgeber for endogenous rhythms? *Naturwissenshaften, 71,* 567–574.

Curtis, R. (1999). Introduction to ionizing radiation. U.S. Department of Labor, Occupational Safety and Health Administration (OSHA). Retrieved from http://www.osha.gov/SLTC/radiationionizing/untrotoionizing/ionizinghandout.html.

De Guire, I. (1988). Increased malignant melanoma of the skin in workers in a telecommunications industry. *British Journal of Industrial Medicine, 45,* 824–828.

Dolk, H., Shaddick, G., Walls, P., Grundy, C., Thakrar, B., Kleinschmidt, I., & Elliott, P. (1997a). Cancer incidence near radio and television transmitters in Great Britain. I. Sutton Coldfield Transmitter. *American Journal of Epidemiology, 145,* 1–9.

Dolk, H., Elliott, P., Shaddick, G., Walls, P., & Thakrar, B. (1997b). Cancer incidence near radio and television transmitters in Great Britain II. All high power transmitters. *American Journal of Epidemiology, 1,* 10–17.

Environmental Protection Agency. (2000). Radiation: risks and realities. Retrieved March 27, 2000 from http://www.epa.gov/radiation/rrpage/rrpage1.html.

Environmental Protection Agency. (2002). Radiation: Risks and realities. Retrieved from http://www.epa.gov/radiation/docs/risksandrealities/index.html.

Environmental Protection Agency. (2004). What is radiation? Retrieved from http://www.epa.gov/radiation/students/types.html.

Environmental Protection Agency. (2005). Radiation frequent questions. Retrieved from http://www.epa.gov/iaq/radon/radonqa1.html#faq8.

Garland, F., Garland, C., Gorham, E., & Young, J. (1990). Geographic variation in breast cancer mortality in the United States: A hypothesis involving exposure to solar radiation. *Preventive Medicine, 19,* 614–622.

Goldhaber, M., Polen, M., & Hiatt, R. (1988). The risk of miscarriage and birth defects among women who use visual display terminals during pregnancy. *American Journal of Industrial Medicine, 13,* 695–696.

Hardell, L., Holmberg, B., Malker, H., & Paulsson, L. (1995). Exposure to extremely low frequency electromagnetic fields and the risk of malignant diseases: An evaluation of epidemiological and experimental findings. *European Journal of Cancer Prevention, 4,* 3–107.

Hocking, B., Gordon, I., Grain, H., & Hatfield, G. (1996). Cancer incidence and mortality and proximity to TV towers. *Medical Journal of Australia, 165,* 601–605.

International Commission for Non-Ionizing Radiation Protection (2003). ICNIRP statement: Health uses of ultraviolet tanning appliances used for cosmetic purposes. Retrieved 7/01/03 from http://www.icnirp.de/documents/sunbed.pdf.

International Non-Ionizing Radiation Committee of the International Radiation Protection Association. (1994). Video display units—Radiation protection guidance, pgs. 11–12. Geneva, Switzerland: International Labour Office.

Johansson, O., Hilliges, M., Bjornhagen, V., & Hall, K. (1994). Skin changes in patients suffering from so-called "screen dermatitis": A two case open-field provocation study. *Experimental Dermatology, 3,* 234–238.

Kameras, D. (2004). AFA recommends continued prohibition of airborne use of cell phones: Authorities urged to allow time to understand and reduce threats to flight and operational safety. PR Newswire, December 15. Retrieved from http://www.findarticles.com/p/articles/mi_m4PRN/is_2004_Dec_15/ai_n8573028.

Liburdy, R. Sloma, T., Sokolic, R., & Yaswen, P. (1993). ELF magnetic fields, breast cancer and melatonin: 60 Hz fields block melatonin's oncostatic action on ER breast cancer cell proliferation. *Journal of Pineal Research, 14,* 89–97.

Lonn, S., Ahlbom, A., Hall, P., & Feychting, M. (2004). Mobile phone use and the risk of acoustic neuroma. *Epidemiology, 15,* 653–659.

Lotz, W., Rinsky, R., & Edwards, R. (1995). Occupational exposure of police officers to microwave radiation from traffic radar devices. Cincinnati, OH: NIOSH. Retrieved 7/1/03 from http://www.osha-slc.gov/SLTC/radiofrequencyradiation/fnradpub.html#results2.

Mann, J., Lee, R., Aragon, T., & Bhatia, R. (2001). Radiofrequency radiation from broadcast transmission towers and cancer: A review of epidemiology studies, pgs. 1–27. Retrieved from http://www.dph.sf.ca.us/reports/RadioFreqRadRpt032001.pdf.

Mayo Clinic. (2005). Mayo Clinic: Key dates. Retrieved from http://www.mayoclinic.org/about/keydates.html.

Microwave News. (1997). Physical characteristics and possible biological effects of microwaves applied in wireless communication. A report on non-ionizing radiation. Workshop held in Rockville, MD, February 7, 1997. Retrieved from http://www.microwavenews.com/FDA_Workshop_Abstracts.html.

Milham, S. (1988). Increased mortality in amateur radio operators due to lymphatic and hemotopoietic malignancies. *American Journal of Epidemiology, 127,* 50–54.

Moulder, J. (2000). The electric and magnetic fields research and public information dissemination (EMF-RAPID) program. *Radiation Research, 153,* 613–616.

Muller, H. (1927). Artificial transmutation of the gene. *Science, 66,* 84.

Murray, K. (1984). Hazard of microwave oven to transdermal delivery system. *New England Journal of Medicine, 16,* March, 721.

Nordenberg, T. (2000). Cell phones and cancer: No clear connection. FDA Consumer, 34, 19-21, 23. Retrieved March 8, 2001 from http://www.fda.gov/fdac/features/2000/600_phone.html.

Pavlicek, W., Geisinger, M., Castle, L., Borkowski, G., Meaney, T., Bream, B., & Gallagher, J. (1983). The effects of nuclear magnetic resonance on patients with cardiac pacemakers. *Radiology, 147,* 149–153. Retrieved from http://radiology.rsnajnls.org/cgi/content/abstract/147/1/149.

Reiter, R. (1994). Melatonin suppression by static and extremely low frequency electromagnetic fields: Relationship to the reported increased incidence of cancer. *Reviews on Environmental Health, 10,* 171–186.

Repacholi, M., & Greenebaum, B. (1999). Interaction of static and extremely low frequency electric and magnetic fields with living systems: Health effects and research needs. *Bioelectromagnetics, 24,* 133–160. Retrieved from http://www3.interscience.wiley.com/cgi-bin/jissue/55002432.

Ryder, A. (1997). *Light measurement handbook.* Retrieved July 1, 2003, from http://www.intl-light.com/handbook.

Sait, M., Wood, A., & Sadafi, H. (1999). A study of heart rate and heart rate variability in human subjects exposed to occupational levels of 50 Hz circularly polarized magnetic fields. *Medical Engineering and Physics, 21,* 361–369.

Scarry, E. (1998). The fall of TWA 800: The possibility of electromagnetic interference. Retrieved from http://www.physics.ohio-state.edu/~wilkins/writing/Assign/topics/twa800-emi.htm.

Sheynkin, Y., Jung, M., Yoo, P., Schulsinger, D., & Komaroff, E. (2005). Increase in scrotal temperature in laptop computer users. *Human Reproduction, 20,* 452–455.

Stevenson, D., & Kerner, J. (1992). Effects of microwave radiation on anti-infective factors in milk. *Pediatrics, 89,* 667–669.

Szmiglielski, S. (1996). Cancer morbidity in subjects occupationally exposed to high-frequency (radio frequency and microwave) electromagnetic radiation. *Science of the Total Environment, 180,* 9–17.

University of Louisville. (2005). Welcome to the MRI page. Retrieved from http://www.louisville.edu/~jcschw02/Welcome%20to%20the%20MRI%20Page.htm.

Unknown author. (1995). Do cellular phones cause headaches? *Microwave News,* November/December, 7–12.

Volkrodt, W. (1989). *Electromagnetic pollution of the environment.* In Krieps, R. (Ed.). *Environment and health: A holistic approach,* pgs. 71–76. Aldershot, England: Grower Publishing Company.

Weiss, M. (1983). The video display terminals—Is there a radiation hazard? *Journal of Occupational Medicine, 25,* 100.

Wertheimer, N., & Leeper, N. (1987). Possible effects of electric blankets and heated waterbeds on fetal development. *Bioelectromagnetics, 7,* 13–22.

World Health Organization. (2005). Electromagnetic fields and public health: Intermediate frequencies (IF). Information sheet, February. Retrieved from http://www.who.int/peh-emf/publications/facts/intmedfrequencies/en/.

World Health Organization. (2005). What are electromagnetic fields? Retrieved from http://www.who.int/peh-emf/about/WhatisEMF/en/.

Zubkova, S. (1996). Adaptive changes in the body upon exposure to electromagnetic radiation. *Biofizika, 41,* 917–922.

ASSIGNMENTS

1. Select information about radiation exposure and determine health risks to you and other citizens residing in your area.

2. Distinguish between the two types of radiation, their sources, and their risk to human health.

3. Find information about the Nuclear Regulatory Commission and nuclear power plant sites on the Internet. Summarize your findings and include the Web site URL where information was found.

4. After determining the amount of exposure you and members of your family have to electromagnetic radiation, determine potential dangers and ways that it could be reduced.

5. Take a stance on how you feel about the interstate transportation of nuclear waste to dumping sites and finding new locations for low-level radioactive waste.

6. Contrast the health effects of light to the negative effects of light.

7. Determine the difference between RF, IF, and ELF fields according to sources and potential health effects.

8. Search the literature to see what the radioactive exposure and potential health effects are for a CT scan and an MRI scan.

9. Call local cellular phone companies, radio stations, or television stations to find out where their microwave towers are located.

10. Keep a weekly log of the time you spend using a microwave, computer, and a cellular phone. Find a Web site that helps determine your exposure to electromagnetic radiation.

SELECTED ENVIRONMENTAL LAWS

1968 ***Comprehensive Radiation Health and Safety Act (PL 90-602)***

Established the regulation of hazardous waste management, set up performance standards to control emissions from ionizing radiation-emitting products, microwaves, radio frequencies, laser lights, sonic, infrasonic, and ultrasonic devices. Established requirements for notification by manufacturers of defects, repairs, or replacements. Required codes for reporting listed electronic products and electronic product radiation warnings. Charged the responsibility for determining the harmful effects of products and foods charged with radiation from the Public Health Service Bureau of Radiological Health to the Food and Drug Administration.

1969 ***National Environmental Policy Act (NEPA) (PL 91-190)***

Declared a national policy encouraging harmony between man and the environment, efforts to prevent or eliminate damage to the biosphere, enrich the understanding of ecosystems and natural resources, and establish a Council on Environmental Quality. Amended by PL 94-52 (1975), PL 94-83 (1975) and PL 97-258 (1982).

1997 *Electric and Magnetic Fields Research and Public Information Dissemination Program Act (PL 105-23)*
Extended the Electric and Magnetic Fields Research and Public Information Dissemination Program, a joint DOE and NIEHS venture for 1 year.

Health Physics
Health Physics Society Journal
Journal of Nuclear Biology and Medicine
Nuclear News
Nuclear Safety
Radiation and Environmental Biophysics
Radiation Protection Management
Radiological Protection Bulletin
RadWaste Magazine

ADDITIONAL READINGS

Alen, E. L. (1998). *Radiation biophysics,* 2nd edition. Englewood Cliffs: Prentice-Hall.

Ashton, J., & Laura, R. (1998). *The perils of progress: The health and environment hazards of modern technology and what you can do about them.* New York: Zed Books, Ltd.

Draganic, I., Dragonic, Z., & Adloff, J. (1993). *Radiation and radioactivity on earth and beyond.* Boca Raton, FL: CRC Press, LLC.

Eisenbud, M., & Gesell, T. (1983). *Environmental radioactivity.* Bethesda, MD: National Council on Radiation Protection and Measurements.

Environmental Protection Agency. (1994). *A citizen's guide to radon,* 2nd edition. Indoor Air and Radiation (6604J) 402-K92-001. Washington, DC: U.S. Government Printing Office.

Knoll, G. F. (1989). *Radiation detection and instrumentation,* 2nd edition. New York: John Wiley & Sons, Inc.

Ryder, A. (1997). *Light measurement handbook.* Retrieved from http://www.intl-light.com/handbook.

Valkovic, V. (2000). *Radioactivity in the environment.* New York: Elsevier.

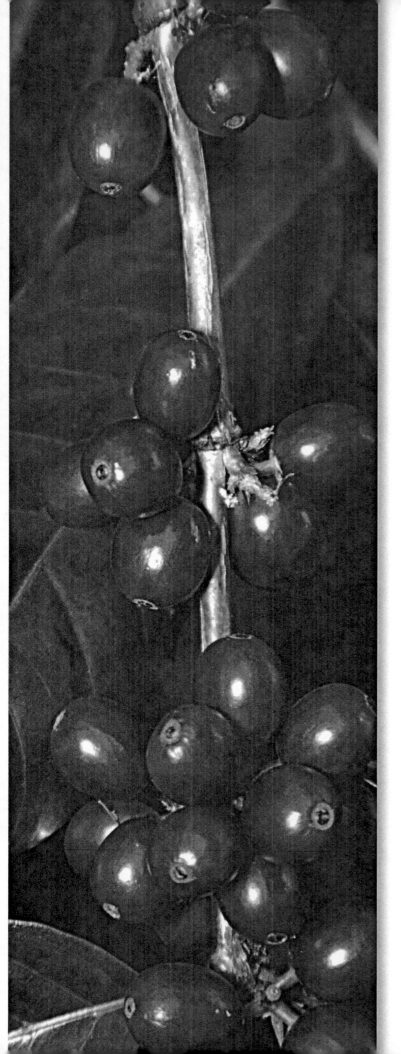

Food Safety Concerns

13

You are what you eat.

American proverb

To eat is a necessity, but to eat intelligently is an art.
La Rochefoucauld

OBJECTIVES

1. Name five federal laws protecting the quality of food.

2. Explain the contributions of Typhoid Mary and Upton Sinclair to food safety.

3. Provide an overview of several food-borne illnesses.

4. Describe the measures taken to assure food quality by food inspectors.

5. List the pros and cons of food irradiation.

6. Explain what is meant by the term organically grown.

7. Tell what consumers should look for on food labels to ensure quality and low exposure to harmful substances.

8. List substances or ingredients that may cause problems for individuals with food sensitivities.

9. Explain concerns about using hormones and antibiotics to produce meat.

10. Provide an overview of the potential for genetically engineered foods.

11. Differentiate various types of food recalls.

Introduction

ood safety has always been a concern and measures have been taken to improve food quality and preservation for quite a long time. The qualities of each food ingredient, their shelf life, the presence of contaminants, the preparation of foods, and the storage of foods are all very important. For the United States, the Food and Drug Administration (FDA) has the primary responsibility for inspecting and protecting the quality and safety of foods. The best scientific strategies are used to determine the risk and technologies to reduce risk. The incidence of food-borne illnesses is just one indicator that food safety should be addressed, particularly when a greater number of quantities of food are processed by several handlers. The knowledge of human behaviors and the consequences of these actions is also important. With just one error, many people can become ill from one food source, making it a public health and environmental health concern.

Efforts Toward Food Quality

n 1906, the Pure Food and Drug Act called for the inspection of foods and drugs for adulteration and mislabeling. Until then, substances such as borax, salicylic acid, and formaldehyde were used in foods, drinks, and medicines, as **adulterants** to "stretch" a product and increase profits. In 1907, 28 food inspectors were hired to inspect milk for the addition of water and chemicals, a common problem at the time. This was followed by the inspection of unprocessed foods such as eggs, poultry, and oysters because of poor refrigeration facilities in many establishments. Inspectors looked for sanitation, the health of company employees, and use of chemical preservatives and coloring. In 1937, one of the most tragic mass poisonings occurred when diethylene glycol was used as a solvent to make Elixir Sulfanilamide. One hundred and five patients died from its use (Wax, 1995). In response, Congress passed the 1938 Federal Food, Drug, and Cosmetic Act, requiring the proof of safety before a drug is released, for consumer protection. The law gave the FDA authority to confiscate adulterated drugs and determine the safety of new drugs. Three amendments to the law followed: the Pesticide Amendment of 1954, Food Additives Amendment of 1958 (PL 85-929), and Color Additives Amendment in 1960.

[handwritten margin note: When food law changed 1938]

Food-Borne Illnesses

ach year **food-borne illnesses** cause an estimated 76 million illnesses, 325,000 hospitalizations, and 52,000 deaths nationwide (CDC, 2002). Food-borne illnesses result from fecal **contamination**, improperly prepared foods, and infected food handlers. Meat, milk, eggs, and produce can be brought home from the store with fecal contamination. It is referred to as the "fecal-oral route" of transmission, when discussing illnesses associated with fecal contamination of food or water. Fecal contamination can occur through either sewage-contaminated water, improper meat processing procedures, or improper cooking.

Adulterant
An impure or inferior substance.

Food-borne illnesses
Sicknesses caused by pathogens that contaminate food.

Contamination
The act of soiling, corrupting, or infecting by contact or association; to make inferior or impure; to make unfit for use by the induction of unwholesome or undesirable elements.

Digging Deeper

HEALTHY PEOPLE OBJECTIVES 2010 RELATED TO FOOD SAFETY

10-1 Reduce infections caused by key food-borne pathogens (*Campylobacter* species, *E. coli*, *Listeria monocytogenes*, *Salmonella* species, *Cyclospora cayetanensis*, Postdiarrheal hemolytic uremic syndrome, congenital *Toxoplasma gondii*)

10-2 Reduce outbreaks of infections caused by key food-borne bacteria (*E. coli* and *Salmonella*).

10-3 Prevent an increase in the proportion of isolates of *Salmonella* species from humans and from animals (cattle, broilers, and swine) at slaughter that is resistant to antimicrobial drugs (Fluoroquinolones, third-generation cephalosporins, Gentamicin, Ampicilliin).

10-4 Reduce deaths from anaphylaxis caused by food allergies.

10-5 Increase the proportion of consumers who follow key food safety practices.

10-5.1 Improve food employee behaviors and food preparation practices that directly relate to food-borne illnesses in retail food establishments.

10-6 Reduce human exposure to organophosphate pesticides from food.

1785 Massachusetts passed the first comprehensive food adulteration law in the United States.
1850 Lemuel Shattuck's report for Massachusetts recommended control of *adulterated* food.
1862 Congress established the U.S. Department of Agriculture.
1906 The Pure Food and Drug Act prohibited mislabeled and adulterated foods, drinks, and drugs. The Federal Meat Inspection Act passed.
1917 The U.S. Food Administration (USDA) was established to supervise the food supply for World War I. The USDA issued the "five food group" dietary recommendations.
1924 Iodine was added to salt to prevent goiter.
1927 Food, Drug, and Insecticide Administration established.
1930 The Food, Drug, and Insecticide Administration was renamed the Food and Drug Administration (FDA).
1941 The FDA created standards for the enrichment of flour and bread with B-complex vitamins and iron.
1946 The National School Lunch Program was established.
1948 The Food Additives Amendment Act prohibited use of a food additive until safety was established by the manufacturer. The Delaney Clause prohibited carcinogenic additives. The Generally Recognized As Safe (GRAS) list was established.
1965 The Food Stamp Act was passed by Congress.
1967 Congress passed the first major meat inspection law requiring states to have inspection requirements at least equal to federal requirements.
1972 The Women, Infants, and Children (WIC) program was established. Amendments to Older Americans Act of 1965 established meal programs for senior centers and home delivery.
1984 The U.S. Surgeon General developed strategies for promoting breastfeeding.
1989 The National Academy of Sciences released a document describing the role of pesticides in agriculture and food safety.
1991 The FDA completed a study on America's dietary intake of pesticide residues.
1992 The use of and procedures for food irradiation was federally endorsed. The Food Guide Pyramid was published.
1993 The federal policy on pesticides was reversed in favor of "integrated pest management" with beneficial insects and crop rotation recommended.
1994 New food labels informing consumers of nutritional content of foods was required.
1996 The Food Quality Protection Act regulated pesticides to minimize risk to children.
1997 President Clinton announced a new "early warning system" called the Food Safety Initiative to help stop food-borne disease outbreaks.

Bacillus is a spore-forming bacterium found in soil, on vegetables, and in many raw and processed foods. Food poisoning results when foods are prepared and held before serving without adequate refrigeration. Foods most likely to contain *bacillus cereus* include cooked meat and vegetables, boiled or fried rice, vanilla sauce, custards, soups, and raw vegetable sprouts. Two types of illness have been attributed to the consumption of foods contaminated with *B. cereus*. The first is characterized by abdominal pain and diarrhea 4 to 16 hours after eating. The second is characterized by an acute attack of nausea and vomiting without diarrhea that occurs within 1 to 5 hours after consumption.

Campylobacter jejuni is associated with raw milk, sewage-contaminated water, undercooked poultry, nonchlorinated water, raw hamburger, and raw shellfish. It is the most common form of food poisoning in the United States, affecting 9 million people annually, causing approximately 9,000 deaths per year (Schewmake & Dillon, 1998). Campylobacteria are commonly found in the intestinal tracts of animals. The bacteria is easily killed when food is heated to an internal temperature of 160° F (Anonymous, 2005). Symptoms include fever, headache, and muscle pain followed by diarrhea, abdominal pain, and nausea appearing 2 to 5 days after eating the contaminated food. Serious complications can develop such as Guillain-Barre syndrome, arthritis, meningitis, or death (Blaser, 1997).

Clostridium botulinum is associated with home-canned foods, improperly baked potatoes in foil, refried beans, and honey. The harmful toxin produces symptoms of double vision, blurred vision, drooping eyelids, slurred speech, difficulty swallowing, dry mouth, and muscle weakness that may predict fatal symptoms such as paralysis and respiratory failure. *Clostridium perfringens* is not as severe as botulism (U.S. FDA, 1992).

E. coli is associated with meats and poultry, particularly ground meats. It has also been found in juices that have not undergone **pasteurization**, sprouts, lettuce, and other vegetables contaminated with manure. It accounts for 10,000 to 20,000 cases of food poisoning and 50 to 100 deaths per year. In order to decrease the possibility of an *E. coli* infection, produce items should be rinsed and meat should be cooked to 160° F or until there are no traces of pink color and juices run clear. Diarrhea may occur 1 to 3 days after consumption. Complications from *E. coli* include hemolytic uremic syndrome, thrombocytopenia purpura, seizures, and strokes.

George Soper, a civil engineer, known for his epidemiological analyses of typhoid fever epidemics, investigated typhoid fever outbreaks in New York City. Soper was hired by one of the families to investigate the cause of the family's affliction. Soper ruled out contaminated water and milk, clams, and direct contact as causes for the epidemic. He found that seven families affected with typhoid had one thing in common—the same cook. Mary Mallon, an Irish cook, was the first typhoid fever carrier to be identified and charted in North America. She worked for eight families in the New York area from 1906 to 1907.

Mary Mallon was apprehended in March of 1907 after attempting to throw Soper out of her house. Soper called Dr. Herman Biggs and Dr. S. Josephine Baker to intervene. Dr. Baker was sent to collect specimens from Mary Mallon for analysis. When Dr. Baker arrived, Mallon slammed the door in her face. The next day Dr. Baker returned with several police officers. Mallon ran into the house and was found hiding in a closet. She fought against having blood taken and was forcibly transported in an ambulance to Willard Parker Hospital where blood, urine, and feces were obtained. The blood and urine culture were negative but the stool culture was positive with typhoid bacilli. Health officials did not trust that she would behave in the public's interest and comply with public health codes so she was kept in custody at Riverside Hospital. While in custody, health officials tried to eliminate her infection, but at the time there were no antibiotics so treatment consisted of dietary measures and laxatives. Because the bacteria was not eliminated, Mallon concluded that the doctors did not know what they were doing.

Two years after her apprehension, she unsuccessfully sued for release. In 1910, it was decided that she had been retained long enough and was freed after 2 years and 11 months of incarceration. Mary was released with orders to take up a different occupation other than cooking and to return every 3 months to the laboratory for testing. The new health commissioner found work for her in a laundry, but she ignored her conditions of release and returned to cooking. Mallon disappeared and more than 5 years later, epidemiologists tracked her down when another typhoid outbreak was traced back to her kitchen. She was sent to North Brother Island, New York and was trained by a physician to work in the hospital laboratory (Leavitt, 1996). She suffered a paralyzing stroke in 1932 and died November 11, 1938. This case is historic because Mary Mallon, known as "Typhoid Mary," was denied her liberty for 26.5 years, in the interest of public health.

In retrospect, health officials only focused on elimination of the disease, rather than teaching Mallon ways to reduce the transmission of the disease by simply washing her hands and not preparing raw food. Judith Leavitt, author of *Typhoid Mary,* believes that Mary's personality contributed to her extreme treatment from health officials. She was Irish, a woman, had a temper, was not a "breadwinner," and did not believe she was a carrier.

Hepatitis A is transmitted in food either through an infected food handler or seafood contaminated by sewage waters. The incidence of food-borne Hepatitis A outbreaks in the United States is low. It is more common in areas where people live in crowded quarters, lack running water, and have poor sanitation. Symptoms include fatigue, poor appetite, fever, vomiting, dark-colored urine, and jaundice. Symptoms usually appear 3 to 4 weeks after exposure.

Listeria monocytogenes is associated with fecal-contaminated milk, processed meats (cold cuts and hot dogs), leafy vegetables, and processed cheeses. The pathogen can survive for long periods of time under adverse conditions and can grow under refrigeration. Only pasteurized dairy products should be consumed. Symptoms include fever, chills, headache, backache, abdominal pain and diarrhea 12 hours to 3 weeks after ingestion. The 10% mortality rate is high.

Norwalk viruses are associated with infected food handlers. Norwalk viruses are almost as common as the common cold. Sources include contaminated water, produce, and undercooked clams and oysters. Symptoms include nausea, vomiting, diarrhea, and some stomach cramping. The illness begins suddenly and the infected person may feel very sick for 1 to 2 days.

Another very common virus- associate w/ cruises

Salmonellosis is associated with poultry, meat, or eggs. To help prevent infection, eggs should be washed before they are cracked. An individual will develop diarrhea, headaches, stomach cramps, nausea, and vomiting within 12 to 24 hours.

Pasteurization
The process of heating milk or juices before they are consumed or processed to make other foods.

Mary Mallon, otherwise known as "Typhoid Mary," was the first healthy carrier of typhoid fever identified in the United States. Mary's case is unique because she was arrested in 1907 and kept in quarantine, violating her civil rights as we know them today.

Mary Mallon was accountable for 47 illnesses and 3 deaths. She was not, however, the most deadly carrier. In 1922, a typhoid fever outbreak occurred in New Jersey, resulting in 87 cases and 2 deaths. One man was responsible for 35 cases and 3 deaths in New York City. This man was not ar-rested and placed in jail. He was employed as a laborer in building construction work and added to a list of carriers. He was required to report to public health officials weekly. Tony Labella, another carrier, caused 122 people to become ill, five of whom died. Labella was isolated for 2 weeks and then released. In 1924, Alphonse Cotils, a New York City bakery and restaurant owner, was identified as a carrier and forbidden to prepare food in his own restaurant. He later appeared in court, guilty of preparing food against orders. The judge let him remain free if he promised not to handle food and to conduct his business over the phone.

Because Mary Mallon and Alphonse Cotils broke health codes after being told of their health status, New York City began to examine the health of food handlers. In 1928, 29 new chronic carriers were identified. It was estimated that 3% of those who had typhoid fever became carriers, creating 90 to 135 new carriers per year. By 1938, 394 typhoid fever carriers were identified.

Sources: Brooks, 1996; Leavitt, 1992; Leavitt, 1996; Marr, 1999; Mendelsohn, 1995.

 Measures to reduce or eliminate the threat of food poisoning include (Kramer and Gilbert, 1989; Reed, 1994):

- Avoid preparing food too far in advance of planned service.

- Avoid holding cooked foods at room temperature.

- Use **quick chill** methods by storing food in shallow containers to cool foods below 45° F within 4 hours of preparation.

- If the food is especially thick (e.g., refried beans), store no more than 3 inches deep.

- Hold or store hot foods above 140° F until served.

- Reheat foods rapidly to 165° F or above.

Shigella is contracted through the fecal-oral route of infection or from eating food contaminated by infected food handlers, sewage-contaminated vegetables, flies, contaminated drinking water, swimming in contaminated water, or changing diapers. Symptoms include acute abdominal pain, watery diarrhea, nausea, vomiting, and fever. Blood or pus is sometimes found in the stool. The illness usually develops 1 to 2 days after consuming contaminated food. It is more severe than most forms of gastroenteritis, producing toxins similar to *E. coli*.

Staphlococcus aureus is normally present on the skin, nose, and throat of most people. It is also found in pus of wounds, acne pimples, and boils. It is associated with infected food handlers and is involved in 20 to 40% of all food poisonings. It is usually associated with foods such as desserts, salads (such as egg salad, tuna salad, chicken salad, potato salad, and macaroni salad), or baked goods (especially custards, mayonnaise, and cream-filled or topped desserts) that are served or stored at room or refrigerator temperature. Foods should be kept hot (above 140° F) or cold (below 40° F) during serving time. Leftovers should be refrigerated and frozen as quickly as possible. Symptoms develop within 6 to 12 hours and include nausea, vomiting, stomach distention, and diarrhea.

Vibrio vulnificus is a naturally occurring bacteria present in coastal waters. It may be present in uncooked shellfish, primarily oysters, clams, and mussels. The FDA estimates that 5 to 10% of all shellfish are contaminated with the bacterium (Food Safety Net, 1999). This can usually be detected, especially if foam is present when the shell is open. It is always best to steam the shellfish until the shell opens completely or it can be deep fried. Symptoms include fever, chills, nausea, vomiting, diarrhea, abdominal pain, and stupor. Vibrio bacteria are responsible for many food-borne illnesses including *Vibrio cholerae* (cholera) and *Vibrio parahaemolyticus*.

Food Handling

The handling of food products is very important to prevent food-borne infections. Animals raised for food consumption have *Campylobacter, E. coli,* and *Salmonella* in their gastrointestinal tracts. There are multiple ways animal products can be contaminated. Processed meats pose the greatest dangers of food-borne illnesses because they are handled more. In 1906, the Meat Inspection Act created meat inspection procedures. In 1967, a new act required states to uphold standards for meat production at the same level as government authorities. The slaughtering, cold storage, freezing, smoking, and pickling of fresh meats is inspected by the U.S. Department of Agriculture (USDA) (Figure 13-1). Meat is graded according to its quality.

Poultry and red meats frequently are contaminated with food-borne pathogens (Zhao et al., 2001). In a recent study, the majority (70.7%) of chicken samples ($n = 184$) were contaminated with *Campylobacter* (Zhao et al., 2001). Safe handling and cooking of poultry meats is essential to prevent food-borne illnesses. The primary bacteria concerned with red meats is *E. coli.* When the meat of several animals is ground together, the possibility of contamination increases. Contaminated meat often looks and smells normal, so the contamination often is undetected until large numbers of people are infected. In 1982, *E. coli* made headlines when several people became sick and small children died from eating meat from a Jack-in-the-Box restaurant in Washington. As a result of that and subsequent outbreaks, President Clinton proposed a $43 million Food Safety Initiative designed to reduce food-borne illness by strengthening and improving food safety practices and policies (FDA, 1999). The President's Council on Food Safety was established to make recommendations. In 1998, the USDA implemented new regulations for major meat and poultry slaughter and processing plants, establishing Hazard Analysis and Critical Control Points (HACCP). This was followed by putting HAACP regulations into effect for seafood, and by developing plans to apply regulations to the production of fruits, vegetables, eggs, and egg products. In addition, Food-borne Diseases Active Surveillance Network (FoodNet) sites at state health departments were established to track cases of food-borne infection by building a national "fingerprinting" database of bacterial DNA. The result was PulseNet, a computerized database of bacterial DNA subtypes. The National Antimicrobial Resistance Monitoring System (NARMS) was also developed to improve our ability to detect emerging bacteria resistant to antibiotics. Federal agencies are actively involved in supporting and promoting the Fight BAC! campaign, launched by the public/private Partnership for Food Safety Education.

Fish is processed much like beef products, held just above freezing for 2 weeks to enhance the flavor of the meat. Shellfish such as raw or undercooked oysters, clams, and mussels have the highest risk of transmitting seafood illnesses. Clams and oysters process 15 to 20 gallons of water per day, thus storing bacteria and viruses if they are grown in polluted waters. Forty-eight states have

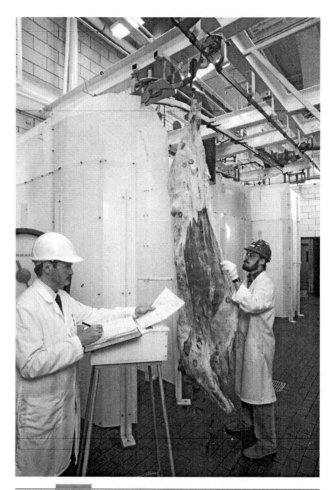

FIGURE 13-1 **Checking Washed Carcasses for Microbes** The U.S. Department of Agriculture has an important role in determining the quality and safety for meat.

fish advisories regarding mercury contamination from waters polluted by power plants, industrial sites, and incinerators. Other contaminants include PCBs, chlordane, dioxins, and DDT.

Milk, eggs, and dairy products can contain food-borne pathogens from infected animals. Milk products must be filtered and cooled immediately after milking. Milk should also be pasteurized to destroy disease-causing pathogens. After pasteurizing, milk should be cooled and bottled. Milk sales are monitored in grocery stores, dairy farms, and health food stores so that the products are not sold after their expiration date. On July 1, 1999, the Clinton Administration announced two new measures to improve the safety of shell eggs in order to reduce the number of illnesses and deaths associated with outbreaks of *Salmonella enteritidis* (SE). The FDA published the first

Quick chill
The method of putting food in shallow containers for quick cooling in the refrigerator.

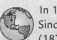
In 1906, Upton Sinclair (1879–1968) shook the meat industry with his book *The Jungle*, revealing unhygienic practices in Chicago's stockyards and meat-packing plants. Confirmed by public health inspectors, public alarm led to the enactment of the 1906 Pure Food and Drug Act. In 1967, Sinclair was invited by President Lyndon B. Johnson to witness the signing of The Wholesome Meat Act, designed to eliminate loop holes in meat-inspection regulations.

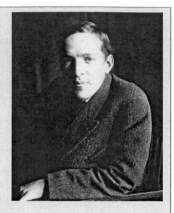

Food Code to encompass recommendations for all types of retail level establishments in 1993 and has published revisions of it in 1995, 1997, and 1999.

Food Irradiation

The concept of food **irradiation** to kill bacteria was developed in 1886 when it was determined that X-rays could kill bacteria (Wills, 1986). The practice began in 1905 when radiant energy was used to preserve food by eliminating spoilage microorganisms. In 1921, X-rays were used to kill *Trichinella spiralis* nematodes in pork. The first commercial food irradiation was in 1937 in Germany, when spices used in sausages were sterilized, using irradiation technology. After World War II, there was rapid growth of nuclear technology. Nuclear reactors produce an excess of high energy neutrons that convert to unstable radioactive isotopes more penetrable than X-rays. The development of food irradiation, using gamma rays, X-rays, or electron beams, emerged with the growth of the nuclear industry. Since the 1970s, the National Aeronautics and Space Administration (NASA) has used irradiation for foods consumed by astronauts (Wood and Bruhn, 2000). Irradiation is used for security checks at airports, destroying bacteria in cosmetics, and to sterilize the anthrax found in U.S. mail in 2001 (Brennand, 1995).

The first use of irradiation for controlling foodborne pathogens in the United States began in 1983, restricting the use of spices and vegetable seasonings (Steele, 2001). The use was extended for pathogen control to dry enzyme preparations in 1985, to raw pork in 1986, to raw poultry in 1992, to beef and lamb by 1997, to refrigerated and frozen raw meat and meat

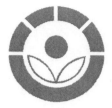

FIGURE 13-2 **Radura Label** This label is found on irradiated foods to warn consumers.

products by 2000, and ground hamburger by 2002 (Frenzen et al., 2000; International Food Information Council, 2003).

Food irradiation is also called "cold pasteurization" or "irradiation pasteurization" (Morehouse, 1998). Extremely short wavelengths of radiation from Cobalt 60, Cesium 137, X-rays, or high-energy electron beams penetrate food and the molecular structure of the food is disrupted. According to the International Food Information Council, irradiated food is safe because the food moves through the energy field but never touches the energy source (IFIC, 2003a). The use of a microwave is also considered irradiation. Microwave radiation has short waves that selectively heat water in food, causing the food to cook. Conventional heat radiation has long waves and is generated from grilling or cooking food. Pathogens, worms, and other parasites are killed by the heat.

Irradiation kills or inactivates *E.coli 0157:H7, bacillus cereus, clostridium botulinum, Listeria monocytogenes, salmonella, staphylococcus aureus, campylobacter jejuni, Cyclospora,* and *toxoplama gondii.* Not all microorganisms on food are vulnerable to irradiation. Insects, parasites, and bacteria are sensitive to irradiation, but viruses, spores, cysts, toxins, and prions are not. An amendment to the Food and Drug and Cosmetic Act of 1958 considered irradiation as a food additive, regulated by the FDA. The FDA approves ionizing radiation sources and doses, the nutritional adequacy of foods, and food safety. Facilities where foods are irradiated are also regulated by the National Environmental Policy Act of 1969 (Shea, 2000). The FDA requires the labeling of irradiated foods with the Radura logo (Figure 13-2) (FSIS, 1998).

Concerns about food irradiation include:

1. food quality, such as changes to the **glycemic index** of foods

2. destruction or alternation of vitamins (especially **antioxidants**) in foods that protect against cancer and heart disease and are relatively sensitive to radiation

3. loss of **nutrients** because irradiated foods can be stored longer

These concerns are outweighed, however, by the fact that not all foods in the American diet are irradiated. In

Digging Deeper WHAT CONSUMERS KNOW ABOUT FOOD SAFETY

A study commissioned by the U.S. Department of Agriculture in 1998 and conducted by the Research Triangle Institute in North Carolina revealed that there are shortfalls in consumer knowledge and actions regarding food safety. Approximately 76 million people in the United States contract food-borne illnesses annually. Pathogens are responsible for most of them (CDC, 2005). The report found that safer food handling practices have improved in the last few years, including checking expiration dates. However, consumers still skip safety measures such as proper hand washing and properly defrosting meat and poultry. One reason for this is that most consumers get their information from food labels, packaging, and television or radio news. After listening to the media, consumers appear more confident about the safety of meat and poultry than they did before 1996. Many consumers believe that most food-borne illnesses are caused by food processors and food handlers in restaurants, believing that the risk of food-borne illnesses is higher outside the home. In fact, experts estimate that half of all *Salmonella* cases result from unsafe handling of food at home. Sources: CDC, 2005; Consumer Information Center, 2005.

---

fact, irradiated foods account for a very small portion of foods on the market. Part of the reason is because of the cost. It costs more to transport them to and from irradiation units, use the special handling techniques to irradiate them, and put on the special Radura labels (Frenzen et al., 2000).

There are some concerns about harm to children and the elderly and the regulation of companies that irradiate food. Early studies warned of potential harm to animal health showing tumors, reduced growth rates, lower birth weights, kidney damage, changes in white blood cells, and genetic damage (Barna, 1979). Researchers found that children in India who were fed irradiated wheat developed cells with an abnormal number of chromosomes that increased as the exposure increased (Bhaskaram and Sadasivan, 1975). However, other laboratories have failed to demonstrate that irradiation causes mutations in humans.

In spite of indications that it may be harmful, food irradiation is endorsed by the American Dietetic Association, American Medical Association, United Nations Food and Agriculture, World Health Organization, and other public health agencies.

Consumer attitudes toward irradiation of foods are favorable, depending on what they know. In a study by CDC's FoodNet, only half of consumers were willing to buy irradiated products and only one-fourth were willing to pay more for them (Frenzen et al, 2000). Once consumers understand that irradiation helps kill pathogens and extend the **shelf life** of foods, they are more likely to approve of it. In fact, in similar studies, findings were that consumers were more likely to endorse the purchase of irradiated foods than they were 10 years prior. Consumers expressed more concern for pesticide and animal residues, growth hormones, food additives, bacteria, and naturally occurring toxins than for irradiation (Rippel, 2002; Johnson et al., 2004).

 The term *radiation* is commonly used to cover a wide spectrum of energy. Radiation leads to the formation of ions, known as "ionizing radiation." Ions dissociate into "free radicals," which are extremely reactive chemically and alter biological structures such as chromosomes, proteins, enzymes, nucleic acids, lipids, and carbohydrates. It kills cells by fragmenting DNA and lowering biochemical reactions (Steele, 2001). In low doses it is used to kill parasites, in medium doses it is used to reduce cooking time and extend the shelf life of foods, and in higher doses, it is used to sterilize meat, poultry, and seafood as well as disinfect herbs, spices, and teas (Morehouse, 1998). Irradiation is desirable because it does not substantially alter the nutritional value of foods and is no more harmful than a dental x-ray.

Irradiation
The use of radiation to destroy harmful bacteria and insects before food is sold.

Glycemic index
A numerical index given to a carbohydrate-rich food based on the average increase of serum glucose levels after the food is consumed.

Antioxidants
Substances that inhibit oxidation or reactions promoted by oxygen.

Nutrients
A substance providing nourishment.

Shelf life
The length of time a product may be stored without becoming spoiled or unsuitable for consumption.

Food Purchase Selections: Let the Buyer Beware!

The source of foods is important, but hard to control if purchased from a grocery store. Most foods sold in the United States are grown in the United States, but some foods are imported. The country of export is important because some foods grown in other countries are contaminated with DDT (banned in the United States), other toxins, or contaminated land or water. At "health foods" stores, sometimes unpasteurized products are for sale. Many **organic** products have a short shelf life. Be careful about buying foods from bulk, because they are more likely to have contaminants in them from insects and vermin. A certain amount of food contaminants, such as hair, feces, dirt, and other particles are acceptable, according to the FDA because they do not cause food-borne illnesses. Consumers should give careful thought to the foods they select to take home or consume away from home. Fast food establishments, restaurants, bakeries, coffee shops, and outdoor vendors are required by law to follow food regulations, but they are not always consistent. Some health departments rate restaurants based on past performance and inspections. These ratings are not always available when a consumer frequents the restaurant.

Food Additives

Over 2,800 food additives are used to modify the appearance, flavor, texture, or storage properties of foods. **Enhancers** are added to improve the quality, flavor, and texture of food or food preservatives. Food **additives** used to enhance the quality of food often enrich the food with nutrients such as iodine, thiamine (vitamin B_1), riboflavin (vitamin B_2), niacin (vitamin B_{12}), iron (ferrous sulfate), or iodine. Flavor enhancers include monosodium glutamate (MSG) and spices such as salt, pepper, garlic, cinnamon, cloves, mustard, ginger, and nutmeg. **Emulsifiers** such as propylene glycol; stabilizers such as agar-agar, bean gum, and guar gum; or thickeners such as pectin and gelatin enhance the texture of foods. Benzol peroxide is used to bleach food and carotenes are added for a yellow color.

> Foods should not be purchased if the packages are torn or leaking. Bent cans are also not a good idea because contaminants may leach into the food. Do not buy foods after the expiration date has expired. Meat packages that have a cloudy or "bulging" appearance may be an indication of bacteria.

Sugar, salt, vinegar, ascorbic acid (vitamin C), and potassium permanganate are used to preserve food. Ascorbic acid is added to meat to give it a fresh, red color. BHA and BHT, nitrites, and sulfites are also used to preserve food. As a result of the Delaney Clause of 1958, food additives have been regulated by the FDA. It is always a good idea to read the label, particularly if a member of the family has any food sensitivities.

Food Sensitivities

Some individuals, particularly those with allergies of any kind, are sensitive to food products. Some individuals are allergic to foods such as eggs, wheat, milk, nuts, soy, shellfish, or food additives such as sulfites and MSG. Sensitivity to sulfites and monosodium glutamate are described because they are food additives.

SULFITES

Sulfur-based preservatives, or *sulfites,* have been used around the world for centuries to inhibit oxidation (browning) of light-colored fruits and vegetables, prevent melanosis (black spot) on seafood, discourage bacterial growth as wine ferments, condition dough, bleach food starches, and maintain the stability and potency of some medications. Sulfites are safe for most people, but asthmatics and other sensitive individuals may experience harmful side effects (Papazian, 1996). One in 100 people are allergic to sulfites, particularly those with asthma. Sulfites are known to induce a severe reaction in 1.7% of asthmatics (IFIC, 2003b) and 5% of those people who have asthma have severe reactions. Foods most likely to cause immediate problems are those on which sulfites are sprayed (such as lettuce) or a beverage (such as beer or wine). The most severe reaction occurs when the sulfites are part of the food itself. Sulfites are found in a variety of cooked and processed foods (including baked goods;

FOOD ADDITIVES	
Antioxidants	BHA, BHT, propyl propyl gallate
Emulsifiers	Lecithin, monoglycerides, diglycerides, sorbitan monostearates, polysorbates
Humectants	Sorbitol, glycerol, propylene glycol
Preservatives	Sodium propionate, sodium benzoate, propionic acid
Bleaching agents	Benzoyl peroxide, chlorine, nitrosyl chloride
Sweeteners	Sorbitol, mannitol, xylitol, corn syrup

condiments; dried and glacéed fruit; jams; gravy; dehydrated, pre-cut or peeled "fresh" potatoes; molasses; shrimp; and soup mixes), beverages (such as beer, wine, hard cider, fruit and vegetable juices, and tea), and dried fruits. Because sulfites were harmful and perhaps dangerous to some individuals, the FDA took regulatory actions in 1986 to ban the use of sulfites on raw fruits and vegetables and require that product labels indicate sulfating agent used at 10 ppm or higher in the products (as in dried apricots, canned vegetables, maraschino cherries, and guacamole). FDA regulations do not require managers of food service establishments to disclose whether sulfites were used in food preparation.

MONOSODIUM GLUTAMATE

Monosodium glutamate (MSG) is used in foods as a flavor enhancer. It is found in many foods served in restaurants, and also can be found in processed meats, frozen entrees, ice cream, frozen yogurt, some crackers, breads, canned tuna, and quite often in low-fat and no-fat foods. Many individuals are sensitive to the glutamate properties in it, especially asthmatics.

MSG is an amino acid with less sodium than table salt. In 1968, a physician described a collection of symptoms he allegedly experienced after eating Chinese food. At the time, MSG was commonly used in soups at Chinese restaurants to enhance the flavors. He coined the symptoms "Chinese Restaurant Syndrome." His symptoms included numbness at the back of the neck and a feeling of pressure in the face and upper chest muscles (Kwok, 1968). Others reported burning sensations, flushing, and headache. Since then several double-blind studies have been conducted indicating that the symptoms may be histamine reactions unrelated to MSG. As a result of these studies, MSG is now considered to be a safe food additive. To assure those who experience sensitivity to

MSG, labels require that it be listed if it is used as an ingredient (IFICF, 2001).

The "MSG complex syndrome" symptoms include burning sensation in the back of the neck, forearms, and chest; numbness in the back of the neck, radiating to the arms and back; a tingling, warmth, or weakness in the face, temples, upper back, neck, and arms; facial pressure or tightness; chest pain; headache; nausea; rapid heartbeat; bronchospasm; drowsiness; and weakness. Symptoms occur within 1 hour after eating MSG on an empty stomach or without other food. A reaction is most likely if the MSG is eaten in a large quantity or in a liquid, such as a clear soup.

Questionable Ingredients

ood substitutes such as cyclamates, aspartame, olestra, and others have been criticized as creating long-term health concerns (National Cancer Institute, 1997). Cyclamates and saccharin were associated with bladder cancer in laboratory animals and were taken off the market at one time. Cyclamates are also associated with high blood pressure, genetic damage, and testicular atrophy. Aspartame has been associated with ir-

---

Organic
The production of food or material with animal or plant materials, but without the use of pesticides.

Enhancers (as in food enhancers)
Something added to food to increase or improve value, quality, desirability, or attractiveness.

Additives (as in food additive)
Something added to enhance food to improve flavor, appearance, or to extend shelf-life.

Emulsifier
To stabilize in a liquid form.

Consider the Cost GREEN STORES

In most communities, a number of merchants sell all-natural products, organic foods, and environmentally friendly products. In addition, there are often farmers markets where fresh produce can be purchased. There are co-ops in which members pay a fee so that food items can be purchased in bulk, in their raw or natural form, or from local people. Milk, cheese, honey, and homemade items are just some of the items local farmers may bring to the market. Some may offer herbs that can be used for cooking and medicinal purposes. Some may sell clothing, bags, rugs, wall hangings, and other products made with jute, cotton, and other natural materials. Some may sell books on how to relax, cook vegetarian dishes, use natural substances for self-treatment, and exercise. Some sell hypoallergenic and biodegradable products. Some may sell food items that are not available in local grocery stores such as rice milk, soy milk, and other food alternatives. Some sell personal hygiene products such as deodorants, lotions, toothpaste, ointments, and others made from natural products or do not contain ingredients suspected to cause harm. There are usually cleaning products that are less harmful than what is normally found in other stores. There may be plants that are noted for their air-cleaning, low-maintenance, medicinal, or space-saving properties. Co-ops require that members help package bulk products or work in the store to keep costs down.

ritability, mood disorders, and sleep problems in some individuals; other reported side effects include headaches and heart palpitations (Pivonka & Grunewald, 1990). Acesulfame-K has been associated with cancer and insulin production in laboratory animals. Consumer demand advocated for reintroduction of the products. Olestra, a synthetic fat-substitute has caused gastrointestinal problems in users and efforts to market it have been reduced, although the product is still available.

MEATS

Meats that are cured, such as bacon or ham, contain sodium nitrate which converts to nitrosamines, a carcinogenic compound. Nitrosamines are also found in meats smoked or grilled on a charcoal grill; residues from the smoke attach to the meat. Liquid "smoke" products can be used instead of grilling but these also have substances that may be harmful to some people. It is a good idea to eat grilled foods only occasionally.

TABLE 13-1 Non-nutritive Sweeteners

Sugar Substitute	Brand Names	Sugar Equivalent	Uses	Cautions
Saccharin	Sucaryl, Sugar Twin, Sweet 'N Low, Sweet Magic	200 to 700 times sweeter than sugar	Diet soft drinks, baked goods, and tabletop sweetener in restaurants	Saccharin is a sulfonamide known to cause dermatological reactions in those who are allergic to sulfa drugs, especially children. Side effects include itching, blotchy skin discolorations, eczema, photosensitivity, prurigo, wheezing, nausea, diarrhea, tongue blisters, tachycardia, fixed eruptions, headache, increased urination, or sensory neuropathy.
Aspartame	NutraSweet, Equal, Spoonful, Natra Taste	160 to 220 times sweeter than sugar	Beverages, breakfast cereals, desserts, chewing gum, and a tabletop sweetener	Some people experience side effects that include nausea, burning with urination, and headaches. It will cause dangerously high levels of phenylalanine in people with **phenylketonuria (PKU)**.
Sucralose	Splenda	600 times sweeter than sugar	Baked goods, soft drinks, chewing gum, frozen dairy desserts, fruit juices, and gelatins	
Acesulfame-K	Sunette, Sweet One	200 times sweeter than sugar	Used in dry mixes and chewing gum. It can be used in baked goods, frozen desserts, candies, and beverages	
Neotame		7,000 to 13,000 times sweeter than sugar	Baked goods, soft drinks, chewing gum, gelatins and puddings, confections and frostings, jams, jellies, processed fruits, and fruit juices	Similar side effects to aspartame.

Sources: American Dietetic Association. (1998). Position statement: Use of nutritive and nonnutritive sweeteners. *Journal of the American Dietetic Association, 98,* 580.

Earles, J. (2003) Sugar-free blues. Everything you wanted to know about artificial sweeteners. Article from *Wise Traditions in Food, Farming, and the Healing Arts,* quarterly magazine of the Weston A. Price Foundation. Retrieved from http://www.westonaprice.org/modernfood/sugarfree_blues.html.

University of Iowa Health Care. (2003). Sugar substitutes. HIL File NUTR4838.RF2 VRS# 6979. Retrieved from http://www.uihealthcare.com/topics/nutrition/nutr4838.html.

PRODUCE

Some produce items may have pesticide residues, particularly those with porous skins such as peaches, strawberries and raspberries (Figure 13-3). Because of this residue, it is a good idea to wash all produce before serving. In some cases, peeling the skin may be the best way to remove all pesticide residues. There was much debate regarding the risk of pesticide residues on food. Under the Federal Food, Drug, and Cosmetic Act (FFDCA), the Environmental Protection Agency (EPA) was responsible for establishing tolerances for pesticide residues in or on foods. Under the Delaney Clause, pesticides are considered a food additive with some risk of cancer in humans or animals, and should not be permitted. Because it was estimated that the risk was one in a million, the risk was considered to be "negligible" (Vogt, 1992). There was debate concerning the effects of pesticide residues on young children because they consumed larger amounts of food per body weight (EPA, 1988). The outcome was the development of the Food Quality Protection Act of 1996, setting tolerance levels for children and pesticide residues (NCSE, 1996).

Hormones in Meat

For some time, growth hormones have been permitted to hasten accelerated weight gain in cattle and chickens. In the 1970s, diethylstilbestrol (DES) was given to chickens and cattle. The chemical was said to have "chemically castrated" cattle, enabling them to grow faster. DES was also used as a drug in human medicine (Gandhi & Snedeker, 2000). Because of concerns about the effects of DES on the offspring of women who used it, DES was outlawed for veterinary use in the mid-1970s.

The hormones approved for use in the United States include estradiol, testosterone, progesterone, trenbolone acetate, and zeranol. The FDA approved these hormones because they believed no physiological effect could be expected in individuals consuming meat from hormone-treated livestock. Testosterone and progesterone are produced by humans as part of normal functioning and maturation of every mammal. No monitoring is done for the naturally occurring hormones. The FDA maintains that because humans produce some of these hormones (also known as anabolic steroids), themselves, the amount of hormones from food is insignificant. Trenbolone acetate and zeranol are synthetic hormones. The FDA required extensive testing to determine tissue residue tolerance levels before they were approved for use. The Food Safety and Inspection Service (FSIS) of the USDA conducts the National Residue Program to prevent the marketing of animals containing unacceptable levels of animal drugs, pesticides, and other chemicals.

> *Phenylketonuria*
> A condition in which a person's mind does not work properly due to an accumulation of the amino acid phenylaline.

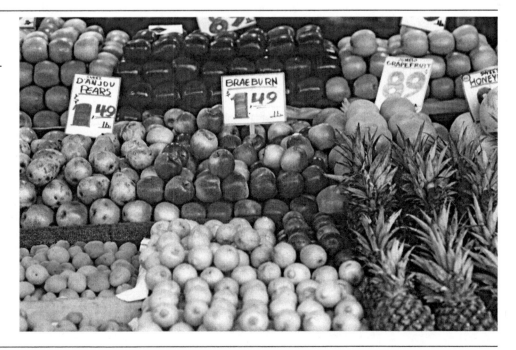

FIGURE 13-3 Produce Section of the Grocery Store Produce can be brought in from many countries. It is a good idea to wash before eating.

The environmental concern regarding hormone use in meat-producing animals is the hormone content in the excrement. Researchers from Munich, Germany reported that the manure of Holstein cattle (Figure 13-4) receiving trenbolone hormones contained 10% of the hormones they were given. They also observed how long it took to breakdown in the manure and that drugs resisted bacterial breakdown until the manure was spread over fields and dried. Studies were conducted from water sites downstream from feedlots in Nebraska, reporting estrogenic and androgenic pollutants at downstream sites, which were sometimes two to four times that of the upstream site (Soto et al., 2004). Researchers found that fathead minnows in the waters had significantly reduced head and testis size. Effects on minnows for 21 days of exposure to trenbolone in a laboratory setting revealed tubercles on the heads of female minnows, normally observed only in males. The females also produced less eggs (Raloff, 2002). Similar findings were observed when elevated blood concentrations of egg-yolk protein were found in female turtles at nearby ponds, creating superfemales (Irwin et al., 2001). These findings have generated concerns about finding pharmaceuticals in runoff as well.

Antibiotics in Meat

antibiotics are used on meat-producing animals to prevent the onset or progression of a disease when animals are cultivated in close quarters and to enhance weight gain (Gustafson & Bowen, 1997). This practice began in 1985 and has been monitored because of consumer concerns. The problem with giving animals antibiotics is that the drugs can create resistance to antibiotics by consumers of the meat. However, the risk is no greater than when physicians overprescribe antibiotics to humans or people fail to complete an antibiotic regimen on their own. Another

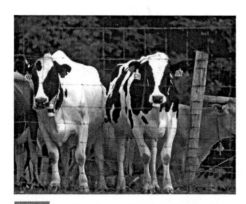

FIGURE 13-4 **Cattle to Be inspected for Mad Cow Disease** Bovine spongiform disease (BSE) can be found where cattle are fed bonemeal.

concern is that people allergic to certain antibiotics, such as sulfa drugs may have adverse reactions from consuming meat from treated animals. As a general rule, animals should not be slaughtered within 60 to 90 days after given the antibiotic. Meat from slaughtered animals is tested prior to being packaged and sold. Additionally, pathogens in meat are becoming antibiotic resistant.

Genetically Engineered Foods

cientists have been cross-breeding and creating hybrid seeds for many years. The process of biotechnology has recently begun genetic engineering to produce plants that are easier to grow and less susceptible to insects and other pests. Less pesticides and herbicides are needed, giving support to being more environmentally friendly (Charman, 2002). Approximately 70 to 75% of all processed foods in America contain **genetically engineered** ingredients. Foods that have been genetically engineered include canola, radicchio lettuce, corn, cotton, papaya, potato, soybean, tomato, yellow crookneck squash, sugar beets, and rice. Corn and soybeans are the most frequently engineered crops. Some of the corn and soybeans are used to make vaccines and antibiotics, but most of it is fed to livestock.

Genetic engineering involves introducing the DNA from another plant (called a *transgene*) into a host plant using bacteria or a *gene gun* (FDA, 2003). The genetically engineered plants are used to develop pest-resistant plants, plants with increased nutritional value, plants for vaccines and antibiotics, and to make some plants more **nutrient dense**. The genes from a soil bacterium and two genes from a daffodil are inserted into rice to create golden rice with beta-carotene. It is hoped that countries dependent on rice as a staple food will experience less vitamin A deficiency because of this process. Genetically engineered products are regulated by the EPA and USDA.

Genetically engineered foods are being sold without extensive research because they fall under the 1938 Food, Drug, and Cosmetic Act stating that any product made up of proteins, fats, and carbohydrates with a safe history does not need to be approved by the FDA prior to being sold. To date the only concern about consuming genetically engineered foods is food allergies. Individuals allergic to peanuts may be allergic to a food item genetically engineered with peanut genes. A 50% increase in allergies to soy products has been reported since 1998 from the same genetically engineered soybean source (Keeler, 2001). The FDA does not require that the product be labelled unless the product may cause an allergy in some individuals, and that requirement is voluntary. At this time, it is difficult for consumers to know whether or not they are purchasing a product made with genetically engineered foods. Potential long-term effects of genetically

Vegetarians do not eat meat products, but do eat some animal products such as milk, yogurt, cheese, and eggs. Vegans are strict vegetarians who do not eat dairy, eggs, or meat products. Some vegetarians do not eat meat because they cannot tolerate the idea of potential mistreatment or slaughtering of animals. Others simply cannot afford the extra expense of a meat-eater's diet. Some vegetarians adhere to recommendations by their religious beliefs and others simply enjoy eating a healthier diet. The average American consumes more meat than needed for the daily nutritional requirements for protein. Nonmeat sources of protein

(incomplete proteins) combined together form a complete protein containing the same amino acids as meat. Protein can be found in grains, soy products, legumes (lentils, beans, and peanuts), nuts, seeds, and many fruits and vegetables. Vegans must be very conscientious in order to get the protein they need. Most people combine these sources with dairy or egg products to boost the protein content of their meals. An example of how foods can be combined together to form a complete protein are as follows:

Bagel and cream cheese
Cereal and milk
Nacho chips and cheese dip

Pasta or macaroni and cheese
Peanut butter on toast
Red beans and rice
Rice and peas
Tortillas and beans

The advantages to eating a nonmeat diet include less weight gain because there is less fat in vegetable products than meat products, particularly red meat. In addition, there is less cholesterol. Certain vegetable sources of protein, such as soybeans, have additional health benefits such as phytoestrogens that help prevent osteoporosis and cancer of the breast and prostate (Halstead, 2003).

In 1990, chocolate chip cookies promoted as weight loss aids and a partial cure for colon cancer were recalled by the FDA. Review of the cookies revealed that they contained twice the calories, half the fiber, and five times the fat declared in the labeling.

In April of 2001, a preterm male infant died from *E. sakazakii,* a bacterial infection that was traced back to his infant formula, made from a powdered product (Himelright et al., 2002). The FDA routinely tests powdered infant formulas now.

In 2000, Mission Foods recalled 300 yellow corn products, including corn tortillas made from corn meal produced by StarLink (Anonymous, 2000; FDA, 2000). The tortillas were made from a genetically modified hybrid yellow corn containing Cry9C, which is approved by the EPA for animal and industrial use, but because of allergen sensitivity, not human consumption. The problem arose when farmers purchasing StarLink seed comingled the seeds, thereby producing the genetically modified corn materials.

Food recalls are issued in the event of a possible health hazard. The recalls are classified according to the following levels:

Class 1 recall = Reasonable probability that use of the product will cause serious adverse health consequences or death.

Class 2 recall = Use or exposure to the product may cause temporary or medially reversible adverse health consequences or when the probability of serious adverse health consequences is remote.

Class 3 recall = Use or exposure to the produce is not likely to cause adverse health consequences.

Market withdrawal = The product is withdrawn by the manufacturer for minor violations that would not be subject to FDA legal action.

Food Recalls

ood is inspected by two different agencies, the USDA and the FDA. The Food, Drug and Cosmetic Act of 1938 authorized the FDA to recall a product if it poses a risk to human health. The FDA recalls nonmeat items and the USDA recalls meat and poultry items. Oftentimes the food recalls are voluntary. The Food Safety and Inspection Service of the USDA oversees

engineered products have not been studied and is an area worthy of additional research.

There is also concern because genetically engineered plants are hardier than the average plant. In Canada, for example, the genetically engineered canola plant pollinates and reproduces in such a manner that it is known as a "super-weed," requiring stronger herbicides to keep them under control. To control the possibility of bioinvasion, biotechnologists are develping "terminator" plants that produce seeds that will not germinate. Some plants are being developed that do not develop normally unless they are sprayed with a special chemical to reduce the possibility of bioinvasion.

Genetically engineered
To alter the genetic material by changing genetic processes.

Nutrient dense
Having the quality of more nutrients per gram; raw foods have more nutrients than processed foods.

all recall activities. Foods are recalled if they are contaminated with infectious agents or if they contain potential allergens (such as nuts) or undeclared ingredients.

Food Perishability

lthough microorganisms are found in fresh foods, some bacteria, yeast, and molds are helpful. For instance, bacteria in yogurt aids the digestive system. Fungi are used to make bread, beer, wine, cheese, or vinegar. Still excessive amounts of bacteria, produced when the proper conditions of air, temperature, and moisture are present, can be harmful. When bacteria is allowed to grow, food will spoil and rot. The longer a food is stored, the more likely it will spoil. Fruits and vegetables are more likely to spoil when the outer surfaces are removed. Foods have a shelf life that is a normal range when the product can be stored and consumed safely. In order to extend the shelf life, food can be refrigerated, frozen, dried, or preservatives can be added. The shelf life of any food is dependent upon three things: temperature, moisture, and oxygen. When one of these things is altered, the shelf life of foods can be extended.

During the French Revolution, Napoleon offered a reward to anyone who could develop a way to preserve food longer for military troops. Nicholas-Francois Appert, a French chef, developed a technique known as *canning* in 1809. The process involved heating foods, placing them in a jar, and heating the jar until a seal was formed. This method prevented oxygen from getting to the food. When the container cools, a vacuum is sometimes created inside the jar that further removes the air that bacteria need to grow. Before consuming a canned item, make sure that the seal is not broken. If the seal is broken, the food has been contaminated by air and should be thrown out.

Foods can also be preserved by adding salt or sugar to prevent bacterial growth. Cooking foods in sugar syrup causes **plasmolysis** due to a process known as *osmosis*. Soaking foods in a salt *brine* solution is known as *pickling*. This process draws the water out of the food so bacteria cannot grow.

Preparation of items for freezing is also important. It is important to minimize the growth of microorganisms. **Blanching** foods means to put a fresh food item, usually a vegetable, into a pot of boiling water briefly until the color brightens to kill bacteria before freezing. Other ways to preserve food include drying or *desiccation*, which removes moisture from foods so bacteria cannot grow. To dry foods, fresh items must be used and not allowed to ripen before drying. Foods that can be dried include fruits, vegetables, milk, eggs, and meat. It is best to store dried foods in an airtight container or package. They may also be placed in the refrigerator to preserve them longer, particularly in hot climates.

Food Storage

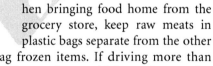hen bringing food home from the grocery store, keep raw meats in plastic bags separate from the other foods. Double bag frozen items. If driving more than 30 minutes to get home, keep cold items in a cooler with ice. Unload the bags immediately and refrigerate cold items.

REFRIGERATION

Foods with a short shelf life should be refrigerated or frozen. Refrigeration and freezing is often called *cold storage*. Cold storage does not kill all bacteria or molds; it only slows the growth of microorganisms. Refrigerator and freezer temperatures are important. The temperature inside a refrigerator should be 40° F or below. The temperature inside a freezer should be 0° F.

Most produce items should be kept in the refrigerator to prolong shelf life. Bananas may be an exception because the skin turns brown when it is exposed to cold temperatures. Items such as lettuce, onions, celery, and carrots can be kept in a drawer in the bottom of the refrigerator, often referred to as a crisper. Some produce items may be kept in the refrigerator 1 to 3 weeks. Potatoes should not be stored in the refrigerator because the cold makes them become more **starchy**.

The most common type of food contamination is contamination with human excrement. This occurs when a person does not wash their hands properly after using the bathroom and then handling food. Hands should be washed carefully after using the bathroom or diapering a child or handling items that may have been touched by other individuals. Doorknobs, dishes, and money are just some of the items that can transfer bacteria and viruses from one person to another. Food must be prepared by those who are disease-free, understand how to prevent cross-contamination, and by those who practice good hand-washing techniques.

It takes from 15 to 30 seconds for a proper hand-washing technique. Hand washing with hot soapy water is essential. Fingernails and wrists need to be washed as well as the hands. In order to estimate how much time needed to wash your hands, sing "Happy Birthday" or another simple song. There is no substitute for hand washing. Hand sanitizers may offer some protection when no water is available, but they should only be used in those circumstances. Hand sanitizers contain alcohol and evaporate easily, but they do not necessarily kill germs.

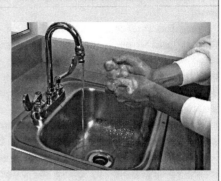

To prevent illness from *E. coli* or *Salmonella,* meat should be refrigerated or frozen immediately after bringing it home from the store. Refrigeration will extend the shelf life of dried foods, but it should still be used within a reasonable amount of time. Milk can be kept in the refrigerator for 1 week and 1 to 3 months in the freezer. Ground meats (beef, turkey, veal, pork, and lamb) and fish can be kept for 1 to 2 days and frozen for 3 to 4 months. To prevent freezer burn, meats may need to be wrapped with foil or placed in a plastic freezer bag even though they are already in a package. Other fresh meats (beef, pork, and poultry) can be kept for 3 to 5 days in the refrigerator. Fresh eggs can be kept in the refrigerator for 3 weeks. Hard-cooked eggs can be kept for 1 week. Raw egg yolks and whites can be kept 2 to 4 days and frozen for up to 1 year. Frozen dinners can be kept in the freezer for 3 to 4 months. Frozen meats should be used within 4 to 6 months.

Foods can be refrozen after they have been partially thawed (for instance, during a power outage). The general guideline is that foods should still have ice crystals in them and the temperature should be below 40° F. If the power has been off less than 2 hours, the contents of the refrigerator are within the desirable temperature range as long as the refrigerator door remains closed. In the event of a longer power outage, it may be necessary to remove items (such as milk, dairy products, meats, fish, poultry, eggs, gravy, stuffing, and leftovers) to a cooler with ice. A freezer that is half full should be cold up to 24 hours and a full freezer should keep cool for 48 hours if the door is kept closed.

PANTRY

The pantry or cupboards should be kept clean. Foods that do not require refrigeration need to be kept cool (between 50° to 80° F), dry, and dark. Light deteriorates the quality and shelf life of many foods. Always use older food items first. Unopened canned and bottled foods can be kept up to a year. How long a dry food product can be stored depends on whether it is opened and its fat content. Fats can become rancid in a relatively short period of time. Granulated sugar and most spices can be kept for up to 2 years. Breads with no preservatives can be kept in the refrigerator for 2 to 3 weeks and up to 2 to 3 months in the freezer. Once foods have been opened, they should be kept in airtight containers or plastic bags to reduce exposure to air, moisture, and insects.

Sanitation Principles

t is important to prepare clean foods, to use clean utensils, and to avoid **cross-contamination**. The consumer does not often think of cans

Plasmolysis
The shrinkage of a living plant or bacterial cell caused by loss of water through osmosis.

Blanching
Heating a food, usually a vegetable, for a short period of time to destroy surface bacteria and other pathogens; the process is usually used prior to canning or freezing food.

Starchy
Containing starch.

Cross-contamination
The act of contaminating one food with the pathogens of another.

or jars as being contaminated, but when they sit on shelves and pass through many different environments, it is possible that they have been contaminated by insects and vermin. It is always a good idea to wash cans and jars before opening them. The can opener should be clean so that old food particles do not fall into the newly opened food.

Stainless steel is considered the best cooking utensil. Pottery and copper utensils may contain lead. Some cleaning solutions used to shine silver or copper items may leave a toxic residue. Baking soda or salt can be used to remove food residues on pots and pans without any toxic effects.

Cross-contamination occurs when one type of food comes in contact with another type of food. This problem most often occurs when meat residues are transferred to vegetables by using the same cutting board. When using the same cutting board for meats and vegetables, the cutting board should be cleaned with soap and water between uses (Figure 13-5). The best type of cutting board is glass or a strong plastic, one that is not easily marred with cuts where bacteria can be trapped and grow. It is always a good idea to use a bleach and water solution after using the cutting board to kill any bacteria in the cracks. Counters and sinks should be cleaned with soap and water and a diluted bleach solution to assure that they are properly sanitized. The best way to dry dishes is to allow them to dry in the dishwasher or air dry. Towels used to dry dishes should not be used for drying hands.

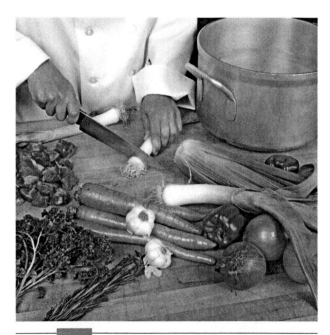

Food Preparation

THAWING FOODS

Meats, fish, shellfish, poultry, and vegetables often have bacteria that is dormant when frozen. As food thaws, bacteria growth can occur. The preferred method of thawing these foods is in the refrigerator at or below 40° F. If the packages are sealed, thawing in cold water is acceptable. Many foods can be thawed more quickly in the microwave oven on the "defrost" setting. Breads, pastries, and fruits can be thawed at room temperature. All foods must be used immediately after they are defrosted.

PRECOOKED FOODS

Many produce items are packaged for convenience and to prolong their shelf life. Although the package may say "ready to eat," one should not assume that foods do not need to be inspected, washed, or cooked. Produce should always be rinsed to remove pesticide residues, pathogens, and decaying portions if the skin cannot be removed. Perishable items should be kept cold in ice baths or in the refrigerator before they are served. Lettuce can be washed and then spin dried with a container designed specifically for that purpose or dried by pressing the leaves with a paper towel.

HEATING FOODS

It is not a good idea to eat raw or undercooked eggs. Heating and cooking foods usually kills everything except staphylococcal toxins. The center of the food must be 145° to 180° F (60° C). The process of pasteurization cooks the food just long enough to kill the bacteria without destroying the taste, nutritive value, or digestibility. Meat should always be cooked thoroughly to be certain that bacteria are destroyed (Table 13-2). The best way to tell whether meat is "done" is by using

TABLE 13-2 Safe Temperatures

145° F	Beef, lamb, and veal steaks and roasts
160° F	Ground beef, pork, veal, lamb, pork chops, ribs, roasts, and egg dishes
165° F	Ground turkey and chicken, stuffing, casseroles, and leftovers
170° F	Chicken and turkey breasts
180° F	Chicken and turkey, whole bird, legs, thighs, and wings

a food thermometer. The food thermometer should be placed in the thickest part of the food, away from bones and fat. The temperature of the meat varies with the type of meat.

When microwaving, cook, rotate, stir, and cover to promote even cooking. Do not use plastic wrap over microwave foods unless it is specifically designed for microwave use, as in frozen dinners. It is important to make sure food is evenly cooked and for the correct amount of time. Have the microwave oven checked for leaks. Inspect the seals and hinges around the door to make sure they are secure and airtight. Do not open the door while the oven is on. Avoid microwaving pre-packed microwavable foods in disposable containers or with plastic wrap. When cooking, use glass or ceramic containers, not plastic containers unless the container is specifically made for microwave use.

There is some evidence that microwaving foods may not necessarily kill harmful bacteria found on foods. In Alaska, an outbreak of *Salmonella* food poisoning was associated with eating roast pork that was reheated with a microwave. The meat was flown in from Seattle, Washington, and people took the meat home, then reheated it. Of the 30 people who ate the preheated meat the 10 who used a microwave to reheat the meat became ill. None of the 20 persons using a conventional oven or skillet to reheat the meat became ill (Gessner & Beller, 1994).

Serving Food

ot foods should be served hot and cold foods should be served cold. Hot cooked food should be kept at 140° F. Cold foods can be kept in an ice water bath or refrigerator prior to serving. Picnic foods should be kept in a cooler with a cold pack or ice. The cooler should be kept in the shade and the lid should be opened as infrequently as possible. When food is reheated, it should be cooked to 165° F. Microwaving food does not always heat food all the way through the center.

Storing Leftovers

apid cooling means cooling a heated food as quickly as possible so that bacteria does not have an opportunity to grow. Food should be cooled within 1 hour after it is served and no more than 4 hours after it is cooked. Placing food in a shallow container helps cool the food quicker than keeping it in a deep container. A food thermometer can help determine whether food is properly cooled. Leftovers should be used within 4 days.

Restaurant Inspections

ublic institutions (such as hospitals and schools) and restaurants where food is prepared and served are subject to food inspections by local health departments. Some health departments rate restaurants in terms of food storage, cleanliness, food preparation, and employee training. Some have Web sites listing results from the establishment's last food inspection.

Inspectors generally inspect the structure for cleanliness and proper food storage. Water sources are checked to be sure that they are safe and accessible for proper hand washing. Dishwashing, drying equipment, and procedures are checked to assure proper sanitation. Food

Phthalate
A monoester used in plastics and other consumer items that can break down and get into the gastrointestinal system or bloodstream.

Plasticizers
Any of various substances added to plastics or other materials to make or keep them soft or pliable.

preparation, food serving, and waster management techniques are also observed. The following is a list of things food inspectors look for.

- Structure of the facility
  Cracks in storage and food preparation areas
  Cleanable surfaces
  Screens on windows
  Good ventilation
  Good lighting
  No grease build-up

- Water supply
  Potable water
  Hot and cold running water
  Toilet facilities with self-closing doors
  Soap
  Paper towels or dryers
  No cross-contamination of water supplies

- Equipment and supplies
  No cracks
  No food build-up on can openers and other appliances
  Chemicals stored away from food areas
  Utensils stored where they cannot be contaminated
  Food stored 6 inches off the ground

- Proper temperature controls for food storage
  Refrigerated between 36° to 45° F

- Proper temperature for sanitizing utensils, silverware, glassware, and dishes
  Dishes must be "sanitized" at 170° to 180° F
  Washed for 40 seconds under pressure at 140 gal/min at a temperature of 150° F
  Rinsed for 10 seconds at 180° F

- Waste management techniques
  Waste is kept in airtight containers above the ground
  Trash is picked up at least twice per week

- Approved food sources
  Food is obtained from "approved" sources
  No home-canned foods
  Minimal amount of food handling

- Food serving practices
  Minimal amount of food handling
  "Sneeze guards" on buffets
  Surveillance to reduce contamination

- Hand washing and utensils/dishes
  Soap and paper towels for staff
  Cracks and chips in glassware and dishes

Food inspections provide a valuable public health service. Food is inspected for quality, storage, equipment, preparation, and sanitary techniques of cooks and servers. Restaurants must pass food inspections in order to keep their license. Retail food stores and bakeries must also pass food inspection requirements. Most of the time, consumers complain about food safety in restaurants. If a complaint is filed, health inspectors can make an unscheduled visit and send a written warning if necessary.

Because home kitchens are not inspected, they are more likely to be the cause of food poisonings. Food safety is no longer a part of school curriculums so public health departments and cooperative extension services are the usual source of food safety information. Wise consumers, however, would seek information from one of these sources regarding any questions they have.

Summary

ood is an important component of health. The proper production, handling, and preparation of food is a public health and an environmental health issue. Sanitarians, food service inspectors, and many others play an important role in identifying potential hazards, warning the public, and promoting advancements that can reduce the incidence of food-borne illnesses.

REFERENCES

American Dietetic Association. (1998). Position statement: Use of nutritive and nonnutritive sweeteners. *Journal of the American Dietetic Association, 98,* 580.

Anonymous. (1999). Women in American History: Sara Josephine Baker. *Encyclopedia Britannica.* http://search.eb.com/women/articles/Baker_Sara_Josephine.html.

Anonymous. (2000). Mission Foods recalls all yellow corn products. *High Plains Journal.* Retrieved from http://www.hpj.com/archives/nov00/1016missionrecallmrjmlhtm.htm.

Anonymous. (2005). Cook foods adequately. Department of FSHN, Washington State University. Retrieved from http://foodsafety.wsu.edu/consumers/displayTopic.asp?id=2\.

Barna, J. (1979). Compilation of bioassay data on the whole-someness of irradiated food items. *Acta Alimentana, 8,* 205.

Bhaskaram, C., & Sadasivan, G. (1975). Effects of feeding irradiated wheat to malnourished children. *American Journal of Clinical Nutrition, 28,* 134.

Blaser, M. (1997). Epidemiologic and clinical features of *Campylobacter jejuni* infections. *Journal of Infectious Diseases, 176,* Supplement 2, S103–S105.

Brennand, C. P. (1995). Ten most commonly asked questions about food irradiation. Idaho State University. Retrieved March 7, 2003 from http://www.physics.isu.edu/radinf/food/htm.

Brooks, J. (1996). The sad and tragic life of Typhoid Mary. *Canadian Medical Association Journal, 154,* 6915–6916.

Bryd-Bredbenner, C. (2002). Food safety: An international public health issue. *The International Electronic Journal of Health Education.* Retrieved 5/5/2003 from http://www.aahperd.org/idjhe/template.cfm?template=current/may72002.html.

Centers for Disease Control (2002). Foodborne illness. Retrieved March 8, 2003 from http://www.cdc.gov/ncidod/dbmd/diseaseinfo/foodborneinfections_t.htm.

Centers for Disease Control. (2005). *Escherichia coli O157:H7* Frequently Asked Questions. Retrieved from http://www.nbc5.com/news/1567576/detail.html.

Centers for Disease Control. (2005). Foodborne illness, pg. 5. Retrieved from http://www.cdc.gov/ncidod/dbmd/diseaseinfo/files/foodborne_illness_FAQ.pdf.

Charman, K. (2002). Genetically engineered food: Promises and perils. *Mother Earth News, 194.*

Consumer Information Center. (2005). How to help avoid foodborne illness in the home. Retrieved from the Federal Citizens Information Center at http://www.pueblo.gsa.gov/cic_text/food/foodborn/foodborn.htm.

Earles, J. (2003). Sugar-free blues. Everything you wanted to know about artificial sweeteners. Article from *Wise Traditions in Food, Farming, and the Healing Arts,* quarterly magazine of the Weston A Price Foundation. Retrieved from http://www.westonaprice.org/modernfood/sugarfree_blues.html.

Environmental Protection Agency. (1988). Regulation of pesticides in food: Addressing the Delaney paradox policy statement. *Federal Register, 53,* 41104.

Food and Drug Administration. (1992). Clostridium perfringens. *Bad bug book: Foodborne pathogenic microorganisms and natural toxins handbook.* Center for Food Safety and Applied Nutrition.

Food and Drug Administration. (August 31, 1995). Monosodium glutamate. *FDA Backgrounder.* Retrieved February 18, 2003 from http://www.fda.gov/opacom/backgrounders/msg.html.

Food and Drug Administration. (1999). Healthy People 2000: Status report, food safety objectives. Food Safety and Inspection Service, Centers for Disease Control and Prevention. Retrieved from http://www.cfsan.fda.gov/~dms/hp2k.html#key.

Food and Drug Administration. (2000). Recalls and food corrections, Foods – Class II. FDA Enforcement report, November 1, 00-44. Retrieved from http://www.fda.gov/bbs/topics/enforce/ENF00666.html.

Food and Drug Administration. (2003). Genetic engineering fast forwarding to future foods. Retrieved March 4, 2003 from http://www.fda.gov/bbs/topics/consumer/geneng.html.

Food Safety and Inspection Service. (1998). This year: Food safety hits high gear. *The food safety educator, 3.* Retrieved from the Consumer Education and Information division of the Food Safety and Inspection Service of the U. S. Department of Agriculture, Washington, DC.

FoodSafetyNET. (1999). Safer fresh food is closer than you think. Press release, April 26, 1999. Retrieved from http://archives.foodsafetynetwork.ca/fsnet/1999/4-1999/fs-04-26-99-02.txt.

Frenzen, P., Majchrowicz, A., Buzby, B., Imhoff, B., and the FoodNet Working Group. (2000). Consumer acceptance of irradiated meat and poultry products. *Agriculture Information Bulletin, 757,* 1–8.

Gandhi, R., & Scnecker, S. (2000). Consumer concerns about hormones in food. Program on Breast Cancer and Environmental Risk Factors. Retrieved from http://envirocancer.cornell.edu/Factsheet/Diet/fs37.hormones.cfm.

Gessner, B., & Beller, M. (1994). Protective effect of conventional cooking versus use of microwave ovens in an outbreak of Salmonellosis. *American Journal of Epidemiology, 139,* 903–909.

Gustafson, R., & Bowen, R. (1997). Antibiotic use in animal agriculture. *Journal of Applied Microbiology, 83,* 531–541.

Halstead, C. (2003). Dietary supplements and functional foods: Two sides of a coin? *American Journal of Clinical Nutrition, 77,* 1001S–1007S.

Himelright, I., Harris, E., Lorch, V., Anderson, M., Jones, T., Craig, A., Kuehnert, M., Forster, T., Arduino, M., Jensen, B., & Jernigan, D. (2002). Enterobacter sakazakii infections associated with the use of powdered infant formula, (Tennessee, 2001). *MMWR Weekly, 51,* 298–300.

International Food Information Council. (2001). Glutamate and monosodium glutamate: Examining the myths. *IFIC Review,* November issue. Retrieved from http://www.ific.org/publications/reviews/upload/Glutamate-and-Monosodium-Glutamate.pdf.

International Food Information Council. (2003a). Questions and answers about food irradiation. Retrieved from http://www.ific.org/publications/qa/irradiationqa.cfm?renderforprint=1.

International Food Information Council. (2003b). Food sensitivities, allergies, and intolerances: Separating fact from fiction. Food Insight, July/August newsletter. Retrieved from http://www.ific.org/foodinsight/2003/ja/foodsensfi403.cfm.

Irwin, L., Gray, S. & Oberdörster, E. (2001). Vitellogenin induction in painted turtle, *Chrysemys picta,* as a biomarker of exposure to environmental levels of estradiol. Aquatic Toxicology, 55, 49.

Johnson, A., Reynolds, A., Chen, J., & Resurreccion, A. (2004). Consumer attitudes towards irradiated food: 2003 vs. 1993. *Food Protection Trends, 24,* 408–418.

Keeler, B. (2001). A nation of lab rats. *Sierra, 86,* 45.

Kramer, J., & Gilbert, J. (1989). *Bacillus cereus* and other *Bacillus* species. In M. P. Doyle (Ed.), *Foodborne Bacterial Pathogens,* p. 21–70. Marcel Dekker, Inc., New York.

Kwok, R. (1968). Chinese Restaurant Syndrome. *New England Journal of Medicine, 17,* 796.

Leavitt, J. (1992). "Typhoid Mary" strikes back: Bacteriological theory and practice in early 20th century public health. *ISIS: Journal of the History of Science in Society, 83,* 608–629.

Leavitt, J. (1996). *Typhoid Mary: Captive to the Public's Health.* Boston, MA: Beacon Press.

Marr, J. (1999). Typhoid Mary. *Lancet, 353,* 1714.

Mendelsohn, J. (1995). "Typhoid Mary" strikes again. The social and the scientific in the making of modern public health. *ISIS: Journal of the History of Science in Society, 86,* 617–618.

Morehouse, K. (1998). Food irradiation: The treatment of foods with ionizing radiation. Retrieved January 20, 2003 from http://www.cfsan.fda.gov/`dms/opa-fdir.html.

National Cancer Institute. (1997). Cancer facts: Artificial sweeteners. Retrieved February 17, 2003 from http://cis.nci.nih.gov/fact/3_19.htm.

National Council for Science and the Environment. (1996). Pesticide legislation: Food Quality Protection Act of 1996 (PL 104-170) II. CRS Report for Congress, 96-759 ENR. Retrieved from http://www.ncseonline.org/nle/crsreports/pesticides/pest-8a.cfm#Protecting%20Infants%20and%20Children%20from%20Pesticide%20Residues%20in%20the%20Diet.

Papazian, R. (1996). Sulfites: Safe for most, dangerous for some. *FDA Consumer, 30.* Retrieved from http://www.fda.gov/fdac/features/096_sulf.html.

Pivonka, E., & Grunewald, K. (1990). Aspartame or sugar-sweetened beverages: Effects on mood in your women. Journal of the *American Dietetic Association, 90,* 250.

Raloff, J. (2002). Hormones: Here's the beef. *Science News,* Jan. 5. Retrieved June 30, 2002 from http://www.findarticles.com/cf-0/m1200/1_161/82512511/.

Reed, G. (1994). Foodborne illness (Part 4): Bacillus cereus gastroenteritis. *Dairy, Food, and Environmental Sanitation, 14,* 87.

Rippel, B. (2002). Consumer knowledge about food safety revealed. *Consumers' Research Magazine,* March. Retrieved June 2, 2003 from http://www.consumeralert.org/pubs/research/CRMarch02.htm.

Sagon, C. (2002). The new standards: What does organic really mean? *Washington Post,* October 9.

Shea, K. & the Committee on Environmental Health. (2000). American Academy of Pediatrics: Technical Report: Irradiation of Food. *Pediatrics, 106,* 1505–1510. Retrieved from http://pediatrics.aappublications.org/cgi/reprint/106/6/1505.

Shewmake, R., & Dillon, B. (1998). Food poisoning: Causes, remedies, and prevention. *Postgraduate Medicine,* 103, June 1998. Retrieved from http://www.postgradmed.com/issues/1998/06_98/shewmake.htm.

Soto, A., Calabro, J., Prechtl, N., Yau, A., Orlando, E., Daxenberger, A., Kolok, A., Guillette, L. Jr., Bizec, B., Lange, I., & Sonnenschein, C. (2004). Androgenic and estrogenic activity in water bodies receiving cattle feedlot effluent in eastern Nebraska, USA. *Environmental Health Perspectives,* 112. Retrieved from http://ehp.niehs.nih.gov/members/2003/6590/6590.html.

Steele, J. (2001). Food irradiation: A public health challenge for the 21st century. *Clinical Infectious Diseases, 33,* 376–377.

University of Iowa Health Care. (2003). Sugar substitutes. HIL File NUTR4838.RF2 VRS# 6979. Retrieved from http://www.uihealthcare.com/topics/nutrition/nutr4838.html.

Vogt, D. (1992). The Delaney clause: The dilemma of regulating health risk for pesticide residues. CRS Report for Congress, 92-800 SPR. Retrieved from http://www.ncseonline.org/NLE/CRSreports/Pesticides/pest-3.cfm?&CFID=903438&CFTOKEN=77769066.

Wax, P. (1995). Elixirs, diluents, and the passage of the 1938 Federal Food, Drug, and Cosmetic Act. *Annals of Internal Medicine, 122,* 456–461.

Wills, P. (1986). Radiation treatment of food. *Nuclear Spectrum, 2,* 5. http://www.xenoestrogen.us/index.html.

Wood, O. & Bruhn, C. (2000). Position of the American Dietetic Association: Food irradiation. *Journal of the American Dietetic Association, 100,* 246–253.

Zhao, C., Ge, B., Villena, J., Sudler, R., Yeh, E., Zhao, S., White, D., Wagner, D., & Meng, J. (2001). Prevalence of *Campylobacter* spp., *Escherichia coli,* and *Salmonella* Serovars in retail chicken, turkey, pork, and beef from the Greater Washington DC area. *Applied and Environmental Microbiology, 67,* 5431-5436. Retrieved from http://aem.asm.org/cgi/content/full/67/12/5431.

ASSIGNMENTS

1. Find information on the pathogen *Cyclospora cayetanensis.*

2. Look up information about the absorption of styrofoam container chemicals in food and any potential detrimental effects to human health.

3. Investigate the possibility or development of making plastic food containers from corn rather than petroleum products.

4. Consider food products you consume with an artificial sweeteners such as cyclamates, saccharin, aspartame, or others. Determine how much you consume and any health risks associated with consumption.

5. Check the produce section of three grocery stores to see if consumers are notified of irradiated foods. If there are no signs, ask the produce manager which foods in the produce section have been irradiated.

6. Ask a food inspector from a local health department to come to class and describe how they check restaurants, schools, and health care facilities for food handling violations.

7. Inspect the labels of some of your favorite foods and determine which are food "enhancers" and which are "fillers."

8. Select three Web sites pertaining to food safety and inspections. Write a brief description of the Web site regarding the type of information it contains and contact information.

9. Compare cleanliness of eating areas, food serving areas, restrooms, and observe food handling practices of wait staff and buspeople for two restaurants. Visit one fast food restaurant and one sit-down restaurant and compare.

10. Locate nearest "green store" in your community. Inventory their products and list those you are most likely to purchase in the future.

LAWS

1906 *Pure Food and Drug Act (34 U.S. Stats. 768)*
Enacted laws for the inspection of foods for potential "poisons" and adulterants that might cause harm to human health.

1906 *Meat Inspection Act (34 Stat. 674)*
Authorized the Secretary of Agriculture to order meat inspections and condemn any found unfit for human consumption.

1938 *Food, Drug, and Cosmetic Act (21 USC 301)*
Instituted requirements concerning labeling and false claims on consumable products with attention to the production and marketing of foods.

1958 *Food Additives Amendment, also known as Delaney Clause (PL 85-929)*
Required manufacturers of new food additives to establish safety guidelines, prohibiting approval of any food additive shown to induce cancer in humans or animals. The FDA published the first Generally Recognized as Safe (GRAS) list, containing nearly 200 substances. The 1960 Color Additive Amendment was added later. In 1971, saccharin was removed from the list. In 1977 the *Saccharin Study and Labeling Act* (PL 95-203) was passed by Congress to stop the FDA from banning the chemical sweetener, requiring a label warning that it was found to cause cancer in laboratory animals. In 1996 the *Saccharin Notice Repeal Act* removes the requirement for the saccharin notice on labels.

1967 *Wholesome Meat Act 1967 (PL 90-201)*
Required USDA inspection of all animals when slaughtered and processed into products for human consumption. The purpose was to prevent adulterated or misbranded livestock from being sold as food and to assure that the slaughter conditions were sanitary.

1976 *Fair Packaging and Labeling Act (15 USC 1451-1461)*
Requires consumer products to be honestly and informatively labeled, with the FDA enforcing provisions on foods, drugs, cosmetics, and medical devices.

1977 *The Food and Agriculture Act (PL 95-113)*
Designated the Department of Agriculture as the lead agency for federal agricultural research. Established procedures for coordinating nutrition research in areas of mutual interest between the Department of Health, Education, and Welfare and the Department of Agriculture.

1980 *Infant Formula Act (PL 96-359) and (PL 99-570)*
Amended the Food, Drug, and Cosmetic Act, providing for more stringent control over manufacturing and processing of infant formulas.

1990 *Nutrition Labeling and Education Act (NLEA; 21 CFR 101)*
Requires all packaged foods to bear nutrition labeling and all health claims for foods to be consistent. The law preempts state requirements about food standards, nutrition labeling, and health claims and, for the first time, authorizes some health claims for foods. The food ingredient panels, serving sizes, and use of terms such as "low fat" and "light" are standardized.

1994 *Dietary Supplement Health and Education Act (DSHEA) (PL 103-417)*
Establishes specific labeling requirements and authorizes the FDA to develop good manufacturing practice regulations for dietary supplements. Defined "dietary supplements" and "dietary ingredients," classifying them as food.

1996 *Food Quality Protection Act (PL 104-170)*
Amends the Food, Drug, and Cosmetic Act, eliminating application of the Delaney provision to pesticides.

1996 *Food Quality Protection Act (PL 104-170)*
Amended the Federal Insecticide, Fungicide, and Roden-

ticide Act (FIFRA) and the Federal Food Drug, and Cosmetic Act (Delaney clause) with a new safety standard regarding "reasonable certainty of no harm" applied to the use of pesticides on foods.

1998 *Agricultural Research, Extension, and Education Reform Act of 1998 (PL 105-185)*
Required the Secretary of Agriculture to establish a Food Safety Research Information Office with activities in cooperation with the National Institutes of Health, FDA, CDC, and other public and private institutions.

PROFESSIONAL JOURNALS

American Journal of Clinical Nutrition
American Journal of Public Health
Annual Reviews of Nutrition
Environmental Nutrition
Epidemiology and Infection
FIU Hospitality Review
Food Technology
International Journal of Food Microbiology
Journal of Agricultural & Food Chemistry
Journal of the American Dietetic Association
Journal of the American Veterinary Medical Association
Journal of Applied Bacteriology
Journal of Clinical Microbiology
Journal of Foodservice Systems
Journal of Food Protection
Journal of Nutrition
Journal of Nutritional and Environmental Medicine
Journal of Public Health Medicine
Nutrition and Food Science
Nutrition News
Public Health Nutrition
Reviews of Environmental Contamination and Toxicology

ADDITIONAL READING

Gibbs, G. (1995). *The food that would last forever. Understanding the dangers of food irradiation.* Garden City Park, NY: Avery Publishing Group, Inc.

Leavitt, J. (1996). *Typhoid Mary: Captive to the public's health.* Boston, MA: Beacon Press.

McSwane, D., Rue, N., Linton, R., & Williams, A. (2002). *The Essentials of Food Safety and Sanitation.* Old Tappan, NJ: Prentice-Hall.

National Research Council. (1993). *Pesticides in the Diets of Infants and Children,* Washington, DC: National Academy Press.

Nestle, M. (2003). *Safe Food: Bacteria, Biotechnology, and Bioterrorism.* Berkeley, CA: University of California Press.

Redman, N. (2000). *Food Safety: A Reference Handbook.* Santa Barbara, CA: A B C-CLIO, Inc.

Schlosser, E. (2002) *Fast Food Nation: The Dark Side of the American Meal.* Farmington Hills, MA: The Gale Group.

Schmidt, R., & Rodrick. G. (2003). *Food Safety Handbook.* Hoboken, NJ: John Wiley & Sons, Inc.

Sinclair, U (1995). *The Jungle.* Norwalk, CT: Classics Entertainment International, Inc.

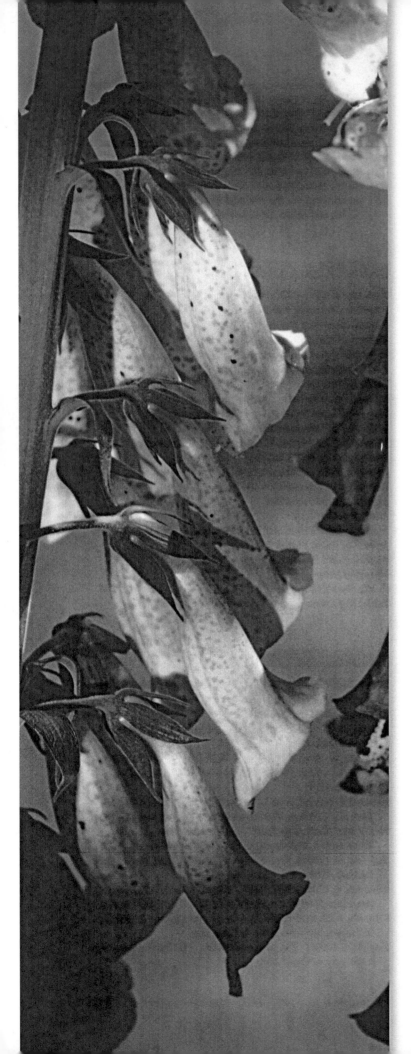

Waste Management

14

Having relied for too long on the old strategy of "out of sight, out of mind," we are now running out of ways to dispose of our waste in a manner that keeps it out of either sight or mind.

Senator Al Gore (1948–present),
from Earth in the Balance *(1992)*

OBJECTIVES

1. Define the terms solid waste, refuse, garbage, rubbish, trash, biosolids, sewage, effluent, and wastewater.

2. Contrast the "old" ways of managing solid waste in communities to the "new" ways they are managed today.

3. Describe hazards associated with land disposal of solid waste.

4. Explain harmful effects of incineration.

5. Describe the management of sewage in municipalities.

6. Provide alternatives to the management of human waste where sewer systems are not available.

7. List steps associated with wastewater management in urban settings.

8. Describe various types of hazardous waste and agencies that regulate hazardous waste storage, transportation, and disposal.

9. Discuss current methods used to dispose of medical waste.

10. List hazards associated with the improper disposal of e-waste.

11. List several laws that regulate the handling, storage, transportation, and clean-up of hazardous waste.

12. List ways that individuals can reduce, precycle, reuse, and recycle waste.

260

Introduction

oday is part of the Disposable Age and consumers are part of a throw away society generating enormous amounts of **waste**. The United States accounts for only 5% of the world population but is responsible for 50% of the world's solid waste (Tilford, 2000). Agriculture, manufacturing plants, mining operations, and power plants produce tons of waste per year. Commercial businesses, building contractors, and homeowners also contribute substantial amounts to the nation's landfills. Waste can be in solid, liquid, or gas form, hazardous or nonhazardous. The management of waste is a major public health problem. Problems associated with solid waste, human waste, wastewater, and **hazardous waste** will be discussed.

What Is Solid Waste?

olid waste consists of materials that no one wants. Solid waste includes **refuse** and items that people throw away. Refuse consists of **garbage**, **rubbish**, ashes, and solids from human activities. Garbage is organic materials from food. *Rubbish* (also known as **trash**) is combustible and noncombustible materials that need to be thrown away. Rubbish consists of unusable paper, plastic, cans, wood, paper, and other products.

Solid waste consists of agricultural, commercial, industrial, and domestic wastes. Half of all solid waste is from agriculture. **Agricultural waste** includes leftover crops and crop residue, spoiled crops, weeds, pesticides, herbicides, animal manure, and animal carcasses. In most cases, agricultural waste is managed by farming operations on land that they own dumping and covering or spreading and plowing it back into the soil. The problem with agricultural waste, particularly chemicals and livestock waste, is that it can pollute nearby surface and groundwater sources, affecting local drinking water supplies. **Commercial waste** consists of materials left over from service industries, construction, and food packaging. **Industrial waste** includes waste generated from mining, power plants, and the manufacturing of products (such as paper, steel, and chemicals). Commercial and industrial waste often contains hazardous material detrimental to human health leaked into groundwater

sources. **Municipal solid waste** (MSW) consists of trash, rubbish, and garbage generated by homeowners and small businesses. Some solid waste generated, regardless of the source, is considered hazardous. It is estimated that the average person uses 4.5 pounds of waste products per day (Tilford, 2000). The United States produces more than 200 million tons of municipal solid waste (MSW) every year (Lawrence Berkeley Laboratory, 2005). Thirty-nine percent of the waste from U.S. homes and offices is paper. Thirteen percent is yard trimmings, 10% is plastics, and 10% is food waste (Tilford, 2000). According to the EPA, 28% of MSW is recycled or composted, 15% burned at combustion facilities, and the remaining 57% disposed of in landfills.

Waste
Objects that are rejected as worthless or unwanted; thoughtless or inappropriate use.

Hazardous waste
Waste that poses a threat to human health or the environment. The EPA defines a substance as hazardous if it is flammable, reactive or explosive when mixed with other substances, is corrosive, or is toxic.

Refuse
Waste material composed of garbage, rubbish, and ashes; products that can be blown out of a landfill like paper products or trash bags.

Garbage
Discarded food or organic matter.

Rubbish
Combustible and noncombustible solid waste generated from people's activities; includes paper, beverage cans, yard trimmings, and many other materials; can include articles difficult to decompose, such as furniture, old refrigerators, and tires.

Trash
Material considered worthless, unnecessary, and offensive; usually discarded or thrown away; parts that have been broken off, stripped off.

Agricultural waste
Leftover crops, crop residue, spoiled crops, weeds, pesticides, herbicides, animal manure, and animal carcasses thrown away as a result of agricultural use.

Commercial waste
Discarded objects from construction, service industries, and food packaging.

Industrial waste
Mining, power plant, and manufacturing products from paper mills, steel mills, and chemical plants that are thrown away.

Municipal solid waste (MSW)
Trash, rubbish, and garbage thrown away by homeowners and small businesses.

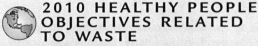

2010 HEALTHY PEOPLE OBJECTIVES RELATED TO WASTE

8-15 Recycled municipal solid waste
Increase recycling of municipal solid waste.

The handling of garbage is one of the biggest expenses of city budgets, behind education, police protection, and fire protection. Improper disposal of waste can cause problems with vermin and insects. Laws have been designed to regulate the management and disposal of waste, the cleanup of **dump** sites detrimental to communities, and minimizing the amount of waste dumped into landfills. Landfills that are poorly constructed or managed can also leak hazardous substances into groundwater supplies.

The first federal law to address the problem of solid waste was the Solid Waste Disposal Act of 1965. This act provided research and technical assistance to state and local planners. In 1970, the Resource Recovery Act was designed to promote the demonstration, construction, and application of waste management and resource recovery systems. The Resource Conservation and Recovery Act of 1976 was designed to regulate the storage, transfer, transportation, and disposal of hazardous substances. This act required states to develop comprehensive plans for the management of nonhazardous (or household) wastes. It also established a system for controlling hazardous waste from the moment it is generated until it is disposed. Finally, it regulated the performance of underground tanks and the development of new methods to prevent, detect, and repair leaks in existing facilities (US EPA, 2005a).

Ways to Dispose of Solid Waste

Prior to the 1800s, it was a common practice to dump garbage and **sewage** out the windows onto the streets. As more people moved to cities to find jobs, it became apparent that a different method was needed to decrease noxious odors and rat populations. Citizens began to use pits for disposal but that practice still attracted flies and other pests. In 1874, **incineration** of municipal waste was used to reduce the volume of trash and garbage, but concerns about the cost and air quality arose. Finally it was determined that waste needed to be transported outside of city limits but asking citizens to do this on their own resulted in open dumping along roadsides and open property. Realizing that waste disposal was becoming a public health concern and a nuisance, city officials in the twentieth century began to set up garbage collection systems (Figure 14-1). Official garbage dumps (now known as *landfills*) were developed with trucks to carry it from urban areas to the dump site (Figure 14-2).

Waste is categorized according to its relative harm to the environment; it is either hazardous or nonhazardous. The term *solid waste* is often used to describe nonhazardous waste. The most common method for disposing of solid waste is land disposal. Over half of solid waste is disposed on land, more than 25% is **recycled** or recovered, and 15% is incinerated (US EPA, 2001).

LAND DISPOSAL

Land disposal consists of landfills, land application, and deep-well injection. Landfills, land set aside for dumping garbage, are the most common.

Landfills

Landfills are popular because this method of waste disposal is cheaper than the others. The method consists of digging a large hole in the ground, dumping solid waste into designated areas, packing it down tightly, and then covering the waste materials with dirt. For this reason,

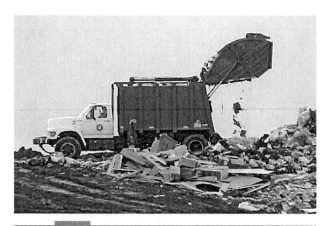

FIGURE 14-1 **Garbage Truck** Residential areas in urban settings need the help of garbage services to remove trash.

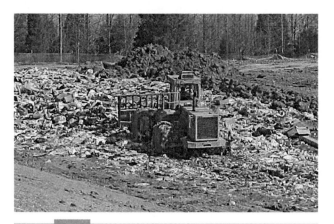

FIGURE 14-2 **Landfill** Landfills must be compacted by heavy equipment.

landfills fill up quickly. Communities relying on landfill disposal must continue to look for additional sites, usually farther away from where the first one was excavated. This is also a problem as no one wants a landfill near their property. As a result, the cost of solid waste management services increase due to increased transportation costs and landfill fees associated with higher construction costs.

Landfills must be built where land is sectioned off in areas with high groundwater tables and sandy **loam** soil. A major concern with the use of landfills is pollution of groundwater. As new landfills are being built, some are installed with multiple liners. **Leachate** migration (liquid materials that leak through liners and penetrate soil) can contain harmful substances. Landfills must be carefully constructed on soil with a vinyl liner over a foundation or base between the garbage and the land (Figure 14-3). There should also be a geologic buffer such as a layer of rock under the liner above the aquifer. There should also be a special collection container where leachate can be diverted. If the liner becomes torn or cracked, garbage residue leaks into the ground, **percolates** through the soil, and enters groundwater supplies. Even the most advanced landfills, however, will eventually leak into surface or underground water (Wadman, 2005).

Concerns associated with landfills are debris that blows onto nearby land and the odor. As garbage decomposes, methane gas is produced. Methane not only causes odors, but it is flammable and can start a fire that can burn for years. The smell of rotting garbage attracts vermin, flies, and other pests to landfill areas. When a new landfill is proposed, residents often protest because of these concerns as well as the increased litter, traffic, and noise. In spite of the disadvantages, landfills will continue to be the primary means of disposing solid waste. The number of landfills is expected to decrease, however, making it necessary to create regional landfills that serve several communities, counties, and even states. Despite this it is necessary to decrease the volume of waste by diverting some of the waste to recycling facilities.

Land Application

Land application means that **sludge** is discharged over large areas of land for drying. After it has dried sufficiently, the material is tilled into the ground and used as fertilizer. There are some objections to this process because biosolids may still contain pathogens that can get onto food raised from this land (Renner, 2002). The pathogens can also become airborne. In most cases, the biosolids are treated and environmental authorities

Mulch
A protective layer of chipped yard waste that is used in landscaping around plants to prevent evaporation.

Dump
The act of unloading waste; an open, unmanaged, illegal disposal site used instead of a permitted landfill.

Sewage
Objects, chemicals, and wastewater poured down the drain or flushed down the toilet.

Incineration
The burning of waste.

Recycle
To collect, separate, process and market materials so they can be used again.

Loam
A rich soil consisting of sand, clay, and decaying organic materials.

Leachate
Rain water or other liquid that percolates through solid waste and dissolves hazardous materials from it, often contaminating ground and surface water.

Percolate
To pass or ooze through.

Sludge
Solids and liquids separated out of wastewater when sewage is treated; usually containing organic matter, pathogens, metals, and chemicals.

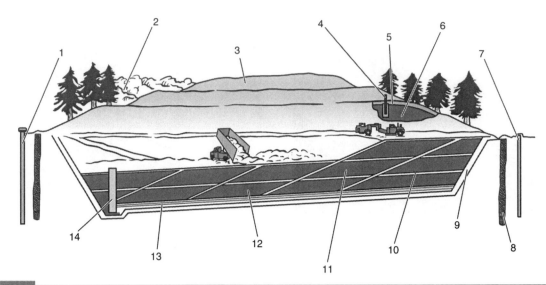

FIGURE **14-3** **Landfill Diagram** (1) Groundwater monitoring well. (2) Screening vegetation. (3) Vegetated and graded slopes to promote runoff and minimize erosion. (4) Gas vent pipe. (5) Vegetated topsoil. (6) Clay cap. (7) Methane gas probe. (8) Slurry wall. (9) Low permeability clay liner. (10) Daily cover. (11) Compacted waste. (12) Granular leachate collection layer. (13) Leachate collection pipe. (14) Leachate sump. Source: http://www.cedarnet.org/bhcswmc/cell.html.

monitor the types of pathogens that should be controlled before the discharge. Other land application methods include spraying **effluent** over the land.

Deep-Well Injection

Deep-well injection is used to dispose of wastes that might harm the public by placing them in a specially designed well that is deep beneath the surface of the ground. On average, injection wells are one-quarter to 1 mile below the ground surface. The sites are carefully selected so that groundwater cannot be contaminated and the rock formations around the well are secure. Hazardous materials, such as solvents, dioxins, and large amounts of heavy metals, organophosphates, and biphenyls, are not permitted in these sites.

INCINERATION

Incineration is used as an alternative to landfills for approximately 15% of municipal solid waste in the United States (Tilford, 2000). Although waste is reduced up to 75% by burning, there are still leftover products such as ash and particulate matter. Trucks dump waste into a pit, the waste is moved to the furnace by a crane, the furnace burns the waste at a very high temperature that heats a boiler producing steam, and the steam generates electricity and heat. Most experts believe that incineration can never be a primary means for garbage disposal because the ash still needs to be transported to a landfill. In addition, poisonous gases (such as dioxin), acid gases (sulfur dioxide and nitrous oxide), and heavy metals (such as mercury) can be emitted when chlorine, paints, fluores-

cent lights, batteries, electronics, aerosols, and other waste products are burned. Pollution-control devices such as scrubbers help to minimize the pollution, but particulate matter is still a problem when burning anything. Scrubbers do not eliminate harmful emissions. In addition, **toxic** materials still end up in the ash that is transferred to the soil.

Ways of Reducing Solid Waste

Landfills are filling quickly and land for new landfills is becoming more difficult to find. Rather than looking for more land to dump waste, the most effective means at reducing solid waste is the source reduction technique. **Source reduction** is fundamentally different and more desirable than waste management or pollution control because it minimizes the accumulation of waste.

The use of disposable items has increased the demand for more landfills. Some countries have responded by encouraging citizens to recycle reusable products. In some cases, money is returned for recycling items. Agricultural and **yard waste** account for a significant amount of land pollution. **Composting** and **vermicomposting** are ways to utilize yard and garden waste and other plant waste to hasten the decomposition process. The resulting **compost** can be used to protect water loss from the soil and to return essential nutrients back to topsoil. In this way, it can be used as a natural fertilizer (DHEC, 1994). In 1996, the EPA observed that solid waste decreased due to source re-

264   ENVIRONMENTAL HEALTH

Approximately 18 to 30% of solid waste hauled to landfills is food and yard waste that can be reused. Yard waste can be recycled for personal use by a method known as *composting*. Composting reduces old yard waste such as grass clippings, tree and shrub prunings, and leaves into mulch and fertilizer for the garden and lawn. Vegetable matter, coffee grounds with paper coffee filters, egg shells, fruits, tea leaves in bags, grass clippings, shrub trimmings, and leaves are deposited into a pile that is watered and mixed periodically to enhance decomposition. Composting can be done on one's property, but it must be done away from the house and neighbors who may complain about the smell. Compost piles can be contained in a plastic garbage bag (with the bottom cut out and holes in the side to let air circulate), a wooden bin, or a wire cage. The following provides guidelines for composting:

1. Find a level spot in the corner of the yard about 3 to 5 square feet.

2. Pile compost materials onto the spot and keep it moist by watering occasionally.

3. Stir with a pitchfork or stick every few weeks to circulate air to stimulate the decomposition process and distribute moisture evenly.

4. If the compost has a bad odor, the pile is too wet and there is not enough air. Turn it and add coarser materials.

5. If the pile becomes dry, add moisture retaining materials such as grass and cover the pile, water it, and then turn it.

6. If the pile is damp, but woody, turn it and mix in fresh grass clippings or fertilizer. Chop up large woody pieces.

7. The compost is done when it becomes a dark, crumbly material that is uniform in texture. The process takes several weeks to 3 to 6 months.

Communities can begin composting projects that collect materials, allow them to decompose, and then "decontaminate" or "refine" the composting product. It can then be bagged and sold. Because of its ability to retain moisture, the decomposed material can be used for landscaping mulch and fertilizer for farms, gardens, or nurseries. Source: South Carolina Department of Health and Environmental Control, 1994.

---

duction. The decrease was largely due to better consumer use of yard trimmings and food scraps through composting, mulching, and other means.

Consumers pay for the packaging on products. Consumers have indicated that they are willing to pay more for packaging that would cause less harm to the environment (Pierce, 2002). This has stimulated a concept known as "green marketing" that emphasizes the benefits of "green design" for product packaging. Product manufacturers also substituted glass containers with plastic and other materials that were lighter and took up less space than traditional packaging materials.

In addition to buying fewer disposable products, **source reduction techniques** include recycling and composting. Interest in recycling began in the 1980s when citizens realized that landfills were filling up and other states would not accept their garbage. The term *recycling* is applied to any item that can be reused. Recycling is a recovery method that reduces the amount of solid waste hauled to the landfill or **incinerator**. Estimates are that at least half of consumer waste can be recycled. Items that can be recycled include paper, glass, cans, and plastic. Paper products can be mixed with rags to make recycled

Effluent
Solid, liquid or gas waste material being discharged into the environment, either treated or untreated; usually used to describe water discharges; can be used for air or other material emitted into the environment.

Toxic
A substance that will cause harm, illness, or death.

Source reduction
Another term for waste reduction; deliberately reduces waste through prudent purchases and product usage.

Yard waste
Grass clippings, shrub prunings, leaves, tree branches, and other discarded organic material from yards and gardens.

Composting
A process of degrading organic matter (such as yard waste, kitchen scraps, and manure) by microorganisms into a humus-like material that is nutrient-rich that can be used as a soil conditioner; this is done in an outside pit or bin set aside for composting waste.

Vermicomposting
The production of compost using worms to digest organic waste.

Compost
A mixture of decomposing vegetable refuse for fertilizing and conditioning soil.

Source reduction technique
Reducing the amount of waste by redesigning products, patterns of production, or consumption; includes reducing packaging, reusing products, or lengthening the life of products to postpone disposal.

Incinerator
A furnace for burning garbage or other refuses.

The most common form of paper to be recycled is newspaper. It is accepted in virtually all recycling centers. Some recycling centers also will accept corrugated cardboard; some will take magazines. Businesses are encouraged to recycle other paper waste by shredding it and placing it in plastic bags for other uses such as use for packing materials.

The Coors Brewery Company was the first to advocate the recycling of aluminum cans. Today nearly 90% of aluminum cans are recycled. A major reason for the success of recycling aluminum cans is the money received for turning them in.

Some states have "bottle laws" that mandate a deposit of 5 to 10 cents on glass beverage containers. When bottles are turned in, the person receives the deposit back.

paper products. Most glass, metal, and plastics are not **biodegradable** and remain intact for many years. Glass can be reused or crushed to make other products. Some states have "bottle deposit" programs in which consumers pay extra for products sold in glass. When the bottles are brought back, the consumer gets their deposit back. Aluminum is the most abundant metal on Earth and has been used to make cans since the 1820s. As a result, quantities of the metal are decreasing. The largest use for aluminum is to make beverage cans. Because soft drink consumption has increased dramatically, aluminum cans contribute substantially to the amount of solid waste generated. Fortunately, aluminum cans can be recycled and used again. More than 40 different types of plastic is generated in the United States creating more plastic than aluminum cans and all other metals combined.

Problems associated with recycling programs include the costs associated with collecting and transporting the product to the transfer sites and to the places where the products can be reused. Most consumers prefer that waste

management companies provide curbside pick-up. Some communities offer recycling collection sites where citizens can transport their garbage and recyclables nearly every day of the week at no charge. Smaller communities with recycling advocates have been creative in recruiting volunteers to help host collection days on certain weekends.

It is best to have recyclable materials pre-sorted to minimize handling. Newspapers are bundled, cardboard boxes are flattened, glass is sorted by color, aluminum cans are separated from tin cans, and plastic is sorted according to number.

Another problem is low demand for recyclable materials. The cost for recycling programs cannot be offset by the sale of the materials. There is a market for automobile batteries, tires, and printer cartridges. Automobile oil can also be reused. Nearly every state has some type of recycling program, and some states have laws requiring residents to recycle. Some states require certain items (newspapers, telephone directories, garbage bags, glass containers and plastic containers) to be made from recycled materials.

Innovative Approaches to Waste Management

ome public power companies are showing an interest in "**green power**"; that is, the use of waste materials as fuel for generating elec-

---

Consider the Cost PERSONAL WASTE MANAGEMENT STRATEGIES

Until the twentieth century, Americans were creative in how they disposed of their waste products. Food scraps were fed to farm animals that produced eggs or meat. Clothes were mended and worn again. Items were passed on to the next generation or to less fortunate people. Rags or scraps were used to make quilts, rugs, and other items. Broken items were repaired. Things that could no longer be used were burned for fuel. On many farms and in

poorer communities and neighborhoods, these practices still apply and there is less waste. In contrast, richer neighborhoods generate volumes of trash because economic buying power provides the means to buy more items other than the essentials. Technological advancements have produced disposable items such as pantyhose, ink pens, food packaging, paper diapers, paper towels, and other items that were not made or meant to be reused. Attracted

to convenience, consumers are drawn to items that do not outlive their usefulness because it is easier to throw them out than to repair them.

The concept of "trash" is conceived according to how one perceives the value or usefulness of an item. Consumers today believe that most items will eventually become worthless or obsolete. As a result, consumers are producing more garbage than ever before.

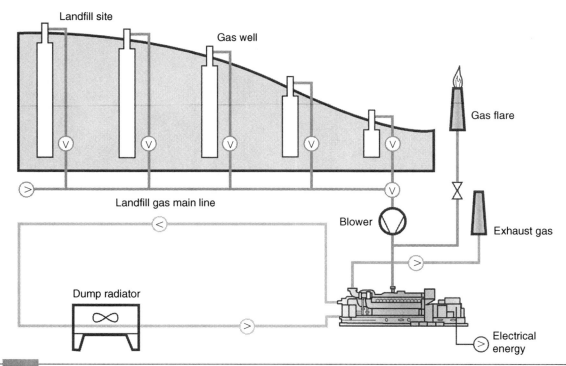

Landfill site

Gas well

Gas flare

Gas flare

Landfill gas main line

Blower

Exhaust gas

Dump radiator

Electrical energy

FIGURE **14-4** **Green Power** "Green Power" is another word for using waste for fuel. Source: GE Mechanical. Used with permission.

tricity (Figure 14-4). This is also known as *waste heat recovery.* Incinerators (known as *waste-to-energy facilities*) burn as much as 250 tons of garbage per day (IWSA, 2005). Some have pollution control devices that minimize particulate matter discharge. The problem with converting trash to energy is the cost associated with it. Because of this, the amount of energy generated from green power is less than 2% of the nation's total energy supply (Chadderdon, 2004).

Another source of green power is the burning of methane gas from landfills. Gas produced by landfills is 50% methane and 50% other gases, including sulfur, which gives landfills their characteristic smell. Methane (CH_4) is a hydrocarbon gas produced from decomposition of organic materials. It is an explosive gas and can be collected from landfills and converted to carbon dioxide, water, and energy to use to fuel engines that provide electricity to household users.

Human Waste

n developing countries where there are no sanitation facilities, human waste (excrement) pollutes the land and water as residents urinate or defecate on the ground, in waterways, in ditches, or in pits. In many urban areas, human waste is disposed in a sewer system.

MANAGEMENT OF HUMAN WASTE IN RURAL AREAS

In rural areas, pit privies (Figure 14-5), cesspools (Figure 14-6), and **septic** tanks are used. A pit *privy,* also known as an outhouse, is a hole dug with a small building placed over it for seating one or two people. The pit privy is moved when it is filled. Pit privies must be built 100 feet away from a water source to prevent contamination of drinking water from private wells. A *cesspool* consists of a large perforated tank surrounded by an absorption bed where solids are digested by bacteria and water is filtered through an open bottom and holes in the sides. Cesspools function according to how many chemicals from the house, such as detergents, bleach, and other cleaners, are discharged into the cesspool.

Biodegradable
Capable of being broken down by microorganisms into simple, stable compounds such as carbon dioxide and water; able to break down or compose easily.

Green power
New term for "refuse-derived fuel"; the incineration of solid waste for fuel.

Septic
Something that contains disease-causing organisms and causes putrefaction.

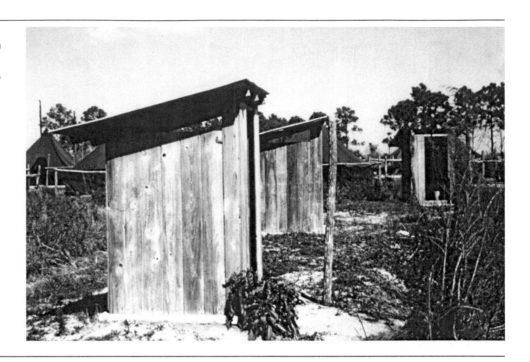

FIGURE **14-5** **Pit Privies on Migrant Farm Camp** In many parts of the United States and other countries, these facilities are used.

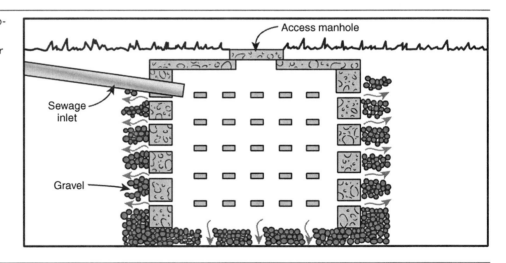

FIGURE **14-6** Cesspools provide one way of managing household sewage when sewer systems are unavailable. Source: G. E. Mechanical, http://www.gemechanical. com/septic101.html. Used with permission.

Labels in figure: Access manhole · Sewage inlet · Gravel

Some rural homeowners and residents living outside municipal boundaries install septic systems to handle human and household waste from the kitchen, bathrooms, and laundry (Figure 14-7). A *septic system* consists of a septic tank made of concrete, plastic, or fiberglass; an inspection port; and an absorption field (sometimes called a drain field) where the effluent flows into the soil. The septic tank is a watertight container made of concrete or fiberglass with a capacity from 750 to 2000 gallons (at least 250 gallons per person in the house) and is buried in the ground with trenches or ditches leading to a drain field (Clemson Extension Service, 1992). The septic tank holds sewage for 24 to 72 hours. During this time, heavier materials settle to the bottom, forming sludge. Lighter particles migrate to the top of **wastewater**, forming a **scum** layer. The middle layer consists of wastewater that flows out of the tank to the drainage field. The wastewater effluent filters through the soil and soil microorganisms break down the organic material. Tanks require periodic cleaning every 3 to 5 years to remove the scum and sludge layers. The frequency of cleaning a septic tank depends on the amount of solids going into the tank. The toilet should not be used as a trash receptacle for facial tissues, feminine hygiene products, condoms, or cigarette butts. Grease and oils should not be poured down the drain. A garbage disposal doubles the amount of solids in the tank so it will need to be emptied more often.

According to the EPA, United States residents produce 4.4 pounds of waste per person per day compared to 2.7 pounds per person per day in 1960 (US EPA, 2004). Responsible consumers are aware of what they consume and what they dispose of. The concept of **enviroshopping** is related to "precycling," or reducing the amount of consumables used, particularly those with excessive or disposable packaging (SWA, 2005). The idea is to think about how the product would be disposed before you buy it. Enviroshoppers want to use products that are necessary, reusable or recyclable, made from plentiful resources or recycled materials, and has a minimal amount of packaging, therefore reducing waste and the need for disposal.

To become an enviroshopper, follow the five "R's" of enviroshopping:

- Reduce the amount of packaging you buy and throw away (also known as *precycling*).

- Reuse packaging when possible.

- Recycle whenever possible.

- Reject packaging that is unsatisfactory.

- Respond to producers and retailers to let them know how you feel about the environment.

Precycling, also known as *source reduction,* is the most important thing an enviroshopper can do to reduce the solid waste problem. If you don't buy a product or bring it into the home in the first place, you won't have to worry about what to do with the waste it leaves behind. Examples of precycling strategies include:

- Take grocery bags back to the store to keep from having to get new ones every time.

- Purchase and use canvas shopping bags to use each time you shop.

- Look for packages that use the least amount of material. Avoid those that have several layers when one layer would do.

- Buy concentrated products, then dilute them at home in a larger reusable container.

- Buy products in the largest quantity possible in one package. Refill smaller spray bottles or dispensers from the large jug.

- Buy items in tubes rather than "pumps" (such as toothpaste).

- Use cloth rather than paper napkins.

- Do not buy large containers of food if you cannot use it up before it spoils.

- Look for products with reusable dishes, rather than paper, styrofoam, or disposables.

- Select loose produce so you can get the pieces you want. Large packages often have bruised or moldy produce you have to buy with the package.

- Eat inside a fast food restaurant to save on extra packaging from the drive-thru.

- Encourage fast food restaurants to use recycled materials.

- Reduce clutter in the home by having a yard/garage sale, or donating items to charity.

- Consider renting an item you may rarely use or repairing items that work as well as a new one.

Sources: Solid Waste Authority, 2005; U.S. Environmental Protection Agency, 2004.

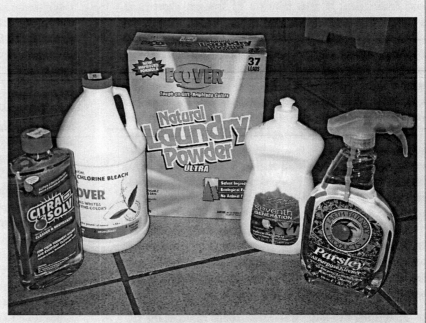

Wastewater
Liquid waste, unclean water that has been used for industrial or household purposes.

Scum
Excess matter that forms on the top of water or other liquid.

Enviroshopping
The practice of purchasing goods and services in the interest of preserving the environment; includes buying recycled products, products with minimal packaging, products that are not harmful, and products that can be recycled.

Precycle
To reduce waste at the source by changing buying habits.

FIGURE 14-7 Septic tanks are an improvement over cesspools because the sewage is dispersed over a larger area away from the building.
Source: G. E. Mechanical http://www.gemechanical.com/septic101.html. Used with permission.

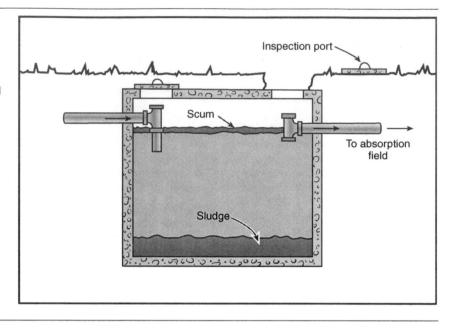

SEWAGE DISPOSAL IN URBAN AREAS

Sewage consists of liquid wastes from homes, businesses, and industries. It also consists of human excrement, garbage disposed down the drain, water, detergents, cleansers, and anything else poured down the drain. It contains debris such as toilet paper, tissues, tampons, condoms, hair, and sand. Sewage may also contain urban runoff from roads, roofs, yards, golf courses, and parking lots. This adds more toxic materials from automobile emissions, pesticides, paint, and other toxic substances. The proper disposal of sewage is important to prevent the spread of disease, protect water supplies, and to return water back to the environment in a safe form. In cities, human waste, water, food, detergents, and household chemicals are routed away from the home through sewer pipes to wastewater treatment facilities.

The management of sewage in cities is usually referred to as *municipal wastewater treatment*. The treatment of wastewater addresses the suspended solids, organic matter, inorganic matter, and bacteria decomposition. Wastewater is treated through several stages.

■ Preliminary treatment removes solids through the use of screens, grit chambers, gravel, or other means to catch floating debris as wastewater flows through the material. The solids are shredded or ground and coarse objects are removed to a landfill. The wastewater then is "shaken up" and exposed to air. This causes some of the dissolved gases (such as hydrogen sulfide) to be released from the water. The wastewater enters a series of long, parallel concrete tanks known as *settling tanks*. Air is pumped through the water to replenish the oxygen supply and to keep organic material suspended while other particles

known as *grit* (sand, coffee grounds, etc.) settle out. The grit is pumped out of the settling tanks and taken to the landfill. This stage of treatment does not reduce suspended solids, **biochemical oxygen demand (BOD)**, bacteria, or toxins. The wastewater still represents a serious environmental and health hazard and is not considered "treated" at this point.

■ Primary treatment occurs when wastewater moves to sedimentation tanks. This stage is sometimes referred to as the *sedimentation stage* because materials sink to the bottom and rise to the top of the tank. Aluminum sulfate or another foaming agent may be added to precipitate suspended solids (grease, oil, plastics, soap, etc.). This is sometimes referred to as the **flocculation stage**. Flocculation tanks have slowly rotating wooden paddles to continuously mix the water and chemicals. The floc is carried to sedimentation tanks where water is retained until it settles to the bottom with the sludge. The scum is skimmed off the surface of the wastewater by slow-moving rakes and thickened before it is pumped to the **digesters** with the sludge. The resulting solids may be kept for 20 to 30 days in large, heated tanks where bacteria breaks down the material, reducing it in volume and odors and killing pathogens. It is then agitated and compressed and sent to landfills or released to drying beds for fertilizer on open land. Conventional primary treatment without the use of chemicals removes 40 to 60% of the total suspended solids and 25 to 40% of the *BOD*. It reduces fecal coliform levels by 45 to 55% and about half of the metals found in water, but little if any of the other toxics.

A lagoon is a shallow pond located at least one quarter mile from residential areas where seepage will not pollute groundwater. A lagoon is a rectangular excavation, at least half an acre in area and from 3 to 5 feet in depth. Organic materials settle to the bottom of the lagoon where bacteria decomposes them into ammonia, carbon dioxide, and water. Algae feed on the solid nutrients and sunlight reduces odors.

Sewage consists of 99% water and 1% suspended bacteria, plant, mineral, and animal material.

The bacteria is both nonpathogenic and pathogenic. The **biochemical oxygen demand (BOD)** is a measure of oxygen required to satisfy oxygen demands of the sewage. A high BOD means the sewage is highly concentrated and large amounts of oxygen is being used by the biochemical actions of the sewage. BOD is as important as pH and temperature to water quality because they all determine whether other organisms, such as fish and other aquatic and plant life, can survive. The BOD represents the amount of dissolved oxygen in the water, essential to fish, aquatic plants, and other wildlife.

BOD is calculated by taking two oxygen readings from the same water sample. The water is placed into two different vials with the same dilution of distilled water. The vials are shaken and an oxygen meter reads the first vial to determine the concentration of oxygen. The second vial is tested 5 days later. BOD is calculated by subtracting the meter reading from the second vial from the meter reading from the first vial.

Water from an exceptionally clear lake might show a BOD of less than 2 ml/liter of water. Raw sewage may have readings in the hundreds. Food-processing wastes may be in the thousands.

■ Secondary treatment is known as *biological treatment* because it uses biological oxidation to break down wastewater pollutants and reduce the BOD. Bacteria and microorganisms are allowed to consume the rest of the organic material. It is also known as the *filtering stage* because trickling filters are used to **aerate** the effluent, reduce the BOD, and activate the sludge to promote the breakdown of organic matter. Trickling filters consist of a bed of coarse stones or plastic covered with bacteria, protozoa, and fungi. Activated sludge treatment occurs in an aeration tank where wastewater is mixed with bacteria-rich sludge to create a mixture that is aerated for several hours. The mixture is transferred to a settling tank where the sludge is routed back to the aeration tank. The effluent flows to a clarifier tank. At the end of this stage, almost all of the fecal coliform bacterium is removed. Much of the metals and organic toxics are also removed from the effluent. The effluent is still harmful to aquatic life because of the high ammonia content.

■ Tertiary treatment includes processes necessary to handle the sewage, depending on the type of problems. After the solids are removed, the wastewater filters through sand, crushed anthracite coal, diatomaceous earth, and sometimes carbon particles to further remove suspended solids and reduce BOD. This is often referred to as the *filtration stage*. This removes almost all the bacteria, reduces turbidity, removes odors, reduces iron, and removes most other solid particles that remained in the wastewater. Phosphates, nitrogen, and carbon must be removed or algae will grow in the water body where it will be stored. Aluminum sulfate or ferrous chloride is used to remove phosphorus. Nitrogen removal is more complex, moving the effluent through towers dis-

tributing it in trays. As effluent falls from the trays, droplets are formed. This enables ammonia gas to escape so chlorination can be more efficient.

■ The *disinfection stage* normally adds chlorine to reduce BOD and odor. Ozone, bromine, hydrogen peroxide, iodine, or UV light exposure can also be used to kill disease-causing pathogens. The **chlorine residual** should be between .25 and .70 ppm. The end product of sewage treatment is

Flocculation stage
A stage of wastewater management when small particles of solids clump together forming a sediment.

Digesters
A vessel in which materials are digested, or converted into an absorbable substance.

Aerate
To expose to the circulation of air, as in raking a compost pile.

Biochemical oxygen demand (BOD)
A measure of oxygen required to satisfy oxygen demands; the amount of oxygen that would be consumed if all the organics in one liter of water were oxidized by bacteria and protozoa.

Chlorine residual
Chlorine remaining in water or wastewater at the end of the disinfection stage that will react chemically and biologically.

water that can be safely discharged into a body of water such as a pond, lake, or lagoon.

■ The final stage of wastewater treatment dumps effluent into receiving waters such as rivers, lakes, or the ocean under the supervision of federal or state agencies. The larger the body of receiving water, the greater the safety factor (Green & Ottoson, 1999).

Sewage treatment costs are paid for by citizens through their water bills. This practice is based on the assumption that the amount of water a household uses is a good indication of how much the household uses sewer services. Cities without adequate sewage systems pose a public health problem. Construction and operation of sewage treatment facilities and effluent disposal are responsibilities of the community. Some communities find it necessary to issue bonds for the construction of a treatment plant. Regulation of sewage treatment plants and disposal of effluents are the responsibility of state officials, and plans for sewage treatment systems must be approved by state engineers. Sewage disposal plant operators must pass state certification examinations.

Scrap Metal and Bulk Waste

crap metal waste comes from discarded automobiles, household appliances, and other items such as bicycles, furniture, televisions, mattresses, chairs, sofas, toys, and more. Automobile salvage yards buy and store scrap iron and other metals. Consumers can often purchase "recycled" items here for less money than new to replace broken parts. Salvage yards are considered an eyesore in most communities and some cities have required owners to erect large fences to make the neighborhood more attractive. Salvage yards also provide shelter for vermin, snakes, and other less desirable animals. Some salvage yards crush the automobiles and transport them to facilities where the metal can be reused. Some appliances, furniture, tires, and bicycles can be repaired and resold (Figure 14-8). If the item cannot be repaired, resold, or used, which is often the case, then the landfill is the last option. Some items have parts with hazardous materials that should be handled appropriately.

Regulating Waste Disposal

aste must be handled carefully to prevent contamination of water supplies and the air. When the Resource Conservation and Recovery Act (PL 94-580) was passed in 1976, the idea was to protect human health and the environment from potential hazards associated with waste disposal. The act provided guidance pertaining to preserving natural resources and energy, waste reduction, and waste management. There were specific regulations for solid waste, hazardous waste, and underground storage tanks containing petroleum products or certain chemicals. There are other acts associated with waste disposal, such as the Clean Air Act Amendments (PL 95-95), Clean Water Act (PL 95-217), and the Safe Drinking Water Act (PL 93-523). These laws call for the preservation of clean air and water. Prior to these laws, it was not uncommon for solid waste to be dumped in the open, discharged into surface waters, or burned.

FIGURE 14-8 **Tire Pile**
Old tires are often discarded rather than recycled. They can be refurbished for resale.

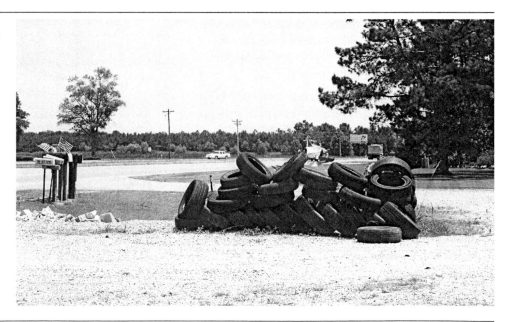

Digging Deeper — HAZARDOUS WASTE REPORTING

The Emergency Planning and Community Right-to-Know Act of 1986 (EPCRA) (PL 99-499) established ways citizens can be aware of toxic releases in their area and prepare for potential disasters. Since 1987, EPCRA has required industrial facilities to manufacturing, mining, electricity production, and hazardous waste treatment facilities to report their production and disposal of toxic waste. According to Sections 311 and 312 of EPCRA, businesses are to report the locations and quantities of chemicals stored on-site to help communities prepare for accidental spills or similar emergencies. Section 313 requires EPA and each state to collect data on releases and transfers of toxic chemicals and to make the data available to the community by publishing the Toxics Release Inventory (TRI). In 1990, Congress passed the Pollution Prevention Act requiring that additional data on waste management and source reduction activities be reported on the TRI.

The EPA has reported a decrease in toxic chemical waste by more than 20% from 2000 to 2001. In 2000, the chemical manufacturing sector decreased toxic waste from 15.7 billion pounds to 10.7 billion pounds, a reduction of 32.2%. The primary metals industry reported the second largest decrease with 27.4%, and the metal mining industry had the third largest decrease with 15.5% (USEPA, 2003). According to the EPA, over 20,000 hazardous waste generators produce over 40 million tons of hazardous waste each year (USEPA, 2004).

Hazardous Waste

*H*azardous *waste* is defined as any waste product that is **ignitable**, corrosive, **reactive**, or toxic. It can be in solid, liquid, or gas form. It is called hazardous because it causes injury, illness, death, and destruction of the environment. Hazardous waste is only a small portion of all waste generated, but the potential for human harm is greater (Figure 14-9). Serious health problems arise when inhaled, ingested, or absorbed. In 2002, the EPA listed more than 500 hazardous wastes.

The EPA distinguishes between large-quantity and small-quantity generators of hazardous wastes. Large-quantity generators are responsible for the production of 90% of all hazardous waste in the United States. The largest producers are chemical manufacturers, followed by petroleum refineries, and metal-processing industries. The remaining 10% comes from small-quantity generators and households.

Ignitable
Ability to catch fire easily; refers to liquid having a low flashpoint or nonliquids liable to cause fires with friction, moisture absorption, or spontaneous chemical change.

Reactive
Producing a heat reaction, and sometimes a gas, as a result of two chemicals being combined; capable of exploding and generating toxic gases when combined with air or water.

FIGURE 14-9 **Hazardous Waste** Hazardous waste must be disposed of properly to minimize the danger of potential exposure.

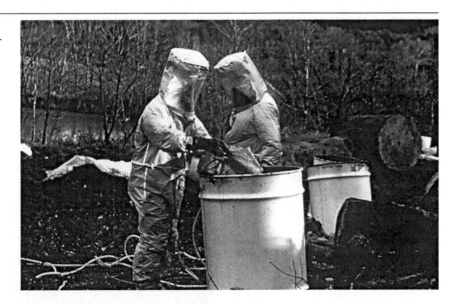

Types of Hazardous Waste

There are many types of hazardous waste including *commercial, household,* **medical waste,** and **e-waste** to name just a few. Hazardous waste is a potential danger to humans, animals, plants, and the land.

COMMERCIAL WASTE

Mining operations produce waste when rock, tailings, and water are discharged. In order to remove minerals, ore, or uranium from the ground, rock has to be removed. Chemicals are also necessary to remove minerals from the ore and become waste products that need to be disposed of properly. Between 96 to 98% of the waste generated from gas and oil drilling is water. The water is either pumped out of the ground or it is mixed with oil.

The water and oil or gas is separated before it is refined for fuel. When water is discharged from agricultural, manufacturing, and other industrial uses, it is often referred to a large pond where it is treated before it is disposed. This is known as **surface impoundment.**

There are other commercial businesses and industries that also have hazardous waste products to dispose. Any business that uses solvents, manufactures pesticides, or makes products with them is likely to have problems disposing of their hazardous wastes. Construction waste is also considered commercial waste (Figure 14-10).

HOUSEHOLD WASTE

There are many products that are used and need to be disposed of that are considered hazardous. Some of the products such as batteries, engine oil, and paint can be recycled. Any product that is corrosive such as cleaning

FIGURE 14-10 Construction Waste
Construction waste is considered commercial waste, a significant source of solid waste in developing communities.

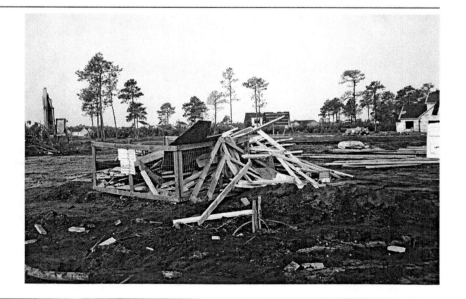

sprays, cleansers, drain uncloggers, or aerosol products have the potential for harm if they are not treated as hazardous waste materials (National Ag Safety Database, 2002). Many recycling centers have proper receptacles for disposing of them. Other communities will host a specific day or week when hazardous household materials can be collected.

MEDICAL WASTE

The EPA defines *medical waste* as any solid waste generated as a result of diagnosis, treatment, or immunization of human beings or animals. Hospitals generate about 15 to 25 pounds of waste per hospital bed, 16 to 20% of which is considered "infectious" (Rutala & Odette, 1989). Medical waste carries pathogens from body fluids such as saliva, semen, vaginal secretions, cerebrospinal fluid, synovial fluid, pleural fluid, peritoneal fluid, amniotic fluids, or any bodily fluid contaminated with blood. Infectious medical waste is suspected to contain pathogens in sufficient concentration or quantity to cause disease in susceptible hosts, especially surgical waste and waste from patients in isolation wards, dialysis patients, and items having contact with infected persons or animals.

Medical waste management policies among health care facilities ensure the correct handling, treatment, storage, and disposal procedures by properly training employees, providing hazardous materials receptacles, and medical surveillance of disposal techniques. Medical waste is sometimes reduced by sterilizing or **autoclaving** surgical and other equipment. Some materials are shredded and disinfected with a sodium hypochlorite (bleach) solution. Other materials are gassed, microwaved, or controlled-air incinerated.

Federal regulations and agencies govern the management of medical and infectious waste and each state may also regulate the management of medical waste. The EPA does not regulate medical and infectious waste as a separate type of waste unless it meets the definition of a hazardous waste. Bulk blood, suctioned fluids, excretions, and secretions may be poured down a sewer drain because there is no epidemiological evidence suggesting that medical waste is any more "infectious" than residential waste. The Department of Transportation, however, regulates shipments of medical and infectious wastes (CDC, 2002). State health department officials can provide information and guidance regarding the selection of contractors disposing of medical and infectious waste. There are no standards for how a contractor would dispose of medical and infectious waste, but the EPA and Centers for Disease Control do have some guidelines. The EPA regulates medical waste treatment procedures that reduce the infectiousness of the waste by destroying microorganisms (US EPA, 1998). Treatment methods include chemical treatment, steam sterilization, incineration, encapsulation, or thermal inactivation. Once treated appropriately, medical and in-fectious waste can be accepted for disposal in a landfill (except incinerator ash with hazardous waste characteristics). Residual ash or grindings from medical and infectious waste must be transported to a permanent disposal facility.

A NEW KIND OF WASTE: E-WASTE

Technological advancements and obsolete equipment have generated a new type of waste known as *e-waste*, or *electronic waste*. This type of waste is usually determined to be a type of hazardous type of waste because some of the components of electronic equipment may contain radioactive products or other materials that can be harmful. Unfortunately, most e-waste cannot be reused. The result is a large amount of bulk waste that must be disposed of in the same way as old appliances or automobiles.

Because some components of e-waste are hazardous, they should be disposed of properly. Computer monitors contain brominated flame retardants in circuit boards, cables, wires, casings, and housings. The chemicals in these materials are similar to PCBs, which are environmental toxins. Picture tubes and display screens in televisions and computer monitors contain lead because no suitable alternative can be found. Computer monitors also have cadmium that causes damage to the nervous system. Back-light systems of computer monitors contain mercury, also damaging to the nervous system.

Regulation and Transportation of Hazardous Waste

ecause of the potential dangers, the handling of hazardous waste requires careful storage, transportation, and disposal. The EPA has

Medical waste
Solid waste generated as a result of diagnosis, treatment or immunization of human beings or animals including laboratory equipment, surgical gloves and instruments, needles, body organs, and fabric stained with body fluids.

E-waste
Electronic waste such as televisions, computers, printers, scanners, and computer monitors.

Surface impoundment
The holding of water to be treated until it is safe for disposal.

Autoclaving
A device used to sterilize reusable instruments.

Unwanted household chemicals become not just garbage, but hazardous waste. Many people do not consider household substances as harmful and innocently dump, pour out on the ground, pour down the drain, bury, or burn hazardous substances. The problem with disposal by any of these methods is that hazardous materials are released into the environment, potentially harming innocent children, neighbors, animals, and plant life. Most hazardous materials are "persistent," meaning that they remain in the air, water, and soil for a long period of time. It only takes a small amount of a hazardous substance to pollute large bodies of surface water and groundwater supplies. It is said that it only takes 1 gallon of oil to ruin 1 million gallons of water.

Hazardous materials include **corrosives**, toxic wastes, ignitable waste, and reactive waste. Batteries contain acid, which is corrosive. Pesticides, cleaning products, paints, photographic supplies, and many art supplies are toxic, causing illness or death. Charcoal lighter fluid, gasoline, kerosene, and nail polish remover are ignitable, catching fire or burning easily.

WHY CAN'T I JUST THROW IT IN THE GARBAGE?

Sanitation workers have been seriously burned, lost their eyesight, and suffered lung damage while compacting hazardous materials unknowingly tossed out with other household garbage. Most landfills are not designed so that hazardous waste cannot burn through their vinyl liner and leak into water supplies. For this and other reasons, many landfills do not accept certain hazardous household products. If they do, they will only accept them if the paint is dried and solid or otherwise harmless.

WHY CAN'T I JUST POUR IT DOWN THE DRAIN OR FLUSH IT DOWN THE TOILET?

Hazardous chemical products can corrode plumbing and pipes in the home. If a home has a septic system, certain chemicals can destroy the bacteria needed to break down organic matter. Other chemicals pass through the septic system to the drain field where it is discharged, staying in the soil and harming animals and plants. Some products have chemicals that react with other chemicals in the septic system, making them more harmful than before. If connected to a municipal sewage system, areas where wastewater is discharged (rivers, lakes, streams, oceans) may become contaminated with the chemical.

WHY CAN'T I JUST POUR IT OUT ON THE GROUND OR BURY IT?

Children, pets, and wildlife can be harmed by hazardous waste. Dogs can die from antifreeze poisoning and often find it when it is spilled or poured onto a driveway or roadway. Anything that is poured on the ground (rain, chemicals, oil, etc.) will filter down into groundwater supplies. Most hazardous materials cannot be filtered out of drinking water even with some of the best water treatment facilities. In addition, when it rains on contaminated soil, the chemicals will erode with the soil into lakes, rivers, streams, and the ocean.

WHY CAN'T I JUST BURN IT?

It is better to let trained professionals burn hazardous waste in specially designed incinerators than to risk harming ones self or violating open-burning laws in the area. Some woods used for decks or outdoor construction are coated with creosote or arsenic that can emit harmful gases into the environment. Aerosol cans will explode if burned.

The best way to dispose of hazardous substances is to use it up, donate it to an organization that would be glad to have it, or save it for a community-wide household hazardous materials collection day. Any place that sells auto batteries must also recycle them, and sometimes they may buy the old battery. Used automotive oil can be taken to a gas station, automotive repair business, or oil-changing business. Old tires are sometimes bought by tire dealerships. Paint, household cleaners, and lawn chemicals are accepted by charitable organizations, churches, theater groups, the local housing authority, or other nonprofit organizations. If you are not sure about how to dispose of something, call the local landfill or solid waste management authority. Some items must be taken to a facility where household waste can be properly disposed. It is a good idea to contact the local waste management or solid waste authority for locations, dates, and times for collection.

The following is a list of hazardous household products and how they normally are disposed:

- Dispose in a landfill
  Cosmetics
  Nail polish (solidified)
  Lawn and garden fertilizer
  Auto body filler (solidified)
  Glue-solvent based (solidified)
  Paint-latex (solidified, not exterior paint containing mildewcides or mercury)
  Paint-oil based (solidified)
  Varnish (solidified)
  Shoe polish

- Save for a community hazardous waste collection day
  Automatic transmission fluid
  Automobile battery
  Batteries (cadmium, alkaline, carbon-zinc, lithium)
  Carburetor cleaner
  Car wax (with petroleum distillates)
  Diesel fuel
  Engine degreaser
  Fluorescent light ballast (those manufactured before 1978 contain PCB)
  Floor care products (solvent-based)
  Fuel oil
  Furniture polish
  Fungicides for the lawn
  Gun cleaning solvents
  Herbicides for the lawn or garden
  Insecticides
  Kerosene
  Lighter fluid
  Metal polish (with petroleum distillates)
  Moth balls and flakes
  Motor oil
  Paint (synthetic auto enamel, model airplane)
  Paint brush cleaner with solvent
  Paint thinner
  Photographic chemicals
  Resins (fiberglass or epoxy resins)
  Rodent poison
  Shoe dye
  Swimming pool chemicals (unmixed)
  Spot remover; dry cleaning solvent
  Turpentine
  Artists' paints, mediums (oils)
  Source: Hammet, 1991.

the primary responsibility for permitting facilities to treat, store, and dispose of hazardous waste. Hazardous wastes are regulated under subtitle C of the Resource Conservation and Recovery Act (PL 94-580). In the United States, 96% of all hazardous waste is treated and stored at the site where it is produced. The remaining waste is handled by commercial waste service companies.

Although one would hope that most producers and users of hazardous waste would dispose of it properly, this has not always been the case. Because improper disposal requires expensive cleanup efforts, the Comprehensive Environmental Response, Compensation, and Liability Act of 1980 (CERCLA; PL 96-510) established funds to clean up abandoned hazardous disposal sites. These funds, known as the Superfund, were intended to be used to cleanup disposal sites posing a risk to groundwater and public health (Figure 14-11). When the Superfund was first created, it was to be used for a few sites in a short period of time. It became clear that many more sites needed attention and that the average cleanup operation took at least 12 years to complete. Funds are still available and the law requires the government to maintain a list of sites posing the highest potential threat to human health and the environment. There are over 1,200 sites on the National Priorities List (NPL). Included are "mega sites" that cost more to clean up than other sites. Cleanup of NPL sites are estimated at $1.5 billion per year. Because of the cost, only a few sites can be cleaned up each year. Those generating hazardous waste are compelled to clean up their own mess, but if funds are not available, CERCLA funds can be used. Responsible parties are to pay back the money but it sometimes means legal action. Only about one fifth of the cleanup costs have been recovered because offenders are unable to pay or disappear.

Methods for handling hazardous waste include reduction, recycling, treatment, incineration, land disposal, and deep-well injection. The reduction approach is applied when manufacturers produce less waste. Waste materials can also be recycled or recovered and reused or sold. A variety of processes can be used to neutralize or destroy toxic compounds. Hazardous waste can also be burned. Hazardous wastes that cannot be reduced, recycled, or burned, must be buried like other materials. Before they are buried, however, they must be treated. Hazardous waste can be placed in a "secure" landfill away from drinking water sources in barrels lined with concrete after it has been evaporated or compacted to reduce the volume and hazardous characteristics.

There are many hazardous waste treatment, storage, and disposal facilities in the United States. However, many states do not provide waste disposal facilities, requiring the waste to be transported from one state to another. At one time, each state had to have a plan for dis-

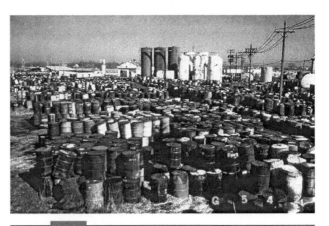

FIGURE **14-11** **Superfund Toxic Waste Cleanup Site** There are many toxic waste sites that are targeted for Superfund cleanup due to limited funding resources.

posing of their hazardous waste. They were not required to have their own facilities, but to belong to a **compact**. Some states have rejected hazardous waste from other states because they do not want to be a dumping ground for other states. The need for hazardous waste facilities is so great that the United States is sending toxic waste out of the country to Mexico, Central America, and South America.

The movement of hazardous waste from one area to another and hazardous waste disposal sites are extremely controversial. Estimates are that nearly 400 million tons of hazardous waste crosses international boundaries, illegally moved to unauthorized disposal sites where regulations are more relaxed and enforcement is overlooked (Yassi, Kjellstrom, de Kok, & Guidotti, 2001). The transportation of hazardous waste poses a major concern because an accident on the road is more likely than a natural disaster exposing hazardous waste from underground. Hazardous waste may be transported by truck, train, or barge. Each transportation order must have a "shipping order" listing the type of waste hauled, proper labels and signs, trained haulers with insurance, and proper registration. Each label contains a symbol and a number so that if an accident should occur, emergency rescue workers are able to identify the materials and take appropriate action.

Corrosives
Products that may eat through living tissue or nonliving items through a chemical reaction; having a pH below 2 or above 12.5.

Compact
An agreement of several states to transport and share storage for low-level radioactive waste in a specific area.

Nuclear Waste

O f the various types of hazardous waste, **radioactive waste** (also known as **nuclear waste**) poses the biggest concern. Radioactive waste in the United States is rated according to two categories: high-level and low-level waste. The disposal of either waste has been highly controversial and there is no consensus on the best way to handle it. Nothing can protect against the risk of exposure to radioactive waste which can exist for thousands of years.

HIGH-LEVEL RADIOACTIVE WASTE

The most dangerous type of radioactive waste is **spent fuel** (also known as **irradiated reactor fuel**) from nuclear power plants. The spent fuel rods have significant amounts of uranium and plutonium with penetrating and toxic radioactivity levels. Some of the fuel rods can be **reprocessed** and the rest must be stored. Nuclear power reactors also generate wastewater when fuel cells are placed in the cooling pond. The water then becomes radioactive and requires special handling. The usual method for disposing of hazardous wastewater produced by large-quantity generators is to store it in deep underground wells.

Another source of high-level radioactive waste is from nuclear weapons that are disarmed or torn apart. However, radioactive waste from nuclear weapons can be converted into fuel for nuclear power plant reactors. Buildings where nuclear materials have been stored must be decontaminated. High-level radioactive waste is characterized by heat generation and a long half-life. Most of the waste is in liquid form and it is stored for a year or more in water tanks or cooling tanks to cool down before being processed for disposal. Once excessive heat generation has subsided, liquid waste is solidified in deep underground stable rock formations that must be safe enough so that the risk to human health or the environment is not likely to occur for thousands of years.

LOW-LEVEL RADIOACTIVE WASTE

Until the 1960s, low-level radioactive wastes were dumped into the ocean. Most radioactive waste is considered "low level" because much of the radioactive properties have already been discharged. Low-level radioactive waste includes waste from nuclear plants such as protective clothing, rags, mops, filters, equipment, tools, and other items used to clean up any spills. Medical facilities also utilize radioactive procedures and need to discard patient items, swabs, injection needles, syringes, human tissue, and laboratory animal carcasses that also are considered low-level radioactive waste. Normally, low-level waste is stored on-site until it has decayed away and can be disposed of as ordinary trash or hauled away to a low-level waste disposal site. Low-level radioactive waste can also be disposed of using near-surface burial or in underground repositories in the United States. This generates concerns about contamination of groundwater, land, and other problems. It takes 10 to 100 years for radioactive waste to decay until it is harmless.

The first commercial site to handle low-level radioactive waste was opened in 1962 and the volume of waste has increased dramatically since then. The Low Level Waste Policy Act of 1980 (PL 96-573) was passed to establish a national system for storage of low-level radioactive waste. The law required each state to find a disposal site and states were encouraged to organize into compacts to develop new waste facilities. For many years, there were only three low-level radioactive waste sites in the United States: Nevada, South Carolina, and Washington. Governors and citizens in these states protested being a dumping ground for the other 47 states. As a result, the Low-Level Radioactive Waste Policy Amendments Act of 1986 (PL 99-240) was passed, making each state responsible for the disposal of low-level radioactive wastes produced within that state. States could either find a disposal site in their state or form a regional compact. Penalties and incentives were formed to encourage states to construct their own sites for low-level radioactive disposal facilities. The Nevada facility closed January 1, 1993 and the only new site was built in Utah in 1995. Until more sites can be built, many nuclear waste generators must store the waste on-site until new disposal facilities are established. As a result, nuclear waste generators have an incentive to minimize the volume of waste and the use of incineration and compacting so the amount of waste is less than it was before.

U.S. government officials and the nuclear regulatory industry have been looking for a location to dispose of nuclear reactor waste for the past 50 years (CBS, 2004). It is currently kept in temporary facilities with cooling ponds and storage buildings in 39 states, accumulating up to 70,000 tons of highly radioactive nuclear waste. For the last 20 years, the Department of Energy and Congress have targeted a facility in Nevada at Yucca Mountain on federal land. While Yucca Mountain is in a desert area, the population in nearby Las Vegas is growing to 1.6 million citizens with 35 million tourists per year. In addition to concerns about potential danger to Nevada citizens if an earthquake should occur, there is concern about the transportation of hazardous waste by truck or rail across the country to the site. The Nuclear Waste Policy Act (PL 97-425) specifies that government activities to build a national used nuclear fuel repository can be reviewed by a court of law. The state of Nevada has challenged the selection of Yucca Mountain as the nation's primary used nuclear fuel repository.
Sources: CBS News, 2004; Nuclear Energy Institute, 2005.

Glass is easy to recycle and saves energy by processing recycled glass compared to making glass from new materials. New glass cannot be completely made from recycled glass, but it can be used for packaging food. All glass can be recycled. It is a good idea to rinse jars out if they do not have the lids on. Many recycling centers ask that lids be removed and sorted according to the type of material used to make the lid (plastic or metal).

Aluminum is 100% recyclable. A pound of recycled aluminum will make a pound of "new" aluminum. If aluminum cannot be separated from other materials, it cannot be reused. Most aluminum cans sold today were made from recycled cans. In order to save space when saving aluminum cans, consumers may crush them.

Corrugated cardboard (often used for moving or storage) and *paper* (office or newspaper) are used to make the grey colored boxes used for cereal boxes or stationary. To save space at home and at the recycling center, flatten the boxes. Some recycling centers ask that newspapers be bound together with twine for easier handling. Some centers ask that colored advertisements inserted into newspapers be removed because they may contain lead or other materials that make recycling difficult or costly.

Steel is easy to recycle because it easily attaches to magnets in order to separate it from other materials. Steel cans (also known as tin cans) can be recycled from food, paint, or aerosol cans. It takes half as much energy to make steel from recycled materials than making it from raw materials (coal, iron, and limestone).

Some *plastics* are more recyclable than others. Plastic containers usually have a number that indicates the type of plastic used; for example, a milk container may be a "2" and a detergent container a "5." Plastics of different types cannot be recycled together, but rather they need to be sorted by resin type. Plastic bottles used to package liter-sized soft drinks can be recycled into fiberfill stuffing, lawn chair strapping, carpet fiber, ski jackets, and erosion control mesh used on new road construction projects. This type of plastic is known as polyethylene terephthalate (PET). The type of plastic used for milk jugs is known as high-density polyethylene (HDPE). It can be used to make agricultural drainage pipes, toys, flower pots, plastic lumber, base cups for soft drink bottles, dish detergent containers, and household cleaner containers. Other plastics can be used to make park benches, fence posts, parking stops, and waterproof "lumber" for piers. Not all recycling centers will accept all types of plastic. It is a good idea to check with the recycling center to see which plastics they accept and if they want the tops removed, the bottles rinsed out, and the types presorted.

Printer cartridges can be recycled through various office supply stores. Some offer incentives such as a free ream of recycled paper in exchange. Some schools encourage families to collect empty printer cartridges because they receive donations for each computer cartridge they turn in. Printer cartridges can be refilled and reused. Offices can receive discounted prices if they use refilled printer cartridges.

Computers and monitors can (and should) be recycled. Computers can be dismantled, melted down for other uses, or parts can be used to repair other computers. Because computers and monitors contain hazardous materials, they should be disposed of through a computer distributor or the original manufacturer. Many computer manufacturers have recycling programs that include pick-up on site or mailing for a minimal fee.

Regulation of Nuclear Waste Storage, Transportation, and Disposal

In 1954, the Atomic Energy Act established the Atomic Energy Commission. Today the Nuclear Regulatory Commission (NRC) regulates the transfer, manufacture, acquisition, possession, and use of any nuclear facility and regulates radioactive materials and their by-products (NRC, 2004). The NRC is required to ensure that radioactive materials and facilities are managed to protect the public and the environment.

Burial and aboveground storage are the primary ways radioactive nuclear waste is stored. In 1982, the Nuclear

Nuclear waste
Radioactive waste generated from the production of nuclear energy; produced by nuclear power plants.

Radioactive waste
Hazardous waste material due to an emitted radiation.

Spent fuel
Nuclear reactor fuel used to the extent it can no longer effectively sustain a chain reaction; also known as irradiated reactor fuel, or depleted fuel.

Irradiated reactor fuel
See spent fuel.

Reprocessed
A special process or treatment to prepare something for reuse; as in extracting uranium and plutonium from spent fuel rods of a nuclear reactor to use as fuel.

Waste Policy Act (PL 97-425) was amended to require an investigation of possible sites for the storage of high-level radioactive waste. The U.S. government has established two locations for long-term nuclear waste. In 1999 the Waste Isolation Pilot Plant near Carlsbad, New Mexico, became the first depository to store **tranuranic waste** from nuclear defense sites. The waste is moved at night to limit the possibility of an accident. The newest site is near Yucca Mountain in Nevada. Most states do not want to harbor high-level radioactive waste, but as nuclear power plants approach the expiration of their licenses, the need for more storage is inevitable. High-level radioactive waste can be sealed in the ground in a mined geologic repository.

Summary

No matter what, consumers will produce waste. The generation, storage, transportation, and disposal of waste is controversial because it affects everyone. Large businesses often receive the most attention for their improper handling of waste products, particularly hazardous or nuclear waste. In truth, waste is an individual responsibility. The less waste generated from purchasing fewer products, the less each one needs to worry about how and where to dispose of it. Federal agencies such as the EPA and NRC regulate waste practices, but laws intended to protect citizens are still being violated.

Tranuranic waste
Also spelled as _transuranic,_ referring to elements such as uranium and plutonium.

REFERENCES

Anonymous. (1994). _Composting._ Columbia, SC: Office of Solid Waste Reduction and Recycling.

CBS News. (2004). Yucca Mountain. Retrieved from http://www.cbsnews.com/stories/2003/10/23/60minutes/main579696.shtml.

Centers for Disease Control. (2002). Issues in health-care settings: Infectious waste: Retrieved March 2003 from http://www.cdc.gov/ncidod.hip/enviro/guide.htm.

Chadderson, L. (2004). (Harness the power of green energy. Retrieved from http://www.greenfeet.net/newsletter/greenpower101.shtml.

Clemson Cooperative Extension Service. (1996). _Enviroshopping: Shopping with concern for the environment._ Pamphlet printed on recycled paper with soy ink. Clemson, SC: Cooperative Extension Service.

Clemson Cooperative Extension Service. (1992). Septic systems: What you need to know. Clemson, SC: Clemson University.

Green, L.W., & Ottoson, J.M. (1999). Community water and waste control, pgs. 443–451. In _Community and population health, 8th edition._ Boston: WCB McGraw-Hill.

Hammett, W. (1991). Disposal of hazardous household waste. HE 368-3. Raleigh, NC: North Carolina State University.

Integrated Waste Services Association. (2005). New Clean Air Act rules for waste-to-energy facilities. Retrieved from http://www.wte.org/m_act.html.

Lawrence Berkeley Laboratory. (2005). Landfill problems. Retrieved from http://esd.lbl.gov/ECO/smart_store/problems.html.

Moeller, D. (2005). _Environmental Health, 3rd edition._ Cambridge, MA: Harvard University Press.

National Ag Safety Database. (2002). Disposal of hazardous household waste. Retrieved from http://cdc.gov/nasd/docs/d001201-d0013/d001236/d001236.html.

Nuclear Energy Institute. (2005). Upfront: Nevada court challenges to the selection of the Yucca Mountain site. Retrieved from http://www.nei.org/index.asp?catnum=2&catid=310.

Nuclear Regulatory Commission. (2004). Who we are. Retrieved from http://www.nrc.gov/who-we-are.html.

Pacific Northwest Pollution Resource Center. (2000). Environmentally preferable purchasing. Retrieved from http://www.pprc.org/pubs/epp/epp_report.cfm.

Pierce, L. (2002). Being 'green': How much does it cost? How much does it Pay? A global commitment to 'environmental stewardship', incessant legislation and consumer opinion. Food & Drug Packaging. Retrieved from http://calbears.findarticles.com/p/articles/mi_hb037/is_200307/ai_n5762138.

Renner, R. (2002). Is sludge safe? *Environmental Health Perspectives, 10*, A667.

Rutala, W., & Odette, R. (1989). Management of infectious waste by U.S. hospitals. *Journal of the American Medical Association, 252*, 12.

Solid Waste Authority. (2005). Recycling: Enviroshopping. Retrieved from http://www.swa.org/Departments/recycling/enviroshopping.htm.

South Carolina Department of Health and Environmental Control. (1994). *Composting*. Columbia, SC: Office of Solid Waste Reduction and Recycling.

Tilford, D. (2000). Sustainable consumption: Why consumption matters. Retrieved from http://www.sierraclub.org/sustainable_consumption/tilford.asp#cost.

U.S. Environmental Protection Agency. (1998). Managing and tracking medical waste. EPA 530-SW-89-021. Retrieved from http://es.epa.gov/technpubs/1/2211.html.

U.S. Environmental Protection Agency. (2001). Municipal solid waste in the United States: Facts and figures for 1999. EPA 530-R-01-014. Washington DC: Office of Solid Waste and Emergency Response. Retrieved from http://www.epa.gov/epaoswer/non-hw/muncpl/mswfinal.pdf.

U.S. Environmental Protection Agency. (2003). 2001 Toxics Release Inventory Data Release: Questions and Answers. Retrieved from http://www.epa.gov/tri/tridata/tri01/external_qanda_for_revision.pdf.

U.S. Environmental Protection Agency. (2004). Basic facts about waste. Retrieved from http://www.epa.gov/epaoswer/osw/facts.htm#hazardous.

U.S. Environmental Protection Agency. (2004). Basic facts: Municipal Solid Waste. Retrieved from http://www.epa.gov/epaoswer/non-hw/muncpl/facts.htm.

U.S. Environmental Protection Agency. (2005a). Basic information: The office of solid waste (OSW). Retrieved from http://www.epa.gov/rcraonline/.

U.S. Environmental Protection Agency. (2005b). Environmentally preferable purchasing: Database on Environmental Information for Products and Services. Retrieved from http://www.epa.gov/oppt/epp/database.htm.

Wadman, M. (2005). Issues of the environment: Landfills and recycling. Retrieved from http://www.necc.mass.edu/MRVIS/MR1_9/start.htm.

Yassi, A., Kjellstrom, T., de Kok, T., & Guidotti, T. (2001). *Basic environmental health*. New York: Oxford University Press, Inc.

ASSIGNMENTS

1. Learn the manufacturer of your personal computer, monitor, keyboard, or mouse and determine the correct course of action for disposal and recycling of the e-waste when you upgrade.
2. Interview someone who has visited a foreign country about how consumers there buy and dispose of items.
3. Determine where the recycling centers are in the area where you live, the hours they are open, and their rules for recycling materials.
4. Select three different states in this country and learn if there are different laws for recycling or using recycled materials.
5. Investigate laws in your state regarding the transportation, storage, and handling of hazardous wastes.
6. Locate the low-level radioactive waste site nearest your home.
7. Visit the nearest landfill site and interview the solid waste manager.
8. Discuss ways you can better manage solid and hazardous waste in your home.
9. Visit a wastewater management facility and observe the stages of processing.
10. Debate how medical waste should be handled by local health care facilities.

SELECTED ENVIRONMENTAL LAWS

1954 *Atomic Energy Act (PL 85-703)*
An amendment to the original Atomic Energy Act (PL 79-585) of 1946 that established the Atomic Energy Commission. Provides for the development and regulation of the uses of nuclear materials and facilities in the United States. Requires that the civilian use of nuclear materials and facilities be licensed and empowers the Nuclear Regulatory Commission to enforce standards to protect public health and safety. A later amendment established liability and compensation for damage caused by nuclear accidents.

1965 *Solid Waste Disposal Act (PL 89-272)*
Provides technical and financial assistance to state and local governments and interstate agencies for the development of solid waste management plans; prohibits open dumping on land; encourages product substitution, recovery, recycling, and reuse.

1970 Resource Recovery Act (PL 91-512)
Established a major research program to develop new and innovative ways of dealing with solid waste. Gave the EPA responsibility for providing technical and financial help to state and local governments to develop resource recovery and waste disposal systems.

1976 Resource Conservation and Recovery Act (RCRA) (PL 94-580)
An amendment to the Solid Waste Disposal Act of 1965 to protect human health and the environment from dangers associated with waste management, including hazardous waste. Amended in 1984 to regulate underground storage tanks.

1978 Uranium Mill Tailings Radiation Control Act (PL 95-604)
Established programs through the NRC to stabilize and control mill tailings at uranium or thorium mill sites to prevent or minimize the diffusion of radon into the environment.

1980 Comprehensive Environmental Response, Compensation, and Liability (CERCLA or Superfund)(PL 96-510)
Requires cleanup of existing disposal sites; address problems of abandoned hazardous waste sites; 1986 amendments established financial responsibility for the sites.

1980 Radioactive Waste Policy Act (PL 96-573)
Gave states the responsibility to dispose of radioactive waste generated within their borders; allowed states to form compacts to locate facilities to serve a group of states.

1982 Nuclear Waste Policy Act of 1982 (NWPA) (PL 97-425)
Requirements for disposal of high-level radioactive wastes including deep geologic disposal of spent nuclear fuel rods removed from commercial nuclear reactors.

1985 Low-Level Radioactive Waste Policy Amendments Act of 1985 (PL 99-240)
Amended the Low-Level Radioactive Waste Policy Amendments to improve procedures for the implementation of compacts providing for the establishment of regional disposal facilities for low-level radioactive waste and other purposes.

1986 Superfund Amendments and Reauthorization Act (SARA) (42 U.S.C.9601 et seq.)
This amendment to CERCLA stressed the importance of permanent remedies and innovative treatment technologies in cleaning up hazardous waste sites, provided new enforcement authorities, increased state involvement, increased the focus on human health problems posed by hazardous waste sites, encouraged greater citizen participation, increased the size of the trust fund to $8.5 billion, and revised the hazard ranking system (HRS) to ensure accurate assessment of the relative risk to human health and the environment by uncontrolled hazardous waste sites to be placed on the national priorities list (NPL).

1987 *Nuclear Waste Policy Amendments Act (PL 100-203)*
This amendment to the Nuclear Waste Policy Act of 1982 (NWPA) narrowed the Department of Energy's repository investigations to Yucca Mountain and canceled the eastern repository.

1990 *The Pollution Prevention Act of 1990 (42 U.S.C. 13101 and 13102)*
Provided controls regarding the production, discharge, and storage of waste products. The measure called for source reduction, recycling, sustainable agricultural practices, and the efficient use of energy, water, and natural resources through conservation efforts.

1990 *Hazardous Materials Transportation Uniform Safety Act (HMTUSA)*
Authorized additional regulations for safe transportation of hazardous materials, required the Department of Transportation to establish training recommendations for public sector emergency response and preparedness teams.

1992 *Federal Facility Compliance Act (PL 102-386)*
Amended the Solid Waste Disposal Act to clarify requirements and sanctions to federal facilities.

PROFESSIONAL JOURNALS

Biocycle: Journal of Composting and Recycling
International Journal of Emergency Management
Journal of the Air and Waste Management Association
Recycling International
Resources, Conservation and Recycling
Waste Management
Waste Management and Research
Water, Air, and Soil Pollution

ADDITIONAL READING

Clemson University Cooperative Extension Service. (1996). *Enviroshopping: Shopping with concern for the environment.* Clemson, SC: Cooperative Extension Service.

Green, L. W., & Ottoson, J. M. (1999). *Community and population health,* 8th edition. Boston: WCB McGraw-Hill.

Moeller, D. (2005). *Environmental health,* 3rd ed. Cambridge, MA: Harvard University Press.

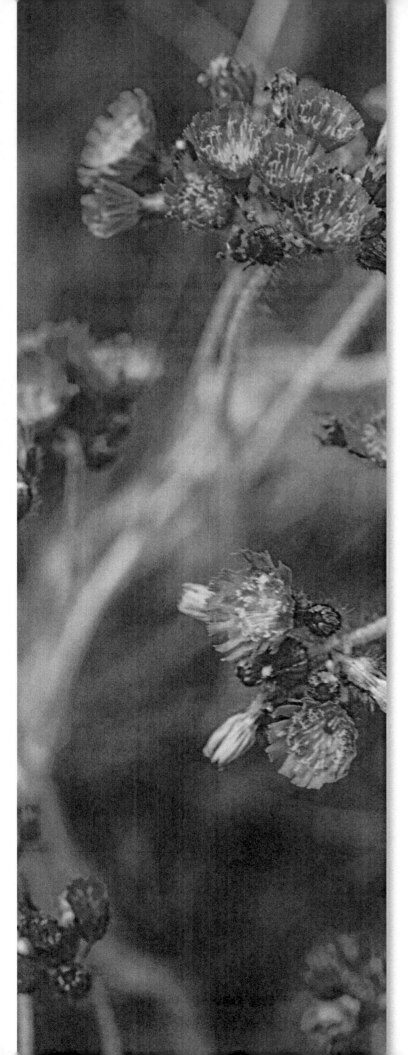

Housing and Indoor Environments

15

The most important work you and I will ever do will be within the walls of our own homes.

Harold B. Lee (1899–1973)

OBJECTIVES

1. Contrast health problems due to outdoor and indoor air pollution.

2. Provide a list of basic housing needs for safety, noise, space, air flow, humidity, temperature, and lighting.

3. Describe why indoor air pollution is more problematic for children.

4. Give the hazards associated with seven indoor air pollutants.

5. Compare health hazards of physical indoor air pollutants such as ETS and radon exposure.

6. Give examples of VOCs.

7. List sources of indoor chemical pollutants.

8. Describe circumstances when mold and mildew are likely to grow.

9. Explain why an individual might be hypersensitive to fragrances and cleaning products.

10. Discuss the effectiveness of air-cleaning devices.

11. Explain how to determine if an illness is SBS.

12. List measures to control indoor pollutants.

Introduction

approximately 90% of a person's time is spent indoors, therefore the indoor environment is just as important as the outdoor environment (U.S. EPA, 2001). Between 30 and 70% of indoor environments have pollution problems. The EPA ranks indoor air pollution as one of the top five environmental risks (IESO, 2002) and reports of indoor environments causing illnesses have increased (Kilburn, 2002). Indoor air is two to five times worse than outdoor air pollution. Indoor air pollution accounts for the vast majority of lung cancer deaths. Nearly 55 million children spend their days in elementary and secondary schools; one out of five schools have unsatisfactory indoor air quality (IAQ) and one in four schools have inadequate ventilation. Children are more susceptible to pollutants than adults. This chapter will discuss basic shelter needs, various types of air pollutants and their effects, and what can be done do decrease risk of indoor air pollution.

Finding a Good Place to Live

americans live in a mobile society, changing jobs several times in a lifetime and relocating to places to find employment. Each city has its own unique characteristics that may promote or interfere with good health. Finding a "safe city" is important. Information about climate, cost of living, unemployment, crime rates, morbidity and mortality rates, and death rates of a community are important. Some cities grow so fast in all directions without regard to how individuals might get to work, whether construction of new schools is necessary, and if citizens will have resources such as grocery stores, gasoline stations, and other services. New housing developments (Figure 15-1) spring up in areas that may have once been landfills, wetlands, or other unusable land. Some developments intrude upon land that was set aside for Native Americans and national parks. Trees, foliage, and native plants are destroyed. The distribution of new developments requires new roads that take up valuable land space. Water and sewer lines must be dug. Power, telephone, and cable lines must also be added. As the new roads become traveled, pollutants from automobiles and litter contaminate the area. Residents use fertilizers, pesticides, and water as if the supplies were endless and the consequences were insignificant.

When searching for a place to live, many people select a region or a city based on the type of climate they prefer. Climate determines many things such as availability of water, potential for flooding, and what type of home would withstand normal and abnormal weather conditions for that area. Climate is affected somewhat by the topography of the land. Coastal regions are more likely to be warm, humid, with occasional hurricanes. Mountainous regions may be cool and dry with ice and snow. Flat lands may have more wind and tornados. Climate determines plant and animal life that must cohabitate with

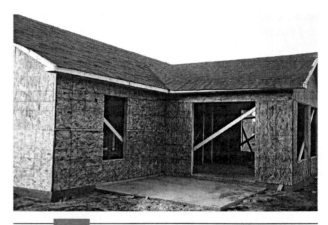

FIGURE 15-1 New homes are constructed very quickly. The workmanship is important to good health and safety.

Digging Deeper — 2010 HEALTHY PEOPLE OBJECTIVES

8-16 Reduce indoor allergen levels (dust mite allergens, German cockroach allergens).

8-17 Increase the number of office buildings that are managed using good indoor air quality practices.

8-18 Increase the proportion of persons who live in homes tested for radon concentrations.

8-19 Increase the number of new homes constructed to be **radon** resistant.

8-20 Increase the proportion of the Nation's primary and secondary schools that have official school policies ensuring the safety of students and staff from environmental hazards, such as chemicals in special classrooms, poor indoor air quality, asbestos, and exposure to pesticides.

8-22 Increase the proportion of persons living in pre-1950s housing that has been tested for the presence of lead-based paint.

8-23 Reduce the proportion of occupied housing units that are substandard.

27-10 Reduce the proportion of nonsmokers exposed to environmental tobacco smoke.

people. Areas with more water will have more plants and animals that can become a problem for residents. Agri-cultural areas will have more domestic animals that may attract insects and bacteria-causing odors.

Unemployment rates usually predict crime rates. As unemployment increases, resources become more valu-able. Robberies, burglaries, rapes, homicides, and acci-dents increase. Most people do not think to look at death rates in a given area, but it is a health indicator that can de-termine insurance premiums and health care costs to con-sumers. An example would be a state with high morbidity and mortality related to obesity or cancer. Both conditions are related to the environment and lifestyles. Communi-ties that do not provide sidewalks for children to walk to school may have increased traffic as parents find it neces-sary to drive them to school or buses become necessary. Narrow roads make it almost impossible for bicycle travel and aggressive driving practices are more dramatic.

Some neighborhoods prohibit pets, motorcycles, mo-tor homes, untrimmed grass, and other things considered by the residents to be "nuisances." There are gated com-munities that permit only residents and their guests to enter. There are neighborhoods where parking an auto-mobile may cost more than the rent.

Basic Shelter Needs

asic human survival needs include water, food, sleep, clothing, shelter, and protection from accidents and disease. Choosing a proper home or apartment or office is important to good health. The World Health Organization (WHO) and the EPA estimate that 30 percent of all buildings worldwide are unfit for human occupation (Evans, 2002).

LOCATION

Any realtor will explain that the three most important things about a residence are location, location, location. A good neighborhood is also important for good health.

In a new neighborhood, there may be frequent con-struction noise and dust. In an older neighborhood, this is less likely unless neighbors frequently create a distur-bance, interfering with sleep and other activities. When planning to live in a condominium or apartment, it would be wise to become acquainted with others shar-ing the same neighborhood or building. The location of highways, by-passes, and other roads influence the type of traffic flow around a home. In areas of high traffic, the building should be shielded from traffic noise by a berm, fence, or other sound-absorbing barrier. Cities often have ordinances pertaining to noise and distur-bances of the peace.

A person should feel safe and secure in their home or office building. Outdoor areas should be well lit, particularly in building entrances and areas where cars are parked. The building should be away from areas littered with rubbish, trash, or garbage. There should be trees for shade, but they should be trimmed for safety reasons.

COMMUNITY GOVERNMENT AND SERVICES

Air quality (Chapter 8), the quality of drinking water (Chapter 9), and means of solid waste disposal (Chap-ter 14) are also important. Storage areas, parks, and pub-lic transportation are important considerations. There must be garbage removal services at least twice per week. Some communities provide this service; others require residents to pay for their own disposal.

The type of services available to communities is often regulated by government officials. There is usually a county or city council or town board. The county pro-vides money for publicly owned land, particularly for stormwater runoff and highways. The city government provides funding for water, sewers, and garbage service. Cities have zoning laws to protect neighborhoods from commercial development. When there is a proposal to change the way an area is zoned, as in constructing a new school or housing development, public hearings provide citizens the opportunity to ask questions or oppose the change.

Digging Deeper · SHELTER NEEDS

Basic physiological needs for shelter concern the following:

- A good supportive structure
- Absence of ionizing radiation and other toxic materials or chemicals
- Insect and rodent protection
- Garbage and sewage disposal
- Noise protection

- Proper lighting
- Comfortable temperature
- Reasonable humidity
- Adequate ventilation

Basic psychological shelter needs include:

- Protection from crime and drugs
- Cleanliness

- A socially supportive community
- Adequate space for household members
- Privacy
- A calming environment where one can retreat from daily hassles

THE STRUCTURE

A good supportive structure is one that meets building codes and public health codes, and is maintained properly. A good foundation, roof, and exterior walls will protect the homeowner and family from outdoor elements for many years. The standard used by architects and construction engineers in the construction of new buildings is the International Building Code 2003. This is updated and many already-existing homes may not meet the code. Local building codes also dictate how homes should be constructed. Inspect basements and foundations for cracks that may allow **radon**, rodents, or insects to enter the building. Walls and ceilings should be well insulated to maintain desired indoor temperatures and noise levels. If walls are painted, nontoxic (lead-free) latex paint should be used. Floors should be covered with tile, linoleum, or carpeting. Indoor plumbing should be free of any problems such as leaks or stoppages. If living in a condominium or apartment building, there should be sound-proofing between floors.

THE LIVING SPACE

Living space should be large enough to meet spatial and privacy needs of household members. According to the Housing and Urban Development guidelines (see reference to NCEH, 1976), a residence must be a minimum of 400 square feet. Adequate living space is determined by the number of people residing in the home with 150 square feet allowed for the first occupant and another 100 square feet per additional occupant (CDC, 1979). Minimum ceiling height is 7 feet. If there is a sloping ceiling, at least one half of the floor area must have a minimum height of 7 feet. When an individual requires rest, there should be an area where one can retreat to relax without interruptions from noise or an uncomfortable environment. Each sleeping room should have 70 square feet of floor space for the first occupant and at least 50 square feet for each additional occupant. There should also be at least 4 square feet of floor-to-ceiling height closet space for each occupant.

Areas should be free of clutter with adequate lighting, temperature, humidity, ventilation, and sanitation.

LIGHTING

Natural lighting or daylight should be used as much as possible. All building codes require windows or skylights facing the outdoors in rooms that equal 10% of the total floor area of the residence. This is conducive to good mental health because exposure to light helps with sleep schedules, nutrient absorption, and mood regulation.

Rooms are required to have two electrical outlets to supply power to light fixtures. Hallways and stairs must have at least 10 **foot candles** of light at the stair tread or floor level (CDC, 2002). Incandescent lighting should be used as much as possible. Fluorescent lights may be more cost effective, but they contain gases that are harmful if the tube is broken. Light is measured in foot candles and the intensity of light is measured by **lumens**. How much lighting is best depends upon the type of activity and room. A 60-watt bulb supplies 17.5 foot candles of light or 600 lumens for a clear bulb and 800 lumens for a frosted bulb. A 75-watt bulb provides 20.5 foot candles and a 100-watt bulb provides 50.3 foot candles. For reading, sewing, or watching television, the intensity from a 60-, 75-, or 100-watt bulb is about the same, but the less watts used, the less energy used. Energy-efficient bulbs are available and should be used. Never use a bulb requiring more watts than the fixture can support such as a 100-watt

Radon
An odorless, radioactive gas found in the soil and areas where uranium is found.

Foot candle
A unit of measure of the intensity of light falling on a surface, equal to one lumen per square foot.

Lumen
A unit of light used to rate the output of a lamp (bulb).

bulb in a 60-watt maximum socket. In work areas, better lighting may be more desirable. Candles, particularly the scented kind, are a source of indoor pollution.

TEMPERATURE

The APHA-CDC Recommended Housing Maintenance and Occupancy ordinance states that room temperatures should be at least 68° F, 36 inches above the floor (CDC, 2002). Because floor temperatures are usually cooler and ceiling temperatures are much warmer, measurements can be taken at the seating level 30 inches above the floor and at breathing levels five feet above the floor. Temperatures can be lower for working (64° to 70° F) for optimal productivity and for sleeping (60° to 65° F) to promote restful sleep.

HUMIDITY

Humidity is important because the growth of **fungi** and **mildew** proliferate in humid environments. Indoor air humidity should be between 30 to 50%. A ceiling fan will remove some humidity because it helps moisture evaporate. Air conditioning will remove even more humidity. Where humidity is more than 60% and both fans and air conditioners are being used, a dehumidifier may be used, particularly in damp basements, kitchens, or bathrooms. In drier climates or during the winter when indoor air is heated, a humidifier is helpful to keep respiratory passages moist for good health.

VENTILATION

Air indoors should be clean, fresh, and invigorating. Whenever possible, outdoor air should be used to freshen an otherwise stale atmosphere from closed windows and doors. Windows provide access to outdoor air and help ventilate noxious and stale odors. In homes, ventilation fans should be installed in kitchens and bathrooms.

Air movement is important in regulating room temperature and humidity. Air movement should be 500 feet per minute in all rooms or sufficient enough that the total air in a building is turned over 2 to 6 times per hour (CDC, 1979). It is best if large buildings have a forced air system. This is sometimes difficult in buildings and homes with many hallways and rooms with closed doors. Ventilation standards for office buildings set by the American Society of Heating, Refrigerating, and Air Conditioning Engineers (ASHRAE) are 15 to 60 cubic feet of outside air per minute per person. If air circulation is hampered by partitions, partitions should be raised 6 inches off the floor.

SANITATION

Good lighting and ventilation are important to good sanitation for indoor environments. The water supply is also important to clean and sanitize. Water should flow at a minimum rate of 1 gallon per minute from each fixture. The minimum temperature for hot water is 120° F. Chapter 13 provided information about food safety. Chapter 14 provided information about cesspools, septic tanks, drainage, disposal of hazardous materials, and trash removal.

Indoor Air Pollution

Indoor pollution is a concern in home, school, and occupational settings. Prior to the 1970s, the average building completely recycled indoor air with fresh air. Since the 1970s energy crisis, buildings have become tighter to be more energy efficient. A closed building keeps toxins, such as passive smoke, circulating. Chemicals are everywhere in buildings from cleaning agents to synthetic carpets and other home building materials. WHO estimates that 30% of new or remodeled office buildings worldwide are plagued by indoor pollution (Lyles et al., 1991).

Exposure to toxic elements indoors is unavoidable. Indoor pollution levels can be up to 2 to 3 times, and up to 100 times higher than outdoors, and may be responsible for over 10,000 deaths each year. Harmful substances can be found in indoor air, building materials, walls, floors, basements, furniture, bedding, clothing, cleaning products, solvents, pesticides, and room deodorizers. Unfortunately, the human body can be a reservoir for toxic materials. Headaches, allergies, depression, and chronic respiratory problems indicate that toxins are in the air as well. Indoor air pollutants can be classified into three types: physical, chemical, and biological.

Physical Indoor Air Pollutants

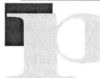

Physical air pollutants include asbestos, **environmental tobacco smoke (ETS)**, and radon.

ASBESTOS

Asbestos is a naturally occurring mineral found throughout the world. It is made up of minerals such as amosite, chrysotile, tremolite, actinolite, anthophyllite, and crocidolite. It is woven into fibers that are not affected by heat or chemicals and do not conduct electricity. Asbestos was first used to make candlewicks burn longer. It has been used for insulation, brake linings, floor tiles, roofing paper, potholders, paints, plastics, cement, and caulking compounds. Asbestos can be found around fireplaces, around joints in plumbing, and materials used to soundproof walls and ceilings. Asbestos crumbles easily in the hand.

Because of its carcinogenic properties, asbestos was one of the first substances regulated as a hazardous air pollutant. The problem with asbestos is that it breaks into small particles that suspend in the air for long periods of time. Problems can arise from even brief asbestos exposure. When inhaled, the particles penetrate respiratory tissues and remain in the body for many years. It may take from 10 to 40 years before symptoms of an asbestos-related condition appear. Smokers have an even greater increased risk of asbestosis (scarring of the lungs), lung and throat cancer, malignant mesothelioma (cancer in the chest or abdomen), and nonmalignant pleural disease. Most people suffering from these diseases were construction workers, ship and boat builders, and plumbers. It is generally agreed that there is no safe level of asbestos exposure.

Many school buildings built from 1946 to 1973 contain asbestos. The effects of asbestos dust are especially harmful to children. The Occupational Safety and Health Administration (OSHA) has set limits on human exposure to asbestos. In 1986, the Asbestos Hazard Emergency Response Act (AHERAA) required inspection of all schools for asbestos. Asbestos removal must be carefully done by trained experts (Figure 15-2). Asbestos abatement includes encapsulating the fibers with a polymer sealant to prevent fiber release, a nonpermeable barrier enclosing the asbestos area off from other areas, and wetting down the asbestos for removal and disposal. Workers in office buildings and schoolchildren should be protected by not being in the building when asbestos is removed.

ENVIRONMENTAL TOBACCO SMOKE (ETS)

In most areas of the country, cigarette smoke is found in office buildings, restaurants, drinking establishments, and in homes. ETS (also known as *second-hand tobacco smoke*) consists of side stream smoke and mainstream smoke. *Side stream smoke* refers to the smoke emitted between puffs of a burning cigarette, pipe, or cigar. *Mainstream smoke* is the smoke exhaled by the smoker. Both types of smoke are harmful. ETS contains approximately 40 carcinogens and thousands of other chemicals including mutagens, poisonous gases such as carbon monoxide, and chemical compounds such as benzene, formaldehyde, and polonium.

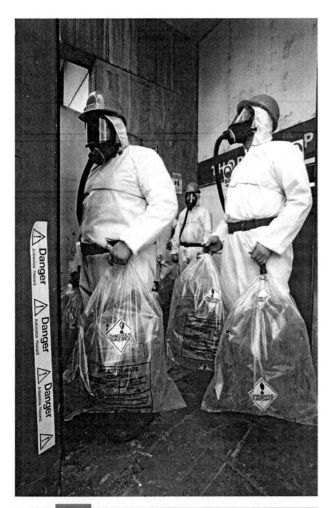

FIGURE 15-2 **Asbestos Removal** The abatement of asbestos from school buildings, offices, and homes must be done by licensed professionals.

Humidity
A measure of water vapor content in the air.

Fungi
Another word for mold. Fungi reproduce by generating spores that become airborne and begin to grow after landing on a moist surface.

Mildew
A black mold that decomposes organic matter.

Environmental tobacco smoke (ETS)
That which is smoked and exhaled and is allowed to burn.

EFFORTS TO STOP ETS
Many American workplaces do not allow smoking indoors and many employers do not hire smokers. Most states restrict smoking in public places such as government buildings. Many states restrict smoking in private workplaces. Some business owners are reluctant to establish nonsmoking policies because they are afraid that business will decrease. In fact, a study of Texas businesses with a ban on smoking reported no difference in business (Martin, 1999; Ruggless, 2002). For materials to help businesses develop and implement no-smoking policies, call 1-800-LUNG-USA (1-800-586-4872). The best action to prevent smoking is to never have started.

ETS is the leading cause of preventable deaths in the United States. ETS causes lung cancer, respiratory tract infections, sinus infections and cancer, heart disease, miscarriage, ear infections, **asthma** exacerbation, and developmental delays in children. ETS can seep into the rooms of nonsmoking tenants. In some areas, "drifting smoke" is considered a nuisance, negligence, harassment, and a fire hazard. Smokers can be sued for damages caused by their inadvertent or neglectful behaviors imposed on others.

The consequences of ETS are numerous. Cigarette smoke is the main cause of lung cancer. Lung cancer is the second leading cause of death in the United States and increases the risk for nine other cancers (American Lung Association, 2000). It is associated with heart disease, asthma, bronchitis, emphysema, ear infections, low birthweight babies, and sudden infant death syndrome (SIDS). In the United States, 27% of homes with children (aged 6 and younger) currently allow smoking, affecting approximately 9 to 12 million children per year (U.S. EPA, 2004). The risk for cancer and other smoking-associated diseases for nonsmokers is also high. The risk is not lowered by smoking "light," "mild," or "low tar" cigarettes. In fact, studies have shown that when smoking these types of cigarettes, smokers often inhale more deeply while smoking them.

RADON

After environmental tobacco smoke, radon is the second leading cause of lung cancer in all individuals and the leading cause of lung cancer in nonsmokers. It can also cause emphysema and pulmonary fibrosis. When radon is inhaled, the DNA in epithelial lung tissue is damaged. If the person inhaling radon is a smoker, their risk is greatly increased. Radon is not detectable by routine medical testing, but can be detected in urine and lung or bone tissue.

Radon is an odorless, radioactive gas formed from the breakdown of uranium found in rocks and soil. Radon has a radioactive half-life of about 4 days, meaning one-half of an amount of radon will decay to other products every 4 days. Some of the radon produced in the soil will move to the surface and enter the air, attaching to dust and other particulate matter. Radon is found at low levels in outdoor air, but is found at higher levels in homes, schools, and office buildings. Radon gas enters a building through cracks in the basement or foundation. Radon is most commonly found in basements, attics, closed-in places with little ventilation, and home with high water tables.

Detection of radon in the home can be accomplished with charcoal canisters, ion detectors, and alpha track monitors available from most health departments or extension agents (Figure 15-3). The best way to rid a building of radon gas is to install a "reverse air flow" system. Cracks can be sealed to prevent radon from entering a building.

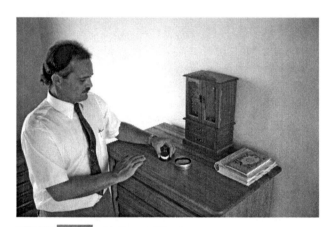

FIGURE 15-3 **Radon Inspection** It is important that consumers know where radon is likely to seep into homes and to use kits available to detect it.

Chemical Indoor Air Pollutants

s stated previously, indoor air pollution is particularly harmful due to exposure of higher concentrations for longer periods of time. Harmful effects of indoor air pollution include allergic responses, asthmatic attacks, and cancer. Children are most at risk. Chemicals contributing to indoor air pollution include carbon monoxide, lead, mercury, pesticides, and **volatile organic compounds (VOCs)**. These chemicals can be found in cleaning products, solvents, pesticides, room deodorizers, and perfumes.

CARBON MONOXIDE

This odorless, colorless gas is a by-product of incomplete combustion or burning. Common sources of carbon monoxide include automobiles running in an enclosed areas, stoves, chimneys, fireplaces, improperly maintained furnaces, gas or kerosene stoves, propane camp stoves, and cigarette smoke. Carbon monoxide attaches to the hemoglobin in red blood cells so oxygen transport cannot occur. As a result, the brain, heart, and lungs are deprived of oxygen. The concentration of carbon monoxide in indoor air is determined by the ventilation available, source, and time it is allowed to accumulate. For example, a common source of carbon monoxide is cigarette smoke. If a roommate or coworker smokes without an open window or ventilation fan that moves the air outdoors, concentrations will become higher with each cigarette that is smoked. Carbon monoxide poisoning can be lethal, depending on the concentration and length of time exposed to it.

Initial symptoms of carbon monoxide poisoning include fatigue, confusion, headache, dizziness, and nausea. Skin color may be pale or cyanotic. Impaired judgment, blurred vision, vomiting, irregular heartbeat, and seizures are an indication of lethal levels of carbon monoxide poisoning. Continued exposure will result in a cherry-red skin color, unconsciousness, coma, and death.

Carbon monoxide is present in any smoky atmosphere, such as a dance club, bar, restaurant, office building, or home where smoking is permitted. Bartenders, waitresses, and club patrons may confuse symptoms of carbon monoxide poisoning such as headaches, dizziness, and nausea with a hangover. The best prevention against carbon monoxide poisoning is to avoid exposure to products that produce smoke or heat.

LEAD

Lead is a heavy metal found in homes in plumbing, pesticides, cooking utensils, ceramic dishes, paint, and gasoline. It is believed to be the oldest known toxic material. Lead is used to solder copper pipes, commonly found in older homes. Usually the lead does not become a problem until the pipes become corroded and break down. You can determine whether copper pipes have been used by observing the pipes under the sink. If porcelain fixtures become stained with a green substance, then the copper is getting into the water supplies. If there is lead solder, the lead may get into the water supply. Lead is also used to create a darker tint for paints. It is also used to make ceramic items fashioned out of pottery.

Asthma
A chronic inflammatory disorder of the airways that causes constriction of the bronchi when mast cells produce.

Volatile organic compound (VOC)
Changing rapidly from a solid or liquid to a vapor at room temperature; liable to change suddenly.

Consider the Cost PREVENT CARBON MONOXIDE POISONING

If gas appliances are used, the pilot lights should be checked to make sure there are no leaks and that the pilot light is burning properly. One rule of thumb for gas fireplaces and gas stoves is to look at the flame. If there is more yellow flame than blue flame, the gas is not burning completely. You can then turn the gas inlet down to burn more efficiently. Another way to prevent carbon monoxide poisoning is to have furnaces inspected every year before turning them on. Changing furnace filters monthly also helps the furnace work more efficiently.

Consider the Cost LEAD SCREENING

Screening for lead in the home can be done with simple home tests, often available free of charge. Tests include: the Frandon Lead Alert kit, 800-634- 2341 and Leadcheck Swabs, 800-262-LEAD.

The effects of lead are cumulative with the worst effects observed among children. Lead poisoning causes neurological and kidney damage, high blood pressure, disrupted blood cell production, and reproductive problems. In 1971, the Lead Poisoning Prevention Act was passed to decrease the use of lead in interior paints. Some paints today still contain lead. When purchasing paint, read the label to make sure it is "lead free."

MERCURY

Mercury is found indoors in paints, particularly those with a metallic sheen. Mercury is also found in older thermometers, barometers, and sphygmomanometers (blood pressure cuffs). It can also be found in thermostats, batteries, and fluorescent bulbs. Mercury is harmful when absorbed through the skin, inhaled, or ingested. More information on mercury was provided in Chapter 5.

PESTICIDES

Chemicals in pesticides and associated problems have already been discussed in Chapter 7. Pesticides are used in buildings and homes around foundations and inside buildings to control pests. Pesticides such as chlordane, aldrin, and dieldrin continue to show up in older homes even though they have been banned for nearly two decades.

Pesticides indoors must be applied by a certified specialist who has special training regarding the type, dosage, and use of each pesticide. Exposure to pesticides indoors is harmful because much high concentrations build over time because they are not biodegradable. Some pesticide specialists ask that pets and small chil-

---

Medical treatment for lead poisoning includes oral **chelating agents** such as dimercaptosuccinic acid (DMSA) or dimercaptopropane-I sulfonate (DMPS). A chelator is a substance known to remove metals and minerals from the bones. A urine test is taken before and after taking the chelator. Ethylenediaminetetracetic acid (EDTA) may also be used to keep lead from redepositing in the brain. EDTA and the vitamins/minerals normally lost through this process are administered intravenously for 3 to 4 hours over several months. Dialysis can also be used to detoxify patients with blood-borne wastes and malfunctioning kidneys. To find a physician trained to administer chelation technique, contact the American College for Advancement in Medicine at 714-483-7666 or 23121 Verdugo Drive, Suite 204, Laguna Hills, California 92653.

---

dren be removed from the home for at least 8 hours after spraying. It is a good idea to leave screened windows open to ventilate the house. Other means can be used to control insects besides spraying such as clearing dead vegetation away from the house and keeping storage areas clean and dry.

VOLATILE ORGANIC COMPOUNDS

Volatile organic compounds (VOCs) are gaseous substances released from solids or liquids at room temperature. They are ideal for solvents, disinfectants, and pesticides because they evaporate easily. VOCs can be found in paint, adhesives, solvents, spray cans, cleaning compounds, room deodorizers, copy machine toners, markers, pens, and correction fluids. VOCs can remain in an indoor atmosphere for as long as 6 months. Short-term exposure can cause eye, nose, and throat irritation; headaches; and nausea. Long-term exposure to high levels may cause damage to the liver, kidney, and central nervous system.

Common VOCs include acetone, benzene, formaldehyde, nitrogen dioxide, paradichlorobenzene, perchloroethylene, tolulene, trichloroethylene, and vinyl chloride.

Acetone

Acetone (dimethyl ketone, 2-propanone, or beta-ketopropane) is used to make plastic, fibers, drugs, and other chemicals. It is also used to dissolve other substances and is the main ingredient in solvents such as fingernail polish remover and duplicating fluid.

Benzene

Benzene is a major concern among VOCs because it is a known human carcinogen. The primary sources of benzene include environmental tobacco smoke, stored fuels and paints, and automobile emissions. Benzene levels can be reduced by eliminating smoking within the home, having maximum ventilation while painting, and discarding paint and fuels that are not used immediately.

Formaldehyde

Formaldehyde is a pungent gas that is water soluble and colorless at room temperature. It is a carcinogenic substance considered to be one of the most hazardous compounds to human health. Formaldehyde is used to manufacture plastics, resins, paint, glue, rubber, textiles, explosives, insulation, and building materials. It is also used in adhesives and photographic chemicals. Formaldehyde irritates the respiratory tract, eyes, skin, and, with continued exposure, body organs. Some occupations are related to formaldehyde exposure more than others, especially those that involve wood products, solvents, copy machines, and correction fluids. Laboratory personnel also are more frequently exposed to formaldehyde.

Paradichlorobenzene

Paradichlorobenzene is commonly used to control moths, molds, mildew, and to deodorize restrooms and waste containers. At room temperature, paradichlorobenzene (p-DCB) is a solid with a strong odor (like moth balls). When exposed to air, it changes to a vapor that acts as the insect killer and deodorizer. P-DCB is a known carcinogen. High exposures will cause dizziness, headaches, and liver problems. Workers breathing high levels of p-DCB have reported painful irritation to the nose and eyes.

Perchloroethylene

Perchloroethylene is a chlorinated hydrocarbon, the chemical most widely used in dry-cleaning fluids and solvents. In laboratory studies, it has been shown to cause cancer in animals. Studies indicate that people breathe low levels of this chemical where dry-cleaned goods are stored and as they wear dry-cleaned clothing. If dry-cleaned goods have a strong chemical odor when picked up, do not accept them until they have been properly dried. If goods with a chemical odor are returned on a regular basis, choose a different dry cleaner. All professionally dry-cleaned clothes should be aired out before brought into the house and placed in the closet.

Toluene

Toluene is a clear, colorless liquid that comes from crude oil and the tolu tree. It is used as a solvent in making paints, paint thinners, fingernail polish, lacquers, adhesives, rubber, and in some printing and leather tanning processes.

Trichloroethylene

Trichloroethylene (TCE) is a nonflammable, colorless liquid with a somewhat sweet odor and a sweet, burning taste. It is used mainly as a solvent to remove grease from metal parts, but it is also an ingredient in adhesives, paint removers, typewriter correction fluids, and spot removers for dry cleaning. It remains in water a long time.

Vinyl Chloride

Vinyl chloride gas is formed when other substances such as trichloroethylene and tetrachloroethylene are broken down. It has a mild, sweet odor. Vinyl chloride is also used to make polyvinyl chloride (PVC), which is used in plastic products such as pipes, coating for wire and cables, and packaging materials. Large exposures can lead to severe liver damage and ballooning of fingertips.

OTHER TOXIC INDOOR AIR POLLUTION SOURCES

Other common chemicals are found in the home that may be harmful to those who have chemical sensitivities. These indoor air pollutants include ammonia, chlorine, hydrofluoric acid, and nitrogen dioxide.

Ammonia

Ammonia is a common ingredient in household products such as glass cleaner and floor cleaners. It has a pungent odor that is easy to recognize. Ammonia can irritate respiratory passages and should not be inhaled in its nondiluted form.

Chlorine

Chlorine is used as a bleaching and disinfecting agent. The main ingredient of household bleach is sodium hypochlorite, a strong alkaline. Chlorine granules, often used to disinfect swimming pools and spas, are corrosive

---

Chelating agent
A substance known to remove toxic metals and minerals from human bone.

if they touch the skin. Chlorine gas, used for the same purpose, is also very corrosive.

Hydrofluoric Acid

Hydrofluoric acid (HF) is the active ingredient in many household rust removers. It is highly corrosive and can cause intense pain and damage to tissues and bones if it comes in contact with the skin.

Nitrogen Dioxide

Nitrogen dioxide (NO_2) gases are a mixture of nitrogen and oxygen. Nitrogen oxides are formed naturally when fossil fuels are burned, when silage ferments, and during electric welding, electroplating, and engraving. A common source of nitrogen dioxide comes from gas stoves, kerosene heaters, and furnaces.

disease resulting in an infection, a growth, or an allergic response. All molds release spores that get into the respiratory tract. They also release characteristic odors and are sometimes referred to as **microbial volatile organic compounds (MVOCs)**. The most dangerous types of molds have **mycotoxins** that are especially harmful to sensitive individuals. Mycotoxins trigger inflammation and immune response, causing fluid accumulation, hyperactive immune responses, and tissue scarring. In addition, molds cause allergies and worsen respiratory conditions such as asthma (Zureik et al., 2002).

Indoor molds can be found in many places such as under kitchen cabinets and around bathtubs, toilets, and faucet fixtures. They can also be found on walls, behind walls, and in ventilation ductwork. *Stachybotrys chartarum* is the most common of indoor molds, found in straw, gypsum board, paper, canvas, and jute. It has a greenish-black color.

Biological Indoor Air Pollutants

iological agents are living organisms, usually microscopic in size, that cause illnesses. Biological agents can be found indoors in virtually any room. Where there is moisture, there will be **mold** and mildew. Where there are plants, animals, and humans, there will be pollen, pet dander, and dust mites. Biological agents include mold, mildew, dust, pollen, and pet dander.

MOLDS

Molds are a fungus that can be found almost anywhere, as long as there is oxygen and moisture. Indoors molds can be found on wood, paper, carpeting, food, under wallpaper, and in insulation. Modern building materials, such as drywall (as opposed to plaster used in older homes), provide a good medium for mold growth. Mold growth is prevalent in areas with high humidity and warm weather. It is most often seen during the summer months. Mold problems occur from roof leaks, poor landscaping, unvented appliances, and floods (Figure 15-4). Some libraries even have old books that contain mold.

The most common types of mold are *Alternaria* (indoor mold) and *Cladosporium* (outdoor mold), both of which are found where there is plant material, wood, textile, and food. Rotting wood and vegetation is the most common source of outdoor mold. An outdoor mold that is particularly harmful is *Aspergillus fumigatus,* found on dead leaves, stored grain, compost piles, and other decaying vegetation. It is the cause of aspergillosis, an invasive

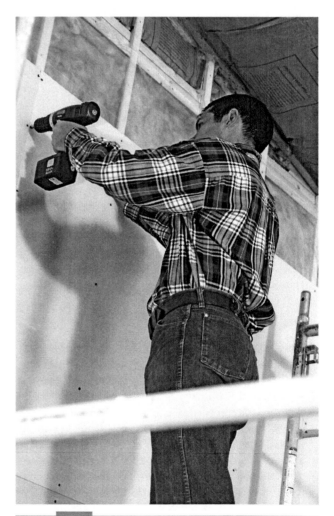

FIGURE 15-4 **Drywall Installation** Drywall is a source of mold if it becomes wet. The type of drywall installed is important as well as the installation process.

Testing for suspected mold growth can be expensive and often is not very accurate. The first assessment is from visual inspection, then air samples are taken. No exposure limits have been set to this date. Regardless of the type of mold, the cleanup procedure is basically the same, although some molds need to be professionally removed. Mold and mildew can be controlled with many different products such as humidity gauges, room air cleaners, dehumidifiers, and electrostatic air filters.

From 1993 to 1994, eight infants in the Cleveland, Ohio, area were hospitalized for bleeding lungs. After returning home, they were later rehospitalized. The Centers for Disease Control found that the homes of all eight infants had sustained water damage. *A. fumigatus* triggers allergic reactions in otherwise healthy individuals; *S. chartarum* is the green-black mold known to cause cold-like symptoms, dermatitis, sinusitis, conjunctivitis, poor concentration, fatigue, and exacerbation of asthma. Mycotoxicosis is the name for diseases caused by toxic molds such as acoustic neuromas and sick building syndrome. Symptoms include hearing loss, headaches, memory loss, poor concentration, fatigue, sleep disturbances, facial swelling, rashes, nose bleeding, gastrointestinal and other respiratory symptoms (Anyanwu et al., 2002). In 1995, the CDC issued guidelines for toxic molds such as *Aspergillus fumigatus* and *Stachybotrys chartarum*.

SICK BUILDING SYNDROME

When several individuals in the same building experience common symptoms that are not associated with a pattern of any particular illness, and symptoms improve when they leave the building, sick building syndrome (SBS) should be suspected. SBS was first recognized by the World Health Organization in 1982. SBS symptoms occur suddenly for no identifiable reason but are related to improperly designed or maintained heating, ventilating and air conditioning (HVAC) systems. SBS is not limited to older buildings and can occur in newer buildings that have less outdoor air ventilation and usually recycle indoor air. Areas with partitions, hallways, and closed doors are particularly susceptible. Measures can be taken to limit the effects of a sick building, in particular mold and dust removal. Some procedures are costly and may require intervention by public health department officials. If the building is an occupational setting and the building owners are not interested in correcting the problem, OSHA officials can be notified. Many occupational settings have an occupational health nurse, a safety engineer, or an OSHA specialist that will make the report. If there is no such individual, employees can also make the report.

MILDEW

Mildew is a mold that has the capacity to decompose paper, fabrics, wood, paint, glue, leather, or anything coated with the slightest amount of organic matter such as food, grease, and soil. Mildew can be identified by an unpleasant musty odor and dark green or black discoloration. Many people are allergic to mildew. Mildew is a persistent problem in warm, humid climates. It can be controlled by keeping items clean and controlling moisture. Moisture can be reduced by air conditioning, using fans for evaporation, using a dehumidifier, or opening the house when it is dry outdoors.

In small, enclosed areas where humidity cannot be controlled, desiccants—materials with silica gel or alumina that absorb moisture—can be used and placed on a shelf or the floor of a closet. When they become saturated, they will still feel dry and can be used again after heating them in a 300° F for several hours, cooling, and then replacing them in the closet (Kline & Redmann, 1995).

DUST

Dust allergy is one of the most commonly overlooked allergies. The cause of the problem is not the dust itself, but the microscopic dust mites that feed on dead human skin found in carpeting, draperies, bedding, and upholstery (NIAID, 2003). Dust mites are especially prevalent in the bedroom. The mattress, box springs, and pillows should be encased in zippered, dustproof covers. Although most people use vacuum cleaners to control house dust, much of the dust is either driven into the carpeting or air as the machine moves around.

It is a good idea to have ductwork in ventilation and furnace systems cleaned as the need arises. According to the National Air Duct Cleaners Association (NADCA), to determine whether the ductwork needs cleaning, remove the register, hold a mirror at a 45° angle, and shine a flashlight into the ductwork. The home also can be tested for dust mites with a device that attaches to the end of the vacuum. The dust sample is emptied into a petri dish and sent to a laboratory to determine the type and concentration of the mites to see if professional cleaning is necessary.

Mold
A fungus found indoors or outdoors where there is oxygen and moisture; some are harmful to humans.

Microbial volatile organic compounds (MVOCs)
Compounds responsible for the characteristic fungi smell from mushrooms or molds.

Mycotoxins
Toxic substances produced by fungi; cause of mycotoxicosis.

POLLEN

In North America, the main producers of pollen are weeds, trees, and flowers. Of the weeds, ragweed produces the most pollen (Spencer, 2001). Broadleaf trees such as oak, ash, elm, hickory, pecan, and boxelder produce pollen that easily blows in the wind. Pine pollen is less of a problem because it is heavier and tends to fall straight down to the ground. Pampas grass, goldenrod, and marigolds are plant pollen-producers. Pollen presents a problem indoors when windows are left open during the spring and fall pollen seasons. It can also be brought into the house by pets and anyone having contact with grass, trees, or other plants.

PETS

As much as one might love their pets, they contribute to indoor pollution. Hair, dander, saliva, urine, feces, fleas, litter boxes, bedding, and so forth contribute to the air quality of the home. If someone in the home is allergic to any of these things, it is best to keep the pet outside. Pet food, however, should be kept inside to avoid attracting other animals such as mice, rats, raccoons, skunks, and other wildlife. If it is not possible to keep your pet outdoors, they should be groomed and bathed regularly.

Allergens

Increasingly more individuals experience allergic sensitivities or impaired immune systems. Each person's body and immune system tolerates toxins and allergens in varying degrees. Exposure to some substances results in allergic sensitivities or an impaired immune system (Figure 15-5). An allergic reaction is common to those with a family history of asthma or allergies. When an **allergen** comes in contact with receptor sites in the eyes, mouth, and nose, the cells stimulate **histamine** production. Histamine triggers inflammatory reactions such as headaches, jitteriness, inability to concentrate, sneezing, coughing, itchy or watery eyes, fever,

and sometimes, skin rashes. Common allergies include contact with dust, pollen, and molds.

Asthma is an allergic reaction occurring as bronchial tubes constrict. Mast cells produce a thick, white mucus that further obstructs the airway. The individual usually begins coughing and then wheezes as the airway becomes constricted. It is relieved by corticosteroids and other medicines prescribed by an allergy specialist or pulmonologist.

Hypersensitive Individuals

Some individuals are more sensitive than others to various indoor pollutants; they seem to detect any type of fragrance and have a negative response to it. Although perfumes, colognes, aftershaves, and lotions seem relatively harmless, they also contain VOCs. Sensitive individuals may also react to fragrances in cleaning products, laundry detergents, dryer sheets, toilet paper, fabric softeners, and facial tissues. The condition has several different names (Hoffman, 1993):

Allergic Hypersensitivity Induced by Chemicals (AHIC)

Chemical Sensitivity (CS)

Environmental Illness (EI)

Multiple Chemical Sensitivity (MCS)

The 20th-Century Illness

Toxicant Induced Loss of Tolerance

Universal Reactor Syndrome

No matter what it is called, the individual experiences an antibody reaction and are considered allergies. Sensitive people reach a saturation point earlier than others and suffer from exposure at minimal levels. The Department of

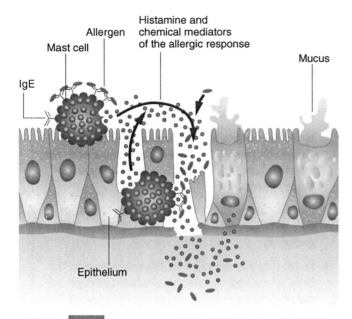

FIGURE 15-5 An allergen (a substance from a pet, plant, insect, or other organism) binds to antibody proteins (IgE) on mast cells. This triggers the release of histamines and other inflammatory substances that characterize the allergic response.

Housing and Urban Development and the Social Security Administration has recognized this illness as a genuine disability since 1990 (NYCAP, 2005). Exposure to environmental toxins may account for a variety of common disease symptoms such as fatigue, headaches, allergies, depression, joint and muscle pain, and respiratory illnesses. Fatigue is usually the first symptom of toxic overload because toxins damage cell membranes, disrupt enzyme pathways, and stress the body as it tries to detoxify.

Unless a radioallergosorbent test is administered, blood tests often miss toxic materials and often show normal conditions in the blood. The determination of chemical sensitivity or allergies must be made by an allergy specialist. Sometimes liver function abnormalities can be detected. Skin patch tests and breath tests can also be used. The most sensitive test for heavy metals is hair analysis, but even that is not 100% reliable. Individuals with persistent allergies should consult an allergy specialist.

Indoor Air Treatments

nyone can develop a sensitivity to indoor air pollutants. The best defense against indoor air pollutants is to prevent the accumulation of indoor air pollutants with good cleaning practices. Indoor air treatments consist of removing carpet and installing wood floors, removing plants and animals, removing window blinds and curtains, installing a centralized

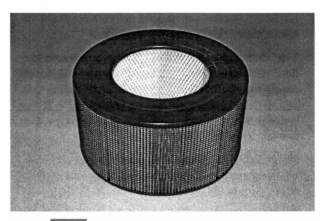

FIGURE 15-6 HEPA Filter The HEPA filter removes smaller dust particles than standard ventilation units.

vacuum system in a new home, using electrostatic furnace filters, changing or cleaning the furnace filter once per month, and using air cleaning devices with a high-efficiency particulate air (HEPA) air filter (Figure 15-6). Normal filters remove large particles indoors, but HEPA filters catch smaller particles. A HEPA filter captures particles less than 0.3 micron. The HEPA filter was developed by the Atonomic Energy Commission during World War II to capture radioactive dust particles from the air and protect the human respiratory system.

Reducing the Effects of Indoor Pollution

ndoor air treatments consist of removing carpet and installing wood floors, removing plants and animals, installing a centralized vacuum system in a new home, and removing venetian blinds and curtains or cleaning them weekly. If a person cannot remodel, there are things that can be done to reduce the effects of indoor pollution from biological and chemical agents.

▪ The most helpful solution is to not allow smoking indoors. If the smoker chooses to smoke outdoors,

Allergen
Foreign substance that can cause an allergic reaction.

Histamine
Chemicals (amines) released by the body when antibodies encounter an allergen.

HEPA air filter
An abbreviation for high efficiency particulate air filters. In order to be classified this way, the filter must allow no more than 3 particles out of 10,000 to penetrate the filtration media.

provide a place where they do not sit next to the entrance that will draw smoke indoors.

- The second most helpful solution is to improve indoor ventilation. Have a heating, ventilation, and air conditioning (HVAC) specialist evaluate the air flow and make recommendations on improving it. If that is not possible, install ventilation fans or ceiling fans that circulate the air.

- Dust weekly, especially if the house is vacuumed often. A vacuum cleaner spews dust in the air while it draws dirt out of carpeting. Use a soft cloth sprayed with a mild dusting agent and wash it immediately after using. A vacuum cleaner can be helpful in cleaning out air ducts where dust has accumulated.

- Remove the sources of indoor air pollution such as animals, pets, blinds, rugs, and other "dust collectors."

- Use HEPA or electrostatic filters and replace furnace filters each month while the furnace is in use.

- Consider air-cleaning devices such as mechanical air-filtering devices, electrostatic precipitators, and hybrid air cleaners that utilize two or more techniques. Air cleaners are not solutions to indoor air quality problems, but can be useful to some extent when used in addition to effective source control and adequate ventilation. The value of any air cleaner depends upon its basic efficiency, proper device for the type of pollutant to be removed, the amount of noise and other pollutants generated, proper size and installation of the device relative to the amount of air space needing cleaning, and faithful maintenance.

- Substitute nontoxic cleaners for toxic ones.

- Reduce dust with vacuum cleaners designed with HEPA filters. Common household vacuums spew it back into the air.

- Do not store food in ceramic, crystal, or porcelain containers that may have a glaze containing lead.

- Buffer the body with nutrients such as calcium, vitamin D, protein, magnesium, copper, chromium, vitamin C, and the B vitamins that boost the immune system.

- Consider increasing your intake of antioxidants such as bright-colored fruits and vegetables and green tea.

- Reduce the consumption of fat, a substance in the body where toxic substances (including drugs) are stored.

To learn more about environmental toxins, contact the Human Ecology Action League (HEAL). Watch for vendors catering to those concerned about environmental toxins such as the Nutritional Ecological and Environmental Delivery System (NEEDS).

Summary

For most individuals, indoor air quality is as important, or more important, as outdoor air quality because individuals generally spend more time indoors than outdoors. The indoor air environment should be a consideration when looking for a place to work and to live. Environmental health special-

---

Digging Deeper   BEWARE OF ION AND OZONE GENERATORS

Some individuals recommend ion generators to clean the air. Ion generators charge the particles in a room so that they are re-suspended in the air, attracted to walls, floors, tabletops, draperies, and occupants. Some devices have a collector to attract charged particles back to the unit. Although ion generators may remove small particles (such as tobacco smoke) from the indoor air, they do not remove gases or odors and may be ineffective in removing large particles such as pollen and house-dust allergens. Although some have suggested that these devices provide a benefit, no controlled studies have confirmed this effect.

Unfortunately, some air-cleaning devices, particularly ion generators, produce ozone, a lung irritant. A toxic gas, ozone does not remove particles from the air, takes many months or years to react with airborne chemicals (e.g., formaldehyde), and is harmful to humans. Ozone worsens chronic respiratory diseases and the ability of the body to fight respiratory diseases. Ozone indoors is the same as ozone outdoors. Under certain conditions, ion generators and ozone-generating air cleaners can produce levels of this lung irritant significantly above levels

considered harmful to human health.

The Food and Drug Administration has set a limit of 0.05 parts per million of ozone for medical devices. Although ozone can be used in reducing odors and pollutants in unoccupied spaces (such as removing smoke odors from homes involved in fires), the levels needed to achieve this are above those generally thought to be safe for humans. Even following the manufacturer's suggestions, ozone generators produced exceptionally high levels. Filters or electrostatic precipitators are safer methods to clean indoor air.

Source: US EPA, 2003.

ists often find themselves addressing indoor air quality issues. Space, temperature, and humidity are major considerations. Exposure to indoor air pollutants such as asbestos, ETS, radon, lead, mercury, VOCs, pesticides, carbon monoxide, nitrogen dioxide, and corrosive chemicals can negatively impact health. Biological pollutants such as molds, mildew, dust, pollen, and pets also contribute to indoor air pollution. Infants, children, and individuals with multiple chemical sensitivity are most susceptible to health problems. Measures can be taken to reduce exposure to and health problems posed by indoor air pollution.

Consider the Cost — SOME THINGS JUST DON'T MIX

When cleaning indoors, be very careful not to mix cleaning chemicals together. When ammonia and bleach are mixed together, a toxic chlorine gas forms that can cause serious respiratory illness.

Consider the Cost — REDUCING HAZARDOUS SUBSTANCES IN THE HOME

Every home has a supply of potentially hazardous waste. As much as 100 pounds of hazardous waste can be found in each home. Household products (chemicals and solvents) containing toxic ingredients can be found in kitchens, bathrooms, basements, utility sheds, garages, and workshops. Cleaning products for the house, car, or yard can be flammable, corrosive, reactive, or toxic. Risks associated with hazardous products are according to type, quality, age, exposure, and vulnerability of the person using them. The challenge for consumers is to reduce the number of hazardous products in the home. Strategies include:

- Use a squeegee to remove water from shower walls immediately after showering to prevent soap scum deposits.

- Reduce the need for hazardous products by cleaning surfaces and floors at least once per week. Bathe pets once per week or every other week to eliminate fleas. Insects are discouraged if there are no food or water available.

- Open windows to air out the home to avoid the need for room deodorizers or air fresheners.

- Prevent the need for harsh cleaners by lining areas that are likely to accumulate spills or build-up. A sheet of aluminum foil in the bottom of the oven will reduce the need for an oven cleaner. A screen over a drain will catch food and hair so that a

drain cleaner is not needed. Pour grease into an empty can and put it in the garbage rather than pouring it down the drain.

- Clean spills as soon as they occur rather than waiting until they harden. This reduces the need to purchase specialty cleaners that are more toxic and harmful to surfaces. If a surface becomes scratched, it will get dirty faster and stain deeper, making it difficult to clean and keep clean.

- Purchase multipurpose cleaners to reduce the number of cleaners used. Determine what the best type of product and packaging is for your use (aerosol, pump spray, powder, liquid, or solid).

Enviroshoppers buy less hazardous products. A list of green cleaning product names might include:

Earth Friendly Products (http://www.ecos.com)

Ecover (www.ecover.com)

Planet Inc. (www.planetinc.com)

Seventh Generation (www.seventhgen.com)

Simple Green (www.simplegreen.com)

Eco-friendly Cleaning Products

White distilled vinegar for disinfecting and deodorizing

Lemon juice for dissolving grease and polishing metals and wood

Baking soda for cleaning and deodorizing

Washing soda (stronger alternative to baking soda)

Borax is effective against mold and some insects

Essential oils have numerous cleaning properties

Nontoxic Cleaners

Salt as an abrasive

Baking soda, activated charcoal, and borax for freshening the air and articles

White vinegar for molds and disinfecting

Olive oil, lemon oil, mineral oil, or beeswax to polish furniture

Equal parts of baking soda and white vinegar to flush and clean drains

ALTERNATIVES TO COMMERCIAL PRODUCTS
Cleaning products can often be made from inexpensive items already in the home. Most homemade products are safer than commercial products. Items already used in the home reduce the need to store additional bottles of cleaners. You can also control the strength of the products you make. It may take more time for homemade products to work, and you may need to scrub harder than with commercial products.

COMPLETELY SAFE WINDOW CLEANER

2 tablespoons vinegar

1 quart of warm water

Mix ingredients and put in a spray bottle. Spray on the surface and wipe with a soft, lint-free cloth.

NONTOXIC WINDOW AND MIRROR CLEANER

4 tablespoons ammonia

1 quart warm water

Mix ingredients and put in a spray bottle. Spray on surface and wipe dry.

NONTOXIC AND FAST-DRYING MIRROR CLEANER

½ cup rubbing alcohol

1 teaspoon ammonia

1 teaspoon liquid detergent (not soap)

1 gallon water

2 drops of blue food coloring (optional)

Mix together. Put in a spray bottle. Spray on surface and wipe dry.

TUB AND SINK CLEANER

2 teaspoons borax

4 tablespoons of distilled white vinegar

3 to 4 cups of hot water

Mix the borax, vinegar, and hot water together. Pour into a refillable spray bottle. For stronger cleaning power, add ¼ teaspoon of liquid soap.

NONTOXIC TUB, SHOWER, SINK, AND TOILET DISINFECTANT

3–5% hydrogen peroxide in a spray container

White or cider vinegar in a spray container

Spray the area to disinfect with hydrogen peroxide and spray vinegar over that. You can also wash your hands and vegetables with this solution.

ALL-PURPOSE CLEANER

4 tablespoons baking soda

1 quart of warm water

Dissolve the baking soda in warm water. Apply to surface with a sponge. Rinse with clear water.

STRONGER ALL-PURPOSE CLEANER

Directly apply baking soda to a damp sponge. Rinse with clear water.

NONTOXIC ALL-PURPOSE CLEANER

1 tablespoon ammonia

1 tablespoon liquid detergent

2 cups of water

Mix ingredients and put in a spray bottle. Spray on surface. Wipe. Rinse with clear water.

TOILET BOWL CLEANER

Sprinkle 2 tablespoons baking soda into the toilet bowl. Add ¼ cup vinegar. Scour with a toilet brush.

TOILET BOWL DISINFECTANT

Pour ½ cup of liquid bleach into the toilet bowl. Let stand for 30–45 minutes. Scrub with a toilet brush (being careful not to splash). Flush.

DRAIN CLEANER

Once a month, dump ¼ cup of baking soda, followed by ¼ cup of vinegar to clean the drain. One cup of bleach will also work well.

For slow drains, mix 1 cup salt with 1 cup soda and pour it down the drain. Add 1 cup of vinegar. Pour 2 quarts of boiling water over all.

For clogged drains, first try using a plunger ("plumber's helper"). If that does not unclog the drain, use a flexible metal snake (rented or purchased). Thread it down the clogged drain and push the clog away.

FURNITURE POLISH/CLEANER

Most dust or sticky residue on furniture can be cleaned with a damp cloth and dried immediately. Furniture with an oil finish needs an oil-based cleaner. To make an oil-based cleaner or furniture polish, combine

2 cups mineral oil

6 drops lemon extract (optional)

Put in spray bottle, shake, and spray.

LIME DEPOSIT REMOVER

Soak paper towels in vinegar and apply the paper towels to the lime deposits. Leave them on for approximately 1 hour. When the deposits have softened, use a Teflon scrubber to remove them. If all of the deposits are not removed, repeat the process.

ALUMINUM COOKWARE CLEANER

To remove burned on food residue inside of pots or pants, combine 1 tablespoon cream of tartar and 2 cups of water. Bring the solution to a boil inside the pan and simmer for 10 minutes. Scrub the pan to remove as much as possible. If some residue remains, repeat the process. Wash and dry as usual.

CHROME AND STAINLESS STEEL CLEANER

Dip soft cloth in undiluted white vinegar. Wipe surface.

BRASS CLEANER

Make a paste of 1 tablespoon lemon juice and 1 teaspoon baking soda. Apply to the surface and rub with a soft cloth. Rinse with water and dry.

For tougher cleaning, make a paste of lemon juice and cream of tartar about the consistency of toothpaste. Apply to the surface and leave on for five minutes. Wash with warm water. Dry with a soft cloth.

OVEN CLEANER

Sprinkle water on oven surface. Apply baking soda. Rub using a Teflon scrubber. Wipe off scum with a damp sponge. Rinse well and dry.

For crusted surfaces, warm the oven to 250° F. Turn off the oven. While the oven is still warm, sprinkle or spray water on the spill, then lightly sprinkle salt on it. When the oven cools down, scrape the spill away and wash the area clean.

CARPET CLEANER/ DEODORIZER

Sprinkle baking soda on the carpet (covering the area lightly) before vacuuming.

ROOM FRESHENER

Purchase fresh oranges, lemon, limes, or grapefruit. Grate the peel into an attractive container and place in the room to freshen.

ENVIRONMENTALLY FRIENDLY PERSONAL CARE PRODUCTS

Many personal care products are in cans. Aerosol cans require a flammable ingredient to expel it from the can. There may also be a halocarbon or CFC substance used to propel the liquid. Whenever possible, purchase solid antiperspirant or deodorant and purchase spray products in a pump, rather than as an aerosol.

There has been some debate about the potential carcinogenic effect of sodium laurel sulfate, the product used to create foam or lather, in shampoos and other bath products. Read the label of the product to see if you can find one that does not contain sodium laurel sulfate. Expect that the product will not lather as much as the product you used to buy.

BABY POWDER

To reduce moisture, dust the area (armpits, skin folds, or perineum areas) lightly with corn starch.

HAIR RINSE TO REMOVE SOAP RESIDUE

¼ cup of white vinegar

1 cup of water

This mixture will remove soap scum and that "gummy" feeling from hair. After rinsing the soap out of hair, pour this mixture over the hair, massage it into the scalp, and rinse thoroughly with cool water. The cool water adds more "shine" to the hair.

TOOTHPASTE

1 teaspoon baking soda

Dash of salt

1 drop mint flavoring

or

Unsweetened green tea (contains fluoride)

MOUTHWASH

Green tea

SKIN ASTRINGENT

1 teaspoon glycerol

1 teaspoon rubbing alcohol

1 cup water

1 drop tea tree oil (for oily skin only)

Apply to a cotton ball and wipe on skin. Use sparingly around the eyes because tea tree oil can be very strong.

REDUCING THE INCIDENCE AND PREVALENCE OF MOLD

The following can lessen the probability and productivity of molds indoors:

- Ventilate the house periodically. Tightly closed homes encourage mold growth.

- Fix leaky plumbing and leaks as soon as possible.

- Watch for condensation and wet spots. Fix moisture problems as soon as possible. Clean and dry wet or damp spots within 48 hours.

- Develop a mold-killing cleaning solution with ¼ cup of bleach and 1 gallon of water. Spray on the surface and let it sit for 7 minutes. Be sure that the surface color would not be damaged by the bleach.

- Clean shower stalls, tubs, the toilet tank, and bathroom ceilings with mold-killing solutions. Do not carpet the bathroom because it absorbs moisture.

- Remove carpeting in the bedroom.

- Place a vinyl cover with zippers over the mattress.

- Use an air conditioner (which dehumidifies air) or a dehumidifier in the summer. Spray the air filter with mold disinfectant when cleaning.

- Keep indoor humidity between 35 to 50% by monitoring with a humidity gauge.

- If the home is older with paneling and wallpaper that have not been removed for some time, check for mold and remove if necessary.

- Remove old newspapers, books, and magazines; they harbor molds and dust.

- Remove house plants, especially those that appear to be growing mold in the potting soil.

- Clean the refrigerator out monthly. Empty the water pans under self-defrosting refrigerators.

- Clean the garbage cans weekly.

- If one room is a particular problem, an air cleaner with a HEPA filter may help.

- When outdoors, avoid cutting grass or raking leaves. If you must do these things, wear a face mask.

Sources: Berthold-Bond, 1994; Clemson University Cooperative Extension Service, 2003; Dad & Tarcher, 1997; Hammer, 1988; Hammett, 1992; Logan, 1997; Steinman & Epstein, 1995.

REFERENCES

American Lung Association of New York. (2000). Lung cancer. Retrieved from http://www.alahv.org/bookfiles4/lung_cancer.html.

Anyanwu, E., Campbell, A., & High, W. (2002). Brainstem auditory evoked response in adolescents with acoustic mycotic neuroma due to environmental exposure to toxic molds. *International Journal of Adolescent Med Health, 14*, 67–76.

Berthold-Bond. (1994). *Clean and green: The complete guide to non-toxic and environmentally safe housekeeping.* Ceres Books.

Centers for Disease Control. (1979). Health and sanitary elements of a housing inspection. In Basic Housing Inspection. Retrieved from http://www.cdc.gov/nceh/publications/books/housing/housing.htm#CONTENTS.

Centers for Disease Control. (2002). Health and safety elements of a housing inspection. Retrieved from http://www.cdc.gov/nceh/publications/books/housing/cha3.htm.

Clemson University Cooperative Extension Service (2003). Reducing hazardous products in the home. Booklet. Printed on recycled paper with soy ink.

Dad, D., & Tarcher, J. (1997). *Home safe home: Protecting yourself and your family from everyday toxics and harmful household products.* J. P. Tarcher.

Evans, K. (2002). *The environment: A revolution in attitudes.* Farmington Hills, MI: The Gale Group, Inc.

Hammer, M. (1988). Alternatives that are relatively free of toxic effects. Pamphlet HE 3149. Gainesville, FL: University of Florida.

Hammett, W. (1992). Reducing hazardous products in the home. Pamphlet HE 368-2. Raleigh, NC: North Carolina State University.

Indoor Environmental Standards Organization. (2002). Standards and Newsletter. Retrieved March 26, 2003 from http://www.iestandards.org.

Kilburn, K. (2002). Janus revisited, molds again. *Archives of Environmental Health, 57*, 7–9.

Kline, J., & Redmann, L. (1995). Mildew: How to prevent and remove mildew. HE Leaflet 73. Clemson, SC: Clemson University Cooperative Extension Service.

Logan, K. (1997) *Clean house, clean planet: Clean your house for pennies a day, the safe, nontoxic way.* Pocket Books.

Lyles, W., Greve, K., Bauer, R., Ware, M., Schramke, C., Crouch, J., Hicks, A. (1991). Sick building syndrome. *Southern Medical Journal, 84*, 65–71, 76.

Martin, D. (1999). Smoking ban has not hurt restaurants, analysts say. *New York Times, 148*, B7.

National Center for Environmental Health. (1976). Health and Sanitary Elements of a Housing Inspection. *Basic housing inspection.* Atlanta, GA: Centers for Disease Control and Prevention, Environmental Health Services Division. Reprinted in 1979. Retrieved from http://www.cdc.gov/nceh/publications/books/housing/cha3.htm#chapter03.

National Institute of Allergy and Infectious Diseases. (2003). Airborne allergens: Something in the air. Publication 03-7045. Retrieved from http://www.niaid.nih.gov/publications/allergens/airborne_allergens.pdf.

New York Coalition for Alternatives to Pesticides. (2005). Multiple chemical sensitivity (MCS)—A disorder triggered by exposures to chemicals in the environment. Retrieved from http://www.crisny.org/not-for-profit/nycap/mcs.htm.

Ruggless, R. (2002). Texas study finds anti-smoking laws don't hurt business at local restaurants. *Nation's Restaurant News.* Retrieved March 23, 2003 from Http://www..findarticles.com/cf_0/m3190/19_36/85932647/print.jhtml.

Spencer, C. (2001). Pine pollen not the cause of spring allergies. Master Gardener Column for the Week of May 21, 2001, Brunswick County Extension Service. North Carolina State University and NC A & T State University. Retrieved from http://www.ces.ncsu.edu/brunswick/mastergardener/mg010521.html.

Steinman, D., & Epstein, S. (1995). The *safe shoppers bible: A consumers guide to non-toxic household products.* John Wiley & Sons.

U.S. Environmental Protection Agency. (2001). Healthy buildings, healthy people: A vision for the 21st century. Office of Air and Radiation (6609J) 402-K-01-003. Retrieved from http://www.epa.gov/iaq/hbhplindex.html.

U. S. Environmental Protection Agency. (2003). *Ozone generators that are sold as air cleaners: An assessment of effectiveness and health consequences.* Retrieved 6/4/2003 from http://www.epa.gov/iaq/pubs/ozonegen.html.

U. S. Environmental Protection Agency. (2004). Take the smoke-free home pledge. Retrieved from http://www.epa.gov/iaq/ets/pledge/index.html.

Zureik, M., Neukirch, C., Leynaert, B., Liard, R., Bousquet, J., & Neukrich, F. (2002). Sensitization to airborne molds and severity of asthma: Cross sectional study from European Community respiratory health survey. *British Medical Journal, 125*, 411–415.

ASSIGNMENTS

1. Based on the suggestions from this chapter, make a list of your basic shelter needs and your comfort needs.

2. Look at the ingredients in various products found in your home. You may need to look at labels on carpeting, insulation, household cleaning chemicals, and other items for potentially harmful substances.

3. Ask a firefighter to visit the class regarding items in the home that are flammable and that can accelerate a fire.

4. Change your furnace filter and vacuum cleaner bag.

5. Compare three different air-cleaning devices regarding cost, efficiency, the cost of a replacement filter, warranty, and effectiveness.

6. Debate whether individuals should be asked to stop smoking or wearing perfume indoors.

7. As a class project, investigate student support for a nonsmoking campus.

8. Invite a public health official to tell about sick buildings, lead poisoning, or asbestos abatement.

9. Investigate the harmful effects of indoor air pollution in schools on children.

SELECTED ENVIRONMENTAL LAWS

1971 *Lead Poisoning Prevention Act (PL 91-695)*
Provided $30 million in grants to states over 3 years to treat victims of lead paint poisoning and develop methods for removing lead paint from homes.

1976 *Toxic Substances Control Act (TSCA)*
Authorized the EPA to secure information on existing and new chemical substances and control those that caused unreasonable risk to public health or the environment. This act was later amended with specific mandates for asbestos (see AHERA in 1986), radon, and lead.

1986 *Asbestos Hazardous Emergency Response Act (AHERA-Title II of TSCA) (PL 99-519)*
Established asbestos abatement programs in schools and required the EPA to determine the potential health danger from exposure. Later amended by the Asbestos School Hazard Abatement Reauthorization Act (ASHARA) (P.L. 101-637) in 1990 creating standards for persons conducting asbestos inspections and abatement activities in schools, commercial buildings, and public buildings.

1988 *Indoor Radon Abatement TSCA Title III (PL 100-551)*
Directed the EPA to set standards for controlling radon levels in new buildings and assist states in developing radon abatement programs. Called for areas of the country with elevated levels of indoor radon to be identified.

1992 *Lead-Based Paint Exposure Reduction Act (PL 102-550)*
Provided for exposure studies, determination of lead levels in products, monitoring, abatement, training, and certification for abatement workers. Provisions of the act included exposure studies, determination of lead levels in products, establishing state programs for monitoring and abatement, and training and certification requirements for lead abatement workers.

SELECTED PROFESSIONAL JOURNALS

Building Design and Construction
Environmental Health Journal

ADDITIONAL READING

International Code Council. (2002). *International building code 2003.* Country Club Hills, IL: International Code Council.

Kearns, T. (2001). *Environmentally-induced illnesses: Ethics, risk assessment and human rights.* Jefferson, NC: McFarland & Company, Inc.

National Academy of Sciences. (1993). *Indoor allergens: Assessing and controlling adverse health effects.* Washington, DC: National Academy Press.

National Center for Environmental Health. (2005). *Basic housing inspections.* Retrieved from http://www.cdc.gov/nceh/publications/books/housing/housing.htm.

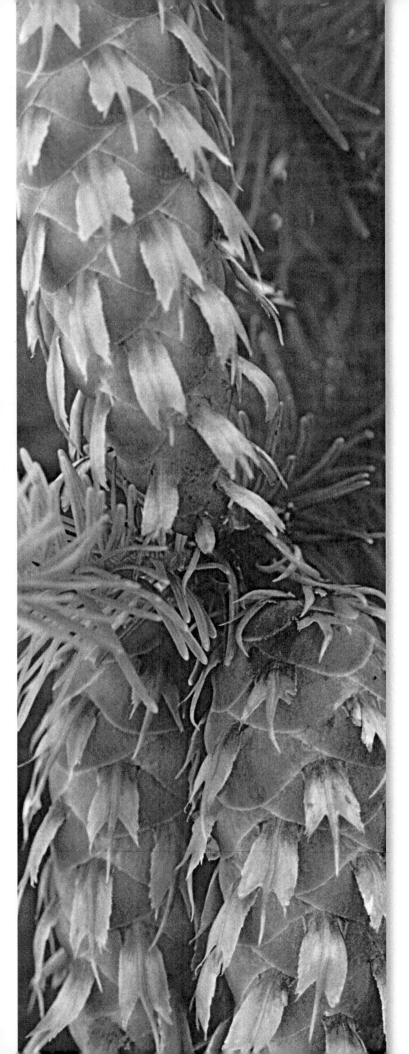

16

Injury and Safety Issues

These are not acts of God, they are failures of machinery and negligence and failures of people.

Hugh DeHaven (1942–present)

OBJECTIVES

1. Summarize the contributions of Johann Peter Frank, Hugh DeHaven, John Gordon, Ross McFarland, William Haddon, John Stapp, and Ralph Nader to the study of automotive safety.

2. Explain what is meant by the term accident prone.

3. State the three phases of an accident described by Haddon.

4. Describe four laws aimed at reducing morbidity and mortality due to accidents.

5. Provide a historical account of the establishment of government agencies and other safety organizations.

6. List types of intentional injuries and define them.

7. Describe ways that individuals can reduce their risk of accidental injuries.

8. List the typical unintentional injuries related to product safety, and to home, school, and recreational activities.

9. List the various types of mechanical and psychosocial hazards and the typical relationship of the two types.

10. Explain why the study of mechanisms of injury contributes to accident prevention.

Introduction

ore than 400 Americans die every day of injuries from motor vehicle crashes, firearms, poisonings, suffocation, falls, fires, and drowning. Many more are injured but don't die. Most people experience a significant injury at one time or another in their lives. The total societal cost of motor vehicle crashes alone exceeds $150 billion annually (Healthy People 2010). Such injuries are a major public health problem, because of health care costs, disabilities, and life lost for those who are injured. To explore how this frightful carnage might be lessened, this chapter reviews the history of accident evaluation, the major concerns about environmental safety, and the efforts of various agencies to enhance environmental safety.

History of Injury Prevention

or centuries accidental deaths and injuries were ascribed to being in the wrong place at the wrong time, or just the cost of doing business. As early as 1788, though, Johann Peter Frank, a German physician and proponent of public health, suggested that accident-prevention activities should be part of comprehensive public health programs. He had in mind efforts to teach or motivate citizens to act safely. At the time, the United States was primarily rural, and an emphasis on individual responsibility for accident prevention made sense. The public attributed unintentional injury to human error. As people moved to cities, however, accidental death and disability statistics rose, and this explanation was not enough.

Digging Deeper — OBJECTIVES RELATED TO INJURY PREVENTION, HEALTHY PEOPLE 2010

With the goal of reducing injuries, disabilities, and deaths due to unintentional injuries and violence, the Healthy People Consortium—an alliance of more than 350 national membership organizations and 250 state health, mental health, substance abuse, and environmental agencies—established a number of objectives related to injury prevention:

- Reduce hospitalization for nonfatal head injuries.

- Reduce hospitalization for nonfatal spinal cord injuries.

- Reduce firearm-related deaths.

- Reduce the proportion of persons living in homes with firearms that are loaded and locked.

- Reduce nonfatal firearm-related injuries.

- Extend state-level child fatality review of deaths due to external causes for children aged 14 and under.

- Reduce nonfatal poisonings.

- Reduce deaths caused by poisonings.

- Reduce deaths caused by suffocation.

- Increase the number of states and the District of Columbia with statewide emergency department

surveillance systems that collect data on external causes of injury.

- Increase the number of states and the District of Columbia that collect data on external causes of injury through hospital discharge data systems.

- Reduce hospital emergency department visits caused by injuries.

- Reduce deaths caused by unintentional injuries.

- Reduce nonfatal unintentional injuries.

- Reduce deaths caused by motor vehicle crashes.

- Reduce pedestrian deaths on public roads.

- Reduce nonfatal injuries caused by motor vehicle crashes.

- Reduce nonfatal pedestrian injuries on public roads.

- Increase use of safety belts.

- Increase use of child restraints.

- Increase the proportion of motorcyclists using helmets.

- Increase the number of states and the District of Columbia that have

adopted a graduated driver licensing model law.

- Increase use of helmets by bicyclists.

- Increase the number of states and the District of Columbia with laws requiring bicycle helmets for bicycle riders.

- Reduce residential fire deaths.

- Increase functioning residential smoke alarms.

- Reduce deaths from falls.

- Reduce hip fractures among older adults.

- Reduce the number of drownings.

- Reduce hospital emergency department visits for nonfatal dog bite injuries.

- Increase the proportion of public and private schools that require use of appropriate head, face, eye, and mouth protection for students participating in school-sponsored physical activities.

- Reduce the number of homicides.

- Reduce the occurrence of developmental disabilities.

Source: Healthy People Consortium, Healthy People 2010.

It was not until the early 1900s that research on accidents became of general interest, primarily among automobile makers and insurance companies (Figure 16-1). Injury research focused on identifying high-risk situations, high-risk individuals, and high-risk behaviors. It became apparent that individuals did not adequately understand injury risks, so prevention strategies addressed the individual. From 1915 to the 1940s, psychologists emphasized the importance of emotional **antecedents** to life events, meaning that emotional states growing out of early experiences caused some people to have accidents. It became accepted that some individuals might be *accident-prone*.

James J. Gibson, a psychologist, was instrumental in changing preconceptions about accident causes. Before his work, it was thought that accidents are random events for which no one but the victim is responsible. Gibson, focusing on the accident itself, defined an accident as an "uncontrolled, unplanned release of transfer of energy." He identified five agents causing injuries: kinetic or mechanical energy, chemical energy, thermal energy, electrical energy, and radioactive energy (Gibson, 1961).

The view that some people are accident-prone dominated safety research for 50 years, even though studies could never determine a particular type of individual more accident-prone than another. Psychological interventions did not appear to work for those who often experienced accidental injuries. Moreover, most researchers focused only on single causes of accidents. In truth, accidents usually have multiple causes. Accidental injuries are often a product not only of human error, but also of product design, mental or physical impairment, environmental conditions, and other factors specific to the accident.

The first attempt to look at more than one factor causing an accident was Hugh DeHaven (1895–1980). A pilot in World War I, DeHaven wanted to know why he was able to walk away from a serious crash. He began research in crash investigation with demonstrations, "survivability" research, and crash testing (DeHaven, 1942). He was later dubbed the "father of crashworthiness research." As a result of his work, better designs in automobiles, seat-belt restraints, and air bags have been developed for the purpose of reducing the severity of injuries in aircraft and automobiles (National Safety Council, 1987).

Dr. John Stapp, a colonel in the Air Force, was also a pioneer in investigating safety harnesses for pilots, which has had application to auto safety belts. Stapp conducted experiments for the U.S. Air Force on the biomechanics of acceleration/deceleration at high speeds. He is known for strapping himself into a rocket sled with a shoulder harness to test the ability of the harness to withstand extreme energy transfer forces. Because of his research, in 1967 Stapp was loaned by the Air Force to the National Highway Traffic Safety Administration as a scientist. When he retired from the Air Force in 1970, Stapp took a faculty position in the Safety and Systems Management Center of the University of California, and later consulted with the U.S. Surgeon General and National Aeronautics and Space Administration (NASA). He also formed the Stapp Foundation, which holds annual Stapp Car Crash Conferences of automotive engineers, trauma surgeons and others to explore the nature of fatal car crashes.

Dr. John E. Gordon (Figure 16-2) studied the distribution and causes of injury events as one would study infectious diseases. Gordon was a colonel in the military during World War II and studied nonbattle injuries during war, practices, and on leave. Gordon believed that **epidemiology**, the study of disease patterns, was a fruitful approach to studying accidents (Gordon, 1949). He regarded the potential agents of injury (from the agent, host, and environment model) as unlimited; that in fact the host, agent, and environmental factors all contribute to an accident. (Cook & Gordon, 1976.) He also noted strategies to prevent injuries (Table 16-1).

ERGONOMICS

After World War II, the field of **ergonomics** was born: "... a body of knowledge about human abilities, human limitations, and other human characteristics that are relevant to design. . . . [It] is the application of human

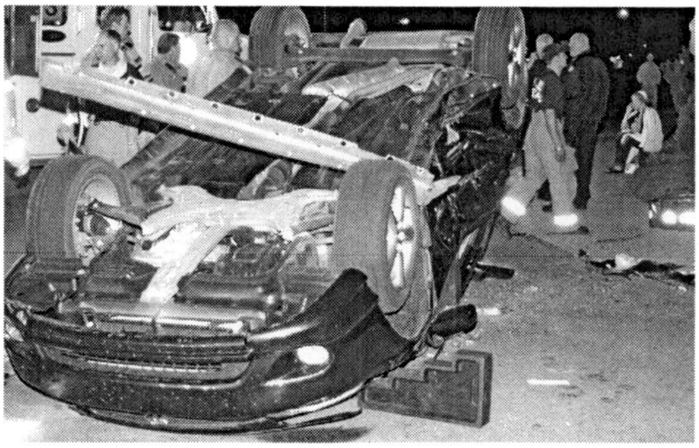

FIGURE 16-1 Rollover automobile accident.

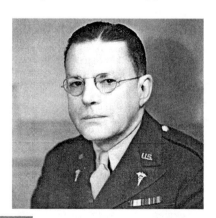

FIGURE 16-2 **Dr. John E. Gordon** Epidemiologist of injury prevention.

factors information to the design of tools, machines, systems, tasks, jobs, and environments for safe, comfortable, and effective human use" (Chapanis, 1991).

Ross McFarland, a psychologist and trainer of aviation medicine specialists, documented the fact that U.S. military service losses from highway crashes exceeded those from plane crashes. He applied the concept of ergonomics by demonstrating, for example, that the design and placement of the gear shift in trucks prevented drivers from moving their legs quickly from the accelerator to the brake to avoid a crash (McFarland, 1957).

WILLIAM HADDON

Dr. William Haddon, Jr., an engineer and public health physician for the New York State Health Department, believed the best way to reduce the incidence and severity of accidents was to study the **kinetic energy** involved. Haddon suggested that injury or damage resulted from interactions in three phases of the accident (Table 16-2):

1. Pre-injury phase, when control of energy expenditure is lost.

2. Injury phase (lasting less than one second), when energy is transferred to people and causes damage.

3. Post-injury phase, when attempts are made to repair the damage and regain physiological homeostasis.

Haddon studied injuries from motor-vehicle accidents by looking at the crash sequence. Haddon argued that there are circumstances before a collision that determine whether or not the crash will happen. The crash itself transfers energy and influences the likelihood for and severity of injury. The events occurring after a crash, such as medical care and response time for an ambulance, determine the outcome.

Haddon's injury-prevention programs emphasized prevention or limitation of energy buildup; control of circumstances of energy used to prevent unintended release; modification of the energy transfer phase to limit damage; and improvement of emergency, definitive, and rehabilitative care.

Haddon's work represented the first epidemiological study for injury research, including relative risk and interaction of contributory factors (Haddon et al., 1961; McCarroll & Haddon, 1962). His model is still used today. Haddon's textbook, *Accident Research* (1964), was a milestone in developing injury research as a science. He is remembered as the "father of injury **epidemiology** and injury control" (Haddon, Suchman, & Kline, 1964).

RALPH NADER

In the 1950s, Ralph Nader began to draw attention to the design of automobiles (Figure 16-3). His 1959 article "The Safe Car You Can't Buy" declared that automobile makers were designing cars for style, cost, and performance while ignoring the number of accidental injuries, disabilities, and deaths. In 1965, he published a book, *Unsafe at Any Speed,* which focused attention on environmental aspects of the pre-crash and crash phases of automobile accidents. The book targeted General Motors'

Antecedent
That which occurs before something happens.

Epidemiology
Study of all the factors affecting the appearance or disappearance of a disease or pathogen.

Ergonomics
The study and modification of human and environmental interactions.

Kinetic energy
Energy associated with force and motion.

Ross A. McFarland (1901–1976) is regarded as the father of human factors in aviation safety. Author of the classic *Human Factors in Air Transport Design,* several other books and hundreds of articles, he was also a consultant to many federal agencies and corporations. In the 1930s and 1940s, McFarland was a researcher at the Fatigue Laboratory at Harvard University, and in 1947 he joined the faculty of the Harvard School of Public Health. His research included studies of the effects of substances such as alcohol, tobacco, and carbon monoxide on human performance; dark adaptation and visual thresholds; anoxia and high altitude physiology; stress and fatigue in pilots and other flight personnel; the physiological and psychological characteristics of airplane pilots; human factors in air and ground vehicle design; health and safety in air and ground transportation; accident prevention; and circadian rhythms in air travel.

TABLE 16-1 Strategies to Prevent Auto Accident Injuries

Host	Agent	Environment
Use seat belts and child safety seats.	Add safety features to autos, such as airbags.	Change roads to have such safety features as good lighting, guardrails, clear sightlines, and separate lanes for cars, bicycles and pedestrians.

Source: Moore, J. D., & Gardner, L. W. (1994). Saving children's lives: Preventing childhood injuries. *North Carolina Public Health Forum*, Vol. 3, No. 1, p. 14.

TABLE 16-2 Factors Affecting the Three Phases of an Accident

	Pre-crash	Crash	Post-crash
Human Factors	Braking	Personal protective equipment	Crash research
	Licensing		Education/Training
	Education/training		Evaluation
	Crash-avoidance skills		
	Attitude toward safety		
	Motorist physical impairment		
	Alcohol/substance impairment		
	Telecommunication distractions		
	Rider risk recognition and judgment		
	Concurrent exposure data collection		
Vehicle Factors	Horns	Vehicle safety equipment	Automated collision notification (ACN) system
	Braking	Personal protective equipment	Crash research
	Intelligent transportation systems/Intelligent vehicle initiative		
	Conspicuity		
	Vehicle design		
	Passenger/loads		
	Vehicle equipment		
	Vehicle modifications		
	Motorcycle performance		
	Vehicle safety equipment		
Environmental Factors	Intelligent transportation systems	Road furniture	EMS response
	Regulation	Other vehicle design	
	Enforcement		
	Road hazards		
	Natural hazards		
	Driver distractions		
	Other vehicle design		
	Lane position/sharing		
	Road design, maintenance		
Social Factors	Enforcement		Transportation safety community attitude
	Rider peer pressure		Medical community attitude
	Motorist awareness		
	Insurance incentives		
	Motorcycle retail advertising		
	Transportation safety community attitude		

Source: Haddon, W., Suchman, E. A., and Klein, D., eds. (1964). *Accident research: Methods and approaches.* New York: Harper & Row.

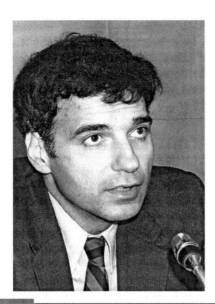

FIGURE 16-3 **Ralph Nader** Advocate for consumer product safety.

sporty Corvair, whose faulty rear suspension system made it possible to skid violently and roll over. The main cause of car injuries, Nader said, was not the "nut behind the wheel" so often blamed by the automakers, but the engineering and design deficiencies of the car itself, making it uncrashworthy. Nader also drew attention to the fact that some manufacturers were hiding information about product safety.

In 1971, Nader founded the NGO Public Citizen as an umbrella organization for his projects. Today, Public Citizen has more than 150,000 members and numerous researchers investigating congressional, health, environmental, and economic issues. Public Citizen is credited with helping to pass the Safe Drinking Water Act and Freedom of Information Act, and prompting creation of the Occupational Safety and Health Administration (OSHA), Environmental Protection Agency (EPA), and Consumer Product Safety Commission (CPSC).

THE RISE OF PUBLIC HEALTH INITIATIVES

During the 1950s and 1960s, the W.K. Kellogg Foundation, a nonprofit organization that gives out grants in health and education, funded several demonstration projects in public health departments. Public health nurses, health educators, and sanitarians were trained to facilitate behavioral changes among persons at risk of injury. Public health activities aimed at injury control were initiated in the U.S. Public Health Service's Division of Special Health Services. The division included programs in radiological health, tuberculosis, air pollution, and chronic diseases.

In 1956, the Division of Accident Prevention was added to address highway and nonhighway safety concerns. State and local health departments began to evaluate and educate drivers, identify populations with a presumed high risk of injury and counsel them on safe behaviors, and teach mothers to keep harmful things away from young children. A second role of the Division of Accident Prevention was to promote and financially support research into safety. In 1967, the National Highway Safety Bureau (NHSB) was formed, with William Haddon as director.

In the 1970s, the Johnson administration created the Consumer Product Safety Commission to study ergonomic factors in safe product design. Also in the 1970s, emergency medical services were expanded to reduce the incidence of deaths due to accident trauma. Standards for emergency medical technicians (EMTs), equipment, vehicles, services, and the development and designation of trauma centers for specialty care were quickly developed. Funds were also made available for small communities to purchase ambulances and train emergency medical technicians. By the 1980s, federal funding for nonhighway safety research had ended, but substantial improvements in highway safety had been gained. The National Highway Safety Bureau became the National Highway Traffic Safety Administration (NHTSA).

In 1985, a committee chaired by Dr. William Foege published *Injury in America,* a report providing an overview of all injuries, not just motor vehicle injuries (Committee on Trauma Research, 1985). It was apparent that the Haddon model was applicable to all types of injury. When determining cause-and-effect relationships, it was apparent that intention was less significant than other factors. The frequency and circumstances of abuse and suicide attempts, which had been ignored by the

1. The lawsuit against General Motors was ultimately decided by the high court of New York, whose opinion in the case expanded the privacy rights that can be remedied in tort. (See *Nader v. General Motors Corp.,* 307 N.Y.S.2d 647 N.Y. 1970.)

public health community, began to receive attention. Conclusions and recommendations from the report also stated that no single agency should have the authority or responsibility for coordinating injury research and programs. Congress provided funding for injury control research to the Centers for Disease Control, and established the National Center for Injury Prevention and Control to study the results of violence as well as accidents. In 1992, the American Public Health Association reestablished its injury control section, disbanded in the 1970s.

Intentional Injuries

Intentional injuries are those that result when one person intends to harm himself/herself or another person. Intentional injuries include homicide, suicide, and domestic violence. With intentional injuries, injuries are judged to be purposely inflicted.

SUICIDE AND HOMICIDE

Suicide rates are difficult to measure because it is not always apparent when death is self-inflicted. Suicide rates are very high among young people in industrial countries, particularly Japan, China, Europe, and the United States. Homicide statistics are more accurate and precise. According to the FBI, by 2002 the murder rate in the United States had fallen to its lowest level in three decades—6 homicides per 100,000 persons. Nearly half of all deaths from firearm injuries are victims of homicide. Homicide is the third leading cause of death for children aged 5 to 14 years, an increasing trend in violent deaths of children. More than 80% of infant homicides are the result of fatal child abuse committed by parents (Overpeck et al., 1998).

ABUSIVE BEHAVIOR

Violent and abusive behavior leading to intentional injury includes domestic violence, physical assault, rape, burglary, mugging, and car jacking. Domestic violence is very common. **Assault** can be physical or verbal. Physical assault (or battery) occurs when another person is physi-

cally injured by another. Verbal assault is a threat that implies future harm to another person. **Rape** is assault, but with forced sexual intercourse. **Statutory rape** is intercourse with a minor under the age of 21. All these acts are against the law and grounds for arrest and prosecution.

Unintentional Injuries

The term *unintentional injury* implies circumstances that could not be avoided, errors in judgment, poor health, or lack of physical ability to prevent harm. Unintentional injuries can be the result of a fall, drowning, fire, or most automobile crashes. Unintended injuries are often a product of human error, product design, impairment, environmental conditions, and other factors specific to the event. Unintentional injuries are the leading cause of death for individuals under the age of 45 and the fifth leading cause of death for the entire U.S. population (Committee on Trauma Research, 1985).

MOTOR VEHICLE ACCIDENTS

We are all potential victims of motor vehicle accidents, whether as driver, passenger, or pedestrian. Motor vehicle accidents are the most common cause of death for people aged 15 to 24 (Figure 16-4). Teenagers account for 10% of the U.S. population but 15% of the deaths from motor vehicles (McFarland & Moore, 1957). Those aged 75 and older have the second highest rate of motor vehicle–related deaths. Motor vehicle crashes are also the most common cause of serious injury. Even if a motor accident is not fatal, major head, spinal, and other injuries from one can be permanently disabling.

Driving Under the Influence

Nearly 40% of traffic fatalities are related to driving under the influence. The highest intoxication rates in fatal crashes in 1995 were recorded for drivers aged 21 to 24 years. Young drivers who have been arrested for driving while impaired are more than four times as likely to die in future alcohol-related crashes (Centers for Disease Control, 1999).

Consider the Cost | **PROTECT YOURSELF FROM INTENTIONAL HARM**

People are injured or killed by malefactors, so it is important that you, especially if you are a woman, take steps to protect yourself. Be conscious of your whereabouts, avoid unfamiliar areas at night, walk with a group or an escort, and have some measure of self-protection (such as a can of pepper spray) so you can get away. Never leave your keys in your car, keep your car locked, and keep valuables in the trunk of your car.

Many states require driver education or use of a temporary license for a probationary period. In states with "zero tolerance" laws, if an underage person is caught driving under the influence of drugs or alcohol (DUI or DUIA), that person's license can be revoked until graduation from high school, time must be spent in jail, and a fine must be paid, no matter the blood alcohol concentration (BAC).

For those who can legally drink alcohol, the legal BAC limit is either 0.08 or 0.10, depending on the state of residence. But DUI or DUIA means "under the influence," no matter what the BAC, so the risk of arrest is there. Most drivers are not stopped unless they are driving erratically or have violated a traffic law. Many people do not know that medications such as antihistamines can make a driver drowsy, impairing judgment. The label stating "do not operate heavy machinery" refers to automobiles as well as earthmovers.

Other Causes of Motor Vehicle Accidents

Heavy traffic, construction, distractions, inexperienced drivers, inconsiderate or impaired drivers, and aggressive driving are just some of the causes of motor vehicle accidents. Many urban areas have traffic delays that irritate drivers in a hurry. Many drivers are distracted by activities inside their car such as crying children, talking on cell phones, eating, drinking, or adjusting dashboard controls. Some drivers are irritated by other drivers who do not signal, cut in front, run through a stop light, or show disregard for other drivers. Aggressive driving means exceeding the speed limit, tailgating, frequent lane changing, verbal abuse or making rude gestures to another driver, and disobeying traffic signs. This kind of driving behavior can lead to dangerous confrontations with other drivers, called *road rage*. Road rage occurs when one driver physically assaults another driver or car. It is not a good idea to get in a fight with someone while you are in your car.

There are several things that can be done to decrease the potential for a motor vehicle accident. Your vehicle should be in good condition and your driving behaviors should be dictated by road conditions and the amount of traffic. Speed should always be within the speed limit, and less if there is fog, rain, snow, or ice on the road. Tailgating is a very bad habit, as well as not looking far enough down the road to anticipate problems. The **"two-second rule"** means two seconds should pass when you approach the same point as the car in front of you. This provides enough time to stop suddenly if the need arises, preventing a rear-end collision.

Wearing Seatbelts and Using Child Restraints

The saying that "seatbelts save lives" is true. Seatbelts hold the driver in place to manage the vehicle in a sudden situation, prevent ejection from the vehicle, and protect the person from hitting objects inside the car (Figure 16-5). Consistent use of safety belts and not driving while impaired by drugs or alcohol are two of the most effective ways to reduce the risk of death and serious injury in mo-

> **YEARS OF POTENTIAL LIFE LOST**
> When a person dies before the age of 65, some years of potential life have been lost. The Centers for Disease Control and Prevention, National Center for Health Statistics (1999), calculates the **years of potential life lost** (YPLL) for each accidental death. Today, unintentional injury and violence account for about 30% of all years of productive life lost before the age of 65, exceeding losses from heart disease, cancer, and stroke combined.

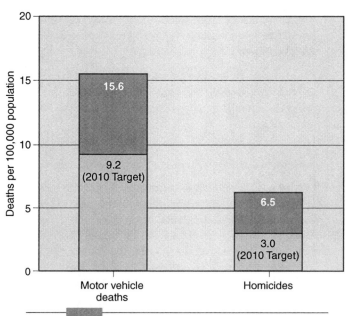

FIGURE 16-4 U.S. motor vehicle deaths and homicides, 1998. Source: National Vital Statistics, CDC.

Assault
A threat that implies future harm to another person, or causing physical injury to another person.

Rape
Assault with forced sexual intercourse.

Statutory rape
Sexual intercourse with a minor under the age of 21.

Years of potential life lost
The number of productive years lost as a result of premature death caused by accident injuries.

Two-second rule
A precautionary measure to avoid rear-end collisions by remaining two seconds behind the vehicle in front of you. Watch the vehicle in front of you pass a stationary object, then count two seconds before your car reaches the same object.

Most accidents can be avoided by getting enough sleep, allowing more than enough time to get to your destination, obeying traffic rules, being courteous to other drivers, using defensive driving strategies, and not driving under the influence of drugs or alcohol, and not tailgating. Tailgating is a common cause of rear-end collisions. When following another vehicle, you must have enough room to stop if the vehicle ahead brakes suddenly.

The rule of thumb for following another vehicle is known as the two-second rule: There must be at least two seconds of stopping distance, no matter what the speed. In order to determine this, you would time the vehicle in front of you by a landmark like a light pole or an intersection, counting two seconds ("one one thousand, two one thousand") to be sure you do not get to the intersection less than two seconds after the vehicle. If you do, you will need to slow down until there are two seconds between you and the vehicle ahead.

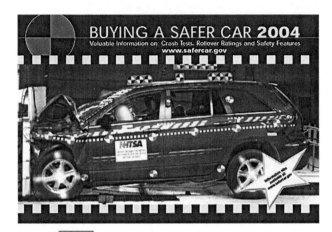

FIGURE 16-5 **Test Dummies after a Crash** Today all vehicles are tested for safety.

tor vehicle crashes. Passengers should always be encouraged to fasten seatbelts and wear them appropriately over the chest and hips. The safest place for children is usually in the back seat. Children weighing more than 40 pounds should be in a car seat facing forward. Car carriers for smaller infants should face rearward.

Home Safety

Injuries in the home occur from falls, poisonings, fires, firearm discharge, and misuse of power equipment. Most of these injuries are preventable. The most susceptible are children and older adults. Homes with young children should be baby-proofed.

- Falls account for the majority of accidental deaths in the home. Falls occur when hallways and stairs are not well-lighted, when rugs are not secure, and when spilled liquids have not been cleaned up.

- Cabinets containing hazardous materials should be locked and out of a child's reach.

- Matches and lighters should be kept in a safe place.

- Homeowners should be sure that electrical cords are not frayed, that outlets are not overloaded, and there are smoke detectors and fire extinguishers in the home.

- Flammable materials should be stored in original containers in a cool, dry place.

- Never store a substance in a container that is not properly labeled or missing instructions on what to do in the event of a spill.

- Keep electrical cords wrapped in such a way so that children do not become entangled in them.

- Power equipment should be well maintained, have protective shields, and be used with protective equipment such as goggles and gloves.

- Kitchen appliances, lawnmowers, and other equipment should only be operated after reading the instructions and observing a skilled user.

- Golf carts, tractors, go-karts, 4-wheelers or all-terrain vehicles (ATVs), and other powered devices should be operated only by an adult or under the supervision of a responsible adult.

- Guns should be kept in a hidden place in a locked cabinet. Adolescents and children should not use BB guns or pellet guns unless under the supervision of an adult.

U.S. Gun Control Efforts

Efforts to restrict possession of firearms is a controversial issue in the United States. Proponents of gun control point to high homicide and accidental death rates from misuse of firearms, criminal or otherwise. Defenders (including the National Rifle Association) assert their interpretation of the second amendment to the U.S. Constitution[2] as a legal defense of unfettered ownership and possession.

2. "A well regulated militia, being necessary to the security of a free state, the right of the people to keep and bear arms, shall not be infringed."

Here is a brief history of the laws concerning gun control:

1939 The U.S. Supreme Court upheld a law prohibiting private ownership of a sawed-off shotgun.

1968 The Gun Control Act of 1968 (PL 90-618) was passed prohibiting the sale of rifles by mail and sale of guns to minors, felons, or addicts.

1986 The U.S. Congress eased some of the restrictions imposed by the 1968 Gun Control Law.

1993 The increasing incidence of gun-related crimes in the United States prompted passage of The Brady Handgun Control Act (PL 103-159) named for James Brady, the press secretary severely wounded in the 1981 assassination attempt on President Ronald Reagan. The act provided for a waiting period before someone could buy a handgun, and a national criminal background check system that gun dealers had to contact before selling or otherwise transferring possession of a firearm.

1994 The Violent Crime Control and Law Enforcement Act of 1994 (PL 103-322) banned the manufacture, sale, and possession of certain assault weapons.

Product Safety

Consumer products cause more than 20 million injuries each year in and around the home (Committee on Trauma Research, 1985). Some of the injuries, particularly to children, result in death. The Consumer Product Safety Commission (CPSC) was created in 1972 because an unacceptable number of consumer products presented an unreasonable risk of injury. The CPSC has the authority to issue standards for more than 15,000 consumer products. The CPSC recalls hazardous products, bans further production of them, and requires safety labels and instructions. The CPSC is also responsible for enforcing the Federal Hazardous Substances Act, the Poisoning Prevention Packaging Act, the Flammable Fabrics Act, the Refrigerator Safety Act, and the Child Protection and Toy Safety Act.

School Safety

Schools have taken measures to assure the safety of children before, during, and after school. A major concern is the safety of students before they get on and after they get off a bus, particularly if they must cross a street in the process. Crossing guards assist children crossing busy intersections. Playgrounds are supervised. School nurses assist with assessing and treating injuries. Schools have been designated as "drug-free zones" where penalties are greater for drug-related crimes committed on school grounds. Programs are in place for many schools to reduce violence and bullying. Students are taught decision-making, assertiveness, and safety skills to avoid harm. At the present time, however, school buses are exempt from requiring passengers to wear seat belts.

Playground Hazards

The most important part of a playground is the surface it is built on (Figure 16-6). Playground equipment is legally considered an "attractive nuisance," which means that children gravitate toward it and can get hurt on it. Playground equipment should be constructed of safe materials. Beware of wooden playground equipment; the wood may be treated with arsenic (a wood preservative and termite deterrent). Arsenic is most toxic when it has been ingested. It is always a good idea to wash hands and skin thoroughly after touching the wood (ATSDR, 2005).

The most dangerous piece of equipment for all ages is the merry-go-round. As the merry-go-round picks up speed, it acts like a centrifuge, causing a person who does not hold on tightly to fall off. A child falling off can get trapped underneath and kicked or knocked about. For this reason, most playgrounds do not have this piece of equipment.

Another potentially dangerous piece of playground equipment is the teeter-totter. When one person decides to dismount suddenly from a teeter-totter, the unsuspecting other person is suddenly jolted, which can injure the spine. Hands and fingers have also been lost by getting caught in the fulcrum of the teeter-totter frame.

Swings are also potentially dangerous because someone may inadvertently walk in front of or behind the swing.

The most dangerous piece of equipment for children under the age of six is the slide (Moore & Gardner, 1994). Children do not always slide down a slide feet first. If a slide is attractive, children will often climb up the slides or on the outer part of the slide. If the ladder on the slide has large steps, a child may put a foot through or lose footing and fall.

The most dangerous piece of equipment for children over the age of six is a climber (jungle gym, monkey bars, etc.). The temptation to hang upside down or knock someone else off is just too great for some children.

Recreational Activity and Safety

More than half of all Americans live in urban areas. One of the most important factors in choosing an area to live is recreational opportunities. Many people have migrated to the mountains, lakes, rivers, and coastal areas, hoping to combine work with pleasure.

Recreation as we know it today is a reflection of three historical movements: the conservation movement, the urban parks movement, and the recreation movement. The conservation movement was based on a wise and balanced use of natural resources. The beginning of this movement was marked by the U.S. Congress passing legislation to give Yosemite Valley to the state of California as

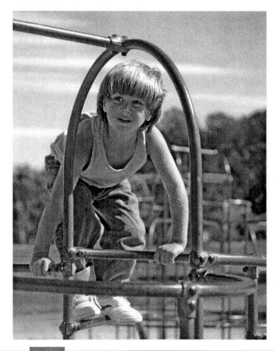

FIGURE 16-6 Playground.

a national park in 1864. In 1958, Congress created the Outdoor Recreation Resources Review Commission and the Land and Water Conservation Fund, and passed three pieces of legislation: Federal Wilderness Act (1964); Wild and Scenic Rivers Act (1964); and National Trails Systems Act (1968).

The urban parks movement was a response to the effects of industrialization and immigration on a rapidly growing urban population. It originated in 1885 when the Massachusetts Emergency and Hygiene Association created the "sand gardens" of Boston, an early version of public playgrounds for children. In 1892, Jane Addams provided a playground at Hull House in Chicago for children of immigrant tenement dwellers. The recreation movement arose from private and philanthropic sources specifically aimed at social reform, rather than from government. The park and recreation movement expanded after World War II in response to population growth, large incomes, and new housing developments.

WALKING, JOGGING, AND BIKING

Although it is common knowledge that pedestrians have the right of way, not all drivers are able or willing to yield it. Thus, pedestrian accidents are frequently fatal. When walking, jogging, or biking, the safest path is one away from traffic. When jogging through wooded areas or public parks, jog with a friend (Figure 16-7). If you jog daily, take a different route each day. Make sure that others

know where you are going and how long you will be gone. Carry a cell phone or carry coins for a pay phone in the event of an emergency.

In areas where you must travel on a road, pedestrians and joggers/runners should proceed against the traffic. Make sure that you are visible to drivers. Wear brightly colored clothing with reflective materials for night. Cross the street at intersections. Train children to obey traffic rules and yield to motorists. Remember that many drivers are not cautious or even aware of others on the road.

Bikers should ride in single file. When riding a bicycle, be sure to wear a helmet. Travel with the traffic as you would if you were driving a car. Obey all traffic signals and signal your turns. Wear brightly colored clothes and travel on roads with wide shoulders or on paths.

HORSEBACK RIDING

It is a good idea to have horseback riding lessons before attempting to ride a horse. Horses are easily frightened by objects, noise, and sudden movements. All horses can kick, bite, stomp, and trample. Horses should never be ridden without proper equipment in good repair. Even with a trained rider, horses can suddenly bolt, run, rear up, and buck, upsetting the rider. If a foot is caught in the stirrup, a rider can be dragged. In most cases when you are riding a horse from a boarding stable, you will be asked to sign a waiver of liability.

SWIMMING

Most drownings or near-drownings occur when swimmers and nonswimmers swim in unsafe areas (Figure 16-8). When visiting an beach, it is best to swim where there is a lifeguard and obey the guard. Lifeguards sit on tall stands so they can look for riptides and schools of fish. Riptides have powerful undercurrents that can pull you underwater and carry out to sea or down the beach for

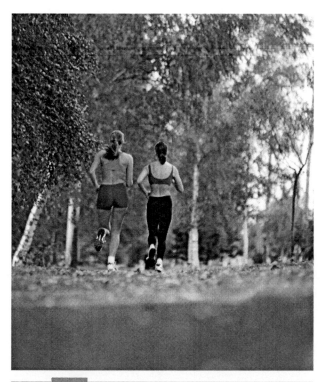

FIGURE 16-7 **Jogging along a street** Joggers need to consider safety factors in rural and urban areas.

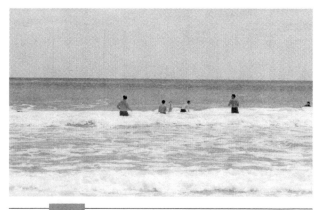

FIGURE 16-8 **Swimmers in the Atlantic Ocean** For the safety of everyone, people should swim where lifeguards are on duty.

long distances. Schools of fish usually indicate that larger fish that feed on them, such as sharks, are in the area.

Do not talk to lifeguards while they are working because they usually have many people to watch at one time. In areas without lifeguards, you swim at your own risk. If you are not a good swimmer, wear a flotation device or stay in shallow water. Whether swimming in a pool or a lake, diving is always considered dangerous. No matter where you swim, it is better to jump in feet first than head first. Always swim with someone who can keep track of you. Rescue equipment, such as a ring buoy or personal flotation device, should always be within reach.

Oceans and lakes may look clean, and the water look safe for swimming most of the time, but sometimes it contains disease-causing organisms. Swimming or playing in unsafe water may result in sore throats or diarrhea, or more serious illnesses. The most frequent sources of disease-causing microorganisms are sewage overflows, stormwater runoff, sewage treatment plant malfunctions, boating wastes, and malfunctioning septic systems. Pollution of beach water is higher during and immediately after rainstorms. Stormwater may carry sewage, animal waste, fertilizer, pesticides, trash, and other pollutants from stormwater waste.

The BEACH Act (Beaches Environmental Assessment and Coastal Health Act of 2000, PL 106-284) amended the Clean Water Act to include beach protection provisions. It requires state, tribal, and local governments to develop and implement monitoring and public notification programs for coastal recreational waters. It also requires states to adopt improved water quality standards for pathogens and pathogen indicators.

Public swimming pools are regularly inspected by environmental health inspectors. Most have completed a "pool operator's license" or some type of training to make sure they are knowledgeable about pool maintenance. Swimming pools need to be vacuumed and skimmed regularly to remove decaying matter, dirt, leaves, animals, or feces. The chlorine levels for pools should be maintained at 1.5 ppm of free chlorine with a pH of 7.4–7.5. If these levels are not maintained, the water will become cloudy and bacteria or algae will grow. When swimmers have "red eyes," it usually means there is bacteria and not enough chlorine in the water.

BOATING

The majority of boating accidents occur as a result of alcohol consumption and poor judgment (Figure 16-9). All boats must have life preservers, a throwable personal flotation device, and a means of calling for help, such as a cellular phone or radio to call the Coast Guard.

Boat captains are required to follow regulations stating that you must wear a life jacket while on board. In ocean waters, it is important to keep the size of the wake (the waves made by a boat) low so as not to upset other boats, harm boats tied to a dock, or erode soil from beaches and riverbanks. Jet skis, water skiing, surfing, and other water activities warrant special attention. Jet skiers often travel faster than other boats and it is difficult to judge what the best maneuver might be to avoid an accident. The U.S.

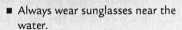

Digging Deeper   WATER SAFETY TIPS

- Always wear sunglasses near the water.

- Always wear sunscreen at least 30 SPF and reapply every hour.

- Spend time in the shade if you burn easily.

- If you plan to be on the beach for a long time, sit under an umbrella.

- Do not shave before swimming in an ocean, lake or river; harmful bacteria can get into small cuts in the skin.

- Do not go into the ocean with a wound or any blood that might lure dangerous fish.

- If you see jellyfish lying on the beach, avoid the water, because the live ones in the water can sting you.

- Make sure that others with you are aware of your swimming abilities or limitations.

- Follow the advice of lifeguards.

- Ease or jump into the water feet first, not head first.

- Supervise your children, even if there is a lifeguard.

- Instruct your children to check with you often and not "drift" away from you.

- Do not fall asleep while your children play in the water.

- Do not allow children to play in warm water streaming from land to water; it may contain untreated sewage.

- Never attempt to swim from one shore to the other or tempt others to do so.

- Shower before entering a public swimming pool, and after swimming in a river, pond, lake or ocean.

- Leave the swimming pool to urinate or defecate.

- Keep babies and toddlers in shallow pools designed for them.

- Leave the area if a thunderstorm or lightning threatens.

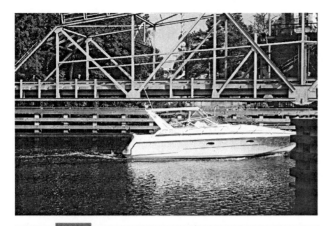

FIGURE 16-9 Boating.

Coast Guard has legal jurisdiction over open waters. In state park facilities, there is usually a park ranger to protect uninformed boaters.

HIKING AND MOUNTAIN CLIMBING

When hiking, climbing, or just enjoying the outdoors, it is always a good idea for someone to know where you are if you do not take someone with you (Figure 16-10). A cell phone is always helpful if you should get into trouble and need help—but don't fail to take other sensible precautions as well. Depending only on a cell phone to get out of avoidable trouble can lead to your being billed several thousands of dollars for a rescue mission.

It is important to keep up with weather forecasts. In the mountains, rainstorms are more likely to occur in the morning, and lightning is always a danger. Be prepared for chilly evenings in high altitude. Food and water supplies are very important. Hydration becomes a problem at higher altitudes and in desert areas. When ascending heights, take your time and take frequent rest breaks to help your body become acclimated to changes in atmospheric pressure and altitude. Eye protection is very important.

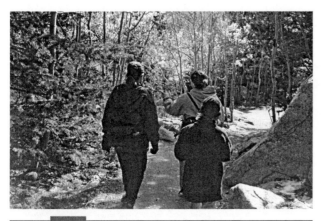

FIGURE 16-10 Hiking.

Equipment should be appropriate for the activity and well maintained. Before starting out on an activity, make sure you are with an experienced individual. Encounters with wild animals are infrequent but can be dangerous, especially during mating season. It is best not to disturb them; find an alternate route.

USING ALL-TERRAIN VEHICLES

GoKarts, ATVs, and motorcycles all look safe, but they can travel extremely fast over rough terrain. Operators of these vehicles should have training, wear safety belts, and always wear a helmet. Some outdoor areas have barbed wire and other hazards that are difficult to see from a distance. Operators should have training and a license. For this reason, many states prohibit operation of these vehicles unless the person is 16 years or older.

SKIING, SNOWBOARDING, AND SNOWMOBILING

Dangers associated with snow activities can often be avoided with proper training. Ankle, knee, or hip injuries are common among even the most experienced of skiers (Figure 16-11). When traveling on snow, it is difficult to

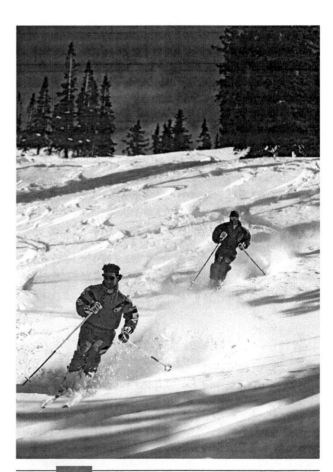

FIGURE 16-11 Skiing.

control the direction and the distance traveled, particularly in snowboarding. Snowboarders often fall several times before they "master" the craft. Snowmobile injuries result from excessive speed, failure to use a helmet, and alcohol consumption.

Activities in cold environments always carry the risk of exposure injury. Conditions that can cause major tissue damage include frostnip and frostbite. Frostnip occurs when an individual has been in a cold environment and ears, nose, face, fingers, and toes become reddened and painful. If the person is not warmed, frostnip can progress to frostbite. Frostbite occurs when ice crystals form under the skin in underlying tissues.

The primary treatment for frostbite is to warm the tissues slowly with warm blankets, clothing, heat, or warm water. Rubbing is a bad idea because it can damage tissues. As the tissue is warmed, the person may experience intense pain and nausea.

Wet clothing or alcohol consumption in a cold environment may lower body temperature to the point of hypothermia. Hypothermia is especially dangerous because a person with hypothermia will become drowsy, lose consciousness, and can freeze to death.

Hunting and Fishing

The oldest forms of recreation in this country are hunting and fishing. Games and parks commissions have officials who survey outdoor areas for poachers, hunting or fishing out of season, killing more game than permitted, and drive-by hunting or fishing with a net. Hunters should complete approved training programs by organizations such as Ducks Unlimited and the Izak Walton Foundation. They should wear orange clothing to be visible to other hunters, and not mistaken for game. All hunters should have permits to hunt in season. Fishermen are also required to have fishing permits. Fish that do not meet size requirements should be thrown back. Deer stands and duck blinds should be carefully constructed so they do not injure the hunter. Hunters and fishermen should always wear insect repellent with DEET. Sunscreen is also a good idea. When hunting or fishing, always carry a first aid kit and be certain others know where you are. Never hunt alone.

Injury Prevention

njuries can be avoided or lessened through anticipation of potential hazards and product design. Hazards raise the risk of an accident if they cannot be avoided, or if they are ignored. Hazards are usually identified as mechanical or psychosocial hazards. Mechanical hazards occur when the transfer of mechanical energy results in immediate or gradually acquired injury. The effects of a car careening out of control, someone falling off a loading dock at work, or a child getting his or her finger crushed in a closing door are examples of mechanical hazards.

Psychosocial hazards, which usually prefigure mechanical hazards coming into play, would include driving or boating under the influence of alcohol or drugs, allowing yourself to be distracted while driving, walking alone down a street in a high-crime area, boating without life jackets or flotation devices, skiing during avalanche season, hiking without taking proper precautions or equipment with you, and so on. Other psychosocial hazards include anger, uncertainty, anxiety, and lack of control, resulting in depression, suicide, substance abuse, violence against others, and psychosomatic diseases. Responses to psychosocial stressors depend in part on the socioeconomic status and role expectations of an individual. Overcrowded and decrepit urban residential areas, disrupted social structures, poverty, physical and mental illness, and social isolation aggravate psychosocial hazards.

Experts examine the **mechanisms of injury** to analyze individual accidents based upon the injuries received. For example, rear-end collisions usually produce back and neck injuries and front-end collisions produce head injuries. As a result products are designed with safety features such as seatbelts, air bags, and headrests to reduce injury from accidents.

Summary

t was commonly thought at one time that accidents are random events for which no one but the victim is responsible. Later, it was assumed that some people are accident-prone. However, with the exception of natural disasters, war, and terrorism, injuries do not occur as random events. Most injuries are predictable and preventable, particularly those resulting from motor vehicle accidents. In 1877 Johann Peter Frank suggested that accident-prevention activities should be part of comprehensive public health programs. James J. Gibson focused attention on the accident itself, rather than on the victim. Hugh DeHaven was the first to view an accident as being caused by more than one factor. John Stapp conducted experiments for the U.S. Air Force on the biomechanics of acceleration/deceleration at high speeds, in researching belt restraints. Dr. John E. Gordon believed that epidemiology was a fruitful approach to studying acci-

Mechanism of injury
Evidence that indicates how an injury occurred.

dents. After World War II, the field of ergonomics was born. Dr. William Haddon, Jr., suggested that injury or damage resulted from kinetic energy interactions and that there were three phases of an accident: pre-injury, injury, and post-injury. In the 1950s, Ralph Nader declared that automobile makers were designing cars for style, cost, and performance, while ignoring the accidental injuries, disabilities and deaths caused by design flaws. Epidemiologists have studied injuries over the years to come up with ways to reduce public harm, and governments have created many programs to address the causes and cure of injuries from auto accidents, accidents at home and at school, and recreational activities.

REFERENCES

ATSDR (Agency for Toxic Substances and Disease Registry). (2005). Arsenic. Retrieved from http://www.atsdr.cdc.gov/atsdrhome.html.

Chapanis, A. (1991). To communicate the human factors message, you have to know what the message is and how to communicate it. *Bulletin of the Human Factors Society, 34,* 1–4.

Cook, E., & Gordon, J. E. (1976). Accidental trauma: Non-battle injury. In: *Preventive Medicine in World War II. In Civil Affairs/Military Government Public Health Activities,* Vol. III, Chapter 7. Washington, D.C., Office of Medical History. Retrieved from http://history.amedd.army.mil/booksdocs/wwii/PrsnlHlthMsrs/chapter7.htm.

Centers for Disease Control. (1999). Achievements in Public Health, 1900-1999 Motor-Vehicle Safety: A 20th Century Public Health Achievement. *MMWR, 48,* 369–374.

Committee on Trauma Research. (1985). *Injury in America: A continuing public health problem.* Washington, DC: National Research Council.

DeHaven, H. (1942). Mechanical analysis of survival in falls from heights of fifty to one hundred and fifty feet. *War Medicine, 2,* 586–596.

Gibson, James J. (1961). The contribution of experimental psychology to the formulations of the problems of safety: A brief for basic research. In Haddon, W., Jr., Suchman, E. A., and Klein, D. (1964). *Accident research: Methods and approaches.* New York: Harper & Row.

Gordon, John E. (1949). The Epidemiology of Accidents. *American Journal of Public Health. 39,* 504–515.

Haddon, W., Suchman, E. A., and Klein, D., eds. (1964). *Accident research: Methods and approaches.* New York: Harper & Row.

Haddon, W., Valien, P., McCarroll, J., & Umberger, C. (1961). A controlled investigation of the characteristics of adult pedestrians fatally injured by motor vehicles in Manhattan. *Journal of Chronic Diseases, 14,* 655–578.

Healthy People Consortium, Healthy People 2010. http://www.healthypeople.gov/.

McCarroll, J., & Haddon, W. (1962). A controlled study of fatal automobile accidents in New York City. *Journal of Chronic Diseases, 15,* 811–826.

McFarland, R., & Moore, R. (1957). Human factors in highway safety. *New England Journal of Medicine, 256,* 390–397, 792–799, 837–845.

Moore, J. D., & L. W. Gardner (1994). Saving Children's Lives: Preventing Childhood Injuries. *North Carolina Public Health Forum,* Vol. 3, No. 1, p. 14.

Nader, R. (1959). "The Safe Car You Can't Buy," *The Nation,* April 1959.

Nader, R. (1965). *Unsafe at any Speed: The designed-in dangers of the American automobile.* New York: Grossman Press.

National Safety Council. (1987). Hugh DeHaven biography. Retrieved August 1, 2003 from http://www.nsc.org/insidensc/shhofi/biodehv.htm.

Overpeck, M., Brenner, R., Trumble, A., Trifilletti, L., & Berendes, H. (1998). Risk factors for infant homicide in the U.S. *New England Journal of Medicine, 339,* 1211–1216.

ASSIGNMENTS

1. Search for Internet Web sites that help determine the safety of the car you are currently driving, or one that you would like to buy.

2. Research the differences between a standard driving course and an advanced hazardous driving course, with emphasis on the physics of control and loss of control under different conditions. Prepare a presentation on the topic.

3. Visit the National Center for Injury Prevention and Control Web site to retrieve specific information related to either an unintentional or intentional injury. Prepare a presentation on that topic.

4. Find an Internet site for the Consumer Product Safety Commission and research the safety record of a particular product you are interested in.

5. Search Web sites that provide information on jobs, training, and other resources pertaining to injury prevention.

6. Invite an orthopaedic surgeon or osteopath to visit the class and discuss the types of injuries common to most auto accidents.

7. Invite a local weatherman to visit the class and discuss the accuracy of storm and other natural disaster predictions.

8. Ask a local emergency services technician or director about the state of emergency preparedness in your community.

9. Read one of the books in the Additional Reading section and discuss it in class.

10. Using the matrix below developed by Dr. William Haddon, determine the best approach to decreasing the number of accidental falls in a home. Discuss each factor in the pre-event, event, and post-event phase of the analysis, then choose the "most important" and "changeable" factors for intervention.

Phase	Human Factor	Equipment Factor	Physical and Socioeconomic Environment Factor
Pre-event			
Event			
Post-event			

SELECTED ENVIRONMENTAL LAWS

1964 Federal Wilderness Act (PL 88-577)
Provides criteria for determining suitability of areas for designation as part of the National Wildlife Refuge and National Park Systems and the National Forest System, and establishes restrictions on activities that can be undertaken on such areas.

1970 Poison Prevention Packaging Act (PL 91-601)
Established standards for special packaging designed to protect against a risk of illness or injury.

1972 Consumer Product Safety Act (PL 92-573)
Designed to protect against the unreasonable risk of injury associated with consumer products, assist consumers in evaluating the safety of products, develop uniform safety standards to minimize conflicting state and local regulations, and promote research for injury prevention.

2000 Beaches Environmental Assessment and Coastal Health (BEACH) Act (PL 106-284)
Required the EPA to protect people from health risks associated with contaminated recreational waters and noncommercially caught fish by assessing risk and communicating the risks to the public.

SELECTED PROFESSIONAL JOURNALS

Accident Analysis and Prevention
Journal of Safety Research
Journal of Trauma Injury, Infection, and Critical Care
Risk Analysis
Traffic Safety Research Quarterly

ADDITIONAL READING

Baker, S., et al. (1992). *The injury fact book. 2nd ed.* New York, NY: Oxford University Press.

Barss, P., et al. (1998). *Injury prevention: An international perspective epidemiology, surveillance, policy.* New York: Oxford University Press.

Bonnie, R., Fulco, C., & Liverman, C., eds. (1998). *Reducing the burden of injury: Advancing prevention and treatment.* Committee on Injury Prevention and Control, Institute of Medicine.

Christoffel, T., & Gallagher, S., eds. (1999). Overview of landmark injury prevention events in the United States, 1937–1997. In *Injury prevention and public health.* Sudbury, MA: Jones & Bartlett Publishers.

Fox, J. A., & Zawitz, M. W. (1999). *Homicide trends in the United States.* U. S. Department of Justice, Bureau of Justice Statistics.

Hoyert, D., Kochanek, K., & Murphy, S. (1999). Deaths: Final data for 1997. *National Vital Statistics Reports 47,* 19.

Lang, L. (1996). Danger in the dust. *Environmental Health Perspectives, 104.* Retrieved August 1, 2003 from http://ehpnet1.niehs.nih.gov/docs/1996/104-1/focusdust.html.

National Center for Injury Prevention and Control. (1999). Impaired Driving Fact Sheet. Atlanta, GA: HHS, CDC.

National Highway Traffic Safety Administration. (1998). Traffic Safety Facts, 1998. Washington, D.C.: U.S. Department of Transportation.

National Safety Council. (1995). *Accident Facts.* Washington, D.C.: The Council.

Nakayama, K. (1994). James J. Gibson: An appreciation. *Psychological Review, 101,* 329–335.

Waller, J. (1994). Reflections on a half century of injury control. *American Journal of Public Health, 84,* 664–671.

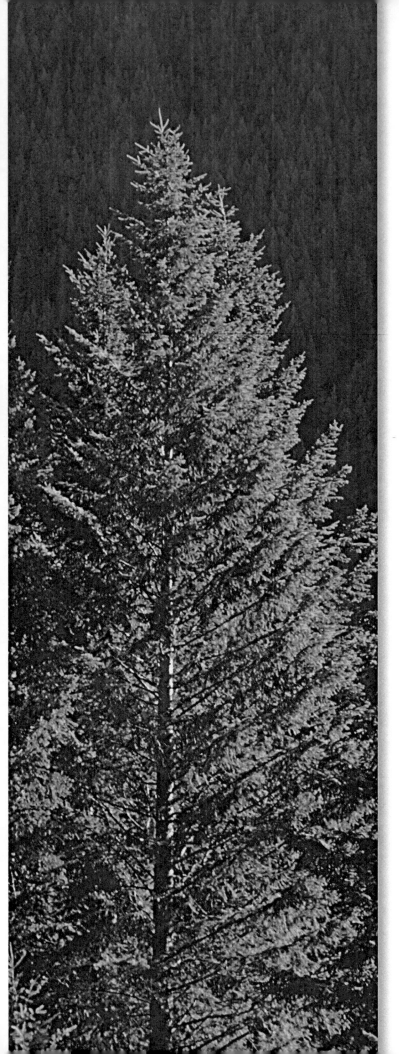

Occupational Health and Safety

17

Nothing will work unless you do.
Maya Angelou (1928–present)

OBJECTIVES

1. Recount the evolution of occupational health and safety standards.

2. Describe three people and their work promoting occupational health and safety.

3. Name three laws critical to the inspection of work facilities, training of workers, and availability of rescue teams.

4. List what type of employers are subject to Occupational Health and Safety Act (OSHA) regulations.

5. List hazardous occupations and explain why they are hazardous.

6. Describe the occupational health concerns for migrant farm workers and their families.

7. Name three lung diseases caused by air contaminants.

8. Give examples of physical, biological, and chemical occupational hazards.

9. Explain the duties and training of an industrial hygienist.

10. Describe the duties and training of safety specialists.

Introduction

Occupational health and safety is a relatively new field, but one of increasing importance due to workplace exposure to various kinds of hazards, both indoors and outdoors. This chapter provides an overview of occupational health and safety hazards, the health problems arising from exposure to and injury from such hazards, and ways the federal government and employers are improving the workplace.

Rise of Occupational Safety and Industrial Hygiene

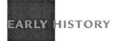

EARLY HISTORY

As revealed by archeological excavations, the first known occupational disease was **silicosis**, found among Egyptian slaves and flint-tool makers (Lechner, 2003). The second oldest occupational disease was probably **pulmonary mycotoxicosis**, associated with the harvesting and storage of grain. Hippocrates (460–370 BCE) wrote of "professional illnesses" caused by lead, sulfur, mercury, and other chemical elements. Pliny the Elder (23–77 CE) reported health risks to those working with zinc and sulfur. He devised the use of animal bladders as respiratory devices against dusts and vapors. In the second century CE,

the Greek physician Galen described lead poisoning and the hazards to copper miners of acid mists.

During the Middle Ages, guilds were formed to help sick and crippled workers and their families. Phillippus Paraclesus (1493–1541) observed occupational illnesses among mining and smelting workers in Austria and Switzerland. In 1473 Ulrich Ellenbog (1440–1499), a German physician, wrote a pamphlet on occupational diseases and injuries among gold miners. Not published until 1524, this is the first known work on industrial hygiene and toxicology. In 1556 the German scholar Agricola described diseases among miners (including silicosis) and suggested preventive measures in his book *De Re Metallica*. He advocated ventilation for miners, and other types of worker protection.

In the 1700s, the Italian physician Bernardo Ramazzini, while observing gastroenteritis among cesspool workers, advocated the idea of studying occupational diseases in the workplace (Franco, 2003). He also wrote about the toxicity of carbon monoxide, lead, mercury, and nitric acid. In 1775, Sir Percival Pott (1713–1788) recognized that chimney sweeps, a large number of them children, had an unusually high incidence of scrotal cancer. The

---

Silicosis
Inhalation of silica or quartz dust by masonry and concrete workers.

Pulmonary mycotoxicosis
A disease from inhaling mold spores from grain, silage and hay; also called "farmer's lung."

Digging Deeper

OBJECTIVES RELATED TO OCCUPATIONAL SAFETY, HEALTHY PEOPLE 2010

- Reduce deaths from work-related injuries.

- Reduce work-related injuries resulting in medical treatment, lost time from work, or restricted work activity.

- Reduce the rate of injury and illness cases involving days away from work due to overexertion or repetitive motion.

- Reduce pneumoconiosis deaths.

- Reduce deaths from work-related homicides.

- Reduce work-related assaults.

- Reduce the number of persons who have elevated blood lead concentrations from work exposures.

- Reduce occupational skin diseases or disorders among full-time workers.

- Increase the proportion of work sites employing 50 or more persons that provide programs to prevent or reduce employee stress.

- Reduce occupational needle-stick injuries among healthcare workers.

- Reduce new cases of work-related, noise-induced hearing loss.

- Reduce the cost of lost productivity in the workplace due to alcohol and drug use.

- Reduce the proportion of non-smokers exposed to environmental tobacco smoke.

- Increase the proportion of work sites with formal smoking policies that prohibit smoking or limit it to separately ventilated areas.

- Establish laws on smoke-free indoor air that prohibit smoking or limit it to separately ventilated areas in public places and work sites.

- Reduce occupational eye injury.

- Increase the use of appropriate ear protection devices, equipment, and practices.

Bernardino Ramazzini, an Italian physician, considered the study of the workplace a necessary tool for discovering the causes, prevention, and treatment of diseases (Franco, 2003). He recommended that starch makers work in open areas to limit their exposure to dust. He suggested that fresh air be forced into mines to expel stale, dust-laden air. He recommended that workers standing for long periods of time or exerting protracted muscular effort be given breaks. He also suggested that workers exposed to loud noises stuff their ears with cotton. He asked workers to refrain from drinking, and sedentary workers to get some exercise. He informed workers of potential hazards and how to protect themselves. He is most famous for his book, *De Morbis Artificum Diatraba* (Diseases of Workers), documenting diseases and their treatment for over 100 occupations.

cause was attributed to ingesting soot. As a result, the British Parliament enacted the Chimney Sweepers Act of 1788, but unfortunately it served only to compensate chimney sweeps for accidents, rather than prevent them. It did, however, make it illegal to employ children under the age of 8 as chimney sweeps.

INDUSTRIAL REVOLUTION

The Industrial Revolution that originated in England and the United States increased the number of mines, factories, and printing plants, also increasing the number of massive injuries and deaths. Unreasonably long hours, intolerable working conditions, poor sanitation, and inadequate housing raised the incidence of occupational diseases. In the 1800s, cotton textile workers experienced **byssinosis**, a lung disease. Sick and dying employees affected output, which made better working

conditions an economic necessity. In England, trade unions to protect workers were not allowed until 1824 (the same time that slavery was abolished in Europe). The English Factory Acts (1833–1878) required inspections, medical certification for children over the age of 9 to work, and decreased use of lead paint, yellow phosphorus (used to make matches), and carbon disulfide (used in manufacturing rubber products) (AIHA, 2005). In the United States, standards for heating, lighting, ventilation, and work hours were adopted from the English Factory Acts. As immigrants moved to the United States in search of better living conditions, competition for jobs increased, leading to declining wages and working conditions.

Child Labor

he Massachusetts Child Labor Act of 1835 was enacted to prevent the employment of young children in industrial settings, but policing powers were not put into effect until 1867 (Figure 17-1). Because child labor was common on farms, and the prevailing opinion was that poor families benefited when their children worked, the law was ignored. Some even considered the child labor laws to be "unconstitutional."

Entire families were often hired. Work days were very long, and families lived in company-owned houses in villages where stores were also owned by the company and goods were overpriced. Even when labor laws were enforced, immigrants were often exploited. They worked long hours for little pay and lived in slums. When photographer Lewis Hine documented gross violations of child labor laws from 1908–1912, publication of his photos fueled the passage of labor reform laws. Employers who did not improve worker conditions found themselves in dis-

---

Digging Deeper   THE MINERS' ANGEL

"I'm not a humanitarian," she exclaimed. "I'm a hell-raiser." Mary Harris "Mother" Jones, who came to be known as The Miners' Angel, was born in Ireland and raised as a U.S. citizen. She was trained to be a seamstress and a teacher. When she was 37, a yellow fever epidemic killed her husband and four children.

Later, after she lost everything in the great Chicago fire, she became involved in the labor movement, attending Knights of Labor meetings. She was called to help with a coal miner's strike

in Virginia and there participated in organizing the United Mine Workers (UMW). She was also a founder of the Industrial Workers of the World (IWW). She was arrested, tried and sentenced to 20 years in prison in 1913, at the age of 83, but later set free. She became involved with the textile workers in Kensington, Pennsylvania, to assist with efforts to create child labor laws. She went on to help the garment workers and streetcar workers strike in New York and the steel workers strike in Pitts-

burgh. At the age of 91, she traveled to Mexico to attend the Pan-American Federation of Labor meeting, an event she called the highlight of her career.

She was a spirited woman, good public speaker, and lived with the workers in tents or shantytowns. She was famous throughout the United States for her support of union workers for better working conditions. She died at the age of 100 and is buried in Illinois, next to the victims of the Virden, Illinois, mine riot of 1889 (Hawse 1999).

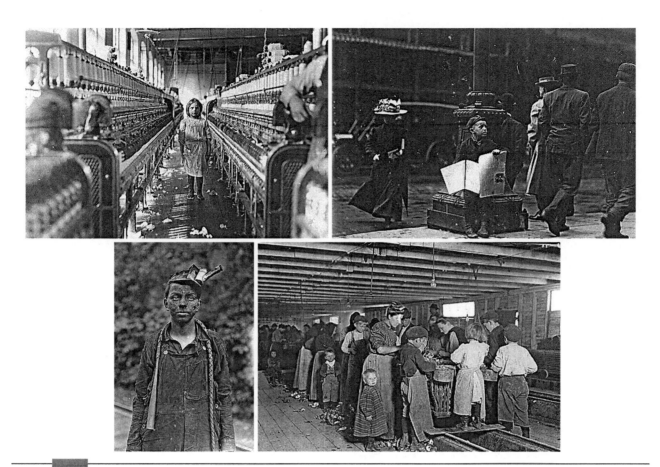

FIGURE **17-1** **Child Workers** (a) Girl in textile mill. (b) Newsboy. (c) Coal miner's son. (d) Girls and women shucking oysters.

pute with labor union leaders such as Mother Jones, who helped workers get the attention of businessmen and government officials (Figure 17-2). Yet today, children still work, in countries and regions with crude living conditions, unskilled workers, and low wages. According to the International Labor Office, in developing countries as many as 250 million children aged 5–14 work.

Byssinosis
A lung disease caused by inhalation of cotton, flax, or hemp dust by mill workers; also known as "brown lung disease."

Plumbism
Lead poisoning.

Occupational Health and Safety Legislation

In 1906, Upton Sinclair's book, *The Jungle*, called attention to the appalling working conditions in meat-packing plants, and aroused concern for the workers (not to mention for the quality of the meat products). In 1908, the first workers' compensation law was enacted, but only for federal employees.

In 1910, the U.S. Public Health Service began to investigate unsanitary conditions and the incidence of tuberculosis among garment workers, along with the incidence of silicosis in coal miners, health hazards associated with the steel industry, lead poisoning from pottery makers, and radiation burns to workers using radium (luminous paint for clocks). Meanwhile researchers also studied occupational diseases such as silicosis, **plumbism** (lead poisoning), anthrax, and benzol poisoning.

In 1910 Dr. Alice Hamilton (1869–1970), credited as the first American specialist in occupational disease and founder of occupational medicine in the United States, studied industrial conditions of felt-hat and lead workers first hand, and provided evidence of toxin exposure to factory managers, mine owners, and state officials.

The first workmen's compensation laws were passed in 1911. In 1913 New York and Ohio established industrial hygiene programs. In 1914, the Office of Industrial Hygiene and Sanitation was created in the U.S. Public Health Service (Figure 17-3). State Bureaus of Mines were established to monitor the working conditions of miners.

The Fair Labor Standards Act, also known as the Federal Wage and Hour Law, was passed in 1938. The

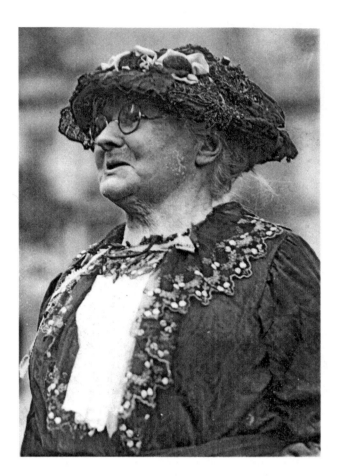

FIGURE **17-2** **Mother Jones** An advocate of workers' rights and union activist.

hours and during vacations in nonmanufacturing, non-mining, and nonhazardous occupations.

The Mines Act, 1952, was enacted by the British Parliament to regulate mine work and safety in India. It provides for worker health and safety, hours of employment, paid leave, and rules and regulations.

In 1970 the Occupational Safety and Health Act (OSHA) was passed and the National Institute for Occupational Safety and Health (NIOSH) was established to conduct research and set standards for worker safety. Since the establishment of OSHA, workplace fatalities, injuries and illnesses in the United States have declined 40%, while the number of workers has doubled.

work week was set at 40 hours, with a minimum wage of 40 cents per hour. The Act prohibited full-time child labor under age 16 and allowed minors 16 and over to work in nonhazardous occupations. Minors over 18 could work in "hazardous" industries. Children aged 14 and 15 could be employed part-time outside of school

Occupational Hazards

here are many occupations in agriculture, construction and manufacturing at risk for deaths, disability and hospitalization due to injuries. Workers most at risk include manual laborers, the users of heavy machines and equipment, those who do heavy lifting and repetitive movement, who work in unsafe working conditions, in extreme heat and cold, and who use unsafe work habits. Construction or logging jobs may involve untrained seasonal workers, and working at unsafe heights or on scaffolding. Construction jobs may also take place in areas of high traffic. Manufacturing jobs may involve working near conveyor belts, presses and other moving equipment. Workers in hospitals and nuclear facilities may be exposed to radiation. In agricultural settings, workers may operate tractors and other large machines to plant, maintain, and harvest crops. Irrigation equipment, pesticides, and fertilizers are additional agricultural hazards. Agricultural equipment and chemicals require special training and protective shielding.

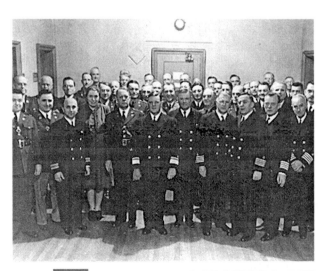

FIGURE **17-3** **USPHS Sanitation Engineers in WWII**

Digging Deeper ALICE HAMILTON

Dr. Alice Hamilton was a pioneer in the field of toxicology. She studied bacteriology and pathology in Germany and pursued postgraduate studies at Johns Hopkins University Medical School. In 1897 she became a professor of pathology at the Woman's Medical School of Northwestern University. She lived in Hull House, founded by social reformer Jane Addams. Living with poor residents of the community, she became interested in the problems workers faced. As certain jobs became more dangerous with the advent of the Industrial Revolution, the study of "industrial medicine" became more important. In 1910 Hamilton was appointed to the newly formed Occupational Diseases Commission of Illinois, the first such investigative body in the United States. For the next decade she investigated a range of issues for a variety of state and federal health committees. She became a leading expert in occupational health, studying occupational illnesses and the dangerous effects of industrial metals and chemicals. She published studies that raised awareness of workplace hazards. She became the first female faculty member at Harvard Medical School in 1919. From 1924 to 1930 she served as the only woman member of the League of Nations Health Committee. She retired as emeritus professor of industrial medicine in 1935. After her retirement, Dr. Hamilton served as a medical consultant to the U.S. Division of Labor Standards, working with the state of Illinois, the U.S. Department of Commerce, and the health committee of the League of Nations. Her publications include *Industrial Poisoning in the United States* (1925), *Industrial Toxicology*

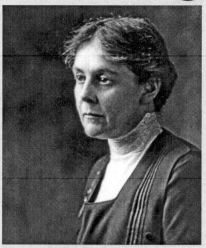

(1934), and an autobiography, *Exploring the Dangerous Trades* (1943). Source: http://www.distinguishedwomen.com/biographies/hamilton-a.html.

AGRICULTURE

Of all the occupations in the United States, agriculture is the most dangerous. Although agricultural workers constituted only 2% of the work force in 1994–1999, they suffered 13% of all occupational deaths (Larson, 2002). Compared to an overall worker death rate of 4.3 per 100,000 workers in the United States, agricultural workers have 22.8 deaths per 100,000 workers (National Center for Health Statistics, 2003). These figures do not just include adults. From 1990–1996, an average of 103 children per year were killed while working on farms (NIOSH, 2001). Many farmers and migrant farmers have children who work. Child labor laws are different in each state. Some states require adult supervision of child workers, others do not.

Every day about 500 agricultural workers suffer lost work-time injuries, some resulting in permanent impairment (National Rural Health Care Association, 1986). Agricultural workers are exposed to heavy lifting, repetitive movement, heat, humidity, pesticides, dust, pollen, molds, parasitic illnesses, and infectious diseases. Agricultural work is also associated with various types of accidents: falling from heights, drowning in ditches, injuries from misusing knives and machetes, and using faulty equipment or vehicles. Exposure to pesticides and the lack of sanitary facilities result in many cases of respiratory problems, skin problems, birth defects, neuropsychological problems, cancer, pesticide poisoning, and death.

MIGRANT WORKERS

Compared to the general population, **migrant workers** and their families have significantly poorer health. The average life expectancy of migrant farm workers is 49 years, compared to the U.S. average of 75 years (National Migrant Resources Program, 1990). The infant mortality rate is also 125 times higher among migrants than U.S.

Migrant worker
A farm laborer who moves from place to place to harvest seasonal crops.

WHO IS AND WHO IS NOT REGULATED BY OSHA

In general, Occupational Safety and Health regulations extend to all employers and their employees in the 50 states, the District of Columbia, Puerto Rico, and all other territories under federal government jurisdiction, including U.S. Postal Service employees. The exceptions are people who are self-employed, farmers who employ only immediate family members, and employees of state and local governments. Compliance with OSHA regulations is governed either by the federal OSHA or an OSHA-approved state occupational safety and health program for government employees. The Occupational Health and Safety Act does not apply to working conditions addressed by the Mine Safety Administration, Department of Transportation, or the Nuclear Regulatory Commission.

citizens. Health problems common among migrant farm workers and their children include respiratory disease, skin infections, chronic diarrhea, vitamin A deficiency, parasitic conditions, and undiagnosed congenital and developmental problems. Accidental injuries, heat-related illness, and chemical poisoning are also highly prevalent (Shotland, 1989; National Rural Health Care Association, 1986).

At least one-third of migrant children work on farms to help earn family income or because there are no child care services available. The health of these children is at high risk from heat-related illnesses and dermatitis, from farm injuries and from pesticide poisoning. A study in New York State found that over 40% of migrant worker children interviewed had worked in fields wet with pesticides and 40% had been sprayed while in the field (Pollack, 1990). Children are more susceptible to pesticide poisoning because their nervous systems and organs are more vulnerable and because they absorb more of it per pound of body weight.

Work Site Hazards

he potential hazards of any work site include air contaminants, exposure to chemicals, microorganisms, radiation, ergonomic hazards,

and stressful working conditions. Outdoor work-site hazards include exposure to physical hazards (heavy equipment, motor vehicles, heat), toxins, and hazardous materials. Workers exposed to any of these hazards on a daily basis have an increased probability of illness, injury, disability, and death.

AIR CONTAMINANTS

Any work process that produces dust that can be inhaled or ingested should be considered hazardous. Air contaminants are usually classified as particulate matter or gas/vapor. The most common particulate contaminants are dust, fibers, mists, and aerosols. The term "mist" refers to a liquid suspended in the atmosphere. Aerosols are a type of mist with smaller liquid particles. Gases and vapors can also be volatile; that is, potentially explosive.

The lungs are very vulnerable to respiratory injury. Occupational lung disease is the number one work-related illness in the United States based on frequency, severity, and preventability. Occupational lung cancer is attributable to inhalation of carcinogens in the workplace such as asbestos, coal, and petroleum-related carbon compounds. Approximately 18,000 lung cancer deaths per year are attributable to inhalation of carcinogens in the workplace (American Lung Association, 2000).

Construction workers, demolition workers, automobile mechanics, shipyard workers, and electricians ex-

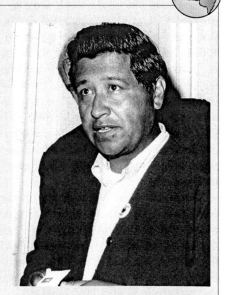

posed to asbestos can develop respiratory conditions such as **asbestosis** several years later. It has been known for some time that coal miners suffer ill effects from inhaling coal dust, often contracting **pneumoconiosis**, or black lung disease. Byssinosis (brown lung disease) is a chronic condition involving obstruction of the small airways, severely impairing lung function. It is caused by inhaling dust from hemp, flax, and cotton processing. **Chalicosis** is a lung disease resulting from the inhalation of copper. Silicosis is common among construction workers from exposure to free crystalline silica in cement, bricks, mortar, sheetrock (gypsum board or dry wall), stucco, bricks, and blasting sand. Welders and ironworkers are often exposed to beryllium and manganese fumes, increasing susceptibility to **nodulation** and **siderosis**.

PHYSICAL HAZARDS

Physical hazards include temperature, light, noise, vibration and radiation exposure. Air temperature can be reduced by installing fans and air conditioning. If the temperature cannot be reduced, frequent breaks and liquids are needed. Noise can be controlled by installing quieter equipment, shielding noisy equipment, or installing mufflers, silencers or baffles. Floors, ceilings and walls can be treated with acoustical material to reflect or reduce the noise. Workstations can be surrounded by partitions to reduce noise. If noise cannot be reduced or avoided, workers can wear hearing protection. Exposure to radiation, including ionizing and non-ionizing electromagnetic radiation, calls for reducing exposure time, increasing distance, and adding shielding for worker safety. This should have been done in the early days of the century to prevent radiation

---

HEAT INJURIES AND ILLNESSES
Illnesses caused by hot, humid environments include heat cramps, heat exhaustion and heat stroke. The primary reason for heat emergencies is the body's inability to cool itself properly. When a person's body temperature rises, the breathing rate increases and the person begins to perspire. Water loss from evaporation and perspiration can result in dehydration and loss of important minerals, called electrolytes, which include sodium, calcium and potassium. A person with cool and sweaty skin should be moved into the shade and given cool liquids to drink if conscious. Cool liquids are absorbed quickly and help cool body temperature. Sports drinks containing sodium and potassium can also help. A person with hot, dry, red skin after being in a hot outdoor environment may have a fever, or may be experiencing heat stroke. The dry skin indicates inability to perspire in order to cool the body. The person should be moved to the shade and cooled down with cool cloths. Do not allow the person to shiver, as it increases body temperature.

burns to clock- and watch-making workers using radium (in the luminous paint) to paint face numbers that would glow in the dark. It was not known at the time that radium is a carcinogen, and many of the workers later died.

CHEMICAL HAZARDS

Chemicals can be inhaled, absorbed, ingested or injected. Chemicals are generally very corrosive and can harm respiratory organs, eyes and skin. When working with chemicals, employers and workers should know exactly what type of substance they are using and what to do in the event an emergency occurs. All containers of chemical substances must identify the substance, and warning labels should never be removed. Chemical laboratories and facilities have shower facilities and emergency procedures in the event of a spill or accident.

Benzene has been used as an industrial solvent for 100 years in the manufacture of detergents, polymers, pesticides, pharmaceuticals and paint. Other sources of benzene are processed food, petroleum products and cigarette smoke. Benzene exposure (benzol poisoning) comes primarily from inhaling vapors but can be absorbed by direct skin contact. Acute exposure to benzene can cause depression of the central nervous system followed by respiratory failure. Acute exposure may also produce pulmonary edema, dermatitis and gastrointestinal irritation. The primary toxic effect of long-term exposure is injury to the blood system, causing aplastic anemia, hemolysis and leukemia. The effects of benzene on exposed workers include chromosomal abnormalities and reproductive damage (Accu-Chem Laboratories, 2005).

Lead is a highly toxic substance. In 2004, 400,000 children under the age of 6 had too much lead in their blood,

---

Asbestosis
A progressive disease that scars lung tissue as a result of chronic exposure to the microscopic fibers of asbestos.

Pneumoconiosis
A respiratory tract condition caused by the inhalation of dust particles in occupations such as mining or stonecutting; when involving coal dust, also known as anthracosis or "black lung disease."

Chalicosis
Lung disease resulting from the inhalation of copper dust.

Nodulation
A node, or collection of cells, forming a bump.

Siderosis
Arc welders' disease.

many exposed in their own homes. For young children under the age of 6, even very low levels of exposure can result in reduced IQ, learning disabilities, attention deficit disorders, behavioral problems, stunted growth, impaired hearing, and kidney damage. At high exposure levels, a child may become mentally retarded, fall into a coma, and even die from lead poisoning.

People are exposed to lead through deteriorating paint, household dust, bare soil, air, drinking water, food, ceramics, home remedies, hair dyes, and other cosmetics. By far the main concern is lead paint found in older housing. The exhaust from leaded gasoline, only recently banned, has deposited lead in the soil over the years, especially near well-traveled roads and highways. Children who play in dirt contaminated by lead can get lead-contaminated soil under their fingernails or on their toys, or they can track it into their homes. Lead can also leach into drinking water from certain types of plumbing (lead pipes, copper pipes with lead solder, and brass faucets).

In adults, lead can increase blood pressure and cause fertility problems, nerve disorders, muscle and joint pain, irritability, and memory or concentration problems. Most adults are exposed at work. House painting, welding, renovation and remodeling activities, smelters, firing ranges, manufacture and disposal of car batteries, and maintenance and repair of bridges and water towers, are particularly risky for lead exposure. A pregnant woman with an elevated blood lead level can easily transfer lead to the fetus, as lead crosses the placenta. In fact, pregnancy itself can cause lead to be released into the bloodstream from the bone, where lead is stored—often for decades—after it first enters the bloodstream (NSC, 1995).

BIOLOGICAL HAZARDS

Biological hazards include pathogens and other living organisms that cause acute and chronic infections. The most common way pathogens enter the body is through a break in the skin or through mucous membrane passageways. Some pathogens enter the body through food, direct contact with sick workers or customers, or contaminated objects. Some illnesses seek hosts that are susceptible because of having been weakened by exposure to another hazard. Laboratory and medical professionals are exposed to biological hazards due to the nature of their work. One fairly common occupational ailment is farmer's lung disease (pulmonary mycotoxicosis), which comes from inhaling mold spores in grain, silage, and hay (Hetzel & Butler, 1996). Another agricultural hazard is exposure to anthrax from the hides of infected animals.

Careful hand-washing practices, mandatory immunizations, skilled handling of needles, proper disposal of contaminated materials, and the use of protective equipment (gloves, masks, gowns) are just some of the techniques used to decrease exposure to biological hazards.

ERGONOMIC HAZARDS

Ergonomic hazards include excessive vibration, noise, eye strain, repetitive motion, and heavy lifting. The hazards may arise from poorly designed work areas, improper equipment, poorly designed tasks, poor body mechanics, or demands for speed in performing a task. Two of the most common ergonomic injuries are lower back pain and **carpal tunnel syndrome**.

When working conditions are evaluated for ergonomic factors, the total physical and psychological demands of the job are reviewed. Workers may be required to lift, hold, push, walk, reach, and perform other physical tasks, so worker tasks are studied for potential muscle, joint, or skeletal problems. Unfortunately some workers may be physically unfit, be inattentive to the task, or use

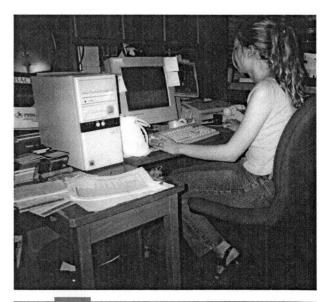

FIGURE 17-4 **A Typical Computer Workstation** It is important to have the chair, monitor height, and keyboard adjusted to the specific needs of the user.

PROTECT YOUR EYES

Worksite activities like welding, dentistry, laboratory work, application of pesticides, and operating power equipment require special measures to prevent eye injuries. Face shields and goggles are recommended. Recreational activities such as swimming, racquetball, and motorcycling require specially fitted goggles or glasses. If a chemical should spill into the face, it is likely to enter the eye. The best way to handle a spill is to rinse the eye with a steady stream of water for 15–20 minutes, or until the eye stops burning. The stream of water should not cause pain or pressure to the eye. The water should flow away from the unaffected eye. If contacts are worn, they should be removed so that chemical material is not trapped under the lens, causing further damage. An ophthalmologist can determine whether further treatment is needed.

improper techniques, resulting in injuries. There are also circumstances where employees may be asked to push themselves beyond normal limits. Fatigue increases worksite accidents no matter what the job.

Attention to **ergonomics** increases worker efficiency, lowers operating costs, uses employees more effectively, and results in fewer accidents and injuries. Workers doing heavy lifting can reduce risk by using special equipment, taking mandatory breaks, or changing the tasks. Desk workers may need to adjust chairs, change the lighting, and adjust computer monitors to reduce strain on the upper and lower back (Figure 17-4).

Industrial Hygienists

ndustrial hygiene has been defined as "that science and art devoted to the anticipation, recognition, evaluation, and control of those environmental factors or stresses arising in or from the workplace, which may cause sickness, impaired health and well-being, or significant discomfort among workers or among the citizens of the community" (Smythe, 1966).

The responsibilities of **industrial hygienists** is to interpret OSHA standards on worker protection from harmful physical agents, toxic chemicals, and biological hazards. They also provide technical assistance and support as well as enforcing OSHA standards in the field. Industrial hygienists use environmental monitoring and analytical methods to detect the extent of worker exposure and employ engineering, work practice controls, and other methods to control potential health hazards.

Most importantly, OSHA and other safety standards require that environmental health specialists post hazard warnings and keep records of employee exposure, medical treatment, and use of personal protective equipment.

Since July 1, 1962, industrial hygienists must be certified by passing written examinations. The qualification for admission to examination is a baccalaureate degree and eight years of full-time practice.

Carpal tunnel syndrome
A repetitive injury that occurs when the tendon sheath of the hands and arms become irritated and inflamed; often seen in cashiers, typists, and assembly-line workers.

Ergonomics
Application of human factors to the design of tools, machines, systems, tasks, jobs and environments to make them safe, comfortable and effective in human use.

Industrial hygienist
A designated employee who anticipates safety problems and takes action to prevent them, while helping improve employee productivity.

Consider the Cost — BUYING ENVIRONMENTALLY FRIENDLY TECHNOLOGY DEVICES

An important consideration when purchasing computer products is to look for the TCO certification. TCO is the Swedish Confederation of Professional Employees, concerned about working conditions and environmentally harmful substances. TCO'92 was the first attempt at a "global environment labeling scheme."

TCO'92 addressed concerns about computer display terminals (monitors) and characteristics such as electrical fields, magnetic fields, energy efficiency, and electrical and fire safety. TCO'95 included all pieces of the complete personal computer, including the display, system unit, and keyboard. TCO'95 standards were upgraded in TCO'99, particularly regarding ergonomic qualities such as design, noise, and heat. It also addressed energy efficiency and ecological concerns regarding the manufacturing process and ecological concerns about disposal and recycling. TCO'93 set standards for specific limits on emissions, energy use, and arrangements for recycling by the manufacturer.

A TCO-certified product is considered environmentally friendly. The four "E"s examined include ergonomics, emissions, energy, and ecology. A TCO-certified device must have the following characteristics:

- Ergonomics. A keyboard that is ergonomically designed. Monitors must have high resolution and a flicker-free image. PCs and printers should produce little noise.

- Emissions. Electrostatic emissions (electrical and magnetic fields) should be minimal.

- Energy. There should be an energy-saving function to reduce heat emissions and to save on energy usage. The energy conservation mechanism must activate after a certain amount of inactivity.

- Ecology. Emissions of brominated and chlorinated flame retardants and heavy metals to the environment should be reduced through recycling arrangements and proper disposal.

Approximately 50% of all computer monitors manufactured in the world are TCO labeled. The first TC laptop/notebook computers were introduced in January of 2003 (Intertek ETL SEMKO 2004).

Safety Specialists

Safety specialists may advise employers to change work practices to minimize employee exposure, inspect equipment on a regular basis, make sure that housekeeping procedures are followed, assure that employees are properly supervised, and restrict the use of food, beverages, chewing tobacco and gum, or applying cosmetics in work areas.

To be effective in recognizing and evaluating job hazards and recommending controls, safety professionals must have training and experience in physics, chemistry, biology, physiology, statistics, mathematics, computer science, engineering, industrial processes, business, psychology, and communication. The usual major field is chemistry, physics or biology, or chemical, mechanical, or sanitary engineering. Additional training in industrial hygiene, toxicology, fire protection, ergonomics, accident investigation and analysis, product safety, construction safety, training methods, and environmental laws are also important. Many safety professionals have advanced training in business management, engineering, radiology, toxicology, and law. All have done advanced study in safety.

Digging Deeper — WORKPLACE VIOLENCE AND SEXUAL HARASSMENT

Workplace violence and sexual harassment can also be a workplace hazard. Avoid being a victim of violence or harassment at work by observing these cautions:

■ Read the company handbook or policy manual, or talk to someone in human resources, to see what your company does to protect employees.

■ Report any threat to human resources or a security guard.

■ Make sure your company has a system for visitors to check in so they do not wander office hallways unaccompanied.

■ If you are in the building where you work during weekend or evening hours, make sure you will be safe.

■ Don't be afraid to ask a coworker to walk you to your car when it is dark outside or the office is closed.

■ If a coworker expresses extreme anxiety or exhibits symptoms of a major depression, notify a supervisor.

■ Take threats from coworkers seriously.

■ In the event of an emergency, call security or 911.

■ Report crimes committed at your work site to authorities.

Digging Deeper — SIGNIFICANT EVENTS IN OCCUPATIONAL HEALTH

1864 Pennsylvania Mine Safety Act (PMSA) passed into law.

1864 First accident insurance policy issued.

1867 First government-sponsored factory inspection program in Massachusetts.

1877 Massachusetts passes a law requiring guards for dangerous machinery.

1902 Maryland passes the first workers' compensation law.

1911 The American Society of Mechanical Engineers (ASME) was founded to develops safety codes for boilers and elevators, as well as develop accident prevention techniques and advance safety engineering as a profession.

1912 A group of engineers representing insurance companies, industry and government meet in Milwaukee to exchange data on accident prevention. This group is now known as the National Safety Council.

1916 The Supreme Court sanctions state workers' compensation laws.

1918 The American Standards Association founded to develop volun-

tary standards. Now called the American National Standards Institute.

1936 The Secretary of Labor, Frances Perkins, calls for a federal occupational safety and health law.

1948 All 48 states have workers' compensation laws.

1966 The U.S. Department of Transportation, the National Highway Traffic Safety Administration (NHTSA), and the National Transportation Safety Board (NTSB) established.

1967 President Lyndon Johnson calls for a federal occupational safety and health law.

1970 President Richard Nixon signs the OSHA law into effect, creating the OSHA administration and the National Institute for Occupational Safety and Health (NIOSH).

1971 First standards adopted to provide a baseline for safety and health protection in American workplaces.

1972 First states (South Carolina, Montana, Oregon) approved to run their own OSHA programs.

2000 Cotton dust and lead standards published.

2000 Permission for workers and OSHA to have access to employer-maintained medical and toxic-exposure records.

2000 First penalties proposed against Union Carbide's plant I West Virginia for violations of occupational safety laws.

2000 Grain-handling facilities standard adopted.

2000 Hazardous waste operations and emergency response standards established.

2000 Standard for occupational exposure to blood-borne pathogens published.

2000 Standard for process-safety management of highly hazardous chemicals adopted.

2000 Asbestos standard updated.

2000 Scaffold standard published.

2000 Standard for ergonomics programs promulgated.

(Occupational Health and Safety Administration, 2000.)

Summary

many accidental injuries, disabilities, and deaths are preventable in the workplace, provided workers are in good condition, working conditions are favorable, and there is proper training. Occupational hazards present several legal issues for employers. Industries considered to be at risk are regulated by OSHA standards. Many businesses have their own occupational safety specialists or industrial hygienists to help determine the presence of hazards and regulate the amount of exposure to hazardous substances for workers.

REFERENCES

Accu-Chem Laboratories (2005). Benzene fact sheet. Retrieved from http://www.accuchem.com/tox/testpanels/datasheets/benzene.htm.

AIHA (American Industrial Hygiene Association) (2005). The development of industrial hygiene as a profession. Retrieved from http://www.aiha.org/ConsultantsConsumers/html/careerworks.htm.

American Lung Association (2000). Occupational lung disease: the number one work-related illness in the United States. Retrieved from http://www.lungusa.org/.

Franco, G. (2003). Bernardino Ramazzini: Father of Occupational Medicine (lectures). Retrieved from www.collegiumramazzini.org/messages/index.htm.

Hawse, M. (1999). Mother Jones: The Miners' Angel. The Wisconsin Laborer. Retrieved from http://www.solidarity.com/wldc/fall1999.htm#Mother%20Jones.

Hetzel, G., and Butler, J. (1996). Causes and symptoms of mold and dust induced respiratory illness. Discussion of farmer's lung disease. Virginia Tech Agricultural Engineering Department. Retrieved from http://www.cdc.gov/niosh/nasd/docs4/va98022.html.

Intertek ETL SEMKO (2004). TCO certification fast facts. Retrieved from http://www.intertek-etlsemko.com/portal/page?_pageid=34,100945&_schema=cust_portal&_dad=cust_portal.

Larson, A. (2002). Environmental/occupational safety and health. *Migrant Health Issues, Monograph No. 2*, 8–13. Retrieved from http://www.cnfh.org/.

Lechner, G. (2003). History of occupational disease. Occupational health committee representative from the Canadian Workers Union. Retrieved 8/1/2003 from http://www.sno.net/caw2301/octhist.htm.

National Center for Health Statistics. (2003). Occupational injury deaths and rates by industry, sex, age, race, and Hispanic origin: United States, 1992–2001. Atlanta, GA: Centers for Disease Control.

National Migrant Resources Program, Inc. (1990). Migrant and seasonal farmworkers health objectives for the year 2000. Document in progress. ED 331 687. Austin, TX: Author.

National Rural Health Care Association. (1986). Occupational health of migrant and seasonal farmworkers in the United States: Report summary. ERIC Documents 292 594. Kansas City, MO: Author.

NIOSH (2001). Agricultural safety information. Retrieved from http://www.cdc.gov/niosh/injury/traumaagric.html.

NSC (National Safety Council) (1995). Lead Poisoning. Retrieved from http://www.nsc.org/library/facts/lead.htm.

Occupational Health and Safety Administration. (2000). Overview of occupational safety and occupational health/industrial hygiene. Retrieved from http://www.osha.gov/SLTC/smallbusiness/sec5.html.

Pollack, S. (1990). Pesticide exposure and working conditions among migrant farmworker children in western New York State. Paper presented at the American Public Health Association Annual Meeting.

Shotland, J. (1989). Full fields, empty cupboards: The nutritional status of migrant farmworkers in America. Washington, DC: Public Voice for Food and Health Policy.

Smythe, H. F. Jr. (1966). The American Board of Industrial Hygiene: History. *American Journal of Public Health.* Vol. 56, No. 7, July, pp. 1120–1127.

U.S. Department of Labor. (2004). The history of Labor Day. Retrieved from http://www.dol.gov/opa/aboutdo/laborday.htm.

ASSIGNMENTS

1. Investigate current occupational health laws that would apply in urban and rural areas.

2. Research the history of occupational health and safety laws.

3. Determine the impact of union workers' strikes on worker conditions in the United States, then discuss whether there would have been a "better" way to get the laws needed.

4. Look up the exceptions to OSHA regulations, and explain the reasons for the exceptions.

5. Report on the ways to make hazardous occupations safe for worker health.

6. Research the health issues of migrant workers in the United States.

7. Research the history of living and working conditions for migrant farm workers. Have they improved in the past half century, and if so, how?

8. Research the epidemiology of occupational lung diseases in the United States.

9. Search for types of occupational illnesses and injuries less common than the ones described in this chapter.

10. Interview an OSHA representative, industrial hygienist, or safety specialist to find out the types of things they must do on the job and the type of training required.

1910 Bureau of Mines Act (PL 61-179)
Created the Bureau of Mines for research and investigation.

1938 Fair Labor Standards Act (*Also known as the Federal Wage and Hour Law*)
Set work week hours and established a minimum wage. Child labor was prohibited for those under the age of 16 except for part-time employment during nonschool hours and vacations in nonhazardous occupations.

1952 The Coal Mine Safety Act (CMSA) (PL 82-552)
Set mandatory safety standards for underground coal mines and more stringent standards for "gassy" mines.

1966 The Metal and Nonmetallic Mines Safety Act (MNMSA) (PL 89-577)
Defined health and safety standards for metal and non-metal mines.

1969 The Construction Safety Act (CSA) (PL 91-54)
Required occupational safety and health standards for employees of the building trades and construction industry working on federally financed or federally assisted construction projects.

1970 Occupational Health and Safety Act (PL 91-596)
Created the OSHA administration and the National Institute for Occupational Safety and Health (NIOSH) with the intention of assuring workplaces free from safety and health hazards such as exposure to toxic chemicals, excessive noise, mechanical dangers, extreme temperatures, and unsanitary conditions.

1971 Noise Control Act (PL 92-574)
Authorized the EPA to regulate noise emissions from railroads and motor carriers and to propose emission standards for these noise sources. The EPA has concluded that an adequate margin of safety required persons to be exposed to no more than a yearly average equivalent sound level of 75 dB for an 8 hour day to prevent hearing loss, and an average equivalent sound level of 55 dB to protect against activity interference.

1977 Federal Mine Health and Safety Act (PL 91-173)
This act put coal and metal/nonmetal mines under the same law, while retaining separate health and safety standards. The Mine Safety and Health Administration (MESA) was moved to the Department of Labor. The law requires four annual inspections for underground mines and two annual inspections for all surface mines. The law created provisions for mandatory training of miners and mine rescue teams for all underground mines.

2000 Federal Coal Mine Safety and Health Act (PL 82-522)
Provides for inspections four times per year, including of surface mines. If mines produce gas, additional inspections are required. Safety standards for all coal mines are included. Fines are mandatory for all violations, includ-

ing criminal penalties for "knowing and willful" violations. The law instituted a training grant program and benefits to miners who are disabled by black lung disease.

2000 Metal and Nonmetallic Mines Safety Act (PL 89-577)
Specifies procedures for developing safety and health standards for metal/nonmetal mines including annual inspections of underground mines, with inspectors issuing violation notices. The law also addresses education and training programs.

2000 Occupational Health and Safety Act (PL 91-596, USC 651)
Assigns to OSHA the principal functions of setting standards and conducting workplace inspections to ensure that employers have complied with standards and are providing a safe and healthful workplace.

SELECTED JOURNALS

American Industrial Hygiene Association Journal
American Journal of Industrial Medicine
Annals of Occupational Hygiene
Applied Ergonomics
Applied Occupational and Environmental Hygiene
Clinics in Occupational and Environmental Medicine
Health Physics
International Archives of Occupational and Environmental Health
Journal of Industrial Ecology
Journal of Occupational and Environmental Medicine
Mine Safety and Health Administration
Occupational and Environmental Medicine
Occupational Hazards
Occupational Health and Industrial Medicine
Occupational Health Safety (online)
Occupational Medicine

ADDITIONAL READING

Leigh, J., Markowitz, S., Fahs, M., & Landrigan. (2000). *Cost of occupational injury and illness.* University of Michigan Press.

Murgueytio, A. (1998). Relationship between lead mining and blood lead levels in children. *Archives of Environmental Health, 53,* 414–424.

U.S. Department of Labor. (2004). Overview of occupational safety and occupational health/industrial hygiene. From http://www.osha-slc.gov/SLTC/smallbusiness/sec5.html.

Weeks, J. (2003). The fox guarding the chicken coop: Monitoring exposure to respirable coal mine dust, 1969–2000. *American Journal of Public Health, 93,* 1236–1244.

Weeks, J. L., Levy, B., & Wagner, G. (1991). *Preventing occupational disease and injury.* Washington, DC: American Public Health Association.

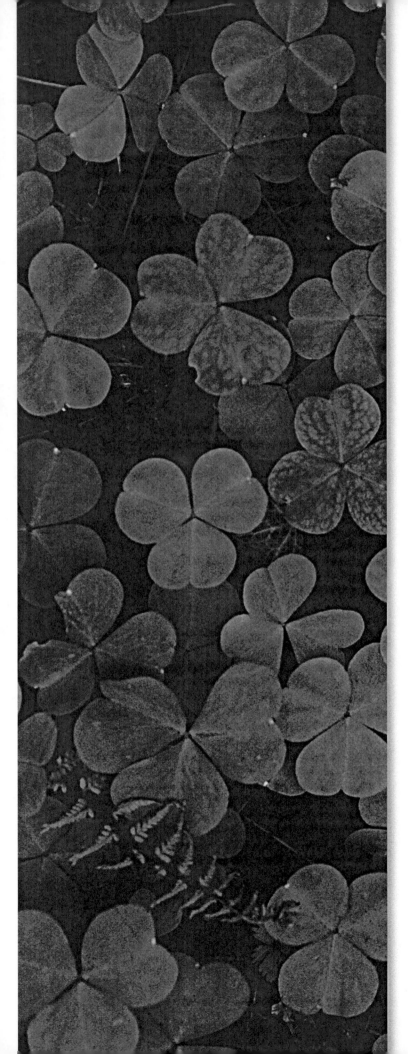

Disaster Preparedness

18

From disaster good fortune comes, and in good fortune lurks disaster.

Chinese proverb

OBJECTIVES

1. Define the term disaster.

2. Name three responsibilities of the National Center for Environmental Health related to disaster epidemiology and preparedness.

3. Describe the effects of climatological disasters.

4. Name various types of natural disasters.

5. Distinguish between climatological and geological disasters.

6. Describe ways to protect yourself and your property from natural disasters.

7. List the various man-made disasters and their effects.

8. Discuss the prevention of man-made disasters.

9. Describe the history of terrorist events since 1984.

10. Describe United States agencies that respond to terrorism and war.

Introduction

disaster is an event that leaves great damage behind and disrupts the lives of many people. Disasters are either natural or man-made. Natural disasters are climatological or geological. There is no area in the United States that can escape the potential of a natural disaster. Man-made disasters include fires, industrial accidents, transportation accidents, **terrorism**, and war. Disaster preparedness is one way we can anticipate the services needed in the event of a disaster.

Goals for Disaster Response

he National Center for Environmental Health (NCEH) and the Centers for Disease Control have responsibilities concerning mitigation of future disasters, disaster preparedness, and tending health needs of people in disaster-stricken areas (National Center for Environmental Health, 1999–2003). The Health Studies Branch of NCEH has the major responsibility for disaster epidemiology at CDC. Goals for the disaster epidemiology program include:

1. Provide service to communities and organizations for preparedness, response, and recovery, including surveillance of deaths, injuries, and illnesses related to a disaster event.

2. Conduct applied research to identify preventable risk factors contributing to disaster-associated morbidity and mortality.

3. Disseminate knowledge of disaster epidemiology (NHEC, 1999–2003).

Climatological Disasters

ecause the weather and climactic changes are always a potential threat, there are more climatological disasters than any other. Climatological disasters include heat waves, drought, hail, tornadoes, hurricanes, tsunamis, and blizzards. Because of global warming trends, more storms have occurred in recent years, and are likely to occur even more frequently in the future.

■ Heat waves and droughts place great stress on humans and animals if they are not able to protect themselves from the effects of the heat, and to have access to sufficient water supplies.

■ Hail damages crops, buildings, homes, and automobiles.

■ When dramatic changes occur in weather, currents of air (e.g., tornadoes and hurricanes) become powerful enough to tear through forests and farmland, rip up homes and businesses, and injure or kill people that stand in their paths.

■ Blizzards pose special problems in mountainous and grassland areas of the United States by freezing power lines and raising the risk of experiencing cold-related injuries and illnesses.

Fortunately, we now have the technology to predict major events fairly accurately, then to warn citizens and to provide rescue services. The U.S. Weather Service, National Oceanic and Atmospheric Administration (NOAA), and many other agencies routinely analyze weather patterns in an effort to warn populations of impending storms so that they may be prepared to deal with them.

HEAT WAVES AND DROUGHT

A heat wave is not usually thought of as a disaster because actions can be taken in advance to reduce its impact on public health. Even so, heat-related deaths totaled more than 8,000 between 1979 and 1999 (CDC, 2002). Heat waves in developed countries increase the need for water and electricity to power air conditioning. In the summer many communities are required by law to conserve water. Droughts have been known to cause disaster emergencies in rural areas, as livestock die and crops fail.

What to Do in a Heat Wave

The problem with a heat wave is that it creates a need for more energy for air conditioners. When this happens, the likelihood of a power outage increases. In order to reduce the need for air conditioning, keeping inside temperatures cooler helps.

■ Raise the air conditioner thermostat to 78 degrees.

■ Use ceiling and room fans to circulate air.

■ Put weatherstripping around doors and windows to keep heat outside and cool air indoors.

■ Close draperies and draw shades during the day to block outside heat.

Disaster
A natural or man-made event that leaves great damage behind and disrupts the lives of many people.

Terrorism
The use of force or violence against persons or property to intimidate or coerce a government or civilian population for the purpose of furthering political or social objectives.

- Use large appliances such as stoves, dishwashers, and washing machines only during the evening hours.
- Turn lights off when not in use.
- Plant shade trees on the south, east, and west sides of the house.

Work outdoors only during the cooler parts of the day. Wear a hat and loose, light-colored clothing and seek shady areas. Avoid drinking alcohol and caffeine, and drink plenty of water.

THUNDERSTORMS, LIGHTNING, AND HAIL

Thunderstorms and rain are more likely to occur during certain months of the year. Thunderstorms are often accompanied by lightning (Figure 18-1). Lightning is a nat-

> ### RECOGNIZING A HEAT-RELATED EMERGENCY
>
> Heat exhaustion can be recognized in someone who is sweating profusely and appears pale. A person who feels dizzy, weak, or overheated should go to a cool place, sit down, and drink water. If the person's skin looks hot and dry, the person is unable to sweat. Body temperature rises, leading to heat stroke. Heat stroke can cause permanent disability and death if not attended to immediately. If you feel a person has heat stroke, move the person to a cooler area, cool them with a water mist, sponge bath, wet sheet, or cool shower. Do not cool them too quickly so as to cause shivering; this is the body's way of increasing internal temperature. Do *not* give the person anything to drink. Call 911 as soon as possible.

ural phenomenon that is good for our environment, releasing nitrogen and replacing it in the soil. But lightning is an electric charge that, if it hits someone, can paralyze breathing, stop a heartbeat, and cause serious burns. Individuals who have been struck or nearly struck by lightning say that the hair on their arms stood up and that they later experienced a severe headache and memory problems. The burns are cauterized from the electric heat and there is no bleeding or oozing, but that doesn't make the injury less painful. There may be an entrance wound and an exit wound. Some individuals will have a "star-like" rash indicating contact with lightning.

At the first sign of lightning, it is a good idea to move out of open areas into a building or motor vehicle. Wet shoes, wet clothing, or standing near a body of water can increase the likelihood of being struck by lightning as water conducts electricity. Holding on to an umbrella, a golf club, a boat, a metal baseball bat, or other metal object is not safe. Coaches and referees should cancel a game rather than risk the lives of athletes and spectators.

Hailstorms occur frequently across the United States. Most hailstorms happen during the spring or fall months. They are localized events, and usually don't cause extensive property damage. However, hail can be about 1.5 inches in diameter, and can cause significant damage to cars, windows, and sides of buildings. When hailstones reach 3 inches in diameter, they can cause major roof damage (Allstate, 2005).

How to Prepare for a Hail Disaster

- Consider replacing your roof covering with roofing material that has received a UL impact resistant classification (UL 2218) of Class 4, meets

FIGURE 18-1 **Lightning Strike** A natural phenomenon, lightning helps bring nitrogen from the atmosphere into the soil. Lightning storms can cause substantial damage.

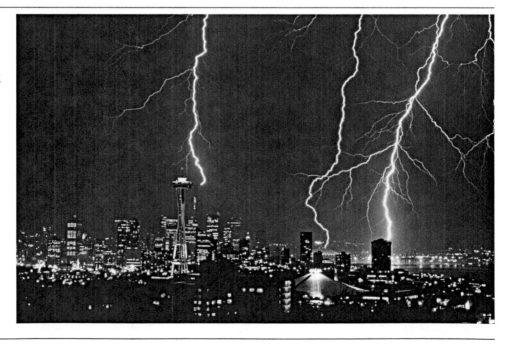

local building code standards, and that requires minimal upkeep and maintenance.

- Listen to weather updates about hail activity.

- Seek shelter immediately if you are caught outdoors—preferably not under a tree.

- Stay indoors until the storm subsides.

- Close drapes, blinds, or window shades for protection from breaking glass.

- Park your vehicle in a garage or under a shelter.

- If driving, pull over to the side of the road—preferably under an overpass or other shelter.

After a hailstorm, assess the damage to your property.

- Check trees, shrubs, and plants around your house.

- Using binoculars, check your roof for damage.

- Check patio covers, screens, windows, and soft aluminum roofs for damage.

- Check vehicles for dents and broken or cracked glass.

- Cover any broken glass in your car to prevent interior damage.

- Cover any broken windows and holes in your roof (Allstate, 2005).

TORNADOES

The most common type of tornado forms from a thunderstorm or hailstorm. Tornadoes can happen any time of the year and at any time of day. In southern states, tornadoes are more likely to occur from March through May. Tornadoes are mostly likely to occur between 3 p.m. and 9 p.m. Some tornadoes appear as a funnel; others may not be seen because of rain or nearby low-hanging clouds (Figure 18-2). The primary dangers associated with tornadoes include property damage, downed electrical lines, and loss of life due to flying debris, collapsing buildings, flash flooding, lightning, and very large hailstones. People most at danger are those in automobiles and in mobile homes.

Tornado Safety

The most important step for anyone in a tornado warning is to listen to the radio. The National Oceanic and Atmospheric Administration (NOAA) provide radios with a warning alarm tone and battery back-up that will turn on automatically and alert you when a tornado watch or warning is issued (Figure 18-3). Most workplaces and schools have emergency plans for tornadoes. Your family should have a plan regarding the safest place to take shelter during a tornado and where to meet when the storm is over.

NATIONAL WEATHER SERVICE MESSAGES

Warnings mean that a certain weather event is *imminent*. Measures should be taken to safeguard life and property *immediately*.

Watches tell you that there is a pretty good chance the event may happen. When a watch is issued, begin making preparations for the upcoming event. Listen to your local

---

Warning
A certain weather event is imminent.

Watch
Good chance a weather event may happen.

FIGURE 18-2 **Tornado in Seymour, Texas** Tornados often occur without advance warning and can cover a large or a small area, bringing devastation in its path.

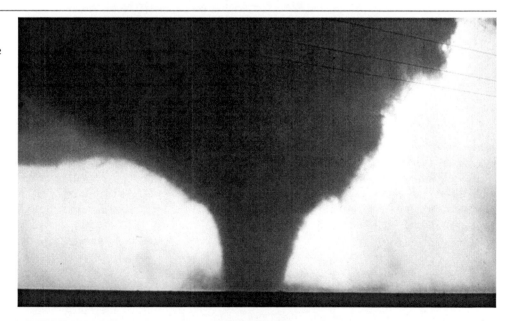

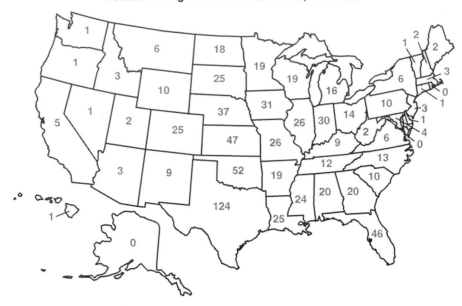

FIGURE **18-3** **Map of Annual Tornadoes by State** Tornadoes are more common in some states than others. Source: National Climatic Data Center. Retrieved from http://www.ncdc.noaa.gov/img/climate/severeweather/small/avgt50as.gif.

Annual Average Number of Tornadoes, 1950-1995

Digging Deeper PROTECT YOURSELF FROM A TORNADO

1. Know where the nearest tornado shelter is and how to get there the quickest way. If you are not in a building with a designated tornado shelter (such as your home), go to a room in the middle of your house without windows or skylights, such as a small bathroom (and close the door), or go into the basement or a crawl space (the best place to be) and close the entrance to that space.
2. Familiarize yourself with the tornado siren signal in your town. These are usually tested once per month (usually first Tuesday). Your town emergency management supervisor or the fire department can provide you

with more information on this. When you hear the siren, it means that severe weather is in your area; go to the tornado shelter with a radio so that you can hear about the weather situation on your local radio station.
3. Know when severe weather is possible in your area by watching the local weather report on TV or the Weather Channel if you have cable TV. When the National Weather Service issues severe weather warnings, they are usually broadcast on TV and on your local radio station. Another possibility is to get a weather radio (a lot of portable radios have

a National Weather Service channel on them) and leave it on the "alarm" setting so when weather alerts or warnings are issued the radio will automatically turn on.
4. If you are outside and a tornado is approaching, go to the nearest substantial building if there is one close by; do not try to outrun the tornado or drive from it. If there is no building nearby, find a low place (roadside ditch, gully, etc.) well away from buildings, your vehicle, and trees (being near a tree poses a danger from lightning), and lie down in the low area with your head covered (Cook, 2004).

---

media to know when warnings are issued. Watches are intended to heighten public awareness of the situation.

Advisories are issued when events are expected to remain below the warning criteria, but still cause significant inconvenience. Advisories are most commonly associated with snow events (National Weather Service).

HURRICANES

The greatest natural disaster in U.S. history occurred when a hurricane struck Galveston, Texas, killing more than 6,000 people on September 8, 1900 (NOAA, 2005).

Fortunately hurricane forecasting, emergency response plans, evacuation procedures, and training of public health workers have improved over the past century and the loss of human life has been greatly reduced. When Hurricane Andrew came through Florida and Louisiana in 1992, the property damage was estimated at $20 billion, but with only 41 deaths (CDC, 2004).

Advisories
Weather events are expected to remain below the warning criteria, but still cause significant inconvenience.

WINTER SEASON

Snow advisory: A snow advisory will be issued when 3–5 inches is expected to fall. Check with your NWS office for local snowfall requirements.

Blowing snow advisory: A blowing snow advisory will be posted for events in which visibility is intermittently ¼ mile or less.

Freezing rain/freezing drizzle advisory: This requires that hazardous driving conditions be taking place and/or up to ¼ inch of freezing rain on tree branches and/or if power lines break.

Winter weather advisory: A winter weather advisory will be issued if conditions warranting two separate winter advisories are met.

Winter storm watch: A winter storm watch may be issued when conditions are forecast to meet the criteria for more than one warning with in the next 36 hours. A watch for a single winter weather event does not exist, for example a wind chill watch or a heavy snow watch. Just the same, if a forecaster thinks there will be significant snow and ice tomorrow, he/she will issue a winter storm watch.

Winter storm warning: A winter storm warning will be issued if conditions are forecast to meet the criteria for two separate warnings in the next 12–24 hours. Example: if you have heavy snow warning conditions along with wind chill warning conditions, a winter storm warning will be issued.

Blizzard warning: A blizzard warning will be issued when the following conditions are forecast to last at least 3 hours. Falling and/or blowing snow frequently reducing visibility to < ¼ mile and sustained winds or frequent gusts > 35 mph.

Ice storm warning: An ice storm warning will be issued if freezing rain/drizzle is occurring with a significant accumulation of ice (more than ¼ inch) or accumulation of sleet (½ inch).

Heavy snow warning: A heavy snow warning will be issued if 6 or more inches of snow is expected in a 12-hour period.

WARM SEASON

Tornado watch: A tornado watch will be issued when conditions are favorable for the development of severe thunderstorms and tornadoes. The Storm Prediction Center (SPC) is the sole agency responsible for issuing a watch. A watch covers several thousands of square miles and generally lasts from two to six hours. Keep an eye on the sky for changing conditions and make preparations in case a weather warning is issued.

Tornado warning: When a tornado warning is issued, tornadoes are occurring and have been spotted or detected by radar. There is imminent danger for people in the area warned. Issued by a local news office, the size of the warning area is generally the size of one or two counties and usually lasts less than an hour. Stay away from windows, doors, and outside walls. Put as many walls between you and the tornado as possible on the lowest floor of your building. If you do not have a basement, seek shelter in an interior bathroom or closet. Get under something sturdy. Protect your head. Stay away from mobile homes. Get out of your vehicle. If there is no safe shelter, lie flat in the nearest ditch or ravine with your hands shielding your head.

Severe thunderstorm watch: A severe thunderstorm watch will be issued when conditions are favorable for development of severe thunderstorms. While not anticipated, tornadoes may occur in the watch area. The Storms Prediction Center (SPC) is the sole agency responsible for issuing a watch. A watch covers several thousands of square miles and generally lasts from two to six hours. Keep an eye on the sky for changing conditions and make preparations in case a weather warning is issued.

Severe thunderstorm warning: When a severe thunderstom warning is issued, tornadoes and/or severe thunderstorms are occurring and have been spotted or detected by radar. The National Weather Service (NWS) defines a severe thunderstorm as having winds 50 kts (58 mph) or hail greater than ¾-inch in diameter (about dime-sized). (A storm that spawns a tornado is obviously also considered severe.) There is imminent danger for people in the area. Issued by a local news office, the size of the warning area is generally the size of one or two counties and usually lasts less than an hour. Stay away from windows, doors, and outside walls. Put as many walls between you and the tornado as possible on the lowest floor of your building. If you do not have a basement, seek shelter in an interior bathroom or closet. Get under something sturdy. Protect your head. Stay away from mobile homes. Get out of your vehicle. If there is no safe shelter, lie flat in the nearest ditch or ravine with your hands shielding your head.

Flood watch: A flood watch will be issued for situations related to widespread general flooding.

Flood warning: A flood warning will be issued when inundation of a normally dry area near a stream or other watercourse is expected, or unusually severe pounding of water expected.

River flood warning: River flood warnings are initiated when a river at a gage site is expected to, or has, exceeded flood stage.

Flash flood watch: A flash flood watch will be issued for serious situations in which life and/or property are in danger. Flash flood watch covers flash flooding, widespread urban and small stream, and headwater flood events.

Flash flood warning: A flash flood warning will be issued in response to a few hours of locally heavy rainfall, a dam or levee failure, or water released from an ice jam rapidly flooding nearby land.

Urban and small stream flood warning/advisory: Urban and small streams flood warnings or advisories are issued when flooding of small streams, streets, and low-lying areas, such as railroad underpasses, and urban storm drains, is occurring.

NONPRECIPITATION EVENTS

Wind chill advisory: Issued when wind chill values are expected to be in the −35°F to −50°F range.

Wind chill warning: Issued when wind chill values are expected to be −50°F or less.

High wind watch: Issued when wind speeds are forecast to meet warning criteria with in the next 24–36 hours.

High wind warning: Issued for sustained wind speeds of 40 mph or greater lasting for 1 hour or longer, or winds of 58 mph or greater for any duration of time.

Wind advisory: Issued for sustained winds 31–39 mph for at least 1 hour; or any gusts to 46–57 mph.

Dense fog advisory: Sense fog advisories may be issued for visibilities ¼ mile or below. These advisories will usually be posted for widespread events, not small local events such as valley fog in the summer.

Heat advisory: A heat advisory will be issued when the heat index is expected to reach 105°F with a nighttime low not below 80°F.

Excessive heat warning: Excessive heat warnings will be issued with a maximum heat index > 115°F and minimum 80°F.

Special heat warning criteria were established for the Chicago metro area after the disastrous July 1995 heat wave. Heat advisories are not issued for Chicago.

Frost advisory: A frost advisory will be issued when widespread frost is forecast during the growing season (temperatures do not necessarily have to be 32°F for frost).

Freeze advisory: A freeze advisory will be issued when widespread temperatures of 32°F or colder are forecast during the growing season (frost may or may not occur).

OPEN WATER/TROPICAL EVENTS

Small craft advisory: A small craft advisory is issued for sustained winds 25–33 **knots** and/or seas > 7 ft within 12 hours.

Gale warning: A gale warning is issued for 1-minute sustained surface winds in the range 39 mph to 54 mph inclusive, either predicted or occurring, not directly associated with tropical cyclones.

Storm warning: A storm warning is issued for 1-minute sustained surface winds of 55 mph or greater, either predicted or occurring, not directly associated with tropical cyclones.

Tropical storm watch: An announcement that a tropical storm poses or tropical storm conditions pose a threat to coastal areas generally within 36 hours. A tropical storm watch should normally not be issued if the system is forecast to attain hurricane strength.

Tropical storm warning: A warning for tropical storm conditions including sustained winds within the range of 39 to 73 mph that are expected in a specified coastal area within 24 hours or less.

Hurricane watch: An announcement of specific coastal areas that a hurricane or an incipient hurricane condition poses a possible threat, generally within 36 hours.

Hurricane warning: A warning that sustained winds 74 mph or higher associated with a hurricane are expected in a specified coastal area in 24 hours or less. A hurricane warning can remain in effect when dangerously high water or a combination of dangerously high water and exceptionally high waves continue, even though winds may be less than hurricane force.

Special marine warning: A special marine warning is issued for a brief/sudden occurrence of sustained wind or frequent gusts > 34 knots, usually associated with thunderstorms (National Weather Service).

As coastal populations grow in the United States, more people face the dangers of a hurricane (Figure 18-4). Approximately 75 million people live within 50 miles of potential hurricane zones today, and the numbers are increasing. Climatologists believe that hurricane activity in the United States will increase because of climatic changes occurring in western Africa. These climactic changes occurred in the decade 1940–1950, leading to three direct hurricane strikes on the United States.

The majority of injuries and deaths during hurricanes are cuts caused by flying class or other debris, puncture wounds from exposed nails, metal or glass, bone fractures, and death by drowning. Hurricanes accompanied by tidal surges or flooding also contaminate water supplies.

Treating Contaminated Water

If a water supply is contaminated with organic matter, it will be cloudy. The water can be strained through a clean gauze or cheese cloth into another container to remove sediment or floating matter. The strained water can be disinfected by boiling vigorously for at least one full minute.

If no electricity is available to boil water, 2 to 6 drops of newly purchased liquid bleach can be added to one gallon of water. The water should be stirred and allowed to stand for 30 minutes before it is used. Water-purifying tablets purchased from a local pharmacy can also be used.

When a Hurricane Threatens

You can improve the odds of your home surviving high winds by taking precautions, but you won't make it hurricane-proof. Nor do these measures guarantee your personal safety.

Take these additional steps to protect yourself and your family as fully as possible:

- Make sure your home is in compliance with building code regulations for areas prone to hurricanes.

- If you can afford it, install hurricane shutters that can be closed when a warning or watch is in effect. Plywood may also be used to protect windows, but you will need to purchase it in advance and have the time to hammer it over windows.

FIGURE 18-4 **Map of Hurricane Activity in the United States** Coastal areas are subject to hurricanes, depending upon ocean currents and global temperatures. Source: U.S. Geological Survey. Retrieved from http://www.usgs.gov/themes/maps5.html.

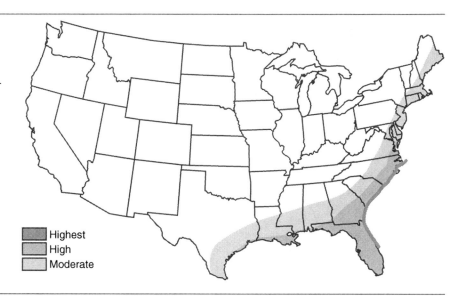

- Highest
- High
- Moderate

- Become familiar with your community's disaster preparedness plans and create a family plan. Identify escape routes from your home and neighborhood and designate an emergency meeting place for your family to reunite if you become separated. Also establish a contact point to communicate with concerned relatives.

- Create an emergency kit.

- Move anything in your yard that can become airborne before a storm strikes.

- If a hurricane threatens, follow weather and news reports so you know how much danger you're facing. Obey evacuation orders from local authorities (Institute for Business & Home Safety 2001).

WINTER STORMS

Blizzards and ice storms are likely to occur during the winter months, and avalanches fall in mountainous regions. Winter storms often down power lines (Figure 18-5). An individual outdoors in cold weather risks frostbite

> **Knot**
> Division of the log's line serving to measure a ship's speed; one nautical mile per hour.

FIGURE 18-5 **Winter Storm Traffic** A major ice storm or blizzard can bring disaster to many if electrical lines are down.

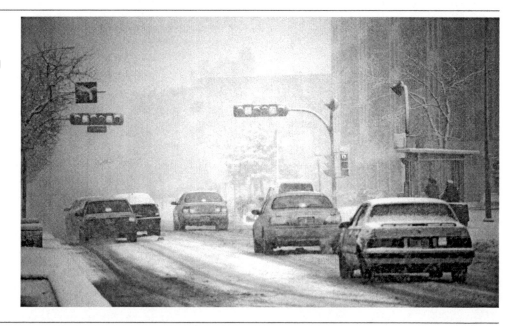

PROTECT YOUR HOME AGAINST HURRICANE DAMAGE

You don't have to be blown away when a hurricane hits. It's never too early to prepare, and you can take several basic steps now to protect your family and your home from disaster.

FIRST THINGS FIRST

Review your homeowner's insurance policy periodically with your insurance agent or company representative to make sure you have sufficient coverage to rebuild your life and home after a hurricane. Report any property damage to your insurance agent or company representative immediately after a natural disaster and make temporary repairs to prevent further damage.

Find out if your home meets current building code requirements for high-wind regions (for example, the Standard Building Code, which is promulgated by the Southern Building Code Congress International, Inc.). Experts agree that structures built to meet or exceed current model building codes' high-wind provisions have a much better chance of surviving violent windstorms.

If you're handy with a hammer and saw, you can do much of the work yourself. Work involving your home's structure may require a building contractor, however, or even a registered design professional such as an architect or engineer.

WHEN WORKING OUTSIDE

- Replace gravel/rock landscaping material with shredded bark.

- Keep trees and shrubbery trimmed. Cut weak branches and trees that could fall on your house.

WHEN BUILDING OR REMODELING

Windows: If you are replacing your existing windows, install impact-resistant window systems, which have a much better chance of surviving a major windstorm. As an alternative to new window systems, install impact-resistant shutters that close over window openings to prevent flying debris from breaking windowpanes.

Entry doors: Make certain your doors have at least three hinges and a dead bolt security lock with a bolt at least one inch long. Anchor door frames securely to wall framing.

Patio doors: Sliding glass doors are more vulnerable to wind damage than most other doors. If you are replacing your patio doors or building a new home, consider installing impact-resistant door systems made of laminated glass, plastic glazing, or a combination of plastic and glass. When a hurricane threatens, an easy, temporary and effective step is to cover the entire patio door with shutters made of plywood or oriented-strand board (OSB).

Garage doors: Because of their size, garage doors are highly susceptible to wind damage. A qualified inspector can determine if both the door and the track system can resist high winds and, if necessary, help replace them with a stronger system. Garage doors more than eight feet wide are most vulnerable. Install permanent wood or metal stiffeners. Or contact the door manufacturer's technical staff for recommendations about temporary center supports you can attach and remove easily when severe weather threatens.

Roofs: If you are replacing your roof, take steps to ensure that both the new roof covering and the sheathing it attaches to will resist high winds. Your roofing contractor should:

- Remove old coverings down to the bare wood sheathing.

- Remove enough sheathing to confirm that rafters and trusses are securely connected to the walls.

- Replace damaged sheathing.

- Refasten existing sheathing according to the proper fastening schedule outlined in the current model building code for high-wind regions.

- Install a roof covering that is designed to resist high winds.

- Seal all roof sheathing joints with self-stick rubberized asphalt tape to provide a secondary moisture barrier.

If you want to give your roof sheathing added protection, but it's not time to reroof, glue the sheathing to the rafters and trusses. Use an adhesive that conforms to Performance Specification AFG-01 developed by APA—the Engineered Wood Association, which you can find at any hardware store or home improvement center.

Gables: Make certain the end wall of a gable roof is braced properly to resist high winds. Check the current model building code for high-wind regions for appropriate guidance, or consult a qualified architect or engineer.

Connections: The points where the roof and the foundation meet the walls of your home are extremely important if your house is to resist high winds and the pressures they place on the entire structure.

- Anchor the roof to the walls with metal clips and straps (most easily added when you replace your roof).

- Make certain the walls are properly anchored to the foundation. A registered design professional can determine if these joints need retrofitting, and a qualified contractor can perform the work the design professional identifies.

- If your house has more than one story, make certain the upper story wall framing is firmly connected to the lower framing. The best time to do this is when you remodel (Institute for Business and Home Safety 2001).

and hypothermia. It is important to dress warmly with several layers of clothing and to stay dry.

Hypothermia occurs when a person's central body temperature is lower than 95° F. It is more likely to occur when a person becomes fatigued outdoors, has on wet clothing, or falls into water. Drinking alcohol, smoking cigarettes, and having a hypothyroidism condition increase the risk. Those who eventually suffer from hypothermia often misjudge how cold it is outside. They become drowsy and may fall asleep, literally freezing to death.

A person suspected of hypothermia may also have superficial or deep frostbite. Superficial frostbite initially occurs in the ears, tip of the nose, fingers, and toes. The area becomes reddened and then very pale. The person may not be able to feel fingers or toes. In the case of cold injuries and hypothermia it is important to remove any wet clothing and warm the individual with blankets and external heat. Do not rub or massage the skin. Do not use direct heat or hot water to warm the person. Give them warm beverages to drink if they are conscious and not nauseated. Never drink alcohol because it causes the body to lose heat.

Geological Disasters

Geological disasters usually result in more deaths and greater economic losses than do climatological disasters. Geological disasters include floods, landslides, avalanches, earthquakes, and volcanic eruptions.

FLOODING

Floods are the most common natural disaster worldwide. Rivers can rise gradually or very rapidly from rapid snowmelt or heavy and repeated rains. Flash flooding accounts for 200 deaths annually (Moeller, 1997). Public health impacts of floods include destruction of homes, soil erosion, and the spread of infectious diseases. Floods contaminate drinking water, disrupt sewer systems and waste disposal, release chemicals from storage tanks, and enhance opportunities for mosquitoes and snakes (Figure 18-6).

LANDSLIDES AND AVALANCHES

Landslides and avalanches often occur in mountainous regions. Landslides are caused by disturbances in the natural stability of a slope of land. Heavy rains following droughts, earthquakes, or volcanic eruptions often precipitate them. Mudslides can be activated by natural disasters. Avalanches occur when loose snow slides down a slope. Broken electrical, water, gas, and sewage lines cause additional concern. Roads and railways can become disrupted. It is important to listen to local weather stations regarding potential dangers.

Hypothermia
State when a person's body temperature is lower than 95° F.

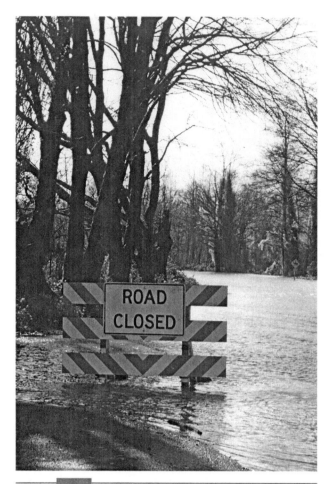

FIGURE 18-6 **Flooded Roadway** Floods bring contaminated water supplies, mold and mud indoors, and harmful disease-causing pathogens.

EARTHQUAKES

Most people in the United States think that earthquakes occur mainly in California. In truth, any area lying over a "fault zone" is at risk (Figure 18-7). Earthquakes have occurred in South Carolina, Montana, and Alaska. Geologists and seismologists have predicted a 97% chance of a major earthquake in the central United States, including Arkansas, Missouri, Tennessee, and Kentucky, before the year 2035. Many earthquakes are minor but they can still interrupt normal living patterns and cause substantial injury.

VOLCANIC ERUPTIONS

Volcanic eruptions include lava flow and intense heat as well as particulate matter diffusion (Figure 18-8). If caught near a volcano during a serious eruption, there is not much you can do to save yourself, but if you are far enough away to survive the blast, you are at risk from the dust. Eruptions of Mount St. Helens in Oregon on May 18, 1980, and Mount Augustine in Alaska on March 27, 1986, raised concerns about the possible adverse health effects of exposure to volcanic dust.

The Mount St. Helens eruption was especially drastic. An earthquake measuring 5.1 on the Richter scale blew out the volcano's north flank, producing a landslide of historic proportions. Almost all life near the volcano disappeared within minutes, and 57 people died. All the trees were flattened in an area of 350 sq km, and towns 400 km away were coated with ash (Palacio, 2005).

The Mount Augustine volcano is an island in Alaska's southern Cook Inlet. It erupted in 1964, 1976, and 1986, which suggests that the next one may come in the mid to

FIGURE 18-7 **Map of Earthquake Hazard Regions in the 48 States** Earthquakes can occur nearly anywhere, but certain areas are more likely to report them. Source: U.S. Geological Survey. Retrieved from http://www.uss.gov/themes/map1.html.

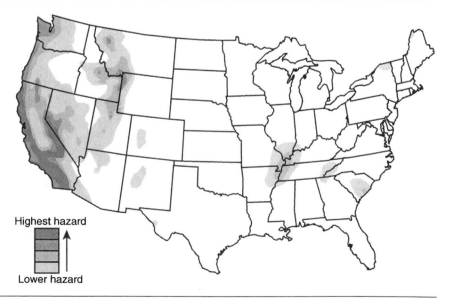

Highest hazard

Lower hazard

FAMILY EARTHQUAKE PLAN

There are several things you should do to prepare for an earthquake—before it happens.

Find the safest place in your home. During an earthquake, stay away from heavy furniture, appliances, large panes of glass, shelves holding heavy objects, and masonry veneer (such as the fireplace). These items tend to fall or break and can injure you. Usually, a hallway is one of the safest places if it is not crowded with objects. Kitchens and garages tend to be the most dangerous. Also, know the safest place in each room. It will be difficult to move from one place to another during a severe earthquake.

Find exits and alternative exits. Always know all the possible ways to exit your house and workplace in emergency situations. Try to discover exits that would only be available to you in an emergency.

Locate shutoff valves. Know the location of the shutoff valves for water, gas, and electricity. Learn how to operate the valves. If you are not sure, contact your utility company.

Provide for the elderly, disabled, persons under medication, and persons who don't speak English. These people may have difficulty moving around after an earthquake. Plan to have someone help them to evacuate if necessary. Also, they may need special foods or medication. Be sure to store several days' supply of these special provisions.

People who cannot speak English often rely on their family or friends for information. If they are separated during an earthquake, they may need help. Prepare emergency information cards for them, written in English, indicating identification, address, and special needs.

Take care of pets. After an earthquake, you should be concerned with your own safety before taking care of your pets. Storing extra food and water for pets is always a good idea. Keep pets in a secure place at home after an earthquake. If you are evacuated, they will not be allowed at the emergency shelter.

Know the location of the nearest police station. Be aware that local fire stations will probably be empty and locked up for days after a major earthquake.

Find shelter and medical care. After a damaging earthquake, emergency shelters and temporary medical centers will be set up in your community. Contact your local and state Office of Emergency Services to find out the plans for your area.

Know your neighbors and their skills. You may be able to help each other after an earthquake. Also know where to go to help in your community after a disaster. It may be days before outside emergency assistance arrives. It is important to help each other.

Plan to reunite with your family. Make a plan on where and how to unite family members. Choose a person outside the immediate area to contact if family members are separated. Long-distance phone service will probably be restored sooner than local service. Remember, don't use the phone immediately after an earthquake, and make local calls only for emergencies.

Plan responsibilities. There will be many things to take care of after an earthquake. Make a plan with your family, friends, and neighbors, assigning specific responsibilities to each person. Remember that it may be difficult to get around after an earthquake, so each person's tasks should be related to where they may be.

Develop a message drop. You need to identify a secure location outside your home were family members can leave messages for each other. This way, if you're separated and unable to remain in your home, your family will know where to go to find you. You don't want to publicize that you are not at home. That is why this location should be secure and discreet, for example, under a paving stone, inside a tin can, in the back yard (Los Angeles City Fire Department, 1997).

SIGNIFICANT EARTHQUAKES IN THE UNITED STATES

1857 Fort Tejeon, California (7.9 on Richter scale)
1872 Owens Valley, California (7.8)
1906 San Francisco, California (7.9)
1933 Long Beach, California (6.4)
1952 Kern County, California (7.5)
1957 Daly City, California (5.3)
1964 Prince William Sound, Alaska (9.2) (strongest in North America)

1971 San Fernando Valley, California (6.6)
1983 Coalinga, California (6.7)
1987 Whittier Narrows, California (5.9)
1988 Loma Prieta, California (6.9)
1991 Sierra Madera, California (5.8)
1994 Northridge, California (6.9)

1999 Bolinas, California (5.0)
1999 Southwest Montana (5.0)
2000 Napa Valley, California (5.2)
2001 Puget Sound, Washington (6.8)
2002 Denali Fault, Alaska (7.9)
2003 San Simeon, California (6.5)
(U.S. Geological Survey, 2005b)

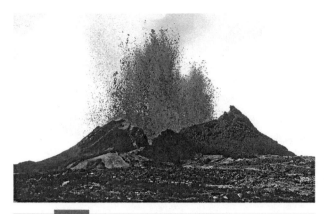

FIGURE 18-8 **Pu'u' O'o Volcano Eruption, Hawaii, 1983**
A volcanic eruption can destroy crops, vegetation, wildlife, homes, and human life.

late 1990s. Ash from an eruption of Mount Augustine disrupts commercial air traffic, including planes flying into Anchorage International Airport. The most destructive hazard is tsunami generated when a huge landslide of debris sweeps from the summit into the sea, as has happened often during the past 2,000 years (USGS, 2005a).

In 1990, NIOSH received a technical assistance request from the Hawaii State Health Department. Of concern was exposure of workers and others to air contaminants from lava and seawater emissions from the Kilaueau volcano that produced detectable amounts of sulfur dioxide, ammonia, carbon disulfide, carbon monoxide, chlorine, hydrofluoric acid, hydrogen sulfide, nitrogen dioxide, and sulfuric acid (CDC, 1986).

Man-made Disasters

man-made disasters are difficult to plan for. U.S. government officials are always on the alert for potential man-made disasters, but not all warnings mean immediate danger to the public. In many cases, the U.S. government succeeds in preventing incidents such as forest fires, industrial incidents, and transportation accidents that might harm U.S. citizens.

FOREST FIRES

Some forest fires arise from natural causes (such as lightning strikes), but most are caused by irresponsible human behavior, such as tossing away lit cigarettes or leaving campfires smoldering. Forest fires can destroy millions of acres of forest land, homes, and businesses, and kill people (Figure 18-9). Fly ash and gases produced from incomplete combustion make it difficult for area residents and animals to breathe. When a major fire occurs, residents must be evacuated to safer locations. Forest fires can last for days, weeks, or several months until the last spark has died. Firefighters from many states are called, many of them volunteers, in an effort to contain forest fires. When forest fires burn out of control, it may take weeks or months of intensive firefighting efforts to get the fire under control. During a major forest fire, homes, lives, wildlife, utility poles, air quality, and gas lines can be destroyed or damaged.

Forest fires are expensive in terms of the manpower hours, firefighting materials, and water needed to fight the fires, and damage the fires themselves cause. The quality of available water may be substantially lowered, making it undrinkable. Water runoff increases sediment in water supplies, encouraging **eutrophication**. Chemicals from fire retardants and foams contain solvents and other chemicals that can also pollute surface water and groundwater sources. When water supplies are tainted with decaying matter, dissolved organic carbon and chlorine react and form **trihalomethane (THM)**, a potentially harmful substance (Chepesiuk, 2001).

INDUSTRIAL ACCIDENTS

Industrial accidents include factory accidents, mining accidents, toxic chemical spills, and nuclear accidents. Potential industrial accidents are reduced by the develop-

Digging Deeper	OTHER MAJOR NATURAL DISASTERS IN THE UNITED STATES	
1888 Blizzard on the East Coast	1992 Hurricane Andrew (Florida, Louisiana, Bahamas); largest insurance loss in history	1996 Hurricane Bertha (coastal North Carolina and the Caribbean)
1900 Hurricane near Galveston, Texas		1999 Hurricane Floyd (eastern North Carolina, souteastern Virginia, east coast of Florida, New England)
1910 Avalanche near Stevens Pass, Washington	1993 Floods in the Midwestern United States	
1925 Tornado through Missouri, Illinois, and Indiana	1995 Heat wave in Chicago, Illinois	
1930s Drought extending from New York to California		2003 Hurricane Isabel (North Carolina) (Dean 2005)

FIGURE 18-9 **Field Fire**

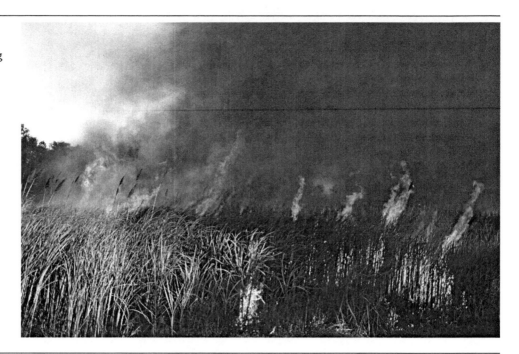

ment and enforcement of regulations governing hazardous sites and materials, and safety devices and procedures for operating machinery.

The International Labour Organization has developed guidelines for preventing industrial accidents. Employers are to keep a documented system of major hazard control for each major hazardous installation that provides for

- identifying and analyzing hazards and assessing risks, including possible interactions between substances.

- safety systems, construction, choice of chemicals, operation, maintenance, and systematic inspection of the installation.

- personnel training, safety equipment, appropriate staffing levels, hours of work, definition of responsibilities, and controls on outside contractors and temporary workers on the site of the installation.

- preparation of effective site emergency plans and procedures, including emergency medical procedures.

- supplying information on potential accidents and site emergency plans to authorities and bodies responsible for the preparation of emergency plans and procedures for the protection of the public and the environment outside the site of the installation (ILO, 1997).

With respect to factory safety, safety devices such as **lockout** and **tagout** systems and the overall design of factory machines are intended to protect machine operators from accidents. Machine designers (engineers) design safety into machines by anticipating ways in which operators can create accidents by negligence or disobedience,

and designing safety systems to prevent such accidents. In current worker's compensation law, employers are exempt from lawsuits for accidents, regardless of cause, but injured employees do receive wages and medical expenses. However, if an accident is attributable to a defect in a machine, the machine's manufacturer can be held legally responsible for product safety (Kamm, 2005).

On March 28, 1979, the reactor core of the nuclear power plant at Three Mile Island in Middletown, Pennsylvania, overheated. As alarms rang and warning lights flashed, the operators did not know what had happened, and did the wrong things. About one-half of the core melted. In a worst case, this would breach the walls of the containment building and release massive quantities of

Eutrophication
Enrichment of a body of water with dissolved nutrients (phosphates), stimulating the growth of aquatic plant life, which usually depletes the dissolved oxygen in the water.

Trihalomethane (THM)
Potentially harmful substance formed when dissolved organic carbon and chlorine react in water supplies tainted with decaying matter.

Lockout
Lock placed on an energy-isolating device to prevent workers from operating a piece of equipment until the lock is removed.

Tagout
Tag placed on an energy-isolating device as a prominent warning of a lockout; should contain the machine operator's name.

- Use fire-resistant or noncombustible materials to cover the roof and exterior structure of the dwelling, or treat wood or combustible material used in roofs, siding, decking, or trim with UL-approved fire-retardant chemicals.

- Use half-inch mesh screen beneath porches, decks, floor areas, and the home itself. Also use this mesh for screen openings to floors, roof, and attic.

- Enclose the undersides of balconies and above-ground decks with fire-resistant materials.

- Clear all flammable vegetation and replace with ornamental landscaping plants that are fire-resistant.

- Plant fire-resistant shrubs and trees. For example, hardwood trees are less flammable than pine, evergreen, eucalyptus, or fir trees.

- Inspect and clean chimneys at least twice a year. Keep the dampers in good working order. Equip chimneys and stovepipes with a nonflammable screen of half-inch or smaller mesh (contact your local fire department for exact specifications).

- Keep a ladder that will reach the roof.

- Regularly clear roof and gutters of pine needles, leaves, or other debris.

- Consider installing protective shutters or heavy fire-resistant drapes over windows.

CREATE A FIRE-SAFETY ZONE AROUND YOUR HOME:

- Clear all combustible material within 10 feet of your home.

- Remove all dry grass, brush, and dead leaves at least 30 to 100 feet around your home. Homes built in pine forests should have a minimum safety zone of 100 feet.

- Regularly rake and remove leaves, dead limbs, and twigs.

- Remove leaves and rubbish from under structures.

- Mow grass regularly.

- Thin a 15-foot space between tree crowns, and remove limbs that are within 10 feet of the ground.

- Remove dead branches that extend over the roof.

- Prune tree branches and shrubs within 10 feet of a stovepipe or chimney outlet.

- Ask the power company to clear branches from power lines.

- Remove vines from the outside walls of the home.

- Clear a 10-ft area around propane tanks and the barbecue.

- Place a screen over the barbecue grill of nonflammable material with mesh no coarser than one quarter inch.

- Stack firewood at least 30 to 100 feet away and uphill from your home.

- Use only safety-inspected and approved wood-burning devices.

- If your home sits on a steep slope, standard protective measures may not be enough. Contact your local fire department or forestry office for additional information.

IF YOUR HOME IS NOT NEAR A COMMUNITY WATER/HYDRANT SYSTEM, MAINTAIN AN EMERGENCY WATER SUPPLY THAT MEETS FIRE DEPARTMENT STANDARDS:

- A cooperative emergency storage tank with neighbors.

- A minimum storage supply of 5,000 gallons on your property.

- Clearly mark all emergency water sources and maintain easy firefighter access to these water sources.

- If your water comes from a well, consider buying and hooking up an emergency generator to operate the pump during a power failure (Allstate, 2005).

---

radiation to the environment. But this did not happen at Three Mile Island. In the months following the accident, thousands of environmental samples of air, water, milk, vegetation, soil, and foodstuffs were collected by various groups monitoring the area. Most of the radiation had been contained and the actual release, which was small, had negligible effects on individuals or the environment (U.S. Nuclear Regulatory Commission, 2005).

On December 3, 1984, a holding tank at the Union Carbide pesticide factory in Bhopal, India, overheated and burst, releasing methyl isocyanate (MIC), a highly toxic gas. MIC, hydrogen cyanide, and at least 65 other gases spread across the city in a cloud, killing more than 5,000 people and turning the leaves of trees black. Nearly two decades after the disaster, survivors continued to suffer neurological disorders, breathlessness, menstrual ir-

regularities, early cataracts, persistent coughing, loss of appetite, recurrent fever, panic attacks, memory loss, and depression. At least 20,000 people have died as a result of the accident, and 15 to 20 more die each month (Organic Consumers Organization, 2001).

TRANSPORTATION ACCIDENTS

Since the introduction of mechanized transportation, large numbers of people have been killed in auto, aircraft, train, and boat incidents. The Department of Transportation, the Federal Aviation Authority, and the Coast Guard investigate each incident to determine causes, and create new standards for the design and maintenance of transportation systems. The design of the Interstate Highway System in the 1950s was especially notable for incorporating new safety features in road design, such as elimination of curves and hills, introduction of over/under intersections, and separation of opposing lanes with medians and median barriers. Both autos and airplanes have been redesigned over the decades to be safer to operate and better protect passengers from accident injury, and boating safety has benefited from improved navigation devices and design of boats and flotation devices.

One all-too-common type of train accident ocurring in recent years are derailments that release toxic chemicals into surrounding communities. In Graniteville, South Carolina, on January 5, 2005, an incorrectly opened train switch diverted a 42-car train with three chlorine tankers onto a siding, where it rammed into another, parked train. The crash released clouds of chlorine gas through the town, killing 9 and injuring 250 people. Officials of the Aiken County Department of Public Safety credited the Homeland Security Department for giving them the equipment, personnel training, and the knowledge to handle the accident, and the Chlorine Institute dispatched an emergency response team to the accident site. Almost all of the 5,400 Graniteville residents were evacuated to the nearby town of Aiken. A new Washington, D.C., effort to ban trains carrying chlorine and other dangerous chemicals past the U.S. Capitol and through the region is gathering momentum after the accident (National Clearinghouse for Worker Safety & Training, 2005).

DISASTER ASSISTANCE

A great many people are harmed by natural disasters, catastrophes, bioterrorism, and war. Federal programs provide assistance to those who have been victimized by floods, tornadoes, hurricanes, and other natural disasters. The Federal Emergency Management Agency (FEMA) works with other agencies, such as the American Red Cross, to provide temporary shelter, food, and supplies in the event of a disaster. FEMA coordinates national efforts to prepare for disasters, respond to them, assist communities in recovery, mitigate potential hazards associated with disastrous situations, and provide funding for disaster assistance. International assistance is available from the Pan American Health Organization and the World Health Organization, if needed.

Terrorism

here are two types of terrorism: domestic and international. Domestic terrorism is committed within national boundaries and not directed from outside the country. International terrorism is conducted by countries or groups whose activities transcend national boundaries.

Terrorist events include the use of biological, chemical, and radiation weapons. Biological agents include anthrax, botulism, bucellosis, cholera, glanders, Nipah virus, plague, psittacosis, Q fever, tularemia, ricin, typhus, smallpox, viral encephalitis (Venezuelan, eastern equine, and western equine), and viral hemorrhagic fevers (**filoviruses** such as Ebola or Marburg; **arenaviruses** such as Lassa and Machupo). Chemical agents include many of the toxic chemicals discussed in Chapter 5 as well as acids, toxins, blister agents/**vesicants**, blood agents, **anticoagulants**, lung/choking pulmonary agents, mustard gas, nerve agents, tear gas, and vomiting agents.

Uses of radioactive materials in terrorist events include the introduction of radioactive material into food and water supplies, destroying a nuclear facility, or exploding a small nuclear device. A so-called "dirty bomb" is a radiological dispersion device combining explosives with radioactive materials in the form of powder or pellets. The blast exposes buildings and people to radioactive material. The primary purpose is to make buildings unusable for a long period of time.

The worst effect of a radiation weapon would be from a meltdown or explosion at a nuclear facility, causing large amounts of radioactive material to be released. A nonterrorist example of what can happen is the Chernobyl disaster in Russia. Nuclear plant workers and citizens living in surrounding areas were injured and exposed or contaminated. A nuclear explosion also results in property damage and people killed from the blast. After a nuclear explosion, radioactive fallout extends over a large region, far from the point of impact, increasing the risk of people developing cancer.

HISTORY OF TERRORIST EVENTS

The attack on the World Trade Center in New York City on September 11, 2001, was part of the worst terrorist attack in the history of the United States, but unfortunately not the only attack. The first bioterrorism attack in the United States occurred in September and October of 1984. In the Dallas, Oregon, area, 751 cases of *Salmonella* gastroenteritis were found to be related to consumption of salad-bar ingredients. Epidemiology studies and the FBI found that members of the Rajneeshee religious cult had contaminated the salad bars with *Salmonella* bacteria to prevent people from voting in the county election so the cult's cho-

Arenavirus
Viruses transmitted to humans from rat excretia, identified by RNA granules in the virion.

Vesicants
Drug or a chemical weapon that causes blistering.

Anticoagulants
Substances that hinder blood clotting.

sen candidates would win. Fortunately no one died. Very little national attention was paid to the event because it occurred in a remote town and it was presumed that such an incident would never happen again. It is significant because it was a bioterrorism event that affected the largest number of people to date (Rubin et al., 2004).

On December 21, 1988, 259 people (including 189 Americans) were killed when PanAm Flight 103, en route from London to New York, suddenly exploded and crashed in Lockerbie, Scotland. On the ground, 11 British citizens were killed and several buildings were destroyed. A British flight commission found evidence of an explosion in the luggage compartment, deemed to be from an intentional explosive device. The luggage belonged to passengers boarding in Frankfort and London. British and U.S. government officials and experts linked the source of the incident to a terrorist organization in the Middle East (Rubin et al., 2004).

On August 14, 1989, President George H.W. Bush formed the Presidential Commission on Aviation Security and Terrorism, calling for a "**zero tolerance**" policy and preparation for retaliatory military strikes against terrorist groups and the countries that harbor them. (Zero-tolerance policies and laws mandate certain responses to presumed offenses, with no allowance made for individual judgments.)

On February 26, 1993, an explosion occurred in the parking garage of the World Trade Center in New York City, the second largest building complex in the world. The explosion killed 7 people and wounded 1,042. FBI and New York Police Department investigators determined that the explosion was in a rented truck loaded with 1,200 pounds of explosives. The bombing was linked to a Palestinian with Jordanian citizenship (Rubin et al., 2004).

A **sarin** gas attack occurred in Tokyo, Japan, on March 20, 1995, in the subway. Members of the AumShinrikyo cult placed open canisters of the nerve gas on five separate cars on three different subway lines. The intent was to kill large numbers of police officers because the cult had learned of a prospective police raid on the cult. The gas affected thousands of commuters; as many as 3,800 people were injured and 1,000 hospitalized. According to a 1999 CDC report, the cult had intended to use large quantities of the gas in the attack, and had experimented with biological agents such as botulism, anthrax, cholera, and Q fever (Rubin et al., 2004).

On April 19, 1995, a truck bomb killed 169 citizens, including 19 children, and injured 500 people in the Murrah Federal Building of Oklahoma City, Oklahoma. The bomb was traced to Timothy McVeigh, Terry Lynn Nichols, and James Douglas Nichols. At the time, the bombing was called the deadliest terrorist event ever committed on U.S. soil. It was an unprecedented attack, planned by heartland Americans (Rubin et al., 2004).

The 1996 Olympic Games in Atlanta, Georgia, were interrupted at 1:20 a.m. on July 27 when a pipe bomb exploded in Centennial Olympic Park. One person was killed and 112 people were injured. In 1998 the Justice Department charged a North Carolina carpenter with the bombing, as well as 1996 bombings at an Atlanta health clinic and night club. He was arrested in 2005 (Rubin et al., 2004).

The bombing of the World Trade Center Towers in New York City and the Pentagon in Washington, DC, on September 11, 2001, was a well-executed attack by foreign terrorists. Approximately 3,300 people died, making this the most deadly single terrorist attack in the world and among the worst disasters, natural or human, in U.S. history.

Later during 2001, anthrax contamination was detected in 21 postal facilities around the country, 20 Congressional buildings in the District, 11 government buildings in Maryland/Virginia, and 6 other facilities around the country. The anthrax attacks affected citizens in Connecticut, Florida, Indiana, Maryland, Missouri, New Jersey, New York, North Carolina, Virginia, and Washington, DC.

As a result of the 2001 events, two executive orders were given, a Homeland Security directive was made, and the Department of **Homeland Security** was formed.

War

Lessons learned from past wars have shown that war motivates the use of any available type of weapon, including **weapons of mass destruction**: the atomic bombing of Nagasaki and Hiroshima to end World War II, the use of Agent Orange in Vietnam to defoliate the countryside and reveal enemy positions, and inspections for and suspicion of WMDs leading up to the second Iraq war. On the positive side, mass trauma training to handle the wounded in battle resulted in the development of the emergency medical system. This system is now nationwide and responds to victims of mass casualties and terrorist attacks.

NATIONAL SECURITY PROTECTION AGAINST TERRORISM AND WAR

National security is important to prevent and manage situations potentially threatening large numbers of people. Whenever there is open hostility, conflict, opposition, or antagonism, or an attempt by one political entity to weaken or destroy another, there is the potential for a riot, terrorism, or war. Acts of terrorism range from threats, assassinations, kidnapping, hijackings, bomb scares, bombings, cyber attacks, and the use of chemical or biological weapons, up to the threat of nuclear weapons. High-risk targets include military and civilian government facilities, international airports, large cities, and high-profile landmarks. Terrorists may also target large public gatherings, or food and water supplies. Bombs and other materials may be sent through the mail. When an event cannot be prevented, government officials must decide the costs and benefits associated with alerting the public to a possible disaster.

The Homeland Security Act of 2002 (PL 107-296) was enacted to create funding and mechanisms for public health officials, the military and emergency personnel to work together to prevent and prepare for potential disasters, particularly those involving biochemical warfare.

Public Health Efforts in Bioterrorism Preparedness and Response

The Centers for Disease Control and Prevention have developed the Bioterrorism Preparedness and Response Program to assist the public, health care providers, military personnel, and public service workers in the event of radiation, chemical, and biological disasters.

Disaster prevention and response plans have been developed in the event of radiation emergencies, bioterrorism (anthrax, botulism, plague, smallpox, ricin), chemical warfare (sarin nerve gas, mustard gas, VX), and weapons of mass destruction. Following are the alert codes developed as a result of the Homeland Security Act:

- **Red** (Severe): Severe risk of terrorist attacks

- **Orange** (High): High risk of terrorist attacks

- **Yellow** (Elevated): Significant risk of terrorist attacks

- **Blue** (Guarded): General risk of terrorist attacks

- **Green** (Low): Low risk of terrorist attacks

Communications systems have been set up to alert public health officials, health care facilities, and emergency personnel of an incident or attack. Citizens are provided warnings and information on how to make a safe shelter out of their homes. Vaccinations, antibiotics, and other medical supplies are stockpiled in the event that large numbers of people require assistance.

Government officials at all levels work together to determine the needs of citizens, reduce risk potential, maintain cooperative efforts between local agencies, and maintain facilities and services.

DISASTER PREPAREDNESS

Responding to public and governmental concerns about safety is a public and environmental health issue that is difficult for any one agency to manage. A primary example of how governmental agencies can work together for the health of populations and communities are efforts to protect and assist citizens in the event of a disaster.

Zero tolerance
Policies and laws that mandate certain responses to presumed offenses, with no allowance made for individual judgments.

Sarin
Extremely toxic and powerful cholinesterase inhibitor used as a chemical warfare agent.

Homeland Security
A national effort to prevent terrorist attacks within the United States, reduce America's vulnerability to terrorism, and minimize the damage to recover from after attacks (2002 Bush Administration definition).

Weapons of Mass Destruction (WMD)
Any weapon or device that has the capacity to cause death or serious bodily injury to a significant number of people; toxic or poisonous chemical, disease organism; or radioactivity.

Digging Deeper   IF YOU NEED TO EVACUATE

- Make arrangements in advance for other housing or a motel. Otherwise, proceed to a shelter.

- Find the official hurricane evacuation route for your location.

- Shut off water and electricity at the main power station.

- Put plastic bags over TVs, lamps, computers, and other items needing protection from moisture.

- Pack dry clothes in plastic bags.

- Store valuables in your empty appliances.

- Let friends and relatives know where you are going.

- Make arrangements at kennels or hotels if you have a pet.

- Leave early, during daylight if possible.

- Lock windows and doors.

- Take with you:

  - important documents and identification.

  - pillows, blankets, sleeping bags, or air mattresses.

  - extra clothing, shoes, and eyeglasses.

  - lightweight folding chairs and cots.

  - items from your disaster survival kit (Institute for Business and Home Safety, 2001).

Each community should have emergency services that are ready to handle extreme situations. A **disaster preparedness** plan ensures immediate response to an event, evacuation procedures for residents, and activities to restore community services. Fire, rescue, police, hospital, and military services must coordinate efforts with utility companies to control the extent to the damage. Public health officials must be involved to provide emergency treatment, clean water, basic sanitation facilities, food, and efforts to dissipate effects of the disaster. National plans help define the responsibilities of personnel in public and environmental health departments and emergency preparedness agencies. Military and civil defense personnel are activated and work with local officials to control traffic and potential crimes.

Communities should also have personnel and communication systems prepared to assist with the detection, reporting, and management of disease outbreaks, injuries, or casualties related to disasters.

Assemble a disaster supplies kit with items you may need if you are advised to evacuate. Store these supplies in sturdy, easy-to-carry containers such as backpacks, duffel bags, or trash containers.

Summary

disaster, natural or man-made, is an event that leaves great damage behind and disrupts the lives of many people. Natural climatological disasters include heat waves, drought, hail, tornadoes, hurricanes, tsunamis, and blizzards. Natural geological disasters include floods, landslides, avalanches, earthquakes, and volcanic eruptions. People living in areas prone to such disasters should prepare for them, and know what to do in the event. Federal programs provide assistance to those who have been victimized by floods, tornadoes, hurricanes, and other natural disasters.

Man-made disasters include forest fires, industrial accidents, transportation accidents, terrorism, and war. Many such disasters are difficult to plan for at the national level, but there are things individuals and families can do to protect themselves. U.S. government officials are always on the alert for potential man-made disasters, but not all warnings mean immediate danger to the public. National security is important to prevent and manage potential situations threatening large numbers of people. The Homeland Security Act of 2002 was enacted to prevent and prepare for any potential man-made disasters. In addition, each community should have emergency services in place and ready to handle extreme situations.

Disaster preparedness
Measures taken by individuals beforehand to be ready to deal with the results of a natural or man-made disaster.

REFERENCES

Allstate Insurance Company, Catastrophe Information Center (2005). How can I prepare for disaster? Hail/Wildfires. Retrieved from http://www.allstate.com/Catastrophe/PageRender.asp?Page=hail.htm.

Centers for Disease Control (CDC). (1986). Epidemiological notes and reports of cytotoxicity of volcanic ash: Assessing the risk for pneumoconoiosis. *MMWR Weekly, 35,* 265–267.

Centers for Disease Control (CDC). (2002). Heat-related Deaths—United States, 1979–1999. *MMWR Weekly July 5, 51(26);* 567–570.

Centers for Disease Control (CDC). (2004). About Hurricanes. Emergency Preparedness and Response. Retrieved from http://www.bt.cdc.gov/disasters/hurricanes/about.asp.

Chepesiuk, R. (2001). Wildfires ignite concern. *Environmental Health Perspectives, 109,* 364.

Cook, D. R. (2004). Tornado Protection. From Ask a Scientist, Newton BBS, DOE Weather Archive, at http://www.newton.dep.anl.gov/askasci/wea00/wea00214.htm.

Dean, C. (2005). Historic Disasters. Retrieved from http://genealogy.about.com.

International Labour Organization (ILO) (1997). Prevention of Major Industrial Accidents, Article 9. Retrieved from www.itcilo.it/en glish/actrav/telearn/osh/legis/c174.htm.

Institute for Business and Home Safety (2001). Protect Your Home Against Hurricane Damage. Retrieved from http://www.ibhs.org/natural_disasters/downloads/hurricane_guide.pdf.

Kamm, L. J. (2005). Industrial Accidents and Product Liability. Retrieved from http://www.ljkamm.com/safety.htm.

Los Angeles City Fire Department (1997). Earthquake Preparedness Handbook. Retrieved from http://www.lafd.org/eqfampln.htm.

Moeller, D. W. (1997). *Environmental health,* revised edition. Cambridge, MA: Harvard University Press.

National Center for Environmental Health (1999–2003). At the turn of the century: Strategic Plan 1999–2003. Centers for Disease Control. Retrieved from http://www.cdc.gov/nceh/publications/stratplan/NCEHstratplan2004_2005.pdf.

National Clearinghouse for Worker Safety & Training (2005). Clearinghouse Report of Related News Stories and Links for the Graniteville, South Carolina Train Accident. Retrieved from http://www.wetp.org/wetp/.

U.S. Nuclear Regulatory Commission (2005). Fact Sheet on the Accident at Three Mile Island. Retrieved from http://www.nrc.gov/reading-rm/doc-collections/fact-sheets/3mile-isle.html.

National Oceanic and Atmospheric Administration (NOAA) Library. (2005). Storm Tales. Retrieved from http://www.history.noaa.gov/stories_tales/cline2.html.

National Weather Service. (2005). Severe weather awareness. Retrieved from http://weather.gov/om/severeweather/index.shtml.

Organic Consumer Organization. (2002). 17 Years After the Bhopal Tragedy, Union Carbide Continues to Evade Responsibility. Retrieved from http://www.organic-consumers.org/toxic/bhopal120601.cfm.

Palacio, Zuli (2005). Mt. St. Helens Eruption. Voice of America. Retrieved from http://www.voanews.com/english/2005-05-10-voa8.cfm.

Rubin, C., Cumming, W., Renda-Tanali, I., & Birkland, T. (2003). Major terrorism events and their U.S. outcomes. Natural hazards research working paper #107. University of Colorado: Natural Hazards Research and Applications Information Center, Institute of Behavioral Science. Retrieved from http://www.colorado.edu/hazards/wp/wp107/wp107.html#seventies.

U.S. Geological Survey (2005a). Cascades Volcano Observatory, Vancouver, WA. Geology of Interactions of Volcanoes, Snow, and Water: Results of Recent Surveys. Retrieved from http://vulcan.wr.usgs.gov/home.html.

U.S. Geological Survey (2005b). Significant Earthquakes in the United States. Retrieved from http://quake.wr.usgs.gov/recent/recent.html.

ASSIGNMENTS

1. Discuss the differences in preventing and preparing for natural disasters and man-made disasters.

2. Describe how you would determine whether you live in a potentially hazardous area where a disaster is likely to occur.

3. Name strategies that could be used to avoid or prepare for a disaster in your community.

4. List several activities and supplies you might need in the event of a disaster.

5. List how would you prepare differently for a hurricane, a tornado, a hailstorm, and a flood.

6. List what you would do following each natural disaster described in the chapter.

7. Locate the local Red Cross chapter and interview a representative concerning disaster training and volunteers needed in your area.

8. Look for disaster preparedness manuals on the Internet or in the public library.

9. Describe how you would modify what is done for homeland security to improve its effectiveness.

10. Investigate and report on your local community's level of preparedness for disasters.

SELECTED ENVIRONMENTAL LAWS

1936 Flood Control and Coastal Emergencies Act (PL 84-99)
Provided for participation of the federal government in solving flooding problems too large or complex to be handled by states or localities.

1974 Federal Disaster Relief Act of 1974 (PL 93-288)
Established the presidential declaration of disasters requiring federal assistance.

1986 Water Resources Development Act (PL 99-662, Section 917)
Established to provide assistance to flood areas and victims.

1988 The Robert T. Stafford Disaster Relief and Emergency Assistance Act (PL 106-390)
Amended the Federal Disaster Relief Act of 1974.

1990 Aviation Security Improvement Act (PL 101-604)
Recommended an assistant secretary of transportation for security and intelligence to oversee aviation safety, and that a federal security manager be assigned to each major airport.

1995 National Defense Authorization Act (PL 103-337)
Repealed the Federal Civil Defense Act of 1950 issuing authority to FEMA to direct, coordinate, guide, and assist states with a comprehensive emergency preparedness system for all hazards in the United States.

1996 Defense Authorization Act of 1996 (PL 104-201)
Enhanced preparedness against terrorism, particularly employment of weapons of mass destruction.

2000 Disaster Mitigation Act (PL 106-390)
Amended the Robert T. Stafford Disaster Relief and Emergency Assistance Act to streamline the administration of disaster relief, to control federal costs of disaster assistance, and to provide impetus for state and local governments to undertake mitigation planning.

2000 Airport Security Improvement Act (PL 106-528)
Directed the Federal Aviation Administrator (FAA) to develop an electronic fingerprint transmission project for criminal history checks for security screeners and other airport personnel.

2002 Homeland Security Act (PL 107-296)
Established a Department of Homeland Security to prevent terrorist attacks within the United States; to reduce vulnerability; to minimize damage; to assist in terrorism recovery; to anticipate chemical, biological, radiological, nuclear and other countermeasures; to increase border and transportation security; and to coordinate emergency preparedness and response systems.

SELECTED JOURNALS

Biosecurity and Bioterrorism
Contingency Planning and Management
Disaster Medicine, Military Medicine
Disaster Recovery Journal
Homeland Security Newsletter
Journal of Pre-hospital and Disaster Medicine
Natural Hazards Observer
NTI Global Security Newswire

ADDITIONAL READING

Barry, J. (1998). *Rising tide: The great Mississippi flood of 1927 and how it changed America.* New York: Simon & Schuster.

Cole, L.A. (2005). *The Anthrax letters: A medical detective story.* The National Academies Press.

Henderson, D. A., Thomas V. Inglesby, T. V., & Tara O'Toole, T. eds. (2005). *Bioterrorism: Guidelines for Medical and Public American Medical Association Press.* Chicago, IL: AMA.

Landesman, L. Y. (2005). *Public health management of disasters: The practice guide.* American Public Health Association.

Levy, B. S., & Sidel, V. W., eds. (2005). *Terrorism and public health.* APHA and Oxford University Press.

Levy, B. S., & Sidel, V. W., eds. (2005). *War and public health, updated edition.* American Public Health Association.

Manning, F. J., & and Lewis Goldfrank, L., eds. (2005). *Preparing for terrorism.* The National Academies Press.

Pan American Health Organization. (2005). *Natural disasters: Protecting the public's health.*

Weinstein, R. S., and Alibek, K. (2005). *Biological and chemical terrorism.* Thieme Medical Publishers.

Weiss, L. D. (2005). *Collision on I-75.* American Public Health Association.

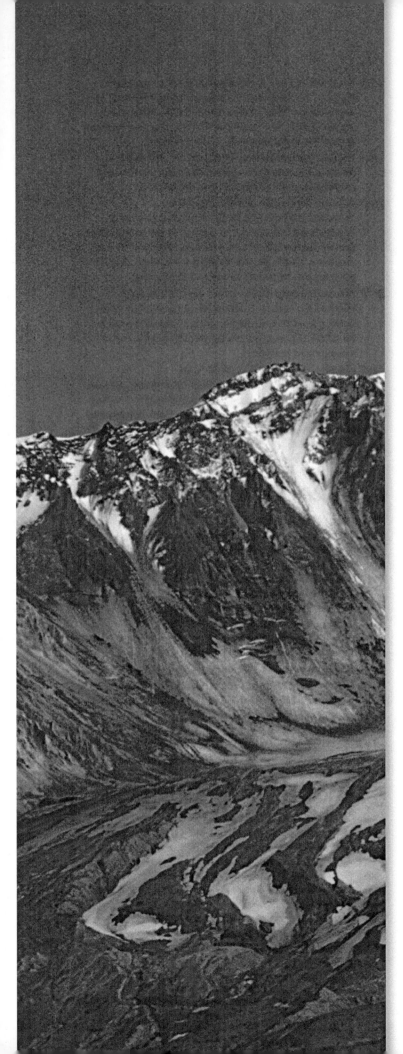

Environmental and Public Health Challenges

Never doubt that a small group of thoughtful, committed citizens can change the world; indeed it's the only thing that ever has.

Margaret Mead

I don't care why someone cares about the environment—only that they do.

Alan Werbach (1997), Sierra Club

OBJECTIVES

1. Review global and United States environmental health issues.

2. List American voter opinions on the environment and governmental interventions.

3. Become familiar with the operating structure of the Department of Health and Human Services and the Centers for Disease Control.

4. Review public health laws and their role in maintaining the environment.

5. Explain how groups involved in the environmental movement can help public health agencies in the quest for a healthier environment.

6. Compare and contrast public health approaches using the microbial, behavioral, and ecological models of disease.

7. Describe the World Health Organization's Healthy City initiative.

8. Explain what is meant by green architecture, green energy, and green transportation.

9. Define sustainable growth.

10. Summarize various local strategies for sustaining the environment.

Introduction

lobal public health issues include uncontrolled population growth, world hunger, natural disasters, bioterrorism, germ warfare, land pollution, air pollution, and diseases. Uncontrolled population growth leads to increased demand for food supplies, destruction of rainforests for pasture and farmland, solid waste disposal problems, and increased use of fossil fuels and increased use of hazardous substances. Environmental changes from global warming are responsible for greater human vulnerability to disease, the emergence of new diseases, and global epidemics.

Increased use of fossil fuels leads to acid rain, drought, and global warming. Increased use of hazardous substances leads to thinning of the ozone layer, decreased biodiversity, and endocrine disturbances. All industrialized and developing countries, including the United States, have a major role to play in sustaining the environment and preventing its demise. In the United States, environmental organizations, laws, and public health agencies strive to make the environment more livable and sustainable. This chapter addresses national concerns and public health efforts to manage environmental health problems. The last part of this chapter addresses state and local issues.

Public Perceptions of the Environment

everal environmental activist and conservation groups regularly poll the public in an effort to see how individuals view the environment. In a 2002 poll conducted by the League of Conservation Voters (2002), it was found that:

- 66% described themselves as environmentalists.

- 60% indicated that current environmental laws are tough enough but not well enforced.

- 41% believe that the environment has worsened in the last 5 years and 38% believe it has remained the same.

- 22% said terrorism is the most important current problem in the United States.

- 12% said the economy is the most important issue facing the United States in the next 25 years.

- 76% said the environmental movement has had the most impact on the nation's public health policies over the years.

In spite of polls showing that Americans believe there are enough laws to protect the environment, few Americans understand that harming the environment is a crime. In 2001, the Environmental Protection Agency filed 482 cases of criminal charges for violating environmental laws. Most of the criminal cases involved industries who violated the Clean Water Act. Some companies are still challenging the laws and expecting leniency because they provide jobs essential to local economies (Environmental Protection Agency, 1986).

Department of Health and Human Services

ow does the federal government address public health issues in the United States? The Department of Health and Human Services (DHHS) has the responsibility for protecting the health of all Americans and providing essential human services (Figure 19-1). The department was created when President Jimmy Carter signed the Department of Education Organization Act (PL 96-88) into law, splitting the former Department of Health, Education, and Welfare (HEW) into DHHS and the U.S. Department of Education. The U.S. Public Health Service, a part of the uniformed service of DHHS, is led by the Surgeon General. With more than 300 programs, it is the largest grant-making agency in the federal government.

Centers for Disease Control and Prevention

major division of Health and Human Services is the Centers for Disease Control and Prevention (CDC). This agency works with states and other partners to provide a system of health surveillance to monitor and prevent disease outbreaks (Figure 19-2). The CDC Division of Environmental Hazards and Health Effects initiated the National Environmental Public Health Tracking Program in 2002 to set up state and national data collection systems. In addition, the system is intended to create a comprehensive program of interventions, monitor the effects of the interventions, create public awareness, and guide research initiatives in all 50 states, the District of Columbia, tribal nations, and U.S. territories. Biological, chemical, biomechanical, and physical agents are analyzed and information sent to the EPA's National Environmental Information Exchange Network. By the year 2010, the tracking program will focus on better environmental health care, legislation, and public awareness.

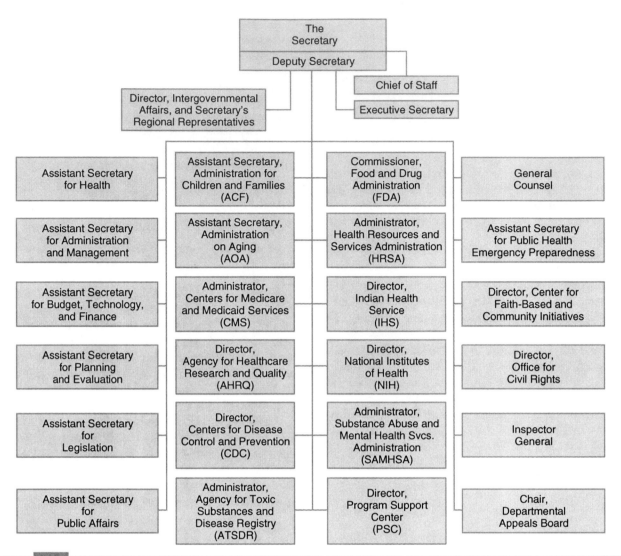

The
Secretary

Deputy Secretary

Director, Intergovernmental
Affairs, and Secretary's
Regional Representatives

Chief of Staff

Executive Secretary

Assistant Secretary for Health	Assistant Secretary, Administration for Children and Families (ACF)	Commissioner, Food and Drug Administration (FDA)	General Counsel
Assistant Secretary for Administration and Management	Assistant Secretary, Administration on Aging (AOA)	Administrator, Health Resources and Services Administration (HRSA)	Assistant Secretary for Public Health Emergency Preparedness
Assistant Secretary for Budget, Technology, and Finance	Administrator, Centers for Medicare and Medicaid Services (CMS)	Director, Indian Health Service (IHS)	Director, Center for Faith-Based and Community Initiatives
Assistant Secretary for Planning and Evaluation	Director, Agency for Healthcare Research and Quality (AHRQ)	Director, National Institutes of Health (NIH)	Director, Office for Civil Rights
Assistant Secretary for Legislation	Director, Centers for Disease Control and Prevention (CDC)	Administrator, Substance Abuse and Mental Health Svcs. Administration (SAMHSA)	Inspector General
Assistant Secretary for Public Affairs	Administrator, Agency for Toxic Substances and Disease Registry (ATSDR)	Director, Program Support Center (PSC)	Chair, Departmental Appeals Board

FIGURE **19-1** **Department of Health and Human Services Organizational Chart** The Department is subdivided into other bureaus according to how they are regulated by the federal government.

Public Health Concerns

The central mission of public health in the United States is to implement protective measures and analyze trends in health, illness, disability, and death. This mission is accomplished by efforts directed at prevention and early detection rather than cure. Preserving the health of the nation has been addressed through organized efforts to consolidate concerns, perceived needs, and professional experiences among experts throughout the United States. The Healthy People Initiative begun in 1979 by the CDC has identified certain major health concerns as "leading health indicators" for the twenty-first century: environmental quality, injury and violence, physical activity,

tobacco use, substance abuse, injury and violence, immunizations, and access to health care. Environmental quality influences the extent to which one is physically active or overweight, mentally healthy, and immune to a disease.

In 2000, the CDC identified future health challenges, asking medical, scientific, and public health communities to address such issues as:

■ Reducing pollution from vehicles, industries, and hazardous waste sites. (The environment will be increasingly challenged by toxic exposures, population growth, continued urbanization, and urban design that hinders healthy behaviors, such as physical activity.)

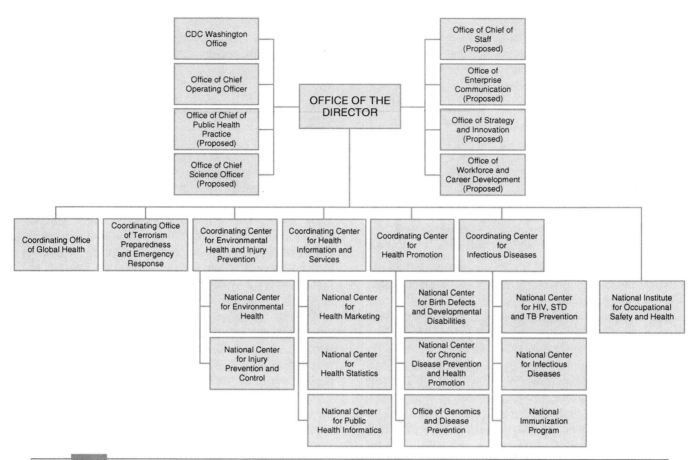

Digging Deeper   WHAT IS THE CDC?

Founded in 1946 to help control malaria, the CDC is a public health agency charged with preventing and controlling infectious and chronic diseases, injuries, workplace hazards, disabilities, and environmental health threats. The CDC employs 9,000 health workers in 170 occupations with a public health focus, including physicians, statisticians, epidemiologists, laboratory experts, behavioral scientists, and health communicators.

The CDC conducts research and applies its findings toward two overall goals:

1. Promoting health and preventing disease, injury, and disability, so

that everyone, especially those at higher risk due to health disparities, may achieve an optimal lifespan with the best possible quality of health in every stage of life.

2. Preparedness, by which people in all communities will be protected from infectious, occupational, environmental, and terrorist threats.

To meet these goals and to respond to disease outbreaks, health crises, and disasters in the United States and worldwide, 3,000 CDC employees work at various locations throughout the

United States, assigned to almost all state health departments, and dispersed to numerous local health agencies. Additional CDC staff are deployed to countries around the globe.

The CDC works in partnership with other agencies within the Department of Health and Human Services and across the U.S. government; with world, state, and municipal governments; with the private sector, health care organizations, academic institutions, and international and U.S.-based nongovernmental organizations (Centers for Disease Control, 2005).

- Responding to new viral, bacterial, parasitic, and other emerging diseases. (Migration and travel, international trade, agricultural practices, and constant microbial adaptation practically guarantee that the world will face more exotic and unusual disease challenges.)

- Reducing the toll of violence in society by targeting communities, schools, workplaces, churches, and the mass media. (Violence has become ingrained in U.S. society and is glorified in virtually every entertainment medium.)

- Using new scientific knowledge and technological advances wisely to decrease and monitor pollution and the use of hazardous substances and fossil fuels.

The DHHS and the CDC have taken primary responsibility for epidemiological surveillance and preventive health programs. Public health is monitored, maintained, and improved through relationships among many federal agencies. These agencies work together through a coordinated effort to monitor, improve, and maintain resources and services for a healthier ecological environment. And it has always been clear that the federal government alone cannot be responsible for all U.S. public health initiatives. Health issues cannot be isolated from such socioeconomic issues as employment, housing, and accessibility to

health care. State and local initiatives to promote economic growth, affordable housing, and quality medical care are essential to a good quality of life.

Environmental Health Laws

aws protecting the environment date as far back as the 1800s. In the United States, environmental laws have three distinct purposes: (1) to protect people and their property, (2) to protect health, and (3) to conserve ecology (U.S. Council on Environmental Quality, 1986). These **public laws** have been translated into **codes** and **statutes** that guide the establishment of **regulations** used by government officials to inspect potential problems, make recommendations, and impose fines for offenders.

Most of the statutes are aimed at controlling businesses and industries because they are easier to monitor and control than individuals. Unfortunately, this strategy is met with resistance because it often contributes to increased overhead and less profit. In addition, environmental regulations require compliance that sometimes interferes with the way a business is run. As environmental laws have become more stringent, businessmen have

---

Digging Deeper   ENVIRONMENTAL LAWS

Environmental laws are federal and state statutes that govern what public health officials do. Most states work with federal agencies to obtain compliance with federal laws. At the local level, statutes are usually called *ordinances*.

Environmental laws provide protection to the environment by requiring:

- Notification of any intended or accidental releases of pollutants or hazardous wastes that need to be reported.

- Regulation of discharge or waste to prevent or minimize the discharge, release, or disposal of wastes and pollutants into the environment.

- Promote the reduction of waste produced and released into the environment.

- Promote the use of less hazardous materials and less packaging.

- Regulate activities that threaten habitats, ecosystems, and resources.

- Reduce risks associated with the transport of hazardous materials.

- Respond to accidental spills and aid in cleanup.

- Provide tax incentives to generate environmentally friendly products and services (Moore 1999).

There are 50 titles under the **Code of Federal Regulations** (CFR). Of them, 18 pertain to environmental health issues:
Title 7 - Agriculture
Title 8 - Aliens and Nationality
Title 9 - Animals and Animal Products
Title 10 - Energy
Title 19 - Customs Duties
Title 21 - Food and Drugs
Title 23 - Highways

Title 24 - Housing and Urban Development
Title 27 - Alcohol, Tobacco Products, and Firearms
Title 29 - Labor
Title 32 - National Defense
Title 36 - Parks, Forests, and Public Property
Title 40 - Protection of Environment
Title 42 - Public Health
Title 44 - Emergency Management and Assistance
Title 47 - Telecommunication
Title 49 - Transportation
Title 50 - Wildlife and Fisheries
(National Archives and Records Administration 2005)

To find out what specific ordinances may apply to your area, you may visit: http://www.municode.com/Resources/online_codes.asp.

pressured government officials to rule in favor of economic growth rather than quality of life. New bills have been introduced to relax environmental protection standards. Most of them have failed to pass, and budget cuts for environmental programs have made it difficult to enforce the laws already on the books.

The Environmental Movement

Environmentalism is founded and driven by science, with **grassroots** participation. Its purpose is to correct damage done to the natural environment by industrial and urban development in order to enhance the natural world, protect human welfare, and provide a **sustainable** economy for future generations. The environmental movement began as an organized effort to create awareness for the need for environmental control by government and citizens. Citizens have shown that when the quality of their air, water, and health of their children is threatened, they can be roused to anger and action. Environmentalists predict that a "new wave of environmentalism" will emphasize the solution of environmental problems through grassroots efforts and improved technology. Social ecologist Brian Tokar (1997) considers morality and relationships between individuals to be crucial to the preservation of environment and society. In order to keep up the momentum of environmentalism aimed at improving the quality of life on Earth, citizens in local communities must become enlightened, educated, and empowered to act.

American environmentalism dates back to colonial times, gaining steam in the twentieth century as concerned citizens expressed their concern about environmental degradation. Environmentalists and **conservationists** called for efforts to preserve forests and wildlife. By the 1960s, the environmental movement had become a part of the Vietnam war protest and the women's movement. Activists and conservationists founded organizations with the goal of maintaining what was good about the environ-

Public law
A law passed by the legislature to be enforced by public agencies.

Code
An interpretation of a public law written as a statute for the purpose of developing regulations and standards; a federal law; United States Code (U.S.C.)

Statute
A law set up by a legislative branch of the government; may include setting up an agency or regulating its authority.

Regulation
A rule that deals with the details and procedures for a regulatory agency to carry out a law.

Code of Federal Regulations
Regulations written by federal agencies to implement laws passed by Congress.

Environmentalism
A social and political movement promoting the preservation, restoration, or improvement of the natural environment and climate.

Grassroots
Operating in or at the local level, usually on political issues.

Sustainable
Using a resource so that it is not depleted or permanently damaged.

Conservationist
Environmental activist whose aim is to preserve nature as we now know it for future generations.

Digging Deeper — THE ENVIRONMENTAL MOVEMENT

Environmentalism is an umbrella concept that has taken various forms. Here are some major examples:

- *Conservation* seeks to protect biodiversity on aesthetic traditional and spiritual grounds.

- *Environmental health* dates to Rachel Carson's writings in the 1960s, and is related to nutrition, preventive medicine, and aging. The natural environment is of interest mostly as an early-warning system for what may happen to humans.

- *Ecology* focuses on Gaia theory, the value of Earth and other relations between human sciences and human responsibilities. Its spinoff, *deep ecology,* is more spiritual but often claims to be science.

- *Environmental justice* seeks an end to economic class–based environmental damage: low-income communities located close to highways, garbage dumps, and factories, where they are exposed to greater pollution and environmental health risk than the rest of the general population, who can afford to live elsewhere (Wikipedia, 2005).

ment and taking action to correct what was bad. Environmental laws restricting pollution emissions were passed and continue to be amended.

No matter how many laws and agencies the government develops to protect our natural resources and our health, efforts would be futile without the aid of U.S. citizens. Often referred to by government officials as "special interest groups," they serve a very important function in bringing environmental health issues to light. The current environmental movement has four camps: **mainstream**, **radical**, conservation, and grassroots (Shabecoff, 2002).

- Mainstream groups seek to work with existing power centers to improve environmental protection by lobbying federal, state, and local governments, political parties, and businesses to reduce pollution, conserve energy, and protect nature. Mainstream groups include the Sierra Club, the Environmental Defense Fund, the Natural Resources Defense Council, the National Audubon Society, the National Wildlife Federation, The Wilderness Society, and the World Wildlife Fund.

- Radical groups seek to make fundamental changes in political and economic systems in order to fight toxic and nuclear contamination and preserve nature. Radical groups include Friends of the Earth, Greenpeace, and Mother Jones.

- Conservation groups aim to preserve nature as we know it for future generations. They include hunting, fishing, and land preservation groups such as Ducks Unlimited, The Nature Conservancy, and the National Rifle Association, and organizations such as the Union of Concerned Scientists seeking to protect the world from nuclear disasters.

- Grassroots organizations tend to be intensely involved in local issues because their health, the health of their families, and their property are immediately at risk. It is estimated that all environmental organizations in this category would consist of 2.5 million members (Adler, 1995; Rosenbaum, 1995).

In recent years the number of environmental organizations have grown rapidly at the international, national, regional, state, and local levels. The memberships of national organizations change according to the economic and political climate, as well as the absence or presence of significant environmental disasters.

Public Health Challenges

The goal of public health agencies is to maintain a healthy population. Public health efforts include organized community efforts for a cleaner environment, reducing the incidence of communicable diseases and infections, and educating professionals and citizens regarding public health needs and strategies. Three models are used as bases for public health prevention and control of disease: microbial, behavioral, and ecological (Gostin et al., 1999). Their interactions are shown in Figure 19-3.

THE MICROBIAL MODEL

In the microbial model or "germ theory" of public health, disease is seen as a product of infection (or exposure to toxic substances), and the job of public health is to identify the pathogen (or toxin) and to eliminate or contain it.

Many public health activities based on this model are thought to be a normal part of life. For example, parents accept routine school vaccinations of their children without protest, and the public expects health de-

Digging Deeper ENVIRONMENTAL MOVEMENT ORGANIZATIONS

Alternatives for Community and Environment (Boston)	Greenpeace USA, Inc.	Orion Society
American Rivers	International Forum on Globalization	Ozone Action
Center for Marine Conservation	Kids Against Pollution (New York)	Rails-to-Rails Conservancy
Ducks Unlimited, Inc.	League of Conservation Voters	Rainforest Action Network
Ecotrust	League of Women Voters of the United States	SeaWeb
Environmental Action, Inc.	National Audubon Society	Second Nature (fosters environmental education at the university level)
Environmental Defense Fund (EDF)	National Environmental Trust	Sierra Club
Environmental Media Services	National Wildlife Federation	Society of Environmental Journalists
Environmental Working Group	Natural Resources Defense Council (NRDC)	Surfrider Foundation
Friends of the Earth	Nature Conservancy	Wilderness Society
Great Lakes United		Zero Population Growth, Inc.
Greater Yellowstone Coalition		

partments to make sure that people handling food in restaurants will not transmit diseases.

But these disease control measures can be controversial. The case of Typhoid Mary (Chapter 13) was an instance when extreme measures were used: A woman was quarantined for the rest of her life. Today, the occasional quarantine of a college dorm for measles inspires no protest; even treating tuberculosis by tracing contacts and isolating patients has been accepted (Coker, 2000). By contrast, many people living with HIV (and their advocates) perceive such measures to be threatening, and oppose them by citing constitutional rights to privacy (Gostin et al., 1999).

The microbial model works well when a particular pathogen causing an illness has been isolated. Public health agencies monitor air, water, food, and land quality so that problems can be appropriately rectified or modified. This model is limited, however, by implying that every disease problem has a single cause.

THE BEHAVIORAL MODEL

The behavioral model recognizes human behavior as an important determinant of health. Here smoking, diet, alcoholism, and a sedentary lifestyle are viewed as invitations to cancer, heart disease, and stroke. In the United States, approximately 400,000 people die each year because they smoke, 300,000 as a result of poor diet and activity patterns, and 100,000 from excessive drinking (Gostin et al., 1999). Behavior can also prevent or cause injuries and accidents (e.g., use of seatbelts, bicycle/ motorcycle helmets, and firearms) and infection (e.g., salmonella and hepatitis).

Focusing on behavior as a primary cause of disease tends to produce three kinds of outcomes: One, the

model is seen as a justification for assigning individual moral responsibility for public health—good health is an individual's reward for virtuous living, and some forms of ill health (e.g., AIDS) are punishment for bad behavior. Two, government penalties for high-risk behaviors (failure to wear a seatbelt or motorcycle helmet, speeding, smoking in offices or restaurants, driving under the influence of alcohol or other drugs), are seen as paternalistic interference with personal choices. Three, health measures aimed at changing individual behavior tend to work by changing the social meaning of the behavior, through requiring behavioral change, or changing beliefs and attitudes (Gostin et al., 1999).

Unfortunately people will engage in wrongful behavior that endangers others if they think they will not be caught, prosecuted, fined, suspended, or jailed. Thus laws and penalties are created to punish such behaviors. People may be required by law to wear seatbelts, not smoke indoors in public areas, or not drive after drinking. The strategy only works when the errant individual feels guilt for not following the rules.

Positive reinforcement works better. When good behavior is rewarded, it will be repeated. But what is a reward for one person may be different for another person. Also, rewards must vary to be effective. And when government promotes sex education, distributes condoms, or exchanges syringes, it implicitly accepts that behavior as inevitable, which some people see as encouraging sex or drug use (Gostin et al., 1999).

THE ECOLOGICAL MODEL

The ecological model of public health disease control regards disease as a harmful interaction between people and their physical environment: Certain social conditions produce unhealthy behaviors or environmental hazards. Public health strategies thus focus on the conditions or hazards. Smoking, for example, is regarded as a consequence of saturation marketing by the tobacco industry and encouragement of smoking by popular culture. Efforts to counteract such promotion include publicity about the health risks of smoking, restrictions on advertising, "sin" taxes, and elimination of tobacco growers' subsidies. Conflict arises when public health regulations targeting ecological causes of injury and disease restrict behavior that people enjoy or that makes producers and distributors money (Gostin et al., 1999).

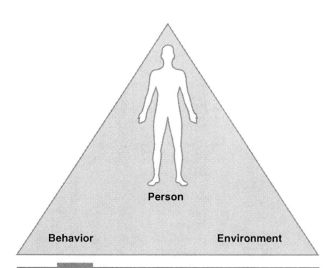

Person

Behavior   Environment

FIGURE 19-3 **Disease Model Relationships** Also known as the "epidemiological model," this structure can be used to find ways to decrease illnesses and accidents.

Mainstream
In the middle; representing the majority view; moderate; working with existing institutions.

Radical
View that extreme changes should be made in existing conditions or institutions.

Public health agencies may also attempt to modify the environment (for example, creating more and better low-income housing or building parks with hiking and biking trails) in an effort to change human behavior, or they may attempt to modify the behavior (for example, screening out individuals who do not meet criteria for assistance).

Urbanization and Local Issues

In the 1800s, the United States population was primarily rural. By 1900, approximately half of the U.S. population was rural (U.S. Census Bureau, 1990). Today, the majority of the U.S. population lives in cities. As rural young and adults migrate to cities in search of jobs, the U.S. working-class population becomes more urban. This creates a strain on water and waste systems originally designed with a smaller population in mind. Living in close quarters in city slums also increases exposure to illegal drug use and violence. If unemployment rises, crime rates, homelessness, and dependence on governmental assistance also rise.

Since the Industrial Revolution began in the 1800s, the spread of industry with its smoke stacks and pollution putting harmful chemicals in air and water has had a deleterious effect on the environment and natural resources. In the United States, each state is responsible for inspecting air, water, and hazardous waste management. State public health employees conduct routine inspections, analyze samples, and keep records that are then reviewed by federal officials. State envi-

ronmental health employees often rely on county and city employees to conduct routine operations and maintenance inspections.

The Healthy Cities Program

The Healthy Cities Program was an effort initiated by the World Health Organization to improve conditions in urban areas worldwide (WHO 1995). The concept is that any city can be a "healthy city" if it is committed to a structure and process working toward improvement of public health. In 1996, 1,000 U.S. cities committed themselves to promoting urban health. Safe Communities Networks and Sustainable Cities networks have also been formed. Housing construction, new transportation systems, and community "clean-up days" are just a few products of these efforts.

To set up a successful healthy city program, city officials, health care providers, community groups, and neighborhood associations work collaboratively to provide health-promotion activities. The first step includes planning and allocation of resources endorsed by local politicians. The plans should have input from local citizens. There should be an office with full-time staff. There should be a decision-making body addressing housing, environment, education, and social services. There should be mediation among industries, city departments, agencies, organizations, and individuals. Urban planning strategies related to transportation and recreation should be addressed. The search for new and innovative ideas should be on-going, including incentives and recognition for those who develop new policies and programs. There

---

Digging Deeper — WHAT MAKES A HEALTHY CITY?

- Clean, safe and high-quality environment (including housing).

- Training of workers so they have the skills needed for technological jobs.

- Economic development plans that include attracting large businesses to their area.

- Diverse employment opportunities so that more residents will have jobs.

- Zoning of subdivisions to attract young families.

- Additional water and sewage systems.

- Additional schools and recreational areas.

- Transportation systems designed to help workers travel between homes and jobs.

- Stable, sustainable ecosystem.

- High degree of public participation and control over decisions affecting health and well-being.

- Meeting basic needs for all residents (water, food, shelter, safety, income, work).

- High health status and low levels of disease.

- Optimum level of appropriate public health and health care services and accessibility.

- Diverse, vital, and innovative city economy.

- Access to a wide variety of experiences and resources with ample interactions.

- Connection with the community's past cultural and biological heritage and with other groups and individuals (World Health Organization, 1995).

should be progress reports that share information and experiences. Each city has its own specific health problems, and actions should be relevant to improving health. Goals should include healthier workplaces, homes, schools, and recreational environments.

The Promise of a Green Future

eveloped and promoted by industrialized countries, such industries as green architecture, green energy, green transportation, and wilderness preservation are among some of the movements expected to grow, particularly as responsible businesses see economic gain in attending to environmental concerns.

GREEN ARCHITECTURE

Green architecture is a term used when environmental goals are considered in designing a new building. The concept is to develop buildings and homes that cost less to build, own, and maintain. Where the building is located, how efficiently it is heated and cooled, and how well waste products are reused or recycled are scrutinized. Buildings can have plywood made of recycled materials, nonpolluting paints, windows that admit sunlight but reduce heat radiation, windows that open for a ventilation, low-flow toilets, roofs with a holding tank so that rainwater can be used for home and garden use, and other features that make them easier on the environment. Architects have gone as far as incorporating the outdoors into buildings with atriums and sky gardens.

It is important to note that that not all building projects can be built in harmony with the environment, and not all individuals residing within them are environmentally aware. As a result, not all builders are enthusiastic about green architecture, particularly those who depend on market demand to sell the homes they build.

GREEN ENERGY AND TRANSPORTATION

Green energy and transportation strategies include developing new machines and seeking alternative fuel sources such as biomass fuel that are energy efficient and friendly to the environment. **Green stores**, sustainable buildings, alternative fuel and hybrid engines, and other innovations are gaining public attention and experiencing increasing demand, often in response to rising oil prices.

Biomass energy—the energy from organic matter—has been in use since people started burning wood to cook food or to keep warm. Today, wood is still the largest biomass energy resource. But many other sources of biomass are available, including plants, residues from agriculture or forestry, and the organic component of municipal and industrial wastes—even the fumes from landfills.

WILDERNESS PRESERVATION

As discussed in Chapter 10, there are many beautiful areas of the United States set aside as national parks for the public to enjoy. It was not always that way. In 1893 President Benjamin Harrison created 13 million acres of forest reserves, including 4 million acres covering much of the High Sierra. During his Presidency (1901–1909), President Theodore Roosevelt established the U.S. Forest Service and the National Wildlife Refuge System. As a result of his efforts, there are now 51 wildlife refuges and 150 national forests in the United States.

In 1916, the Department of the Interior was responsible for 12 national parks, 19 national monuments, and 2 reservations. In order to consolidate management of the national park system, Congress passed the National Park Service Organic Act, establishing the National Park Service for the management and protection of national parks, monuments, and reservations. The law mandated the National Park Service to "conserve the scenery and the natural and historic objects and the wildlife therein and to provide for the enjoyment of the same in such manner and by such means as will leave them unimpaired for the enjoyment of future generations."

Environmental Issues at the Local Level

The political climate of any area has the most significant impact on quality of life where environmental issues are concerned. The structure of government can vary from state to state, making the process of advocating for environmental health complicated. Conflicts may arise between federal, state, and local governments. Conflicts may also arise between states. A primary factor is the economic conditions that affect funding for preventive health measures. An example of this is the most recent use of state officials using tobacco settlement funds to aid programs not related to tobacco prevention or clean air laws for other programs. Another factor is population growth, an indicator of a flourishing economy. Cities that experience such growth usually have more public health

Green architecture
Term used to describe building design that takes environmental goals into consideration.

Green energy
Fuel sources that are energy efficient and friendly to the environment.

Green store
Retail store that sells environmentally sensitive products, such as organic products.

issues. Land usage, new industries, and the need for more housing are usually issues at the meetings of county **council** or city council meetings.

CITY PLANNING AND ZONING

Of major concern to cities experiencing sudden growth is land **zoning**, designating land for certain kinds of use. For example, a person may not locate a business in a residential zone. But neighborhoods change. A person may purchase a home and later find that the neighborhood or street is filling up with commercial businesses because the zoning is lax, or has changed. New roads and highways may require that homes be moved or destroyed. Airports may need more land. Recreational areas may be taken over by industries. Noise, air, and water pollution become problems where they never were before. Each community has its own zoning practices and **ordinances** designed to help citizens with property issues. Citizens may protest rezoning to allow business and industry by organizing and sharing their concerns with governmental officials. Public hearings about rezoning are usually posted in local newspapers so the public has notice of the opportunity to express their concerns.

BUILDING CODES

The construction of safe homes and businesses is an environmental issue. Building codes are intended to preserve the safety of people in buildings and homes. Water availability and drainage are major concerns. Wetlands and forests are sometimes destroyed for new housing subdivisions. Without regulation, homes may be built in a flood zone. Homes built in areas with high radiation content in the soils may mean basements with exposure to radon. Homes built in humid areas must have moisture barriers and other means to control mold growth. In hurricane zones, homes must be built to withstand extreme wind pressures. As more homes are built, more water and sewer lines are needed. Electricity, natural gas, telephone, cable, and other services need to keep up.

PUBLIC HEALTH AND COMMUNITY SAFETY

It is the responsibility of public health workers to determine potential public health risks and notify officials of environmental problems that may affect the health of residents negatively. Public health workers must monitor industries, small businesses, citizens, tourists. and transient populations. Traffic laws, curfews, public intoxication restrictions, and the surveillance of behaviors that might cause harm to others is very important to the safety of a community. In many cases, state police, county sheriffs, and city police cooperate with one another to monitor local businesses, residents, and suspicious activities. There are drug-free school zones, and construction zones where

traffic fines are doubled. As communities grow and crime rates grow, so grows the need for more detention facilities and detoxification facilities. In areas where pedestrian, bicycle, and automobile traffic becomes congested, it may be necessary to conduct a traffic study to determine the need for new bus services, service roads, stoplights, stop signs, and crosswalks.

Sustainable Development

Sustainable development is a term highlighting the inter-dependence of economic development and the environment. It is used to describe approaches to such issues as urban design, transportation, energy conservation, waste treatment, and urban forestry that do not compromise the needs of future generations.

A number of cities in the United States (such as Austin, Texas, Chattanooga, Tennessee, Denver, Colorado, Los Angeles, and Portland, Oregon) are notable for several sustainability initiatives:

- Affordable housing within easy walking distance of a pedestrian-oriented downtown.

- Construction of **greenways** of protected trails for recreational activities.

- Diesel buses for city transportation replaced with electric shuttles.

- Distribution of low-flush toilets to city residents to save water.

- Garden projects for the homeless providing paid jobs and free food for all who participated.

- Green builders constructing homes from recycled materials with passive solar heating systems.

- Old buildings downtown renovated to bring business back to the downtown area.

- Recycling centers created that provide training and jobs for those who would otherwise be unable to find jobs.

Some urban planners dream about building **vertical farms**, urban agricultural complexes located inside skyscrapers, in which a city's sewage and wastewater flow is treated to remove pathogens and toxins and retain nutrients, then recycled to nourish food crops grown in the vertical farm. This idea would change cyclical material flow within cities and reduce effluence. If that happened, rebuilt sanitary systems would be more flexible in meeting urban needs. The development of sustainable cities requires innovation, inspiration, long-term planning, and active citizen participation (Despommier, 2004).

Past Failures

Over 200 years ago our country provided new beginnings for individuals in search of a better way of life. Natural resources were abundant, but lives were hard and short. Diseases wiped out entire towns and populations. Trees were lost, the air became hazy, rivers became polluted, land was ravaged, and what was once a beautiful environment with an unlimited variety of species was threatened or endangered. A little over 30 years ago, the nation was facing an environmental crisis. Garbage floated in our lakes and streams, dead fish washed up on our shores, and rivers actually caught fire. Swimming beaches were closed and public water supplies were declared unfit for human consumption. We have evolved into a nation that has many freedoms, including the freedom to harm ourselves and others. Predictions are that the continued abuse of our environment could result in climactic, genetic, and social changes to the extent that good health will be a precious commodity.

Past Successes

By the early 1970s, public awareness regarding the quality of the environment reached an all-time high, and people demanded action. The U.S. government responded. Laws were passed to regulate the harm that could be done to people and the environment. And local laws, or ordinances, dictated the need for the number and type of workers who serve the public to keep the environment clean and safe.

No single agency or organization has the authority or resources to tackle detrimental human actions. Efforts to control diseases induced by environmental hazards require efforts at the personal, local, national, and international levels. When a problem is understood, support from interest groups is necessary to educate legislators to create policies and funding for preventive and corrective strategies.

City developers and urban developers need to understand how a major project will affect local residents and natural resources. Environmentalists, conservationists, and public health workers cannot do this alone. Major undertakings are required to influence government officials with an eye for economic development, large industries that pollute the environment as they strive to keep operating costs down, and citizens who are uninformed about actual and potential risks. Environmental health efforts are not for the faint of heart.

Future Focus

Without the collaboration and cooperation of government agencies, businesses, special interest groups, and individual citizens, no strategy to improve the environment will be successful. Radical environmentalists have created public awareness of environmental problems, advocated better ways of accomplishing individual and economic goals without compromising environmental quality, and have inspired us to be better citizens. The opportunity to improve environmental quality, our own health and the health of citizens worldwide is available. Leaders lead by example. Followers fol-

---

Council
Group of local residents elected or appointed as an advisory or legislative body.

Zoning
Assignment of use restrictions on incorporated areas where buildings exist or are planned to be built.

Ordinance
A local law regulating human behavior.

Greenway
Area between city street lanes that resembles a park.

Vertical farm
Small farms inside a high-rise city building.

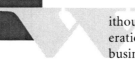

Consider the Cost — EVERYONE HAS A PART TO PLAY IN ENVIRONMENTAL HEALTH

- Environmentalists are concerned about natural ecological systems, wildlife species survival, and effects of humans on Earth.

- Conservationists are concerned about forests, topsoil, distribution of water, and practices that do not harm the environment.

- Public agencies are concerned about adequate housing, diseases, safety, and healthy behaviors.

- All other individuals interested in environmental health monitor the effects of humans on the environment and look for ways to reduce the associated problems.

low good leaders. There is no discounting personal responsibility in return for social and economic gain.

Summary

In the United States, environmental organizations, laws, and public health agencies help make the environment more livable and sustainable. It is apparent from various polls that most Americans are concerned about the environment. The central mission of public health in the United States is to analyze trends in health, illness, disability, and death and implement protective measures for the entire population or sub-populations.

The DHHS is responsible for protecting the health of all Americans and providing essential human services. With more than 300 programs, it is the largest grant-making agency in the federal government. The CDC work with states and other partners to provide a system of health surveillance to monitor and prevent disease outbreaks.

U.S. laws protecting the environment are intended to protect people and their property, protect health, and conserve ecology. These public laws have been translated into codes and statutes that establish regulations and standards used by government officials to inspect potential problems, make recommendations, and impose fines for offenders.

The environmental movement was founded to correct damage to the natural environment, enhance the natural world, protect human welfare, and provide a sustainable economy for future generations. The current environmental movement consists of four groups: mainstream groups, radical groups, conservation groups, and grassroots organizations.

The goal of public health agencies is to maintain a healthy population. In the microbial model or "germ theory" of public health, disease is seen as a product of infection (or exposure to toxic substances), and the job of public health is to identify the pathogen and to eliminate or contain it. Public health models include the behavioral model and the ecological model.

Today, the majority of the U.S. population lives in cities, creating a strain on water and waste systems. The Healthy Cities Program was an effort initiated by the World Health Organization to improve conditions in urban areas worldwide. Any city can be a "healthy city" if it is committed to a structure and process working toward improvement of public health.

Green architecture develops buildings and homes that cost less to build, own, and maintain by paying attention to where the building is located, how efficiently it is heated and cooled, and how well waste products are reused or recycled. Green transportation strategies include developing new machines and seeking alternative fuel sources that are energy efficient and friendly to the environment.

The political climate of any area has a significant impact on its quality of life and environment. A primary factor is the economic conditions that affect funding for preventive health measures.

Sustainable development is urban design, transportation, energy conservation, waste treatment, and urban food production that does not compromise the needs of future generations. It focuses on the inter-dependence of economic development and the environment.

The past 200 years has seen systematic degradation of the environment. By the early 1970s, the public demanded action. Laws and ordinances were passed to keep the environment clean and safe. Future protection depends on the sustained collaboration and cooperation of government agencies, businesses, special interest groups, and individual citizens.

REFERENCES

Adler, J. (1995). *Environmentalism at the crossroads: Green activism in America,* pp. 147–232. Washington, D.C.: Capital Research Center.

Centers for Disease Control and Prevention (CDC). (2000). CDC fact book, 2000–2001. Department of Health and Human Services, Centers for Disease Control. Retrieved from http://www.cdc.gov/maso/pdf/cdc.pdf.

Centers for Disease Control and Prevention (CDC). (2005). About the CDC. U.S. Department of Health and Human Services. From http://www.cdc.gov/about/default.htm.

Coker, R. J. (2000). *From chaos to coercion: Detention and the control of tuberculosis.* New York: St. Martin's Press.

Despommier, D. (2004). The Vertical Farm: Reducing the impact of agriculture on ecosystem functions and services (essay). Department of Environmental Health Sciences, Mailman School of Public Health, Columbia University. From http://www.verticalfarm.com/index.htm.

Environmental Protection Agency. (1986). RCRA orientation manual. Report CPA 530-SW-001. U.S. Environmental Protection Agency, Washington, D.C.

Gostin, L., Burris, S., & Lazzarini, Z. (1999). The law and the public's health: A study of infectious disease law in the United States. *Columbia Law Review,* January 1999, 59–118, 67–77.

League of Conservation Voters (2002). Views on laws protecting the environment. In Presentation, League of Conservation Voters Education Fund. http://www.voteenvironment.org/pdf/2002efpoll.PDF.

Moore, G. S. (1999). *Living with the Earth: Concepts in environmental health science.* Boca Raton, FL: Lewis Publishers. National Archives and Records Administration. Code of Federal Regulations. From http://www.access.gpo.gov/nara/cfr/.

National Archives and Records Administration. (2005). Code of Federal Regulations. Retrieved from http://www.gpoaccess.gov/cfr/index.html.

Rosenbaum, W. (1995). *Environmental politics and policy, 3rd ed.,* pp. 22–27. Washington, D.C.: CQ Press.

Shabecoff, P. (2002). *Earth rising: American environmentalism in the 21st century.* Island Press: Washington, D. C.

Tokar, B. (1997). *Earth for sale.* Cambridge, MA: South End Press.

U.S. Census Bureau (1990). 1990 Census of Population and Housing, Table 4.

U.S. Council on Environmental Quality (USCEQ). (1986, May 27). *40 CFR Part 1502 National Environmental Policy Act Regulations.* Washington, D.C.: U.S. Congress.

Werbach, A. (1997). *Act now, apologize later,* pp. 66–69. New York: HarperCollins.

Wikipedia (2005). Environmental movement. From http://en.wikipedia.org/wiki/Environmentalism.

World Health Organization (1995). *World Health Report.* From http://www.who.int/whr/en/.

ASSIGNMENTS

1. Consult the Code of Federal Regulations home page or a copy of the Federal Register (found in the reference section of a university library) and look up a federal law pertaining to a public health issue. Find the law and print it out. Highlight specific areas relative to environmental health. You may use this search engine to assist you with the United States Code number: http://uscode.house.gov/usc.htm.

2. Pick a city where you would like to live. Research that city for quality of life and environmental information.

3. Find out about past environmental issues in your state.

4. Learn what public health and safety issues are important in your state at this time.

5. Locate a place where you can find state statutes about environmental laws.

6. Search the Internet for organizations and individuals who advocate environmental issues in your state.

7. Search a community Web site for local ordinances on public health and safety.

8. Attend a county council or city council meeting and make a note of environmental issues discussed at the meeting. Observe differences of opinion expressed by various council members.

9. Research and write a critical evaluation of the vertical farm concept.

10. Analyze what your community could do to become a Healthy City.

SELECTED ENVIRONMENTAL LAWS

1969 National Environmental Policy Act (NEPA) (PL 91-190)
The basic national charter for protection of the environment. Establishes policy, sets goals, and provides means for carrying out the policy.

1986 Emergency Planning and Community Right-to-Know Act (EPCRA) (PL 99-499)
Helps local communities protect public health, safety, and the environment from chemical hazards.

1990 Pollution Prevention Act (PPA) (PL 101-508)
Reduces sources of pollution and pollution produced via recycling, and promotes sustainable agriculture.

1998 National Defense Authorization Act (PL 105-85)
Provides U.S. support to specified countries engaging in counter-drug activities.

2000 Public Health Threats and Emergencies Act (PL 106-505)
Provides grants to state and local governments to help them prepare for public health emergencies, including emergencies resulting from acts of bioterrorism.

2001 Homeland Security Act (PL 107-296)
Intended to counter terrorism and improve federal responses to terrorist acts.

2002 Public Health Security and Bioterrorism Response Act (PL l07-188)
Intended to improve the ability of the United States to prevent, prepare for, and respond to bioterrorism and other public health emergencies.

SELECTED PROFESSIONAL JOURNALS

American Journal of Public Health
Atlantic Monthly
EPA Journal
Science
Scientific American
The Nation's Health

ADDITIONAL READING

Ashworth, W. (1986). *The late Great Lakes: An environmental history.* Alfred A. Knopf.

Ayyad, M. A. (2003). Case studies in the conservation of biodiversity: Degradation and threats. *Journal of Arid Environments, 54,* 165–183.

Barnhardt, W. (1987). The death of Ducktown. *Discover, October,* 35–43.

Barton, H., Ed. (2000). *Sustainable communities: The potential for eco-neighbourhoods.* London: Earthscan Publications.

Becker, W. (1994) *Rebuilding for the Future: A Guide to Sustainable Redevelopment for Disaster-Affected Communities.* U.S. Department of Energy.

Bingham, E. (1992). The occupational safety and health act. In Rom, W. N. (Ed.) *Environmental and occupational medicine, 2nd ed.,* pp. 1325–1331. Boston: Little, Brown & Company.

Blaustein, A., Romansic, J., Kiesecker, J., & Hatch, A. (2003). Ultraviolet radiation, toxic chemicals and amphibian population declines. *Diversity and Distributions, 9,* 123–141.

BNA (1993). *Guide to federal environmental laws.* Washington, D.C.: Bureau of National Affairs.

Bright, C. (1998). *Life out of bounds: Bioinvasion in a borderless world.* New York: W.W. Norton.

Council on Environmental Quality (1987). Sixteenth annual report (pp. 4–6). Washington, D.C.: U.S. Government Printing Office.

Evans, K. (2003). *The environment: A revolution in attitudes.* Detroit, MI: The Gale Group.

Findley, R., & Farber, D. (1992). *Environmental law in a nutshell, 3rd ed.* St. Paul, MN: West Publishing Company.

Gompper, M., & Williams, E. (1998). Parasite conservation and the black-footed ferret recovery program. *Conservation Biology, 12,* 730–732.

Gordon, J. (1993). The American environment. *American Heritage, 44,* 30–48.

Gostin, L. (2001) *Public health law: Power, duty, restraint.* Berkeley, CA: University of California Press.

Gostin, L. (2002). *Public health law and ethics: A reader.* Berkeley, CA: University of California Press.

Gostin, L. (2003). *Health and human rights.* Burlington, VT: Ashgate Publishing, Limited.

Hester, R. (1995). *Life, liberty, and the pursuit of sustainable happiness.*

Kaufman, W. (2000). *Coming out of the woods: The solitary life of a maverick naturalist.* Cambridge, MA: Perseus Publications.

Koplan, J., & Fleming, D. (2000). Current and future public health challenges. *Journal of the American Medical Association, 284,* 1696.

Lefebvre R., & Flora J. (1988). Social marketing and public health intervention. *Health Education Quarterly 15,* 299–315.

McCarthy, T. (2002). Let them run wild. Special report: How to save the Earth. *Time Magazine, 160,* A22–A27.

McLeroy K., Bibeau D., Steckler A., & Glanz K. (1988). An ecological perspective on health promotion programs. *Health Education Quarterly 15,* 351–377.

Office of Policy Planning and Evaluation, EPA (1988). Environmental progress and challenges, EPA's update. Publication No. EPA 230-07-88-033. Washington, D.C.: U.S. Government Printing Office.

Reed, P., Wyckoff, P., & Dee, P. (1992). In S. Novick (Ed.), *Law of environmental protection, Vol. 2, Chapter 11.* Deerfield, IL: Clark, Boardman, & Callaghan.

Reitze, A. (1991). A century of air pollution control law: What's worked; what's failed; what might work. *Environmental Law, 21,* 1575–1581.

Schrenk, H., Heimann, H., Clayton, G., Gafafer, W., & Wesler, H. (1949). Air pollution in Donora, Pennsylvania. Epidemiology of the unusual smog episode of October 1948. Washington, DC: U.S. Government Printing Office.

Seigweorth, K. (1943). Ducktown: A postwar challenge. *American Forests, November,* 521–524.

Stokols, D. (1992). Establishing and maintaining healthy environments: Toward a social ecology of health promotion. *American Psychologist 47,* 6–22.

Tilove, J. (1998). Racial generation gap growing. *Sunday Republication, February 22,* B2.

Vass, A. (2002). Over half the world will face water shortages by 2032. *British Medical Journal, 324,* 7349.

Wallace, R. (1950). The miracle of the Copper Basin. *The Tennessee Conservationist, 15,* 8–9.

Wilford, J. N. (1991). The gradual greening of Mt. St. Helens. *New York Times, Oct. 8,* B9.

Witkamp, M., Frank, M., & Shoopman, J. (1966). Accumulation and biota in a pioneer ecosystem of kudzu vine at Copper Hill, Tennessee. *Journal of Applied Ecology, 3,* 383–391.

Index

Photo Credits

p. xviii, © Photodisc; p. 1, © Photodisc; p. 3 (top left), © Photodisc; p. 3 (top right), © Photodisc; p. 3 (middle left), © Photodisc; p. 3 (middle right), © Photodisc; p. 3 (bottom left), © Photodisc; p. 3 (bottom right), © Pavel Filatov/Alamy Images; p. 13 (left), Courtesy of USGS; p. 13 (top right), Courtesy of Gordon H. Rodda/U.S. Fish and Wildlife Service; p. 13 (bottom right), Courtesy USDA APHIS PPQ Archives, www.forestryimages.org; p. 14 (top left), Courtesy of James H. Miller/Forest Service/USDA; p. 14 (top right), Courtesy of APHIS/USDA; p. 14 (bottom), Courtesy of APHIS/USDA; p. 15, © Marc Reech, 2002; p. 17 (top), Courtesy of Stan Butler/NOS/NOAA; p. 17 (bottom), © Photodisc; p. 18, © Photodisc; p. 22, © Photodisc; p. 25, © Flat Earth/ FotoSearch; p. 26, Courtesy of Dr. Edwin P. Ewing, Jr./CDC; p. 27, Kathryn Hilgenkamp; p. 29, Courtesy of Library of Congress, Prints and Photographs Division [LC-USZ62-29808]; p. 31, Courtesy of P. Virot/ WHO; p. 36, © Photodisc; p. 40 (top), © National Library of Medicine; p. 40 (bottom), © National Library of Medicine; p. 41, © National Library of Medicine; p. 42 (left), © National Library of Medicine; p. 42 (right), © National Library of Medicine; p. 52, © Photodisc; p. 54, Courtesy of CDC; p. 54, Courtesy of CDC; p. 59, © National Library of Medicine; p. 60, Courtesy of CDC; p. 62, Courtesy of CDC; p. 63 (top), Courtesy James Hicks/CDC; p. 63 (bottom), Courtesy of CDC; p. 64, Courtesy of CDC; p. 65, Courtesy of CDC; p. 67, © 2002 Charles Stewart and Associates; p. 68, Courtesy of Donald Kopanoff/CDC; p. 70, Courtesy of James Gathany/Anthony Sanchez/CDC; p. 72, Courtesy of Dr. Visvesvara/CDC; p. 78, © Photodisc; p. 84, Courtesy of Edward Baker, MD, MPH/CDC; p. 87, Courtesy of CDC; p. 89, Kathryn Hilgenkamp; p. 94, Courtesy of CDC; p. 98, © Photodisc; p. 100 (left), Courtesy of CDC; p. 100 (right), Kathryn Hilgenkamp; p. 112, © LiquidLibrary; p. 113, by Shirley Briggs. Courtesy of the Lear/Carson Collection, Connecticut College; p. 115, Courtesy of USDA; p. 116 (top left), Courtesy of Clemson University; p. 116 (bottom left), Courtesy of Clemson University; p. 116 (bottom right), Courtesy of Clemson University; p. 117 (left), Courtesy of World Health Organization/CDC; p. 117 (top right), Courtesy of Dr. Dennis D. Juranek/CDC; p. 117 (bottom right), Used with permission from Clemson; p. 118 (top), Courtesy of Eddie Dunbar. Exploring California Insects Program. Quality Nature Displays, Oakland, CA; p. 118 (bottom), Courtesy of Mary S. Blum, University of Georgia; p. 119, Courtesy of USDA; p. 120 (left), Courtesy of Rick Vetter, spiders.ucr.edu, http://spiders.ucr.edu/images/colorloxmap.gif; p. 120 (right), Courtesy of James Solomon, USDA Forest Service; p. 121 (left), Courtesy of PHPPO/DMTS/James Gathany/CDC; p. 121 (top right), Courtesy of Department of Entomology, University of Nebraska-Lincoln; p. 121 (top right), © Dr. David M. Phillips/Visuals Unlimited; p. 122 (left), Courtesy of Jan Ove Rein, The Scorpion Files; p. 122 (right), © Mike Lane/Alamy Images; p. 123 (left), Courtesy of CDC; p. 123 (right), Courtesy of CDC; p. 134, © Photodisc; p. 144, © Photos.com; p. 146, Kathryn Hilgenkamp; p. 150,

© Photodisc; p. 153, © Photodisc; p. 154, Kathryn Hilgenkamp; p. 160, Kathryn Hilgenkamp; p. 162, Kathryn Hilgenkamp; p. 166, Kathryn Hilgenkamp; p. 172, © AbleStock; p. 173 (left), Courtesy of the Aldo Leopold Foundation Archives; p. 173 (right), U.S. Department of Agriculture Photos; p. 175, Courtesy of CDC; p. 177 (top), Courtesy of Theodore Roosevelt Collection, Harvard College Library; p. 177 (bottom), Kathryn Hilgenkamp; p. 178, Kathryn Hilgenkamp; p. 179, Kathryn Hilgenkamp; p. 180, Courtesy of Steve Dutch, University of Wisconsin-Green Bay; p. 182, Courtesy of Gene Alexander/NRCS; p. 185 (left), © Photodisc; p. 185 (right), Kathryn Hilgenkamp; p. 186, Courtesy of A.S. Navoy/USGS; p. 187, Courtesy of CDC; p. 194, © Photodisc; p. 198, Courtesy of Steve Dutch, University of Wisconsin, Green Bay; p. 201, Kathryn Hilgenkamp; p. 203, Photo by Falke Bruinsma (http://photos.innersource.com); p. 204, © AbleStock; p. 206, U.S. Bureau of Reclamation; p. 207, Kathryn Hilgenkamp; p. 208, © Photodisc; p. 210, Courtesy of David Anderson, Centre College; p. 216, © AbleStock; p. 229, © AbleStock; p. 238, © LiquidLibrary; p. 243, Courtesy of USDA; p. 244, Courtesy of The Lilly Library, Indiana University, Bloomington, Indiana; p. 249, © Photodisc; p. 250, Courtesy of USDA/APHIS/Norman Watkins/CDC; p. 253, Courtesy of Kimberly Smith and Christine Ford/CDC; p. 254, © Photodisc; p. 260, © AbleStock; p. 263 (left), Courtesy of Bartholomew County Solid Waste Management District, Columbus, IN; p. 263 (right), Courtesy of Bartholomew County Solid Waste Management District, Columbus, IN; p. 268, Courtesy of CDC; p. 269, Kathryn Hilgenkamp; p. 272, Kathryn Hilgenkamp; p. 273, Courtesy of CDC; p. 274, Kathryn Hilgenkamp; p. 277, Courtesy of CDC; p. 284, © AbleStock; p. 285, Kathryn Hilgenkamp; p. 289, © David Hoffman Photo Library/Alamy Images; p. 290, © David Young-Wolff/ PhotoEdit; p. 294, © Vote Photography/VStock/Alamy Images; p. 297, © Jones and Bartlett Publishers. Photographed by Kimberly Potvin; p. 304, © LiquidLibrary; p. 306 (left), © Shutterstock; p. 306 (right), Courtesy of Office of the Surgeon General, Office of Medical History at www.history. aamed.army.mil; p. 309, © Tramonto/age fotostock; p. 312, Courtesy of National Highway Traffic Safety Administration; p. 314, © Photos.com; p. 315 (left), © Photodisc; p. 315 (right), Kathryn Hilgenkamp; p. 317 (top), Kathryn Hilgenkamp; p. 317 (bottom left), Kathryn Hilgenkamp; p. 317 (bottom right), © Photodisc; p. 322, © AbleStock; p. 324 (a-d), Courtesy The History Place (www.historyplace.com); p. 326 , Courtesy of Library of Congress, The Coolidge Era [LC-USZ62-111391 DLC]; p. 326, Courtesy of National Library of Medicine; p. 327, © National Library of Medicine; p. 328, © AP Photos; p. 330, Kathryn Hilgenkamp; p. 336, © AbleStock; p. 338, © Photodisc; p. 339, Courtesy of National Severe Storms Laboratory/NOAA; p. 343, © AbleStock; p. 346, © Photodisc; p. 348, Courtesy of the USGS; p. 349, © Photodisc; p. 356, © Photodisc.

CPSIA information can be obtained at www.ICGtesting.com
Printed in the USA
LVOW080704070713

341714LV00001B/1/P